CLAIRE B. WILCOX, M.D.
RADIOLOGY

Pleural Diseases

Third Edition

Pleural Diseases

Third Edition

Richard W. Light, M.D.
Professor of Medicine
University of California, Irvine
Chief Pulmonary Exercise Laboratory
Veterans Administration Medical Center
Long Beach, California

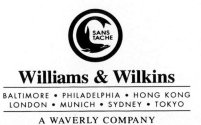

Williams & Wilkins
BALTIMORE • PHILADELPHIA • HONG KONG
LONDON • MUNICH • SYDNEY • TOKYO
A WAVERLY COMPANY

Editor: David C. Retford
Managing Editor: Kathleen Courtney Millet
Production Coordinator: Kimberly S. Nawrozki
Copy Editor: Margaret D. Hanson, R.N.
Designer: Rita Baker-Schmidt
Illustration Planner: Wayne Hubbel

Copyright © 1995
Williams & Wilkins
351 W. Camden Street
Baltimore, Maryland 21201-2436 USA

Accurate indications, adverse reactions, and dosage schedules for drugs are provided in this book, but it is possible that they may change. The reader is urged to review the package information data of the manufacturers of the medications mentioned.

Printed in the United States of America

First Edition 1983
Second Edition 1990

Library of Congress Cataloging in Publication Data

Light, Richard W.
    Pleural diseases / Richard W. Light — 3rd ed.
      p.   cm.
    Includes bibliographical references and index.
    ISBN 0-683-05017-6
    1. Pleura—Diseases.   I. Title.
    [DNLM: 1. Pleural Diseases.   WF 700 L723p 1995]
RC751.L48   1995
617.5'43—dc20
DNLM/DLC
for Library of Congress   94-44122
                                              CIP

                                                97 98 99
3 4 5 6 7 8 9 10

Reprints of chapter(s) may be purchased from Williams & Wilkins in quantities of 100 or more. Call Isabella Wise, Special Sales Department, (800) 358-3583.

This book is dedicated to my constant companion, Judi Despars, who has provided continuous moral support for me while this book was being rewritten.

Preface

The first two editions of Pleural Diseases were well received. Since the Second Edition was published in 1990, there has been a rapid advancement of knowledge concerning pleural diseases. Accordingly, the publishers have requested that I prepare a Third Edition.

As I prepared the Third Edition, I was impressed with how much new information concerning pleural diseases has become known during the past 5 years. Indeed the number of references has been increased approximately 50% since the last edition. Highlights of the changes since the previous edition include the following:

The most profound advance in pleural diseases during the past 5 years has been the advent of video assisted thoracic surgery (VATS) or videothoracoscopy. With modern technology one can view the pleural space as well through the thoracoscope as one could previously with an open thoracotomy. An entire chapter has been added on thoracoscopy and its place in the management of undiagnosed pleural effusions, malignant pleural effusions, complicated parapneumonic effusions, chylothorax, hemothorax, and pneumothorax.

The therapy of malignant effusions is also rapidly evolving. At the time the last edition of this book was published, tetracycline was the sclerosing agent of choice. Now tetracycline is no longer available and much work has been done to find a replacement. The present edition discusses the research behind the recommendation that talc in a slurry, or a tetracycline derivative, be used in this situation.

The therapy of parapneumonic effusions is also changing. In this edition I present a new classification of parapneumonic effusions and empyema, which I believe should simplify the management of these patients. The changes in the management include the use of smaller chest tubes, the earlier use of thrombolytics, and the early use of videothoracoscopy and/or decortication.

There have been several significant changes in the management of patients with pneumothoraces. First, the recommended initial management for most patients with primary spontaneous pneumothorax and iatrogenic pneumothorax is now simple aspiration. The recommended agent for pleural sclerosis in patients with secondary spontaneous pneumothorax is talc in a slurry or a tetracycline derivative. The recommended therapy for patients with persistent air leaks or lungs that do not expand is early videothoracoscopy, with endo stapling of the blebs. It is now recommended that the difficult patient with AIDS and a pneumothorax be sent home with a chest tube and a Heimlich valve, or be subjected to videothoracoscopy.

Since the previous edition of this book, descriptions of several entities that are associated with a pleural effusion have been added. These include the Hantavirus syndrome, the acute respiratory distress syndrome (ARDS), coronary artery bypass surgery, lung transplantation, and liver transplantation. The sections on pleural effusion and pneumothorax occurring in patients with AIDS have been markedly expanded.

It is my hope that the Third Edition of this book will continue to provide a practical, updated reference book for physicians who take care of patients with pleural diseases.

Richard W. Light, M.D.
Long Beach, California

Preface *to the First Edition*

Approximately one million patients develop a pleural effusion each year. Pleural effusions may occur with many different infections or as a complication of pulmonary disease. Additionally, pleural effusions frequently complicate malignant disease, heart disease, liver disease, gastrointestinal disease, kidney disease, and collagen vascular disease. Yet there are no recent books on pleural disease to guide the practicing physician in determining the origin of a pleural effusion or in managing a patient with pleural disease. Moreover, diseases of the pleura receive only superficial treatment in books on pulmonary disease or internal medicine.

This book is intended primarily as a reference book for physicians who take care of patients with pleural diseases. Recent advances in the knowledge of pleural disease make publication of this volume timely. In this one volume, the practicing physician will have a comprehensive discussion of all aspects of pleural disease.

The first three chapters discuss the anatomy, physiology, and radiology of the pleura. The next chapter describes the clinical manifestations of pleural disease and discusses in depth the various diagnostic tests that might be used to establish the etiology of a pleural effusion. In Chapter 5, I present my recommended approach to the patient with an undiagnosed pleural effusion. The following 13 chapters contain discussions of the various disease states that can be associated with a pleural effusion. For each disease, the pathophysiology, clinical manifestations, diagnosis, and management of the pleural effusion are outlined. In Chapters 19 through 21, pneumothorax, hemothorax, and chylothorax are presented, respectively. Pleural thickening not associated with pleural fluid is covered in Chapter 22. The next two chapters are devoted to those procedures used most often in managing patients with pleural disease, namely, diagnostic and therapeutic thoracentesis, pleural biopsy, and tube thoracostomy. The final chapter includes a description of the various drainage systems used with chest tubes.

It is my hope that publication of this book will result in better and more cost-effective management of patients with pleural disease.

Richard W. Light
Long Beach, California

Preface

Acknowledgments

Many individuals contributed to this book. I acknowledge the Medical Media Production Service at the Veterans Administration Medical Center in Long Beach, which is under the supervision of Robert Walker, and provided most of the illustrations for the book. Special credit is due Marian Berman, who created the drawings, and Walter Thill, Carolee Lavarini, and Renee Wright, who did the photography.

I also want to acknowledge Dr. Harry Sassoon, who provided several radiographs for this edition of the book. I am indebted to my companion, Judi Despars, who spent innumerable hours photocopying references and proofreading the text. Lastly, I thank the people at Williams & Wilkins, David Retford, Acquisitions Editor, and Katey Millet, Managing Editor, for their constant support while I was preparing the book.

Contents

CHAPTER 1
Anatomy of the Pleura

The pleura is the serous membrane that covers the lung parenchyma, the mediastinum, the diaphragm, and the rib cage. This structure is divided into the visceral pleura and the parietal pleura. The visceral pleura covers the lung parenchyma, not only at its points of contact with the chest wall, diaphragm, and mediastinum, but also in the interlobar fissures. The parietal pleura lines the inside of the thoracic cavities. In accordance with the intrathoracic surfaces that it lines, it is subdivided into the costal, mediastinal, and diaphragmatic parietal pleura. The visceral and the parietal pleura meet at the lung root. At the pulmonary hilus, the mediastinal pleura is swept laterally onto the root of the lung. Posterior to the lung root, the pleura is carried downward as a thin double fold called the pulmonary ligament.

A film of fluid (pleural fluid) is normally present between the parietal and the visceral pleura. This thin layer of fluid acts as a lubricant and allows the visceral pleura covering the lung to slide along the parietal pleura lining the thoracic cavity during respiratory movements. The space or potential space between the two layers of pleura is designated the pleural space. The mediastinum completely separates the right from the left pleural space. As previously mentioned, only a thin layer of fluid is normally present in this space, so it is a potential rather than an actual space. Many diseases are associated with increased amounts of pleural fluid, however, and a large segment of this book is directed toward an understanding of these diseases.

EMBRYOLOGY OF THE PLEURA AND PLEURAL SPACE

The body cavity in the embryo, the celomic cavity, is a U-shaped system with the thick bend cephalad. The cephalad portion becomes the pericardium and communicates bilaterally with the pleural canals, which in turn communicate with the peritoneal canals.

As the embryo develops, the celomic cavity becomes divided into the pericardium, the pleural cavities, and the peritoneal cavity through the development of three sets of partitions: (*a*) the septum transversum, which serves as an early, partial diaphragm; (*b*) the pleuropericardial membranes, which divide the pericardial and pleural cavities; and (*c*) the pleuroperitoneal membranes, which unite with the septum transversum to complete the partition between each pleural cavity and the peritoneal cavity. This newly formed pleural cavity is fully lined by a mesothelial membrane, the pleura.

When the primordial bronchial buds first appear, they and the trachea lie in a median mass of mesenchyme cranial and dorsal to the peritoneal cavity. This mass of mesenchymal tissue is the future mediastinum and separates the two pleural cavities. In humans, no communication normally exists between the two pleural cavities. As the growing primordial lung buds bulge into the right and left pleural cavities, they carry with them a covering of the lining mesothelium, which becomes the visceral pleura. As the separate lobes evolve, they retain their mesothelial covering. This covering becomes the visceral pleura in the fissures. The lining mesothelium of the pleural cavity becomes the parietal pleura (1).

HISTOLOGY

The parietal pleura over the ribs and intercostal spaces is composed of loose, irregular connective tissue covered by the single layer of mesothelial cells. Within the pleura are blood vessels, mainly capillaries, and lymphatic lacunas. The lacunas are a specialized initial lymphatic shaped like a flat cistern and are located over the intercostal spaces in sheep (2). The mean thickness of the parietal pleura in sheep is 20 to 25 μm, whereas the distance from the microvessels to the pleural space is 10 to 12 μm. Deep to the parietal pleura is the endothoracic fascia. This continuous band of

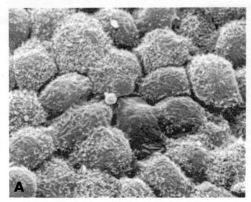 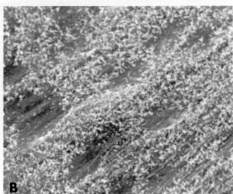

Figure 1.1. Scanning electron microscopic studies of the pleura. **A.** Bumpy pleural surface with cellular borders irregularly depressed. Note that the number of microvilli present on each cell is variable. (Original magnification: ×1300.) **B.** Flattened pleural surface with indistinct cell boundaries and sparse microvilli. (Original magnification: ×1250.) (From Wang NS: The regional difference of pleural mesothelial cells in rabbits. Am Rev Respir Dis 1974;110:623–633.)

dense irregular connective tissue, composed mainly of collagen and elastin, covers the ribs and intercostal spaces and varies in thickness from 75 to 150 μm (2).

The anatomy of the visceral pleura differs markedly from that of the parietal pleura and also varies among species, primarily by its thickness. The dog, cat, and monkey have a thin visceral pleura, whereas man, sheep, cow, pig, and horse have a thick visceral pleura (3). Distinction between lungs with a thick or thin visceral pleura is important physiologically because their blood supply and lymphatic drainage vary whether they are thick or thin. In animals with a thick visceral pleura, the predominant source of blood is the systemic circulation; in those with a thin pleura, the predominant source of blood is the pulmonary circulation (3).

Histologically, a thick visceral pleura is composed of two layers: the mesothelium and connective tissue. Blood and lymph vessels and nerves are located in the connective tissue. Animals with a thick visceral pleura have a layer of dense connective tissue of varying thickness interposed between the mesothelium and the blood vessels (3). This connective tissue layer probably limits the exchange of fluid and particulate matter between the pleural space and the blood vessels and lymphatics in the visceral pleura. In sheep the visceral pleura ranges in thickness from 25 to 83 μm (compared to 10 to 25 μm for the parietal) and the distance from the micro-

vessels to the pleural space ranges from 18 to 56 μm (compared to 10 to 12 μm for the parietal) (2).

Both the visceral and parietal pleura are lined with a single layer of flat mesothelial cells. These mesothelial cells range in size from 6 to 12 μm in diameter (4). By using scanning electron microscopy (5), the pleural surface is found to either be flattened or bumpy (Fig. 1.1). The bumpy areas include most of the visceral pleura and portions of the parietal pleura including the subcostal regions and the pleural recesses. The bumpy areas appear to result from a lack of rigidity of the underlying structures (4).

Scanning electron microscopy also demonstrates that microvilli are present diffusely over the entire pleural surface (Fig. 1.1), but the distribution of the microvilli is irregular. The microvilli are most numerous on the inferior parts of the visceral pleura and the anterior and inferior mediastinum on the parietal pleura. At corresponding regions in the thoracic cavity, more microvilli are present on the visceral than on the parietal pleura. The microvilli are approximately 0.1 μm in diameter, and their length varies from 0.5 to 1.9 μm (4).

The exact function of these numerous microvilli has yet to be defined. At one time it was believed that their presence increased the capacity of the visceral pleura to absorb pleural fluid. This is probably incorrect because recent observations have indicated that the visceral pleura plays a limited role in the absorption of pleural fluid. It is now thought that the most important function of the microvilli is to enmesh glycoproteins rich in hyaluronic acid, especially in the lower thorax, to lessen the friction between the lung and the chest wall (5). Moreover, as mentioned earlier, a thin rim of fluid normally separates the visceral and the parietal pleura. Impingement of the microvilli from one pleural surface into the opposing pleural surface could possibly help to maintain this thin rim of fluid (6), but this is controversial (7).

The mesothelial cells are active cells and are sensitive and responsive to various stimuli. In cell culture mesothelial cells have been shown to produce type I, type II, and type IV collagens, elastin, fibronectin, and laminin, and express intermediate filaments typical of both epithelial cells and fibroblasts (8). Mesothelial cells also express procoagulant activity due to a tissue factor that binds factor VII at the cell surface (9). Mesothelial cells have also been demonstrated to produce growth factor β_1 and fibroblast growth factor (10).

The mesothelial layer is very fragile. At thoracotomy in patients without clinical pleural disease, focal denudation of mesothelial cells is common (11). When the normal layer of mesothelial cells lining the pleura is disrupted, the defect is covered through mitosis and migration of the mesothelial cells (11, 12). When irritated, they retract, but retain continuity with adjacent cells by projections called cellular bridges. Mesothelial cells frequently are dislodged from the pleural surfaces and are thereby free in the pleural fluid. When free in the pleural space, the cells become round or oval (12). Their cytoplasm is rich in organelles. From this state, they may be transformed into macrophages capable of phagocytosis and erythrophagocytosis (12). Such transformed cells frequently have vacuoles in their cytoplasm. Not all the macrophages in pleural fluid evolve from mesothelial cells; some definitely evolve from peripheral blood mononuclear cells, and some may evolve from alveolar macrophages (13). An immunologic role for the macrophages derived from the mesothelial cells has been suggested (13). When mesothelial cells are cultured in tissue culture medium, they undergo a transition into fibroblasts (13).

PLEURAL FLUID

The major considerations in the understanding of pleural fluid are volume, thickness, cellular components, and physicochemical factors.

Volume

Normally, a small amount of pleural fluid is present in the pleural space. The mechanisms responsible for this small amount of residual fluid are discussed in Chapter 2. Although no reliable data on normal human pleural fluid are available, several studies have been done on the pleural fluid in normal animals. Miserocchi and Agostoni carefully measured the volume of pleural fluid in normal rabbits and dogs (14). They found that the rabbits' pleural spaces contained about 1.0 ml pleural fluid, whereas the dogs' pleural spaces contained about 2.4 ml pleural fluid. Sahn and colleagues reported that there was 0.4 ml fluid in the rabbits' pleural spaces (15), but these researchers did not measure the fluid that adheres to the pleural surface and accounts for approximately 50% of the total pleural fluid (14).

Thickness

The small amount of residual pleural fluid appears to be distributed relatively evenly throughout the pleural space. Therefore, the pleural fluid behaves as a continuous system. Albertine and associates studied the thickness of pleural fluid in rabbits by four different methods (7). They found that the average arithmetic mean width of the pleural space was slightly more narrow near the top (18.5 μm) than at the bottom (20.3 μm). Pleural space width in the most dependent recesses, such as the costodiaphragmatic recess, reached 1–2 mm. They were unable to find any contacts between the visceral and parietal pleura. Since the microvilli on the visceral and parietal pleural mesothelial cells do not interdigitate, the frictional forces between the lungs and chest wall are low (7).

Cells

Normal pleural fluid, at least in rabbits and dogs, contains significant numbers of white blood cells and few red blood cells. Miserocchi and Agostoni reported that rabbit and dog pleural fluid contains about 2450 and 2200 white blood cells/mm^3, respectively (14). In the rabbit, 32% of the cells were mesothelial cells, whereas 61% were mononuclear cells and 7% were lymphocytes. In the dog, 70% of the cells were mesothelial cells, 28% were mononuclear cells, and 2% were lymphocytes. Sahn and colleagues also studied normal rabbit pleural fluid and reported a total white cell count of 1500/mm^3 with the differential count revealing 70% monocytes, 11% lymphocytes, 9% mesothelial cells, 8% macrophages, and 2% polymorphonuclear leukocytes (15). The variance in the differential count in these series may be related to the stains used and the definition of mesothelial cells and macrophages.

Physicochemical Factors

A small amount of protein is normally present in the pleural fluid. In rabbits, the protein concentration averages 1.33 g/dl, whereas in dogs, it averages 1.06 g/dl (14). The mean oncotic pressure in the pleural fluid is 4.8 cm H_2O in rabbits and 3.2 cm H_2O in dogs (14). Protein electrophoresis demonstrates that the electrophoretic pattern for pleural fluid is similar to that of the corresponding serum, except that low-molecular-weight proteins such as albumin are present in relatively greater quantities in the pleural fluid.

Interestingly, the ionic concentrations in pleural fluid differ significantly from those in serum. The pleural fluid bicarbonate concentration is increased by 20 to 25% relative to that of plasma, while the major cation (Na^+) is reduced by 3 to 5%, and the major anion (Cl^-) is reduced by 6 to 9%. The concentrations of K^+ and glucose in the pleural fluid and plasma appear to be nearly identical (16). The gradient for bicarbonate persists when the animals are given a carbonic anhydrase inhibitor. When unilateral artificial pleural effusions of distilled water were produced in rats, electrolyte equilibrium between pleural fluid and venous plasma was reached in about 40 minutes, but

the foregoing gradients persisted. The pleural fluid P_{CO_2} is about the same as the plasma P_{CO_2}. Accordingly, in view of the elevated pleural fluid bicarbonate, the pleural fluid is alkaline with respect to the plasma pH (16). These gradients for electrolytes suggest that an active process is involved in pleural fluid formation. The significance of such an active process remains to be defined.

BLOOD SUPPLY

The parietal pleura receives its blood supply from the systemic capillaries. Small branches of the intercostal arteries supply the costal pleura, whereas the mediastinal pleura is supplied principally by the pericardiacophrenic artery. The diaphragmatic pleura is supplied by the superior phrenic and musculophrenic arteries.

The blood supply to the visceral pleura is dependent upon whether the animal has a thick or thin pleura. In general the blood supply to the visceral pleura in animals with a thin pleura originates from the pulmonary circulation, whereas the blood supply in animals with a thick pleura originates from the systemic circulation via the bronchial arteries. Albertine and coworkers have demonstrated in sheep, an animal with a thick pleura, that the bronchial artery supplies the visceral pleura completely and exclusively (3). Because man has a thick visceral pleura, his visceral pleura is probably also supplied by the bronchial artery, but there is still controversy concerning this (17).

LYMPHATICS

The lymphatic vessels of the costal pleura drain ventrally toward nodes along the internal thoracic artery and dorsally toward the internal intercostal lymph nodes near the heads of the ribs. The lymphatic vessels of the mediastinal pleura pass to the tracheobronchial and mediastinal nodes, whereas the lymphatic vessels of the diaphragmatic pleura pass to the parasternal, middle phrenic, and posterior mediastinal nodes.

The visceral pleura is abundantly endowed with lymphatic vessels. These lymphatics form a plexus of intercommunicating vessels that run over the surface of the lung toward the

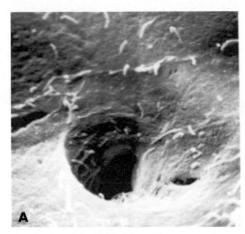
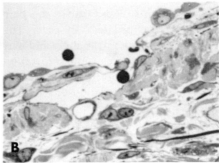

Figure 1.2. Lymphatics of the parietal pleura. **A.** Scanning electron microscopic study of the parietal pleura in the rabbit demonstrating a lymphatic stoma. Microvilli and micropinocytic openings on the mesothelial surface are both much smaller than is the stoma. (Original magnification: ×6500.) **B.** Toluidine blue stain demon-strating a red blood cell at the stoma of a lacuna. (Original magnification: ×1000.) (From Wang NS: The preformed stomas connecting the pleural cavity and the lymphatics in the parietal pleura. Am Rev Respir Dis 1975;111:12–20.)

hilum and also penetrate the lung to join the bronchial lymph vessels by passing in the interlobular septa. Although lymph may flow in either direction, all lymph from the visceral pleura eventually reaches the lung root either by penetrating the lung or by flowing on the surface of the lung. Fluid from the pleural space does not enter the lymphatics in the visceral pleural in man.

The lymphatic vessels in the parietal pleura are in communication with the pleural space by means of stomas that range in diameter from 2 to 6 nm (18) (Fig. 1.2). These stomas have a round or slitlike shape and are found mostly on the mediastinal pleura and on the intercostal surface, especially in the depressed areas just inferior to the ribs in the lower thorax. Few stomas are present in other portions of the parietal pleura (2, 18). The distribution of stomas is similar to the distribution of particulate matter injected into the pleural space (see Chapter 2).

The lymphatic vessels in the parietal pleura have many branches, in some of which are submesothelial, dilated lymphatic spaces called lacunas (Fig. 1.2B) (18). Stomas are found only over the lacunas. At the stoma, the mesothelial cells with their microvilli are in continuity with the endothelial cells of the lymphatic vessels. When red blood cells or carbon particles are injected into the pleural space, they collect around the stomas and in the lacunas and lymphatic vessels (Fig. 1.2B) (2, 18). Therefore, these stomas with their associated lacunas and lymphatic vessels are thought to be the main pathway for the egress of particulate matter from the pleural space (2, 18).

The existence of such stomas in man has yet to be proven definitely. Gaudio and co-workers (4) were unable to demonstrate any such stomas in specimens from 30 patients undergoing thoracic surgical procedures. Peng and associates (11) were able to demonstrate stomas in only two of their nine human specimens. These two studies indicate that if there are stomas in the human pleura, they must be less than abundant.

No stomas are seen in the visceral pleura, and the lymphatic vessels of the visceral pleura are separated from the mesothelial cells by a layer of connective tissue. The lack of stomas in the visceral pleura explains the observation that particulate matter injected in the pleural space is removed through the parietal pleura (see Chapter 2).

INNERVATION

Sensory nerve endings are present in the costal and diaphragmatic parietal pleura. The intercostal nerves supply the costal pleura and the peripheral part of the diaphragmatic pleura. When either of these areas is stimulated, pain is referred to the adjacent chest wall. In contrast, the central portion of the diaphragm is innervated by the phrenic nerve, and stimulation of this pleura causes the pain to be perceived in the ipsilateral shoulder. The visceral pleura contains no pain fibers and may be manipulated without causing unpleasant sensation. Therefore, the presence of pleuritic chest pain indicates inflammation or irritation of the parietal pleura.

REFERENCES

1. Gray SW, Skandalakis JE: Development of the pleura. In: Chretien J, Bignon J, Hirsch A, eds. The Pleura in Health and Disease. Lung Biology in Health and Disease. New York: Marcel Dekker, 1985;30:3-19.
2. Albertine KH, Wiener-Kronish JP, Staub NC: The structure of the parietal pleura and its relationship to pleural liquid dynamics in sheep. Anat Rec 1984;208: 401-409.
3. Albertine KH, Wiener-Kronish JP, Roos PJ, Staub NC: Structure, blood supply, and lymphatic vessels of the sheep's visceral pleura. Am J Anat 1982;165:277-294.
4. Gaudio E, Rendina EA, Pannarale L, et al: Surface morphology of the human pleura: a scanning electron microscopic study. Chest 1988;92:149-153.
5. Wang NS: The regional difference of pleural mesothelial cells in rabbits. Am Rev Respir Dis 1974;110:623-633.
6. Miserocchi G, Agostoni E: Pleural liquid and surface pressures at various lung volumes. Respir Physiol 1980;39:315-326.
7. Albertine KH, Wiener-Kronish JP, Bastacky J, Staub NC: No evidence for mesothelial cell contact across the costal pleural space of sheep. J Appl Physiol 1991;70:123-143.
8. Antony VB, Sahn SA, Mossman B, Gail DB, Kalica A: Pleural cell biology in health and disease. Am Rev Respir Dis 1992;145:1236-1239.
9. Idell S, Zwieb C, Kumar A, Koenig KB, Johnson AR: Pathways of fibrin turnover of human pleural mesothelial cells in vitro. Am J Respir Cell Mol Biol 1992;7:414-426.
10. Bermudez E, Everitt J, Walker C: Expression of growth factor and growth factor receptor RNA in rat pleural mesothelial cells in culture. Exp Cell Res 1990;190:91-98.
11. Peng M-J, Wang NS, Vargas FS, Light RW: Subclinical surface alterations of human pleura. Chest 1994;106: 351-353.
12. Efrati P, Nir E: Morphological and cytochemical investigation of human mesothelial cells from pleural and peritoneal effusions. A light and electron microscopy study. Isr J Med Sci 1976;12:662-673.
13. Bakalos D, Constantakis N, Tsicricas T: Distinction of mononuclear macrophages from mesothelial cells in pleural and peritoneal effusions. Acta Cytol 1974;18: 20-22.
14. Miserocchi G, Agostoni E: Contents of the pleural space. J Appl Physiol 1971;30:208-213.
15. Sahn SA, Willcox ML, Good JT, et al: Characteristics of normal rabbit pleural fluid: physiologic and biochemical implications. Lung 1979;156:63-69.
16. Rolf LL, Travis DM: Pleural fluid-plasma bicarbonate gradients in oxygen-toxic and normal rats. Am J Physiol 1973;224:857-861.
17. Bernaudin JF, Fleury J: Anatomy of the blood and lymphatic circulation of the pleural serosa. In: Chretien J, Bignon J, Hirsch A, eds. The Pleura in Health and Disease. Lung Biology in Health and Disease. New York: Marcel Dekker, 1985;30:101-124.
18. Wang NS: The preformed stomas connecting the pleural cavity and the lymphatics in the parietal pleura. Am Rev Respir Dis 1975;111:12-20.

CHAPTER 2

Physiology of the Pleural Space

The pleural space is the coupling system between the lung and the chest wall and is accordingly a crucial feature of the breathing apparatus. The pressure within the pleural space (the pleural pressure) is important in cardiopulmonary physiology, because it is the pressure at the outer surface of the lung and heart, and the inner surface of the thoracic cavity. Because the lung, the heart, and the thoracic cavity are all distensible, and because the volume of a distensible object depends upon the pressure difference between the inside and the outside of the object and its compliance, the pleural pressure plays an important role in determining the volume of these three important structures.

PLEURAL PRESSURE

If the thorax is opened to atmospheric pressure, the lungs decrease in volume because of their elastic recoil, while at the same time the thorax enlarges. With the thorax open, the volume of the thoracic cavity is about 55% of the vital capacity, whereas the volume of the lung is below its residual volume. With the chest closed and the patient relaxed, the respiratory system is at its functional residual capacity (FRC), which is approximately 35% of the total lung capacity (1). Thus, at FRC, the opposing elastic forces of the chest wall and lung produce a negative pressure between the visceral and the parietal pleura, which is called the *pleural pressure*. This pressure surrounds the lung and is the primary determinant of the volume of the lung. The pleural pressure represents the balance between the outward pull of the thoracic cavity and the inward pull of the lung (1).

Measurement

The pleural pressure can be measured directly by inserting needles, trocars, catheters, or balloons into the pleural space. Direct measurement of the pleural pressure is not usually made because of the danger of producing a pneumothorax or of introducing infection into the pleural space. Rather, the pleural pressure is measured indirectly by a balloon positioned in the esophagus. Because the esophagus is a compliant structure situated between the two pleural spaces, esophageal pressure measurements provide a close approximation of the pleural pressure at the level of the balloon in the thorax (2). Estimation of pleural pressure by means of an esophageal balloon is not without difficulties (2). The volume of air within the balloon must be small so the balloon is not stretched and the esophageal walls are not displaced; otherwise, pleural pressure estimates are falsely elevated. Moreover, the balloon must be short and must be placed in the lower part of the esophagus. Recently it has been demonstrated that reliable measurements of esophageal pressures can be made with micromanometers (3). The use of the micromanometer should circumvent some of the problems associated with esophageal balloons.

Gradients

Only one value for the pleural pressure is obtained when it is estimated by an esophageal balloon. It should be emphasized, however, that the pleural pressure is not uniform throughout the pleural space. A gradient in pleural pressure is seen between the superior and the inferior portions of the lung, with the pleural pressure being lowest or most negative in the superior portion and highest or least negative in the inferior portion (4). The main factors responsible for this pleural pressure gradient are probably gravity, mismatching of the shapes of the chest wall and lung, and the weight of the lungs and other intrathoracic structures (1).

The magnitude of the pleural pressure gradient appears to be approximately 0.50 cm H_2O/cm vertical distance (4). It should be noted that over the past 30 years there have been many studies directed at measuring the pleural pressure gradient and the resulting values have ranged from 0.20 to 0.93 cm H_2O/cm vertical distance (4). The results have been largely dependent upon the method used (4). It appears that the higher values were obtained with catheters that were large relative to the narrow pleural space and accordingly produced distortion of the pleura with subsequent alterations in the measured pressures (4).

In the upright position, the difference in the pleural pressure between the apex and the base of the lungs may be 12 cm or more. Because the alveolar pressure is constant throughout the lungs, the end result of the gradient in the pleural pressure is that different parts of the lungs have different distending pressures. The pressure-volume curve is thought to be the same for all regions of the lungs; therefore, the pleural pressure gradient causes the alveoli in the superior parts of the lung to be larger than those in the inferior parts of the lung. The pleural pressure gradients also account for the unevenness in the distribution of ventilation.

Pleural Liquid Pressure versus Pleural Surface Pressure

There has been a controversy for many years as to whether there are two pleural pressures or one (5). The two different pressures had been proposed to explain a discrepancy obtained when the pleural pressure was measured in two different ways. If the pressure was measured using fluid-filled catheters, the vertical gradient obtained was approximately 1 cm H_2O/cm vertical height. This pressure was designated the *pleural liquid pressure* and was felt to represent the pressure that influenced the absorption of fluid. If the pressure was measured using surface balloons or suction cups, then a gradient of 0.5 cm H_2O/cm vertical height was obtained. This pressure was designated the *pleural surface pressure* and represented the balance between the outward pull of the thoracic cavity and the inward pull of the lung. It now appears that there is only one pressure and that the discrepancies in the pressures arose because of the distortion due to the catheters

as discussed above (4). It should be noted, however, that there is still a school that believes in the two different pressures (6).

PLEURAL FLUID FORMATION

Fluid that enters the pleural space can originate in the interstitial spaces of the lung, the pleural capillaries, the intrathoracic lymphatics, or the peritoneal cavity.

Interstitial Origin

In recent years it has been demonstrated that the origin of much of the fluid that enters the pleural space is the interstitial spaces of the lungs. Either high-pressure or high-permeability pulmonary edema can lead to the accumulation of pleural fluid. When sheep are volume overloaded to produce a high-pressure pulmonary edema, approximately 25% of all the fluid that enters the interstitial spaces of the lungs is cleared from the lung via the pleural space (7). Within 2 hours of starting the volume overloading, the amount of fluid entering the pleural space increases; and within 3 hours, the protein concentration in the pleural fluid is the same as that in the interstitial spaces of the lungs (7). The amount of pleural fluid formed is directly related to the elevation in the wedge pressure. Increases in pleural fluid accumulation only occur after the development of pulmonary edema (8).

The pulmonary interstitial space is probably also the origin of the pleural fluid in patients with congestive heart failure. The likelihood of a pleural effusion increases as the severity of pulmonary edema increases (9). In addition, the presence of pleural effusions is more closely correlated with the pulmonary venous pressure than with the systemic venous pressure (9).

The amount of fluid that enters the pleural space is also increased when there is increased interstitial fluid due to high-permeability pulmonary edema. When increased-permeability edema was induced in sheep by the infusion of oleic acid, pleural fluid accumulated only after pulmonary edema developed (10). In this study there was no morphologic evidence of pleural injury. When pulmonary edema is induced by xylazine (11) or hyperoxia (12) in rats or by ethchlorvynol in sheep (13), the high-protein pleural fluid appears to originate in the interstitial spaces of the lungs. The pleural fluid associated with experimental *Pseudomonas* pneumonia in rabbits originates in the lung (14). It is likely that the origin of the pleural fluid with many conditions associated with lung injury, such as pulmonary embolization and lung transplantation, is also the interstitial spaces of the lung (5).

In experimental studies of hydrostatic and increased permeability edema, a pleural effusion develops when the extravascular lung water has reached a certain level for a certain amount of time (15). The necessary level of edema appears to between 5 and 8 g of fluid/g of dry lung whether the edema is secondary to hydrostatic edema, oleic acid lung injury, or α-naphthylthiourea lung injury (15). With increasing levels of interstitial fluid, it has been shown that the subpleural interstitial pressure increases (16). The barrier to movement of fluid across the visceral pleura appears to be weak, even though the visceral pleura is thick (17). Therefore, once the subpleural interstitial pressure increases, it follows that fluid will traverse the visceral pleura to the pleural space.

Pleural Capillaries

The movement of fluid between the pleural capillaries and the pleural space is believed to be governed by Starling's law of transcapillary exchange. When this law is applied to the pleura

$$\dot{Q}_f = L_p \cdot A[(P_{cap} - P_{pl}) - \sigma_d(\pi_{cap} - \pi_{pl})]$$
(Eq. 2.1)

where $\dot{Q}_f$ is the liquid movement; L_p is the filtration coefficient per unit area or the hydraulic water conductivity of the membrane; A is the surface area of the membrane; P and π are the hydrostatic and oncotic pressures, respectively, of the capillary (cap) and pleural (pl) space; and σ_d is the solute reflection coefficient for protein, a measure of the membrane's ability to restrict the passage of large molecules (18). The σ_d of the canine visceral pleura exceeds 0.80 (18).

Estimates for the magnitude of the pressures affecting fluid movement from the capillaries to the pleural space in humans are shown in

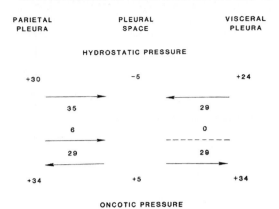

Figure 2.1.   Various pressures that normally influence the movement of fluid in and out of the pleural space in species with a thick visceral pleura, such as man.

Figure 2.1. When the parietal pleura is considered, a gradient for fluid formation is normally present. The hydrostatic pressure in the parietal pleura is approximately 30 cm H_2O, whereas the pleural pressure is about −5 cm H_2O. The net hydrostatic pressure is therefore 30 − (−5) = 35 cm H_2O and favors the movement of fluid from the capillaries in the parietal pleura to the pleural space. Opposing this hydrostatic pressure gradient is the oncotic pressure gradient. The oncotic pressure in the plasma is approximately 34 cm H_2O. Normally, the small amount of pleural fluid contains a small amount of protein and has an oncotic pressure of about 5 cm H_2O (19), yielding a net oncotic pressure gradient of 34 − 5 = 29 cm H_2O. Thus, the net gradient is 35 − 29 = 6 cm H_2O, favoring the movement of fluid from the capillaries in the parietal pleura to the pleural space.

The net gradient for fluid movement across the visceral pleura in man is probably close to zero, but this has not been demonstrated (Fig. 2.1). The pressure in the visceral pleural capillaries is approximately 6 cm H_2O less than that in the parietal pleural capillaries because the former drain into the pulmonary veins. Because this is the only pressure that differs from those affecting fluid movement across the parietal pleura and because the net gradient for the parietal pleura is 6 cm H_2O, it follows that the net gradient for fluid movement across the visceral pleura is approximately zero. It is also likely that the filtration coefficient (L_p) for the visceral pleura is sub-

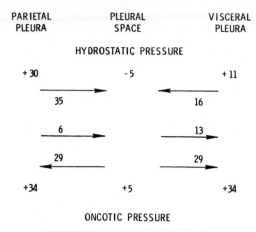

Figure 2.2. Various pressures that normally influence the movement of fluid in and out of the pleural space in species with a thin visceral pleura, such as the dog. See text for explanation.

stantially less than that for the parietal pleura because the capillaries in the visceral pleura are much farther from the pleural space than those in the parietal pleura (20).

The transpleural exchange of fluid is species dependent. Man and sheep have a thick visceral pleura and its blood supply is from the bronchial artery rather than the pulmonary artery (21). However, many species such as the rabbit and the dog have a thin visceral pleura, which receives its blood supply from the pulmonary circulation. In such a situation, as shown in Figure 2.2, the net gradients favor pleural fluid formation across the parietal pleura and pleural fluid absorption through the visceral pleura.

Peritoneal Cavity

Pleural fluid accumulation can occur if there is free fluid in the peritoneal cavity and if there are openings in the diaphragm. Under these conditions, the fluid will flow from the peritoneal space to the pleural space because the pressure in the pleural cavity is less than the pressure in the peritoneal cavity. The peritoneal cavity is the origin of the pleural fluid in hepatic hydrothorax, Meigs' syndrome, and peritoneal dialysis.

Thoracic Duct Disruption

If the thoracic duct is disrupted, lymph will accumulate in the pleural space. When the thoracic duct is lacerated in dogs, sizeable pleural effusions begin to develop almost immediately (22).

Origin of Fluid Normally

The rate of pleural fluid formation in normal sheep is approximately 0.01 ml/kg/hour (23). It appears that in normal individuals the origin of most pleural fluid is the capillaries in the parietal pleural (23). It certainly does not appear to be the interstitial spaces of the lung because the protein level in the interstitial spaces is normally about 4.5 g/dl while the protein level in normal pleural fluid is only about 1–1.5 g/dl. From Figure 2.1 it appears unlikely that it is the visceral pleura. Likewise, both a lymphatic origin and a peritoneal cavity origin appear unlikely. Supporting evidence for this thesis has been provided by Broaddus and coworkers (23). These workers measured the vascular pressures and the pleural fluid protein levels in sheep of different ages. They found that the systemic vascular pressures progressively increased with age while the pleural fluid protein levels progressively decreased with age. They concluded that their findings supported their thesis since higher vascular pressures should produce pleural fluid with lower protein levels (23).

PLEURAL FLUID ABSORPTION

Lymphatic Clearance

From Figure 2.1, one might have the impression that pleural fluid should continuously accumulate because the Starling equation favors fluid formation through the parietal pleura and there is no gradient for fluid absorption through the visceral pleura. Fluid clearance via the pleural lymphatics is thought to explain the lack of fluid accumulation normally. The pleural space is in communication with the lymphatic vessels in the parietal pleura by means of stomas in the parietal pleura. No such stomas are present in the visceral pleura. Proteins, cells, and all other particulate matter are removed from the pleural space by these lymphatics in the parietal pleura (24–27).

The amount of fluid that can be cleared through these lymphatics is substantial. Stewart found that the mean lymphatic flow from one pleural space in 7 patients was 0.40 ml/kg/hour (28), whereas Leckie and Tothill found that the mean lymphatic flow was 0.22 ml/kg/hour in 7 patients with congestive heart failure (29). In both these studies, marked variability was noted from one patient to another. If these results in patients with congestive heart failure can be extrapolated to the normal person, a 60-kg individual should have a lymphatic drainage from each pleural space on the order of 15 ml/hour or 300 ml/day.

Experimental work with sheep, a species with a thick visceral pleura similar to man, suggests that most of the fluid that enters the pleural space in sheep is removed via the lymphatics. Broaddus and coworkers produced artificial hydrothoraces in awake sheep by injecting an autologous protein solution at a volume of 10 ml/kg with a protein level of 1.0 g/dl (30). These investigators found that the hydrothorax was removed almost completely by the lymphatics in a linear fashion at a rate of 0.28 ml/kg/hour. The linearity suggests that the lymphatics operate at maximum capacity once the pleural liquid exceeds a certain threshold volume. Note that the capacity for lymphatic clearance is 28 times as high as the normal rate of pleural fluid formation.

In the foregoing experiments of Broaddus and colleagues, the fluid introduced into the pleural space had an oncotic pressure of about 5 cm H_2O, and from Figure 2.1 one might speculate that if fluids with oncotic pressures other than 5 cm had been introduced, the equilibrium would have been altered such that fluid would enter the pleural space from visceral pleura in animals with high oncotic pressures and would leave the pleural space through the visceral pleura in animals with low oncotic pressures. This does not appear to be the case. Aiba et al. produced artificial pleural effusions in dogs with protein levels ranging from 0.1 to 9.0 g/dl (31). Even when the induced pleural effusion had a protein level of 0.1 g/dl, there was no increase in the concentration of protein with time indicating that the low oncotic pressure did not induce a rapid efflux of fluid out of the pleural space. When the protein concentration of the induced effusions was above 4 g/dl, the concentration of protein in the pleural fluid did gradually decrease with time indicating a net transfer of protein free fluid into the pleural space. The net amount of fluid entering the pleural space even with a protein level of 9.0 g/dl was only 0.22 ml/kg/hour, however. This degree of fluid flux is similar to the lymphatic clearance of 0.22 ml/kg/hour reported in the same studies. Additional evidence supporting a primary role for the pleural lymphatics in pleural fluid absorption comes from the studies of Shinto and Light (32). They did serial thoracentesis on patients undergoing vigorous diuretic therapy for congestive heart failure and reported that the protein and LDH levels in the pleural fluid changed very little over a 24 to 72 hour period, even though the volume of the pleural fluid decreased rapidly. If the fluid had been removed via the capillaries in the visceral pleura, then the protein and LDH concentrations should have increased. These observations strongly suggest that most pleural fluid is removed via the lymphatics in the parietal pleura in species such as man with a thick visceral pleural.

Clearance via Capillaries in Visceral Pleura

Up until the mid-1980s, it was thought that the primary route for the exit of fluid from the pleural space was through the capillaries in the visceral pleural (33). This conclusion was based primarily on experiments in animals with a thin pleura. It is easily seen from Figure 2.2 that in animals with a thin pleura there is a sizeable gradient for the movement of fluid from the pleural space into the capillaries in the visceral pleura. In addition, fluid probably moves across a thin visceral pleura more easily than it moves across a thick pleural membrane. For the reasons cited above, however, it appears that in man almost all pleural fluid is removed via the lymphatics in the parietal pleura. Nevertheless, it should be noted that this view is not accepted by all (34).

The foregoing should not be interpreted to indicate that small molecules do not move across the pleural surfaces. Indeed, water and small-sized molecules exchange easily across both pleural surfaces (35). When hydrothoraces are induced in dogs, the clearance rate for p-aminohippuric acid (PAH) (molecular weight 216) is about 2.0 ml/kg/hour (31). When urea is injected into patients with pleural effusions, its concentration decreases much more rapidly than does that of radiolabeled protein (36). Indeed, the urea clearance rate is several hundred milliliters per hour (36). Because urea and water have comparable molecular weights, one can assume that the rates of exchange for urea and water across the pleural membranes are similar. Therefore, several hundred milliliters of water probably traverse the pleural membranes each day, but the net movement is only a few milliliters because the osmolarity is nearly identical on each side of the membrane.

PATHOGENESIS OF PLEURAL EFFUSIONS

Pleural fluid will accumulate when the rate of pleural fluid formation exceeds the rate of pleural fluid absorption. The main factors that lead to increased pleural fluid formation or decreased pleural fluid absorption are tabulated in Table 2.1. Normally a small amount (0.01 ml/kg/hour) of fluid constantly enters the pleural space from the capillaries in the parietal pleura. Almost all this fluid is removed by the lymphatics in the parietal pleura, which have a capacity to remove at least 0.20 ml/kg/hour. Note that this provides a safety factor of nearly 20.

Table 2.1. General Causes of Pleural Effusions

Increased Pleural Fluid Formation
  Increased interstitial fluid in the lung
    Left ventricular failure, pneumonia, and pulmonary embolus
  Increased intravascular pressure in pleura
    Right or left ventricular failure, superior vena caval syndrome
  Increased pleural fluid protein level
  Decreased pleural pressure
    Lung atelectasis or increased elastic recoil of the lung
  Increased fluid in peritoneal cavity
    Ascites or peritoneal dialysis
  Disruption of the thoracic duct
Decreased Pleural Fluid Absorption
  Obstruction of the lymphatics draining the parietal pleura
  Elevation of systemic vascular pressures
    Superior vena caval syndrome or right ventricular failure

The most common cause of increased pleural fluid formation is increased interstitial fluid in the lung. As mentioned above, whenever the amount of edema in the lung exceeds 5 g/g of lung dry weight, pleural fluid accumulates whether the edema is high protein or low protein (15). This appears to be the predominant mechanism for the formation of pleural effusions with congestive heart failure, parapneumonic effusions, the acute respiratory distress syndrome and lung transplantation.

Increased intravascular pressure in the pleura will also lead to increased pleural fluid formation through its influence on Starling's equation (Figure 2.1). Such increases in pressure can occur with right ventricular failure, left ventricular failure or the superior vena caval syndrome.

Increased protein in the pleural fluid can also lead to increased pleural fluid formation through its influence on Starling's equation (Fig. 2.1). For example, if the protein level in the serum and pleural fluid are identical, then there should be gradients of 35 and 29 cm H_2O from the parietal and visceral pleura, respectively (instead of the normal 6 and 0 cm H_2O) favoring pleural fluid formation. Increased pleural fluid protein levels occur with increased permeability pulmonary edema, hemothorax and with conditions where the permeability of the pleural capillaries is increased. This mechanism is probably not too important since when sheep have a pleural fluid protein level of 9.0 g/dl, the rate of fluid entry into the pleural space is only 0.22 ml/kg/hour (31).

Decreased pleural pressure in the pleural fluid can also lead to increased pleural fluid formation through its influence on Starling's equation (Fig. 2.1). The most common situation in which this mechanism accounts for a pleural effusion is bronchial obstruction leading to atelectasis of a lower lobe or a complete lung. This mechanism is also operable when the visceral pleura becomes coated with a collagenous peel and the lung becomes trapped. In these instances, the pleural pressure can become negative, below −50 cm H_2O (37). It can contribute to pleural fluid accumulation with diseases in which the elastic recoil of the lung is increased.

If there is free fluid in the peritoneal cavity, it will lead to pleural fluid accumulation if there is a hole in the diaphragm. In like manner, chyle will accumulate in the pleural space if there is a disruption in the thoracic duct.

The most common cause of a decrease in the pleural fluid absorption is obstruction of the lymphatics draining the parietal pleura. Normally, the lymphatic flow from the pleural space is about 0.01 ml/kg/hour or 15 ml/day, but the capacity of the lymphatics is about 0.20 ml/kg/hour or 300 ml/day. Lymphatic blockade is probably one of the major factors that contributes to the development of a malignant pleural effusion. Leckie and Tothill studied the lymphatic flow in 8 patients with lung carcinoma and in 6 patients with metastatic breast carcinoma and found that the mean lymphatic flow was only 0.08 ml/kg/hour (29). Obviously, pleural effusions would not have developed in these patients unless excess fluid had also been entering the pleural space. Unless the lymphatic flow is markedly impaired, another factor must be present in addition to lymphatic disease to produce a pleural effusion given the excess capacity of the lymphatics.

Because the lymphatics drain into the systemic venous circulation, elevation of the pressures in the central veins will decrease the lymphatic flow. Pleural effusions develop in sheep when the pressure in the superior vena cava is increased. Allen and coworkers found that pleural fluid accumulated over a 24-hour period when the pressure in the superior vena cava exceeded 15 mm Hg (38). The amount of pleural fluid that accumulated increased exponentially as the pressure was increased. Comparable amounts of pleural fluid accumulated in both pleural spaces. A total of 500 ml pleural fluid accumulated when the pressure was 27 to 28 mm Hg. These workers reported that the larger the pleural effusion, the higher the protein level. They concluded that the pleural effusions developed because of: (*a*) lymph leakage out of the lymphatics that pass through the chest; these include the thoracic duct and the diaphragmatic and pulmonary lymphatics; or (*b*) obstruction of lung or chest wall lymphatics with subsequent leakage of interstitial fluid into the pleural space (38).

WHY IS THERE NO AIR IN THE PLEURAL SPACE?

Because the pleural pressure is negative at functional residual capacity and throughout most of the respiratory cycle, why is there normally no air in the pleural space? Gases move in and out of the pleural space from the capillaries in the visceral and parietal pleurae (39). The movement of each gas is dependent upon its partial pressure in the pleural space, as compared with that in the capillary blood. The sum of all the partial pressures in the capillary blood averages 706 mm Hg (P_{H_2O} = 47, P_{CO_2} = 46, P_{N_2} = 573, and P_{O_2} = 40 mm Hg). Therefore, a net movement of gas into the pleural space should occur only if the pleural pressure is below 706 mm Hg or below −54 mm Hg relative to atmospheric pressure. Because mean pleural pressures this low hardly ever occur, the pleural space normally remains gas free.

If air is discovered in the pleural space, it means that one of three things has occurred: (*a*) a communication exists or has recently existed between the alveoli and the pleural space; (*b*) a communication exists or has recently existed between the atmosphere and the pleural space; or (*c*) gas-producing organisms are present in the pleural space.

When air does enter the pleural space and thereby produces a pneumothorax, its rate of absorption depends upon the difference between the sum of the partial pressures in the pleural space and in the capillary blood. The sum of the partial pressures in the pleural space is close to atmospheric pressure. Because the sum of the partial pressures in the capillary blood is most dependent upon the P_{N_2}, this sum can be rapidly reduced by having the patient breathe supplemental oxygen, which reduces the P_{N_2} of the capillary blood without changing the other partial pressures much. In patients who have small pneumothoraces, administration of supplemental oxygen facilitates the reabsorption of the pneumothorax (40).

HOW IMPORTANT IS THE PLEURAL SPACE?

The pleural space serves as the coupling system between the lung and the chest wall. The thin rim of fluid that normally separates the parietal from the visceral pleura is thought to facilitate the movements of the lung within the thoracic cavity. Therefore, what are the consequences of obliterating the pleural space? Surprisingly, patients with obliterated pleural spaces appear to suffer no significant ill effects. Gaensler studied the pulmonary function of 4 patients before and 6 to 17 months after they had been subjected to pleurectomy (41). The mean vital capacity and maximal breathing capacity were virtually identical pre and postoperatively. Moreover, the ventilation and oxygen uptake on the operated side, as compared to the intact side, were unchanged postoperatively.

Fleetham and coworkers studied regional lung function in 4 men who had undergone thoracotomy for pleurodesis 2 to 9 years previously (42). They found that in all subjects, boluses of xenon inhaled slowly at functional residual capacity were distributed more to the apex and less to the base of the lung on the operated side than on the intact side. These researchers believe, however, that these minor differences were probably not of clinical significance.

Further evidence for the lack of importance of the pleural space is provided by studies of elephants. The pleural space of both Asian and African elephants has been found to be obliterated by connective tissue (33). Whether this observation reflects the normal condition is controversial. Nevertheless, that many of these large mammals function without a pleural space indicates the relative lack of importance of this structure for normal function. The potential pleural space plays a major role in many disease states, however.

Recent experiments in sheep have suggested that the pleural space is important in clearing fluid from the interstitium of the lung. When noncardiogenic pulmonary edema is produced in sheep via the intravenous injection of oleic acid, approximately 20% of the fluid that enters the interstitium of the lung is removed by the lymphatics in the parietal pleura after the fluid crosses the visceral pleura to the pleural space (10). The relevance of this observation to disease in man is yet to be proved. The infrequency of unilateral pulmonary edema in patients with a previous pleurodesis makes one skeptical about the clinical significance of these findings.

PHYSIOLOGIC EFFECTS OF A PLEURAL EFFUSION

The presence of fluid in the pleural space produces restrictive ventilatory dysfunction. When saline solution is instilled into the pleural spaces of dogs, both the FRC and the total lung capacity (TLC) decrease with increasing amounts of saline added to the pleural space (43). When the volume of saline additions were 9, 25, and 45% of the control TLC, the decrease in FRC was about one-third the amount of saline solution added. The other two-thirds of the saline volume must therefore have increased the chest wall volume. This increase occurred predominantly because of downward displacement of the diaphragm. The decrease in the TLC was about 20% that of the added saline volume. Accordingly, there was no decrease in the inspiratory capacity. Most of the volume decrease occurred in the lower lobe; the upper lobe retained its original volume. The esophageal pressure remained unchanged at both FRC and TLC.

In man the presence of a pleural effusion also produces restrictive ventilatory dysfunction and may also adversely affect the diaphragmatic function. Estenne and coworkers measured respiratory mechanics in 9 patients before and 2 hours after removal of 600 to 2750 ml (mean = 1818 ml) of pleural fluid (44). Prior to the thoracentesis the forced vital capacity (FVC) varied from 22 to 51% of predicted. The FRC and static expiratory pulmonary compliance were also low, averaging 61 and 40%, respectively. After thoracentesis, the mean FVC and FRC increased only 300 and 460 ml, respectively. Our group obtained spirometry before and 24 hours after thoracentesis in 26 patients from whom a mean of 1740 ml pleural fluid was withdrawn (45). In these patients the mean vital capacity improved 410 ± 390 ml. Patients in this study with higher pleural pressures after the removal of 800 ml pleural fluid and patients with a smaller decrease in the pleural pressure after the removal of 800 ml pleural fluid had greater improvements in the FVC after thoracentesis.

Estenne and coworkers attributed the relief of dyspnea following thoracentesis to a reduction in the size of the thoracic cage, which allows the inspiratory muscles to operate on a more advantageous portion of their length-tension curve (44). They found that, after thoracentesis, there was a shift in the inspiratory pleural pressure-volume curve such that the maximal pressures generated by the inspiratory muscles at a given lung volume were markedly more negative. The maximal inspiratory pressure (MIP) at TLC was -16 cm H_2O before thoracentesis and improved to -25 after thoracentesis. The highest MIP went from -41 cm H_2O before thoracentesis to -52 cm H_2O after thoracentesis. The downward displacement of the diaphragm by the pleural fluid is probably the primary explanation for these observations.

The PaO_2 is usually decreased and the alveolar-arterial O_2 gradient is usually increased in patients with pleural effusions. It is probable that these changes are due to the underlying lung disease rather than the presence of a pleural effusion. Indeed, blood gases may actually deteriorate following thoracentesis. In one study, arterial blood gases were obtained before and 20 minutes, 2 hours, and 24 hours after therapeutic thoracentesis in 19 patients (46). The mean PaO_2 fell from 70.4 mm Hg before thoracentesis to 61.2 mm Hg 20 minutes after the procedure and remained reduced to 64.4 mm Hg 2 hours after thoracentesis before returning to baseline 22 hours later.

Three separate studies have compared the oxygenation status of patients with pleural effusions when the patients were lying on their sides (47–49). In all three studies there was a small improvement in the oxygenation status when the patient had the lung without the effusion dependent. It was noted, however, in the latter study that patients with severe reduction of their FEV_1 and FVC had a *lower* PaO_2 with the normal lung down, while patients with less severe reductions in their pulmonary function tests had a higher PaO_2 with the normal lung down (49).

It appears that the presence of a pleural effusion may compromise the *cardiac* function of some patients with large pleural effusions. In has been shown in dogs (50) that the induction of a large pleural effusion will lead to right ventricular diastolic collapse and an associated decrease in cardiac output. In dogs with artificially induced bilateral pleural effusions, the occurrence of the right ventricular diastolic collapse occurs when the pleural pressure is about 4 mm Hg (50). Pleural pressures this high are frequently seen in patients with large pleural effusions (37). There have also been two reports of patients with large pleural effusions associated with a compromised cardiac output (51, 52). In both cases, the cardiac output improved after therapeutic thoracentesis. In one of the cases, left ventricular diastolic collapse was documented (52). The frequency of cardiac compromise in patients with large pleural effusions remains to be determined.

Many patients with pleural effusions complain of exercise intolerance; however, a therapeutic thoracentesis does not appear to increase exercise tolerance in many patients. Over the past several years we have performed symptom-limited maximal exercise tests on 25 patients before and 24 hours following a therapeutic thoracentesis during which a mean of 1700 ml pleural fluid was withdrawn (53, 54). Prior to the thoracentesis the exercise tolerance of the patients was markedly limited with a mean maximal workload of only 71 watts. However after thoracentesis the maximal workload tolerated only increased to 78 watts. Only 11 of the patients were able to achieve a higher workload after thoracentesis. There was no significant change in either the hypoxic or hypercapnic drives after thoracentesis. Most of the patients that we studied had malignant pleural effusions and it appeared that general disability due to the underlying disease rather than compromised pulmonary function was responsible for the exercise limitation in many patients.

REFERENCES

1. Ward ME, Roussos C, Macklem PT: Respiratory mechanics. In: Murray JF, Nadel JA, eds. Textbook of Respiratory Medicine. Philadelphia: WB Saunders, 1994;1:90–138.

2. Milic-Emili J, Mead J, Turner JM, Glauser EM: Improved technique for estimating pleural pressure from esophageal balloons. J Appl Physiol 1964;19: 207-211.

3. Chartrand DA, Jodoin C, Couture J: Measurement of pleural pressure with esophageal catheter-tip micromanometer in anaesthetized humans. Can J Anaesth 1991;38:518-521.

4. Lai-Fook SJ, Rodarte JR: Pleural pressure distribution and its relationship to lung volume and interstitial pressure. J Appl Physiol 1991;70:967-978.

5. Broaddus VC, Light RW: Disorders of the pleura: General principles and diagnostic approach. In: Murray JF, Nadel JA, eds. Textbook of Respiratory Medicine. Philadelphia: WB Saunders, 1994;2:2145-2163.

6. Agostoni E, D'Angelo E: Pleural liquid pressure. J Appl Physiol 1991;71:393-403.

7. Broaddus VC, Wiener-Kronish JP, Staub NC: Clearance of lung edema into the pleural space of volume-loaded anesthetized sheep. J Appl Physiol 1990;68: 2623-2630.

8. Allen S, Gabel J, Drake R: Left atrial hypertension causes pleural effusion formation in unanesthetized sheep. Am J Physiol 1989;257(2 Pt 2):H690-H692.

9. Wiener-Kronish JP, Matthay MA, Callen PW, et al: Relationship of pleural effusions to pulmonary hemodynamics in patients with congestive heart failure. Am Rev Respir Dis 1985;132:1253-1256.

10. Wiener-Kronish JP, Broaddus VC, Albertine KH, Gropper MA, Matthay MA, Staub NC: Relationship of pleural effusions to increased permeability pulmonary edema in anesthetized sheep. J Clin Invest 1988;82:1422-1429.

11. Amouzadeh HR, Sangiah S, Qualls CW Jr, Cowell RL, Mauromoustakos A: Xylazine-induced pulmonary edema in rats. Tox Appl Pharmacol 1991;108:417-427.

12. Bernaudin JF, Theven D, Pinchon MC, Brun-Pascaud M, Bellon B, Pocidalo JJ: Protein transfer in hyperoxic induced pleural effusion in the rat. Exp Lung Res 1986;10:23-38.

13. Miller KS, Harley RA, Sahn SA: Pleural effusions associated with ethchlorvynol lung injury result from visceral pleural leak. Am Rev Respir Dis 1989;764-768.

14. Amouzadeh HR, Sangiah S, Qualls CW Jr, Cowell RL, Mauromoustakos A: Xylazine-induced pulmonary edema in rats. Tox Appl Pharmacol 1991;108:417-427.

15. Wiener-Kronish JP, Broaddus VC: Interrelationship of pleural and pulmonary interstitial liquid. Ann Rev Physiol 1993;55:209-226.

16. Bhattacharya J, Gropper MA, Staub NC: Interstitial fluid pressure gradient measured by micropuncture in excised dog lung. J Appl Physiol 1984;56:271-277.

17. Payne DK, Kinasewitz GT, Gonzalez E: Comparative permeability of canine visceral and parietal pleura. J Appl Physiol 1988;65:2558-2564.

18. Kinasewitz GT, Groome LJ, Marshall RP, Diana JN: Role of pulmonary lymphatics and interstitium in visceral pleural fluid exchange. J Appl Physiol 1984; 56:355-363.

19. Miserocchi G, Agostoni E: Contents of the pleural space. J Appl Physiol 1971;30:208-213.

20. Albertine KH, Wiener-Kronish JP, Staub NC: The structure of the parietal pleura and its relationship to pleural liquid dynamics in sheep. Anat Rec 1984;208: 401-409.

21. Albertine KH, Wiener-Kronish JP, Roos PJ, Staub NC: Structure, blood supply, and lymphatic vessels of the sheep's visceral pleura. Am J Anat 1982;165:277-294.

22. Hodges CC, Fossum TW, Evering W: Evaluation of thoracic duct healing after experimental laceration and transection. Veterin Surg 1993;22:431-435.

23. Broaddus VC, Araya M, Carlton DP, Bland RD: Developmental changes in pleural liquid protein concentration in sheep. Am Rev Respir Dis 1991;143:38-41.

24. Cooray GH: Defensive mechanisms in the mediastinum, with special reference to the mechanics of pleural absorption. J Pathol Bacteriol 1949;61:551-567.

25. Courtice FC, Simmonds WJ: Absorption of fluids from the pleural cavities of rabbits and cats. J Physiol 1949;109:117-130.

26. Burke H: The lymphatics which drain the potential space between the visceral and the parietal pleura. Am Rev Tuberc Pulmon Dis 1959;79:52-65.

27. Wang NS: The preformed stomas connecting the pleural cavity and the lymphatics in the parietal pleura. Am Rev Respir Dis 1975;111:12-20.

28. Stewart PB: The rate of formation and lymphatic removal of fluid in pleural effusions. J Clin Invest 1963;42:258-262.

29. Leckie WJH, Tothill P: Albumin turnover in pleural effusions. Clin Sci 1965;29:339-352.

30. Broaddus VC, Wiener-Kronish JP, Berthiauma Y, Staub NC: Removal of pleural liquid and protein by lymphatics in awake sheep. J Appl Physiol 1988;64: 384-390.

31. Aiba M, Inatomi K, Homma H: Lymphatic system or hydro-oncotic forces. Which is more significant in drainage of pleural fluid? Jpn J Med 1984;23:27-33.

32. Shinto RA, Light RW: The effects of diuresis upon the characteristics of pleural fluid in patients with congestive heart failure. Am J Med 1990;88:230-233.

33. Agostoni E: Mechanics of the pleural space. Physiol Rev 1972;52:57-128.

34. Agostoni E, Zocchi L: Starling forces and lymphatic drainage in pleural liquid and protein exchanges. Respir Physiol 1991;86:271-281.

35. Pistolesi M, Miniati M, Giuntini C: Pleural liquid and solute exchange. Am Rev Respir Dis 1989;140:825-847.

36. Nakamura T, Iwasaki Y, Tanaka Y, Fukabori T: Dynamics of pleural effusion estimated through urea clearance. Jpn J Med 1987;26:319-322.

37. Light RW, Jenkinson SG, Minh V, George RB: Observations on pleural pressures as fluid is withdrawn during thoracentesis. Am Rev Respir Dis 1980;121: 799-804.

38. Allen SJ, Laine GA, Drake RE, Gabel JC: Superior vena caval pressure elevation causes pleural effusion formation in sheep. Am J Physiol 1988;255:H492–H495.
39. Magnussen H, Perry SF, Willmer H, Piiper J: Transpleural diffusion of inert gases in excised lung lobes of the dog. Respir Physiol 1974;20:1–15.
40. Northfield TC: Oxygen therapy for spontaneous pneumothorax. Br Med J 1971;4:86–88.
41. Gaensler EA: Parietal pleurectomy for recurrent spontaneous pneumothorax. Surg Gynecol Obstet 1956; 102:293–308.
42. Fleetham JA, Forkert L, Clarke H, Anthonisen NR: Regional lung function in the presence of pleural symphysis. Am Rev Respir Dis 1980;122:33–38.
43. Krell WS, Rodarte JR: Effects of acute pleural effusion on respiratory system mechanics in dogs. J Appl Physiol 1985;59:1458–1463.
44. Estenne M, Yernault J-C, De Troyer A: Mechanism of relief of dyspnea after thoracocentesis in patients with large pleural effusions. Am J Med 1983;74:813–819.
45. Light RW, Stansbury DW, Brown SE: The relationship between pleural pressures and changes in pulmonary function after therapeutic thoracentesis. Am Rev Respir Dis 1986;133:658–661.
46. Brandstetter RD, Cohen RP: Hypoxemia after thoracentesis: a predictable and treatable condition. JAMA 1979;242:1060–1061.
47. Sonnenblick M, Melzer E, Rosin AJ: Body positional effect on gas exchange in unilateral pleural effusion. Chest 1983;83:784–786.
48. Neagley SR, Zwillich CW: The effect of positional changes on oxygenation in patients with pleural effusions. Chest 1985;88:714–717.
49. Chang SC, Shiao GM, Perng RP: Postural effect on gas exchange in patients with unilateral pleural effusions. Chest 1989;96:60–63.
50. Vaska K, Wann LS, Sagar K, Klopfenstein HS: Pleural effusion as a cause of right ventricular diastolic collapse. Circulation 1992;86:609–617.
51. Negrus RA, Chachkes JS, Wrenn K: Tension hydrothorax and shock in a patient with a malignant pleural effusion. Am J Emerg Med 1990;8:205–207.
52. Kisanuki A, Shono H, Kiyonaga K, Kawataki M, Otsuji Y, Minagoe S, Nakao S, Nomoto K, Tanaka H: Two-dimensional echocardiographic demonstration of left ventricular diastolic collapse due to compression by pleural effusion. Am Heart J 1991;122:1173–1175.
53. Shinto RA, Stansbury DW, Brown SE, Light RW: Does therapeutic thoracentesis improve the exercise capacity of patients with pleural effusion? Am Rev Respir Dis 1987;135:A244.
54. Shinto RA, Stansbury DW, Fischer CE, Light RW: The effect of thoracentesis on central respiratory drive in patients with large pleural effusions. Am Rev Respir Dis 1988;137:A112.

CHAPTER 3
Radiographic Examinations

PLEURAL EFFUSIONS

Typical Arrangement of Free Pleural Fluid

Two main factors influence the distribution of free fluid in the pleural space. First, the pleural fluid accumulates in the most dependent part of the thoracic cavity because the lung is less dense than pleural fluid. In essence, the lung floats in the pleural fluid. Second, the lobes of the lung maintain their traditional shape at all stages of collapse, on account of their elastic recoil (1). The shape of a lobe when partially or completely collapsed is a miniature replica of its shape when fully distended.

Bearing in mind that the distribution of fluid within the free pleural space obeys the law of gravity and that the lung maintains its shape when compressed, it is easy to predict the distribution of excess pleural fluid. The first fluid gravitates to the base of the hemithorax and comes to rest between the inferior surface of the lung and the diaphragm, particularly posteriorly, where the pleural sinus is the deepest. As more fluid accumulates, it spills out into the costophrenic sinuses posteriorly, laterally, and anteriorly. Additional fluid spreads upward in a mantlelike fashion around the convexity of the lung and gradually tapers as it assumes a higher position in the thorax.

Based on this pattern of fluid accumulation, the typical radiographic appearance of a pleural effusion of moderate size (~1000 ml) is as follows. In the posteroanterior projection (Fig. 3.1A), the lateral costophrenic angle is obliterated. The density of the fluid is high laterally and curves gently downward and medially with a smooth, meniscus-shaped upper border to terminate at the mediastinum. The layer of fluid is narrower at the mediastinal border than at the costal border; the reason for this difference is that the mediastinal surface of the

lower lobe of the lung possesses less elastic recoil because it is fixed at the hilum and pulmonary ligament (1). In the lateral projection (Fig. 3.1B), the upper surface of the fluid density is semicircular, high anteriorly and posteriorly, and curving smoothly downward to its lowest point approximately midway between the sternum and the posterior chest wall.

Frequently, a "middle lobe step" is observed on the lateral radiograph (Fig. 3.1B). The explanation for the middle lobe step is that as pleural fluid accumulates, the first lobe affected is the lower lobe because it is the most dependent. Therefore, it starts to shrink and to float, but maintains its shape. The middle lobe is unaffected and maintains its full volume. Accordingly, the result is a shrunken lower lobe with a middle lobe that retains its usual size. Radiographically, the fluid is mostly in the posterior part of the chest (Fig. 3.1B).

On the basis of the radiologic appearance, one might surmise that the height of the pleural fluid is greater laterally. The true upper limit of pleural fluid, however, is usually the same throughout the hemithorax (2). The meniscus shape is seen because the layer of fluid is of insufficient depth to cast a discernible shadow when viewed en face (Fig. 3.2).

Radiologic Signs

With the patient in the upright position, fluid first accumulates between the inferior surface of the lower lobe and the diaphragm. If the amount of fluid is small (~75 ml), it may occupy only this position without spilling into the costophrenic sinuses. With this small amount of fluid, the normal configuration of the diaphragm is maintained, and the chest radiograph does not indicate that pleural fluid is present. When more fluid accumulates, it spills over into the posterior costophrenic angle and obliterates that sinus as viewed in the lateral projection (Fig. 3.1B). The normally

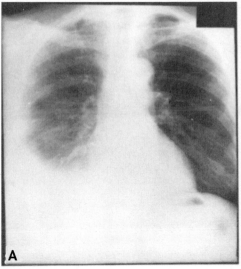

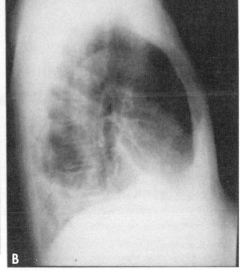

Figure 3.1. Typical arrangement of free pleural fluid. **A.** Posteroanterior view revealing obliteration of the lateral costophrenic angle. Note that in this figure, a small amount of fluid appears in the lateral aspect of the minor fissure. **B.** Lateral view revealing obliteration of the diaphragmatic outline. Note that fluid is present in both major and minor fissures so that the right middle lobe is well outlined.

sharp posterior costophrenic angle is obliterated by a shallow, homogeneous shadow whose upper surface is meniscus-shaped. The pleural line up the posterior thoracic wall is also widened. Any time the posterior costophrenic angle is obliterated or the posterior part of one or both diaphragms is obscured, the presence of pleural fluid is suggested, and further diagnostic efforts should be made. Moreover, if both posterior costophrenic angles are clear and sharp, the presence of clinically significant amounts of free pleural fluid can be nearly excluded.

Increasing amounts of fluid blunt the lateral costophrenic angle of the posteroanterior radiograph. Collins and coworkers injected fluid into the pleural spaces of upright cadavers (3). They demonstrated that at least 175 ml pleural fluid had to be injected before the lateral costophrenic angle was blunted, and in some cases, more than 500 ml pleural fluid could be present without blunting the lateral costophrenic angle. As more fluid accumulates, the entire outline of the diaphragm on the affected side is lost, and the fluid extends upward around the anterior, lateral, and posterior thoracic walls. This fluid produces opacification of the lung base and the typical meniscus shape of the fluid, as demonstrated in Figure 3.1.

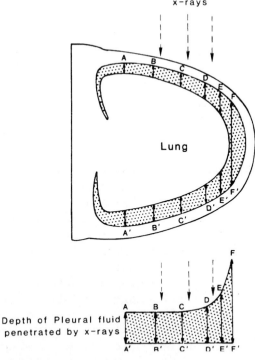

Figure 3.2. Diagrammatic explanation for the meniscus shape of pleural fluid. The distance between the lung and the chest wall is the same around the entire lung. The depth of the fluid when viewed en face AA' to CC' is not sufficient to increase the radiodensity. More laterally at DD' to FF', however, the x-ray beam passes through more and more pleural fluid, so that an increase in density is radiologically evident.

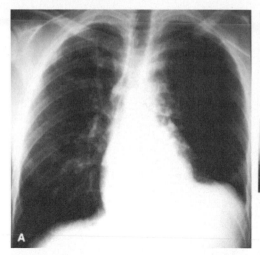

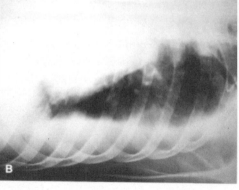

Figure 3.3. Subpulmonic pleural effusion. **A.** Poster-oanterior chest radiograph showing apparent elevation of the left diaphragm with the apex of the apparent diaphragm more lateral than usual. **B.** Lateral decubitus film of this patient showing free pleural fluid. (Courtesy of Dr. Harry Sassoon.)

Subpulmonic or Infrapulmonary Effusions

At times, for unknown reasons, substantial amounts of pleural fluid (over 1000 ml) can be present and may remain in an infrapulmonary location without spilling into the costophrenic sulci or extending up the chest wall. Such pleural fluid accumulations are called subpulmonic or infrapulmonary pleural effusions (Fig. 3.3). Although the posterior costophrenic angle is usually blunted, at times it is perfectly clear (1).

The following radiologic characteristics are common to most cases of subpulmonic effusions (1). The presence of one or more of these should serve as an indication for decubitus examinations to rule out the possibility of a subpulmonic pleural effusion: (*a*) apparent elevation of one or both diaphragms; (*b*) in the posteroanterior projection with subpulmonic effusions, the apex of the apparent diaphragm is more lateral than usual, near the junction of the middle third and the lateral third of the diaphragm, rather than at the center of the diaphragm; (*c*) additionally, the apparent diaphragm slopes much more sharply toward the lateral costophrenic angle (Fig. 3.4); (*d*) if the subpulmonic effusion is on the left side, the lower border of the lung is separated farther from the gastric air bubble than usual; normally, the top of the left diaphragm on the posteroanterior view is less than 2 cm above the stomach air bubble (4); a separation greater

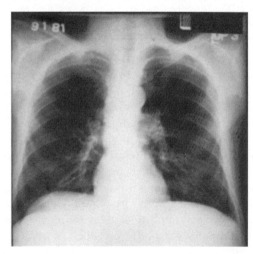

Figure 3.4. Subpulmonic pleural effusion. Note that the right lateral costophrenic angle is clear, but the apex of the right diaphragm is more lateral than usual, and the apparent diaphragm slopes sharply toward the lateral costophrenic angle.

than 2 cm suggests a subpulmonic effusion, but, of course, can also be due to subdiaphragmatic fluid accumulation; if no gastric air bubble is present, the ingestion of a carbonated beverage by the patient will allow evaluation of this sign; and (*e*) in the lateral projection, the major fissure often bows anteriorly where it meets the convex upper margin of the fluid; a small amount of fluid is usually apparent in the lower end of the major fissure at its junction with the infrapulmonary effusion.

Diaphragmatic Inversion

At times the weight of the fluid may cause the diaphragm to become inverted so that its normally convex superior border becomes concave. This inversion occurs almost exclusively with effusions on the left side. Radiologically, the gastric air bubble is pushed inferiorly, and the superior border of the diaphragm is concave upward rather than convex. When viewed under fluoroscopy, such inverted diaphragms move paradoxically with respiration, rising on inspiration and descending on expiration (5). At times, patients with large left pleural effusions suddenly become dyspneic coincidentally with the development of inversion of the left diaphragm. In such instances, a therapeutic thoracentesis is indicated (see Chapter 23). The removal of some of the pleural fluid restores the normal configuration to the diaphragm and rapidly relieves the patient's symptoms (5).

Supine Position

Until this time, I have only discussed the radiologic characteristics of pleural effusions with the patient in the upright position. Many chest radiographs, however, particularly those in acutely ill patients, are obtained with the patient in the supine position. When the patient is supine, pleural fluid gravitates to the posterior parts of the thoracic cavity. Because the pleural fluid is spread over a large area, considerable quantities must be present before any radiographic changes are seen.

The presence of free pleural fluid elicits several signs on the supine radiograph. These include blunting of the costophrenic angle, increased homogeneous density superimposed over the lung, loss of the hemidiaphragm silhouette, apical capping, elevation of the hemidiaphragm, decreased visibility of lower lobe vasculature, and accentuation of the minor fissure (6, 7). None of these signs is present in some patients with a small-to-moderate-sized pleural effusion. In one study (6), none of these radiologic signs was present in 9 of 16 patients with small effusions (defined as measuring less than 1.5 cm on the decubitus radiograph) and in 3 of 13 patients with moderate effusions (defined as measuring 1.5 to 4.5 cm on the decubitus radiograph).

The earliest sign is blunting of the costophrenic angle (6). Subsequently, increased density of the hemithorax, loss of the hemidiaphragm, and decreased visibility of the lower lobe vasculature occur. Apical capping does occur with pleural effusion, but it does not appear to be related to the size of the pleural effusion (6). Elevation of the hemidiaphragm and accentuation of the minor fissure are insensitive signs in that they occur in a minority of patients and they are not related to the size of the effusion (6).

Three characteristics serve to differentiate the increased density due to pleural fluid from that due to a parenchymal infiltrate. First, if the density is caused by pleural fluid, the vascular structures of the lung will be readily visible through the density in a properly exposed film. Any intrapulmonary process that produces a similar density, however, obliterates the vascular structure by the "silhouette effect." Second, if the density is due to pleural fluid, it is usually completely homogeneous. In contrast, infiltrates caused by intrapulmonary processes are usually less homogeneous. Third, air bronchograms are present only if the increased density is due to a parenchymal infiltrate.

Atypical Effusion

The typical arrangement of fluid in the pleural space depends upon an underlying lung free of disease and therefore having uniform elastic recoil. If the lung underlying the effusion is diseased, the elastic recoil of the diseased portion is frequently different from that of the remainder of the lung, and fluid accumulates most where the elastic recoil is greatest. Therefore, an atypical collection of pleural fluid is an indication of underlying parenchymal as well as pleural disease. For example, if disease in a lower lobe increases its elastic recoil, fluid will collect posteromedially. Accordingly, in the posteroanterior projection, the opacity is higher on the mediastinal than on the axillary border, in contrast to the typical appearance in which the opacity is higher at the axillary border. Moreover, the upper surface curves downward and laterally toward the lateral costophrenic sulcus and thereby simulates atelectasis and consolidation of the middle and lower lobes. In the lateral

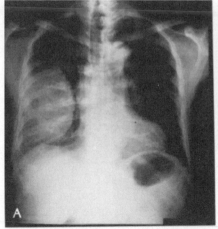

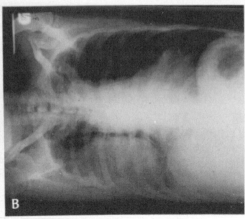

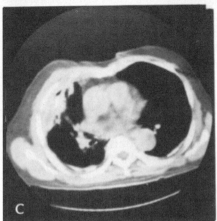

Figure 3.5. Loculated pleural effusion. **A.** Postero-anterior radiograph demonstrating a D-shaped density with base of the D against the right lateral chest wall. **B.** Right lateral decubitus radiograph demonstrating the absence of free pleural fluid in the same patient. **C.** CT scan demonstrating parenchymal involvement adjacent to loculated pleural effusion. This patient has an anaerobic infection of the lung and pleural space.

projection, the upper border of the density roughly parallels the major fissure, beginning high in the thorax posteriorly and running downward and anteriorly to the anterior costophrenic sulcus. For the interested reader, Fleischner has detailed the radiographic appearance of atypical pleural fluid accumulation in disease affecting all the individual lobes (8).

Loculated Effusion

Pleural fluid may become encapsulated by adhesions anywhere between the parietal and the visceral pleura or in the interlobar fissures. Because the encapsulation is caused by adhesions between contiguous pleural surfaces, it occurs most frequently in association with conditions that cause intense pleural inflammation, such as hemothorax, pyothorax, or tuberculous pleuritis. Loculations occurring between the lung and the chest wall produce a characteristic radiographic picture. When

viewed in profile (Fig. 3.5), the loculation is D-shaped, with the base of the D against the chest wall and the smooth convexity protruding inward toward the lung because of compressibility of the lung parenchyma. If the loculation is in the lower part of the thoracic cavity, its lower border may not be visible. Loculation may be differentiated from parenchymal infiltrates by the absence of air bronchograms. A definitive diagnosis of loculated pleural effusion is best established by ultrasound (see the section of this chapter on ultrasound). Because multiple locules are common, the demonstration of one locule should serve as an indication to search for additional locules.

Loculation in the Fissures

The plane of the lung fissures is such that fluid encapsulated in the fissure is usually seen in profile in the lateral view. Fluid encapsu-

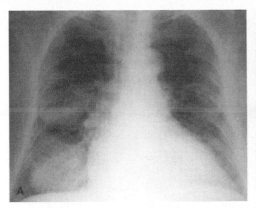 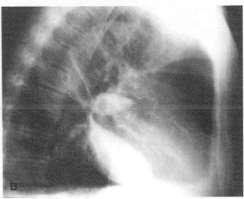

Figure 3.6. Posteroanterior (**A**) and lateral (**B**) radiographs of a patient with congestive heart failure. **A.** Two masslike lesions are visible in the lower right lung field. **B.** The biconvex configuration of loculated fluid in both the major and the minor fissures is evident. With treatment of the patient's heart failure, the lung fields cleared, and the apparent masses disappeared. (Courtesy of Dr. Harry Sassoon.)

lated in a fissure has a profile similar to a biconvex lens. Its margins are sharply defined and blend imperceptibly into interlobar fissures (Fig. 3.6). In some situations, the loculated effusion may simulate a mass on the posteroanterior radiograph. This situation is most frequently seen in patients with congestive heart failure, and because the fluid absorbs spontaneously when the congestive heart failure is treated, these fluid collections have been termed vanishing tumors or pseudotumors. The most common location of these "tumors" is in the right horizontal fissure (9). The distinctive configuration of the loculated interlobar effusion should establish the diagnosis. The disappearance of the apparent mass as the effusion resolves definitely establishes the diagnosis.

At times it is difficult to differentiate encapsulated fluid in the lower half of a major fissure from atelectasis or combined atelectasis and consolidation of the right middle lobe. The following three points help to make the distinction (1). First, if the minor fissure is visible as a separate shadow, the diagnosis of encapsulated fluid is certain. Second, encapsulated fluid does not usually obscure the right heart border; in contrast, middle lobe atelectasis almost invariably does. Third, in the lateral projection, loculated effusions usually have a convex border on one or both sides. When the right middle lobe is diseased, the borders of the shadow are either straight or slightly concave.

Radiologic Documentation

Most of the changes discussed in the previous sections are suggestive rather than diagnostic of the presence of pleural fluid. For example, blunting of the posterior or lateral costophrenic angles can be due to pleural effusion, but it can also be caused by pleural thickening or hyperinflation of the lung. Pleural effusion can obliterate one or both diaphragms on the lateral radiograph, but so can atelectasis or parenchymal infiltrates. Therefore, when the posteroanterior or the lateral chest radiograph suggests a pleural effusion, further radiographic studies are needed to document the presence of pleural fluid. If the pleural fluid is free, lateral decubitus radiographs are recommended. If the fluid is loculated, ultrasound examinations are preferred. The computed tomography (CT) scan is also useful in documenting both free and loculated pleural effusions.

Lateral Decubitus Radiographs

The basis for the use of the lateral decubitus view is that free fluid gravitates to the most dependent part of the pleural space. The patient is placed in the lateral recumbent position with the suspect side dependent. Sufficient radiolucent padding should be placed between the table top and the patient so an unobstructed tangential view of the dependent chest wall can be obtained. The x-ray film should be exposed with a high voltage to

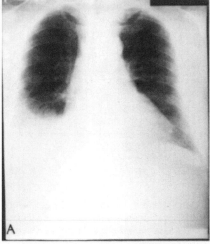
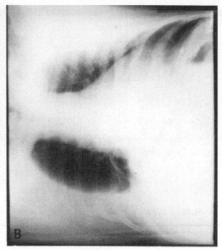
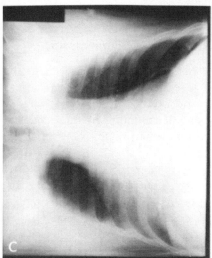

Figure 3.7A. Posteroanterior radiograph demonstrating blunting of the right costophrenic angle. **B.** Right lateral decubitus radiograph of the same patient demonstrating a large amount of free pleural fluid. **C.** Left lateral decubitus radiograph demonstrating that the lower right lung field is clear of parenchymal infiltrates.

ensure that the interface between the fluid and the lung can be identified.

In the decubitus view, free pleural fluid is evidenced by a homogeneous density with a straight horizontal superior border between the dependent chest wall and the lower border of the lung (Fig. 3.7). This appearance is due to the lung floating in the fluid. By injecting fluid into the pleural space of cadavers, Moskowitz and colleagues have demonstrated that as little as 5 ml pleural fluid can be seen on properly exposed decubitus radiographs (10). The amount of free pleural fluid can be semiquantitated by measuring the distance between the inner border of the chest wall and the outer border of the lung (Fig. 3.7): the greater this distance, the more free pleural fluid. Empirically, I have found that when this distance is less than 10 mm, the amount of

pleural fluid is small, and diagnostic thoracentesis is difficult. Accordingly, I rarely attempt a diagnostic thoracentesis when the thickness of the pleural fluid on the decubitus radiograph is less than 10 mm.

Many patients suspected of having pleural effusions have apparent pleural thickening on the posteroanterior chest radiograph. When decubitus views are obtained in such patients, one must compare the distance between the lung and chest wall in the decubitus view to that in the posteroanterior view. If the distance between the lung and the chest wall is not at least 10 mm greater on the decubitus view, the patient does not have a significant amount of free pleural fluid.

In general, bilateral decubitus chest radiographs should be ordered. The film with the suspect side superior is informative because, in this view, the fluid gravitates toward the mediastinum. With the fluid shifted away from the chest wall and the lung, one can more readily assess the underlying lung for infiltrates or atelectasis (Fig. 3.7C). In addition, if the lateral costophrenic angle is blunted on the posteroanterior view and is clear on the decubitus view with the suspect side superior, one can be certain that the blunting is caused by free pleural fluid.

Frequently, when decubitus radiographs are obtained, confusion exists as to which side is down. An arrow is usually seen on the x-ray film, but is the arrow pointing up or pointing down in relation to the patient's position? Four radiologic characteristics allow the interpreter to ascertain the position of the patient when the radiograph was obtained. First, the dependent lung receives a greater percentage of the perfusion and therefore is more radiodense. Second, with the patient in the decubitus position, the abdominal pressure is greater on the dependent side; thus, the diaphragm on the dependent side is pushed higher in the thoracic cavity than the contralateral diaphragm. Third, the radiolucent padding or examination table is often evident outside the thoracic cavity on the dependent side (Fig. 3.7). Fourth, if air-fluid levels are present in the stomach or the intestines, the air will always be on the superior side.

Semisupine Oblique Radiographs

Many patients are too ill or are in too much pain to tolerate decubitus chest radiographs. An alternate procedure that can be used to document free pleural fluid is to obtain oblique chest radiographs with the patient in the semisupine position. The patient assumes a position 45 to 65° backward from the vertical plane. The individual's right side is lowered for separate views of both sides. Then the horizontal radiograph is centered to give a clear view of the dorsal half of the thorax. Films are obtained at full inspiration and full expiration. Pleural fluid is considered to be present when the thickness of the pleural shadow is greater on expiration than on inspiration. In one study the semisupine oblique technique correctly demonstrated the presence of pleural fluid in 38 of 39 patients in whom fluid was demonstrated with decubitus radiographs. Moreover, in only 5 of 73 pa-

tients did the oblique semisupine films suggest fluid when none could be demonstrated by the decubitus technique (11).

Ultrasound

Ultrasound is very useful in the study of pleural disease. It can be used in several different situations, including the following: (a) identification of the appropriate location for an attempted thoracentesis, pleural biopsy, or chest tube placement; (b) identification of pleural fluid loculations; and (c) distinction of pleural fluid from pleural thickening (12). The advantages of ultrasound over CT are the ease and speed with which the examination can be performed, the availability of portable units that can be brought to the bedside of seriously ill patients, the lack of ionizing radiation, the relatively low cost, and the capacity to diagnose and distinguish an associated subphrenic process (12). With ultrasound, one can also assess the thickness of the parietal pleura and identify pleural nodules and focal pleural thickening (13). Lastly, with ultrasound one can determine if there is fusion of the visceral and parietal pleura. Given these advantages, there is no doubt that ultrasound has been under used in the assessment of pleural disease in the United States.

For simplicity, pleural fluid collections with ultrasound can be characterized as echo-free (anechoic), complex septated if there are fibrin strands or septa floating inside the anechoic pleural effusions, complex nonseptated if heterogeneous echogenic material was inside the anechoic pleural effusion, and homogeneously echogenic if homogeneously echogenic spaces are present between the visceral and parietal pleura. In one recent series of 320 patients with pleural effusions, 172 (54%) were anechoic, 50 (16%) were complex nonseptated, 76 (23%) were complex septated, and 22 (7%) were homogeneously echogenic (13). Interestingly, all the patients who had complex nonseptated, complex septated or homogeneously echogenic results had exudative pleural effusions. Patients who had anechoic effusions could have either transudates or exudates (13). The best distinguishing characteristic of a pleural fluid collection on ultrasound is that it changes its shape with respiration (14).

For optimal ultrasonic examination of the pleural space, a high-frequency transducer (e.g., 5.0 or 7.5 MHz) and real-time scanning are preferred (15). The high-frequency transducer improves resolution in the near field so internal echoes in a solid lesion are easier to image which helps distinguish solid lesions from cystic lesions. In addition, near-field reverberation artifacts, which might otherwise obscure fluid close to the skin, are reduced. Real-time scanning is preferred to conventional static scanning because it allows one to assess the changing configuration of pleural fluid with respiration, it is easier to use in the intercostal spaces, and it requires less time to scan large areas (12).

Recently it has been shown that color Doppler ultrasound is superior to real-time gray-scale ultrasound in the identification of pleural fluid (16). With the color Doppler ultrasound, pleural fluid is identified because it provides a color signal. In one report of 51 patients with minimal pleural effusions, color Doppler ultrasound correctly demonstrated color in 33 of 35 (94%) of patients with pleural fluid but was negative in the 16 patients without pleural fluid. In contrast, real-time gray-scale ultrasound identified fluid in all 35 patients with fluid, but also in 5 of 16 patients without fluid (16).

Ultrasonic techniques are useful in identifying the appropriate site for thoracentesis (12, 13, 17). The appropriate site can be identified both in patients with loculated pleural effusions and in those with small amounts of pleural fluid. In addition to identifying the site for aspiration, the appropriate depth for aspiration can also be ascertained, thereby increasing the safety of the procedure. It is important to perform the thoracentesis at the time the fluid is identified by ultrasound. When the skin is only marked at the time of the ultrasonic examination and the patient is sent back to the ward, thoracentesis is frequently attempted with the patient in a different position. In such instances, the relationship between the skin and the pleural fluid is altered, and the thoracentesis may be unsuccessful (17). Of course, the utility of the ultrasonic examination for pleural fluid depends upon the skill and the interest of the ultrasonographer. Performing the thoracentesis in the presence of the ultra-

sonographer will also improve the capabilities of the ultrasonographer.

Computed Tomography

The availability of CT has markedly improved our ability to assess pleural abnormalities radiologically. Pleural abnormalities can be more readily detected and distinguished from lung parenchymal and extrapleural disease by CT than by standard radiographs because these anatomic compartments are distinct on the cross-sectional image with CT (18). Pleural collections or masses tend to conform to the pleural space. As with chest radiographs, the angle of the lesion with the chest wall may help identify whether the lesion is pleural or parenchyma. If the angle of the abnormality with the chest wall is acute, the lesion probably has a parenchymal origin while if the angle is obtuse, the lesion probably has a pleural origin. Sometimes, however, the CT findings are as ambiguous as the radiographs, particularly when there is atelectasis or pneumonia or when a pleural collection forms acute angles with the chest wall.

Free-flowing pleural fluid produces a sickle-shaped opacity in the most dependent part of the thorax posteriorly (Fig. 3.8) (12). Loculated fluid collections are seen as lenticular opacities of fixed position. When free fluid lies in the posterior costophrenic recess adjacent to the diaphragm, it may be difficult to differ-

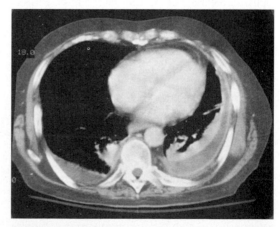

Figure 3.8.   CT scan with contrast demonstrating bilateral pleural effusions, the left larger than the right. Note how the parenchyma on the left is enhanced in comparison to the collection of pleural fluid.

entiate from ascites. Several CT features have been described that aid in the differentiation of pleural fluid from ascites. These are the displaced-crus sign, the interface sign, the diaphragm sign and the bare-area sign (12). With the *displaced-crus sign*, the displacement of the diaphragmatic crus away from the spine by the fluid indicates that the fluid is in the pleural space. In contrast, ascites lies lateral and anterior to the crus. With the *interface sign*, a sharp interface can be identified between the fluid and the liver or spleen and this indicates that ascites is present. This line is much less distinct if pleural fluid is present. With the *diaphragm sign*, fluid that is outside the diaphragm is pleural fluid while fluid that is inside the diaphragm is ascites. With the *bare-area sign*, restriction of ascites by the coronary ligaments from the bare area of the liver indicates that the patient has ascites.

CT is effective at demonstrating abnormalities in the lung parenchyma that are obscured on the conventional chest radiograph by the pleural disease. Chest CT is particularly useful in distinguishing empyema with air-fluid levels from lung abscess, as discussed subsequently. An added bonus with CT is the clear demonstration of bone pathology such as metastases or tuberculosis.

Chest CT is not indicated in all patients with suspected pleural disease. The density coefficients from CT are not specific enough to distinguish among parenchymal lesions, solid pleural masses, or pleural collections of serous fluid, blood, or pus (19). Ultrasonic examinations are preferred over CT when the question is whether pleural fluid is present.

CT examinations of the chest have also provided additional information concerning the effects of a pleural effusion on the underlying lung. Paling and Griffin reviewed the chest CT obtained in the supine position of 46 cases with a moderate or large pleural effusion (20). The volume of the underlying lung, particularly the lower lobe, was reduced in all patients. In only 2 patients, however, was there no atelectasis of the underlying lung. In 19 cases there was segmental collapse of the lower lobe. In 7 cases the atelectatic segment was so large as to produce an appearance initially suggestive of complete collapse of the lower lobe. Recognition that the lower lobe

was at least in part inflated depended on identification of the major fissure anterior to the airless lung, identification of lower lobe bronchi and vessels surrounded by aerated lung on more cephalad sections, and the presence of an identifiable inferior pulmonary vein in normal location within aerated lung. In 25 of 46 cases, the lower lobe collapse involved all except the superior segment, which tended to remain aerated. Recognition of a major degree of volume loss in the lower lobe depended on identification of the bronchial anatomy serving the airless lung and on the loss of an identifiable inferior pulmonary vein, which was buried within the collapsed lung.

CT examinations of the chest have also been used to evaluate the major and minor fissures. In one report 100 CT scans of patients with normal lungs were reviewed to determine the normal characteristics of the major fissures and the minor fissure. Each major fissure was imaged most often as a lucent band, less often as a line, and least often as a dense band. In contrast, the minor fissure was imaged as a lucent area, which was usually triangular with its apex at the hilar region (21).

Magnetic Resonance (MR) Imaging

MR imaging has generated considerable interest as a safe and sensitive technique for imaging human pathologic conditions. The technique basically consists of inducing transitions between energy states by causing certain atoms to absorb and transfer energy. This is accomplished by directing a radiofrequency pulse at a substance placed within a large magnetic field. Measures of the time required for the material to return to a baseline energy state (relaxation time) can be translated by a complex computer algorithm to a visual image. There are two time constants associated with relaxation, called T1 and T2. The T1 relaxation time characterizes a time constant with which the nuclei align in a given magnetic field. In contrast, T2 reflects the time constant for loss of phase coherence of excited spins (22, 23).

With MR imaging the lungs are seen as regions of black signal intensity similar to the black appearance of the lungs on CT. When evaluating the soft tissues, however, several differences are noted. The subcutaneous fat

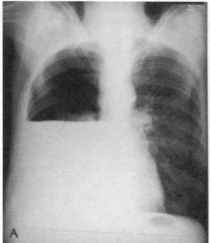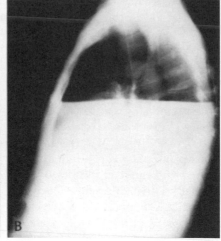

Figure 3.9. Posteroanterior (**A**) and lateral (**B**) radiographs of a patient with a hydropneumothorax. Note that the air-fluid level extends throughout the length and width of the hemithorax. This hydropneumothorax followed an attempted thoracentesis in this patient with a massive right pleural effusion.

on MR has bright signal intensity, compared with the low signal intensity with CT. On MR, the vascular structures including the aorta and main, left, and right pulmonary arteries are seen as regions of signal void (black) distinct from the surrounding mediastinal fat. With noncontrast CT, the vessels and masses have a similar attenuation. The bony structures on MR may be seen as regions of bright signal intensity because of the fat within the marrow or low intensity for cortical bone (23).

Pleural effusions can be identified with MRI. A pleural fluid collection is visualized as an area of abnormally low signal intensity on T1-weighted images, which increases in brightness on T2-weighted images. This characteristic is consistent with the relatively long T1 and T2 values of pleural fluid. With MRI, different types of pleural fluid collections such as transudative fluid, chylothorax, hemothorax or pus may appear somewhat different, but their characteristics are not sufficiently distinct as to be diagnostic. A diagnostic thoracentesis is certainly more definitive and less expensive.

In summary, MR imaging of the chest at the present time is less satisfactory than ultrasound or CT in identifying the presence of a pleural effusion. Presently, there are no definite clinical indications for MR imaging of the chest in the management of patients with pleural disease.

Air-Fluid Levels in the Pleural Space

When both air and fluid are present in the pleural space, an air-fluid level is apparent on radiographs obtained in the erect position (Fig. 3.9). Of course, if the radiograph is obtained with the patient supine, no air-fluid level will be present unless it is a cross-table lateral view. The presence of an air-fluid level in the pleural space indicates that air has gained entry into the pleural space. The differential diagnosis includes bronchopleural fistula from pulmonary infections, spontaneous pneumothorax with pleural effusion, trauma (iatrogenic or noniatrogenic), the presence of gas-forming organisms in the pleural space, and rupture of the esophagus into the pleural space. Air-fluid levels in the pleural space must be distinguished from air-fluid levels in dilated loops of bowel entering the thoracic cavity through a diaphragmatic hernia. Contrast media studies of the gastrointestinal tract are diagnostic in doubtful cases.

It is frequently difficult to distinguish a loculated pyopneumothorax with a bronchopleural fistula from a peripheral lung abscess. This differentiation is important because the former condition should be treated with pleural drainage (see Chapter 9), whereas a lung abscess usually responds to antibiotics and postural drainage alone. Both ultrasound and computed tomography are useful in distinguishing between these two conditions. With ultrasonic examination during hyperventilation, asymmetric motion of the proximal (chest wall-parietal pleura) and the distal (visceral pleura-lung) interface occurs when the process is in the pleural space. If the process is within the lung parenchyma, the proximal and distal interfaces (anterior and posterior walls of the cavity) move symmetrically (24).

The preferred method for distinguishing empyema from lung abscess is chest CT (19). With CT scanning, a pyopneumothorax is characterized by unequal fluid levels on positional scanning that closely approximate the chest wall. The space characteristically has a smooth, regular margin that is sharply defined without side pockets. The appearance of the cavity often changes with variations in the patient's position. In contrast, a lung abscess is typically round with an irregular, thick wall and has an air-fluid level of equal length in all positions. When the patient's position is changed, the shapes of the cavity and of the mass do not change. Frequently, multiple side pockets are adjacent to the main cavity. An additional distinguishing feature is that the larger empyemas displace the adjacent lung and lung abscesses do not (19).

CT is not infallible in distinguishing empyemas from lung abscesses. Bressler and associates reviewed the CT scans from 71 patients in whom the question was whether the individual had a lung abscess or empyema (25). In 5 of the 71 cases, the foregoing morphologic criteria were insufficient to make the distinction. The intravenous administration of a bolus of contrast medium in conjunction with CT was diagnostically useful. The demonstration of vessels within a lesion unequivocally identifies the lesion as parenchymal rather than pleural. Moreover, after administration of sufficient amounts of contrast material, pulmonary parenchyma is enhanced, whereas most pleural lesions show minimal or no enhancement (25).

Another condition that must be differentiated from empyema in a patient with air-fluid levels in the chest is fluid-filled bullae or lung cysts in which the CT findings may resemble those of empyema. On CT scan the fluid-filled cavities have many characteristics of loculated pleural fluid collections including lenticular shape, air-fluid levels of different length on orthogonal views, uniform, smooth inner walls, and mass effect on the adjacent lung. Two features are useful in differentiating fluid-filled cysts from empyema: (*a*) cysts tend to be located in the upper lobes and the air-fluid levels are limited by fissures; and (*b*) one notes the absence of preexisting or coexisting large pleural effusion with fluid-filled cysts (26).

Quantitation of the Amount of Pleural Fluid

It is possible to estimate with some degree of reliability the amount of pleural fluid with either ultrasonography or lateral decubitus chest radiographs. Eibenberger and colleagues (27) recently completed a study of 51 patients who had lateral decubitus chest radiographs and sonography while supine. The thickness of the fluid on the lateral decubitus radiograph and on sonography was measured just cranial to the base of the lung. Subsequent to these studies, the patients underwent therapeutic thoracentesis with removal of all of the pleural fluid. Then the measurements were correlated with the amount of fluid removed with the thoracentesis (Fig. 3.10). It can be seen in Figure 3.10 that the amount of fluid is more closely correlated with the ultrasonic measurement than with the lateral decubitus measurement. Note also that on the lateral decubitus radiograph, a fluid thickness of 30 mm corresponds to a volume of 1000 ml, while on the ultrasound measurement a fluid thickness of 40 mm corresponds to a volume of 1000 ml.

Massive Effusion

When an entire hemithorax is opacified, one should first examine the position of the mediastinum because its position is influenced by the pleural pressures (Fig. 3.11). If the pleural pressure is lower on the side of the effusion, the mediastinum will be shifted toward the side of the effusion (Fig. 3.11*A*). Alternately, if the pleural pressure is higher on the side of the effusion, the mediastinum will be shifted toward the contralateral side (Fig. 3.11*B*). Of course, if the mediastinum is invaded by tumor or other infiltrative processes, it will be fixed, and no shift will be evident on the posteroanterior radiograph.

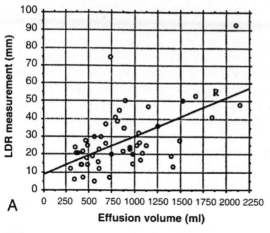

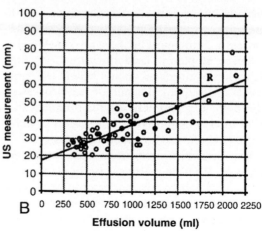

A

B

Effusion volume (ml) Effusion volume (ml)

Figure 3.10. Correlation of actual volume of pleural effusion with (**A**) thickness of fluid on the lateral decubitus radiograph and (**B**) thickness of fluid on sonography. Values are from 51 patients before thoracentesis. The sonographic measurements were more closely corre- lated with the volume of the fluid (r = 0.80) than were the lateral decubitus measurements. (From Eibenberger KL, Dock WI, Ammann ME, et al: Quantification of pleural effusions: sonography versus radiography. Radiology 1994;191:681–684.)

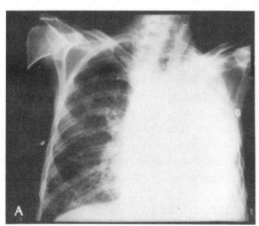

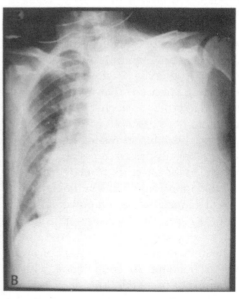

Figure 3.11A. Massive pleural effusion with marked shift of the trachea and mediastinum toward the side of the effusion. This patient had a bronchogenic carcinoma obstructing the left main bronchus. **B.** Massive pleural effusion with marked shift of the trachea and mediasti- num away from the side of the effusion.

When the patient's mediastinum is shifted toward the side of the effusion, the lung under- lying the effusion is usually diseased. In such a case, overexpansion of the contralateral lung produces an enlarged retrosternal clear space on the lateral view. By far the most common cause of this radiographic picture is complete obstruction of the ipsilateral main stem bron- chus by a neoplasm. Therefore, if the mediasti- num is shifted toward the side of the effusion, the initial diagnostic procedure should be bronchoscopy to assess the patency of the bronchial tree. If an obstructing lesion is found, thoracentesis is not recommended because it is unnecessary diagnostically, and it carries an increased risk because of the negative pleural pressure. If no obstructing lesion is found, removal of large amounts (more than 500 ml) of pleural fluid should only be attempted if pleural pressures are monitored (28).

When the patient's mediastinum is shifted toward the contralateral side, an active process in the pleural space has led to the accumulation of pleural fluid. In such instances, not only is the ipsilateral lung completely nonfunctional, but the function of the contralateral lung is also compromised (Fig. 3.11*B*). A therapeutic thoracentesis (see Chapter 23) should be performed immediately to attempt, at least, to restore the mediastinum to midline. The most common cause of massive pleural effusion with mediastinal shift is metastatic disease of the pleura (29), but tuberculosis, cirrhosis, and congestive heart failure may also cause this picture. If the mediastinum is midline in a patient with a massive pleural effusion, the mediastinum is usually invaded by tumor. At times, most of the mediastinum is in the midline, but the tracheal air shadow is shifted. This picture is suggestive of bronchogenic carcinoma (30).

CT scan and ultrasound are both quite useful in evaluating patients with unilateral hemithorax opacification. Yu and coworkers (31) evaluated these two diagnostic modalities in 50 patients with unilateral hemithorax opacification. Either procedure can demonstrate whether the opacification is due to fluid, a tissue mass, or a combination. It is interesting that 9 of the 50 patients in the above series (18%) had no fluid in their pleural space. Both procedures are very effective demonstrating pleural or parenchymal abnormalities while only CT scan effectively demonstrates mediastinal involvement (31).

PLEURAL THICKENING

The pleura may become thickened over the convexity of the thorax and occasionally in the interlobar fissure.

Radiologic Signs

Normally, no line is visible between the inside of the chest wall and the outer border of the lung, but in response to inflammation of the pleura, the lung may become separated from the chest wall by a pleural line. After an episode of pleuritis, the thickness of the pleural line may be 1 to 10 mm. The pleural thickening that follows pleural inflammation results almost exclusively from fibrosis of the visceral pleural surface. The thickening may be either localized or generalized. If the pleural thickening is localized, it most commonly involves the inferior portions of the thoracic cavity because pleural fluid accumulates there. Frequently, with localized pleural thickening, the costophrenic angles are partially or completely obliterated. In such instances, decubitus radiographs (see the foregoing section of this chapter on decubitus radiographs) are indicated to rule out free pleural fluid. The main significance of localized pleural thickening is as an index of previous pleural inflammation.

Following intense pleural inflammation, such as occurs with a massive hemothorax, pyothorax, or tuberculous pleuritis, generalized pleural thickening of an entire hemithorax may occur. This thickening is again due to the deposition of fibrous tissue on the visceral pleura. The thickness of the pleura may exceed 2 cm. Frequently, the inner aspect of this "peel" is calcified, providing an accurate measurement of the thickness of the peel. If the patient is symptomatic and if the underlying lung is functional, decortication (see Chapter 22) may provide symptomatic relief.

Apical Thickening

The pleura in the apex of the lungs sometimes becomes thickened. Although in the past apical pleural thickening was usually attributed to tuberculosis (1), such does not now appear to be the case. Renner and associates studied the apical pleura at autopsy in 19 patients with radiologically visible pleural thickening and found no evidence of tuberculosis in any of the patients (32). The frequency of apical pleural thickening increases with age, and the authors suggested that the apical pleural thickening might be related to the healing of pulmonary disease in the presence of chronic ischemia (32). Apical pleural thickening is frequently bilateral, but can be unilateral (32). Gross asymmetry should raise the suspicion of apical pulmonary carcinoma or Pancoast tumor.

Asbestos-Induced Thickening

Pleural thickening can also result from asbestos exposure (see Chapter 22). In contrast to other types of pleural thickening, the parietal pleura rather than the visceral pleura is thickened following asbestos exposure. The pleural thickening can either be localized, in which case the thickenings are called pleural plaques, or generalized (33). An average of 30 years elapses between the first exposure to asbestos and the appearance of pleural plaques (33). The pleural thickening or plaques associated with asbestos exposure are usually bilateral, are more prominent in the lower half of the thorax, and follow the rib contours (34). The pleural thickening due to asbestos exposure eventually becomes calcified. The calcification ranges from small linear or circular shadows usually situated over the diaphragmatic domes to complete encirclement of the lower portion of the lungs. Computed tomography of the chest is more sensitive than other radiologic procedures in identifying both pleural thickening and pleural calcification due to asbestos exposure (35).

In obese persons subcostal fat may mimic pleural thickening. Typically it appears as a symmetric, smooth, soft tissue density that parallels the chest wall and is of greatest thickness over the apices. In problem cases, subcostal fat can be distinguished from either diffuse thickening or localized plaques with CT. On the CT subcostal fat can be identified as low-density tissue internal to the ribs and external to the parietal pleura (12).

PNEUMOTHORAX

The radiographic signs of a pneumothorax are influenced by two factors (1). First, air in the pleural space accumulates in the highest part of the thoracic cavity because air is less dense than the lung. Second, the lobes of the lung maintain their traditional shape at all stages of collapse. Note that these are the same factors that influence pleural fluid accumulation. The only difference is that with pneumothorax, air rises to the apex of the hemithorax and causes early collapse of the upper lobes of the lung, whereas with pleural effusion, the pleural fluid falls to the bottom of the hemithorax and collapses the lower lobes.

The pleural pressure is normally negative, because of the balance between the inward pull of the lung and the outward pull of the chest wall. If air is introduced into the pleural space, the lung will become smaller, the thoracic cavity will enlarge, and the pleural pressure will increase. If 1000 ml air enters the pleural space, the lung will decrease in volume by about 600 ml while the thoracic cavity will increase in volume by about 400 ml (see Fig. 19.1). The ipsilateral pleural pressure will become less negative, and because the contralateral pleural pressure remains unchanged, the mediastinum will shift toward the contralateral side. The ipsilateral diaphragm will also be lowered on account of the increased pleural pressure and resultant decreased transdiaphragmatic pressure. An enlarged hemithorax, a depressed diaphragm, and a shifted mediastinum do not mean that a tension pneumothorax is present.

Radiologic Signs

A definitive radiologic diagnosis of pneumothorax can only be made when a visceral pleural line can be identified (Fig. 3.12). The visceral pleural line is evident as a faint but sharply defined line separating the lung parenchyma from the remainder of the thoracic cavity, which is clear and devoid of lung markings. Although one might suppose that the partially collapsed lung would have increased density radiologically, it does not for the following reasons. First, blood flow through the partially collapsed lung, which contributes substantially to the density radiologically, decreases proportionately to the degree of collapse. Second, the thorax is a cylinder, and with a pneumothorax, the presence of air both anterior and posterior to the partially collapsed lung decreases the overall density of the lung. The radiologic density of the lung does not increase until the lung loses approximately 90% of its volume. Complete atelectasis of a lung due to pneumothorax is characterized ipsilaterally by an enlarged hemithorax, a depressed diaphragm, a shift of the mediastinum to the contralateral side, and a fist-sized mass of increased density at the lower part of the hilum representing the collapsed lung (Fig. 3.13).

The diagnosis of pneumothorax is usually easily established by demonstrating the visceral pleural line on the posteroanterior radio-

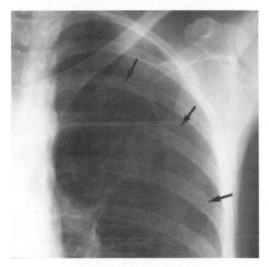

Figure 3.12. Posteroanterior radiograph of a patient with a pneumothorax on the left side. Note the obvious pleural line (*arrows*) separating the lung from the air in the pleural space. The density of the radiograph inside and outside the pleural line is similar. Note also that a bleb (*upper arrow*) is present along the surface of the apical pleural line. This bleb was probably responsible for the pneumothorax. (Courtesy of Dr. Harry Sassoon.)

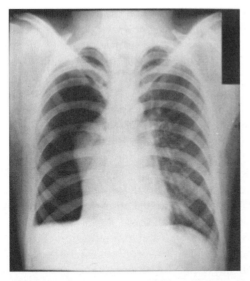

Figure 3.13. Posteroanterior radiograph of a patient with a pneumothorax and complete atelectasis of the right lung.

graph. With small pneumothoraces, however, the visceral pleural line may not be visible on the routine radiographs. In such cases one of the following two procedures can establish the diagnosis: (*a*) radiographs can be obtained in the upright position in full expiration; the rationale is that, although the volume of gas in

the pleural space is constant, with full expiration the lung volume is reduced, and therefore, the percentage of the hemithorax occupied by air increases, making identification of the visceral pleural line much easier; and (*b*) radiographs can be obtained in the lateral decubitus position with the side of the suspected pneumothorax superior; the free air in the pleural space rises, increasing the distance between the lung and the chest wall; additionally, fewer conflicting shadows are seen over the lateral chest wall than at the apex. It appears that the decubitus position is the most sensitive for detecting a pneumothorax. Carr and coworkers (36) obtained conventional chest radiographs and CT scans on cadavers in which varying amounts of intrapleural air had been introduced. They found that the lateral decubitus film was most sensitive (88%) for the diagnosis of pneumothorax, followed by the erect (59%) and supine (37%) views. These researchers reported that the pneumothorax was always detected in the lateral decubitus position when there were more than 40 ml of intrapleural air. In addition, they found that CT scan was no more sensitive than the decubitus views (36).

Pneumothoraces are more difficult to recognize on lateral than on posteroanterior projections. In one series the pneumothorax could not be identified on the lateral projection in 13 of 122 cases (11%) (37). When the pneumothorax is identifiable, the displaced pleural line is more frequently anterior or posterior and is less commonly at the lung apex. In 10% of the cases, an air-fluid level was the only recognizable finding of a pneumothorax on the lateral projection (37).

Skin folds may superficially mimic a pleural line and possibly lead to a misdiagnosis of pneumothorax. A skin fold results in an abnormal edge with a sharp black-white interface laterally, with gradual fading of the density from white to black medially. In contrast, there is no such fading medial to the line with pneumothorax. In addition, lung markings are seen peripheral to the edge of the skin fold, in contrast to the absence of lung markings peripheral to the line of a pneumothorax (38).

It is much more difficult to establish the diagnosis of pneumothorax on a supine radiograph (38). In a review of 88 critically ill patients with 112 cases of pneumothorax, 30% of the cases were not initially detected by the radiologist, and half these cases progressed to tension pneumothorax (39). The most common location for collections of air on the supine film is the anteromedial location because this area is the least dependent pleural recess. The three other locations in which air collects on the supine radiograph are subpulmonically, apicolaterally, and posteromedially. Depending on the size and location of the gas collection, any of the following can be signs of a pneumothorax in the supine position: an exceptionally deep radiolucent costophrenic sulcus, a lucency over the right or left upper quadrant, or a much sharper than normal appearance of the hemidiaphragm, with or without the presence of a visible visceral pleural line above the diaphragm (1). The interested reader is referred to the review article by Buckner and coworkers for details concerning the radiologic appearance of air in these locations (38).

Atypical Pneumothorax

As with pleural effusions, the radiologic appearance of a pneumothorax can be atypi-

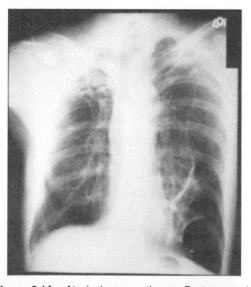

Figure 3.14. Atypical pneumothorax. Posteroanterior radiograph of a patient with old pulmonary tuberculosis and a secondary spontaneous pneumothorax on the left side. Note that the pleural air is seen only in the lower part of the hemithorax because the visceral and parietal pleura over the upper lung had become fused by the old tuberculosis.

cal. If the parenchyma of the lung is diseased such that the lung does not retain its normal shape, the appearance of the partially collapsed lung will be altered. The presence of adhesions between the visceral and the parietal pleura also alters the radiologic appearance of pneumothoraces. Such adhesions are frequently manifested as bandlike structures tethering the partially collapsed lung to the chest wall. Diffuse adhesions between the visceral and the parietal pleura may prevent collapse of an entire lobe (Fig. 3.14).

Clinically and radiologically, it is important to distinguish giant bullae from pneumothoraces because the treatment for the two conditions is different. This differentiation at times is difficult because a large bulla may mimic a large pneumothorax with adhesions. If doubt exists, a CT scan should be obtained because it can unequivocally establish the diagnosis (40).

Tension Pneumothorax

A tension pneumothorax exists when the pressure in the pleural space is positive throughout the respiratory cycle. Because the increased pleural pressure can seriously compromise pulmonary gas exchange and cardiac output (see Chapter 19), it is important to recognize the presence of a tension pneumothorax so treatment can be undertaken immediately. The radiologic diagnosis of a tension pneumothorax is unreliable from plain radiographic films alone. Although it is frequently stated that enlargement of a hemithorax, flattening of the diaphragm, and contralateral shift of the mediastinum indicate a tension pneumothorax, all three signs occur occasionally with nontension pneumothoraces (1). A definitive diagnosis can be established radiologically only by fluoroscopic examination. With a tension pneumothorax, the increased pleural pressure prevents the shift of the mediastinum toward the involved side on inspiration, as occurs with a nontension pneumothorax, and the movement of the ipsilateral diaphragm is restricted (1). In general, however, it is better to insert a needle into the pleural space to ascertain the presence of a tension pneumothorax than to waste time with radiologic procedures (see Chapter 19) (41).

REFERENCES

1. Fraser RG, Paré JAP, Paré PD, Fraser RS, Benereux GP: Diagnosis of Diseases of the Chest. 3rd ed. Volume I. Philadelphia: WB Saunders, 1988.
2. Davis S, Gardner F, Qvist G: The shape of a pleural effusion. Br J Med 1963;1:436–437.
3. Collins JD, Burwell D, Furmanski S, et al: Minimal detectable pleural effusions. Radiology 1972;105:51–53.
4. Vix VA: Roentgenographic recognition of pleural effusion. JAMA 1974;229:695–698.
5. Mulvey RB: The effect of pleural fluid on the diaphragm. Radiology 1965;84:1080–1085.
6. Ruskin JA, Gurney JW, Thorsen MK, Goodman LR: Detection of pleural effusions on supine chest radiographs. AJR 1987;148:681–683.
7. Woodring JH: Recognition of pleural effusion on supine radiographs: How much fluid is required? AJR 1984;142:59–64.
8. Fleischner FG: Atypical arrangement of free pleural effusion. Radiol Clin North Am 1963;1:347–362.
9. Higgins JA, Juergens JL, Bruwer AJ, Parkin TW: Loculated interlobar pleural effusion due to congestive heart failure. Arch Intern Med 1955;96:180–187.
10. Moskowitz H, Platt RT, Schachar R, Mellins H: Roentgen visualization of minute pleural effusion. Radiology 1973;109:33–35.
11. Moller A: Pleural effusion: use of the semi-supine position for radiograph detection. Radiology 1984;150:245–249.
12. McLoud TC, Flower CD: Imaging the pleura: sonography, CT, and MR imaging. AJR 1991;156:1145–1153.
13. Yang PC, Luh KT, Chang DB, Wu HD, Yu CJ, Kuo SH: Value of sonography in determining the nature of pleural effusion: analysis of 320 cases. AJR 1992;159:29–33.
14. Marks WM, Filly RA, Callen PW: Real-time evaluation of pleural lesions: new observations regarding the probability of obtaining free fluid. Radiology 1982;142:163–164.
15. Rosenberg ER: Ultrasound in the assessment of pleural densities. Chest 1983;84:283–285.
16. Wu R-G, Yuan A, Liaw Y-S, Chang D-B, Yu C-J, Wu H-D, Kuo S-H, Luh K-T, Yang P-C: Image comparison of real-time gray-scale ultrasound and color Doppler ultrasound for use in diagnosis of minimal pleural effusion. Am J Respir Crit Care Med 1994;150:510–514.
17. Lomas DJ, Padley SG, Flower CD: The sonographic appearances of pleural fluid. Brit J Radiol 1993;66:619–624.
18. Henschke CI, Yankelevitz DF, Davis SD: Pleural diseases: multimodality imaging and clinical management. Cur Prob Diagnost Radiol 1991;20:155–181.
19. Pugatch RD, Spirn PW: Radiology of the pleura. Clin Chest Med 1985;6:17–32.
20. Paling MR, Griffin GK: Lower lobe collapse due to pleural effusion: a CT analysis. J Comput Assist Tomogr 1985;9:1079–1083.
21. Proto AV, Ball JB Jr: Computed tomography of the major and minor fissures. AJR 1983;140:439–448.
22. Gamsu G, Sostman D: Magnetic resonance imaging of the thorax. Am Rev Respir Dis 1989;139:254–274.
23. Fisher MR: Magnetic resonance for evaluation of the thorax. Chest 1989;95:166–173.
24. Adams FV, Kolodny E: M-mode ultrasonic localization and identification of fluid-containing pulmonary cysts. Chest 1979;75:330–333.
25. Bressler EL, Francis IR, Glazer GM, Gross BH: Bolus contrast medium enhancement for distinguishing pleural from parenchymal lung disease: CT features. J Comput Assist Tomogr 1987;11:436–440.
26. Zinn WL, Nadich DP, Whelan CA, et al: Fluid within preexisting pulmonary air-spaces: a potential pitfall in the CT differentiation of pleural from parenchymal disease. J Comput Assist Tomogr 1987;11:441–448.
27. Eibenberger KL, Dock WI, Ammann ME, Dorffner R, Hormann MF, Grabenwoger F: Quantification of pleural effusions: sonography versus radiography. Radiology 1994;191:681–684.
28. Light RW, Jenkinson SG, Minh V, George RB: Observations on pleural pressures as fluid is withdrawn during thoracentesis. Am Rev Respir Dis 1980;121:799–804.
29. Maher GG, Berger HW: Massive pleural effusion: malignant and non-malignant causes in 46 patients. Am Rev Respir Dis 1972;105:458–460.
30. Liberson M: Diagnostic significance of the mediastinal profile in massive unilateral pleural effusions. Am Rev Respir Dis 1963;88:176–180.
31. Yu CJ, Yang PC, Wu HD, Chang DB, Kuo SH, Luh KT: Ultrasound study in unilateral hemithorax opacification. Image comparison with computed tomography. Am Rev Respir Dis 1993;147:430–434.
32. Renner RR, Markarian B, Pernice NJ, Heitzman ER: The apical cap. Radiology 1974;110:569–573.
33. Hillerdal G: Non-malignant asbestos pleural disease. Thorax 1981;36:669–675.
34. Fletcher DE, Edge JR: The early radiological changes in pulmonary and pleural asbestosis. Clin Radiol 1970;21:355–365.
35. Katz D, Kreel L: Computed tomography in pulmonary asbestosis. Clin Radiol 1979;30:207–213.
36. Carr JJ, Reed JC, Choplin RH, Pope TL Jr, Case LD: Plain and computed radiography for detecting experimentally induced pneumothorax in cadavers: implications for detection in patients. Radiology 1992;183:193–199.
37. Glazer HS, Anderson DJ, Wilson BS, Molina PL, Sagel SS: Pneumothorax: appearance on lateral chest radiographs. Radiology 1989;173:707–711.
38. Buckner CB, Harmon BH, Pallin JS: The radiology of abnormal intrathoracic air. Curr Probl Diagn Radiol 1988;17:37–71.
39. Tocino IM, Miller MH, Fairfax WR: Distribution of pneumothorax in the supine and semierect critically ill adult. AJR 1985;144:901–905.
40. Bourgouin P, Cousineau G, Lemire P, Hebert G: Computed tomography used to exclude pneumothorax in bullous lung disease. J Can Assoc Radiol 1985;36:341–342.
41. Light RW: Tension pneumothorax. Intensive Care Med 1994;106:1162–1165.

CHAPTER 4
Clinical Manifestations and Useful Tests

Normally, the pleural space contains only a few milliliters of pleural fluid. If enough fluid is present to be detected radiologically, it is abnormal. Many conditions can be associated with pleural fluid accumulation (see Table 5.1). When pleural fluid is detected, an effort should be made to determine which of the many conditions listed in Table 5.1 is responsible. In this chapter, the clinical manifestations of pleural effusions are first discussed. Then, the various tests used in the differential diagnosis of pleural effusions are reviewed. In Chapter 5, recommendations are given for a systematic approach to the patient with a pleural effusion.

CLINICAL MANIFESTATIONS

The presence of moderate-to-large amounts of pleural fluid produces symptoms and characteristic changes on physical examination.

Symptoms

The symptoms of a patient with a pleural effusion are to a large extent dictated by the underlying process causing the effusion. Many patients have no symptoms referable to the effusion. When symptoms are related to the effusion, they arise either from inflammation of the pleura, from compromise of pulmonary mechanics, or from interference with gas exchange. Inflammation of the pleura is manifested by pleuritic chest pain. Because only the parietal pleura has pain fibers, pleuritic chest pain indicates inflammation of the parietal pleura. Some patients with pleural effusions experience a dull, aching chest pain rather than pleuritic chest pain. This symptom is very suggestive that the patient has pleural malignancy (1). The presence of either pleuritic chest pain or dull, aching chest pain indicates that the parietal pleura is probably involved and the patient has an exudative pleural effusion.

Ordinarily, the pain associated with pleural disease is well localized and coincides with the affected area of the pleura, because the parietal pleura is innervated mostly by the intercostal nerves. At times, however, pleuritic pain is referred to the abdomen because intercostal nerves are also distributed to the abdomen. A notable exception to the localization of the pain occurs when the central portion of the diaphragmatic pleura is involved. The nerve supply to this portion of the parietal pleura is the phrenic nerve; therefore, inflammation of the central portion of the diaphragm is referred to the ipsilateral shoulder. Pleuritic pain felt simultaneously in the lower chest and ipsilateral shoulder is pathognomonic of diaphragmatic involvement.

A second symptom of pleural effusion is a dry, nonproductive cough. The mechanism producing the cough is not clear. It may be related to pleural inflammation. Alternately, lung compression by the fluid may bring opposing bronchial walls into contact, stimulating the cough reflex.

The third symptom of pleural effusion is dyspnea. A pleural effusion acts as a space-occupying process in the thoracic cavity and therefore reduces all subdivisions of lung volumes. Small-to-moderate-sized pleural effusions displace rather than compress the lung, however, and have little effect on pulmonary function (2). Larger pleural effusions obviously cause a significant reduction in lung volumes, but the improvement in pulmonary function following therapeutic thoracentesis is much less than one would anticipate. We obtained spirometry before and 24 hours after thoracentesis in 26 patients from whom a mean of 1740 ml pleural fluid was withdrawn (3). In these patients the mean vital capacity improved 410 ± 390 ml. Patients in this study with higher pleural pressures after the removal of 800 ml pleural fluid and patients with smaller decreases in the pleural pressure after the removal of 800 ml pleural fluid had greater improvements in the forced vital capacity (FVC) after thoracentesis. Associated parenchymal disease probably explains this small increase in pulmonary function following therapeutic thoracentesis. The degree of dyspnea is frequently out of proportion to the size of the pleural effusion. Either pleuritic chest pain, with the resultant splinting, or concomitant parenchymal disease is usually responsible for the disproportionate dyspnea. When the pleural effusion is large, ventricular filling may be impeded leading to a decreased cardiac output and dyspnea (4). Arterial blood gases usually remain at clinically acceptable levels regardless of the size of the effusion (5), because of the reflex reduction in perfusion to the lung underlying the effusion.

Physical Examination

When the chest of a patient with or suspected of having a pleural effusion is examined, particular attention should be paid to the relative sizes of the hemithoraces and the intercostal spaces. If the pleural pressure is increased on the side of the effusion, that hemithorax will be larger, and the usual concavity of the intercostal spaces will be blunted or even convex. In contrast, if the pleural pressure on the side of the effusion is decreased, as with obstruction of a major bronchus or a trapped lung, the ipsilateral hemithorax will be smaller, and the normal concavity of the intercostal spaces will be exaggerated. In addition, with inspiratory efforts, the intercostal spaces retract. Enlargement of the hemithorax with bulging of the intercostal spaces is an indication for therapeutic thoracentesis to relieve the increased pleural pressure. Signs of decreased pleural pressure are a relative contraindication to therapeutic thoracentesis because the decreased pleural pressure can lead to re-expansion pulmonary edema (6). Of course, in many patients with pleural effusions, the hemithoraces are equal in size, and the intercostal spaces are normal.

Palpation of the chest in patients with pleural effusions is useful in delineating the extent of the effusion. In areas of the chest where pleural fluid separates the lung from the chest wall, tactile fremitus is absent or attenuated because the fluid absorbs the vibrations emanating from the lung. Tactile fremitus is much more reliable than percussion for identifying the upper border of the pleural fluid and the proper place to attempt a thoracentesis. With a thin rim of fluid, the percussion note may still be resonant, but the tactile fremitus is diminished. Palpation may also reveal that the cardiac point of maximum impulse is shifted to one side or the other. With large left pleural effusions, the cardiac point of maximum impulse may not be palpable. In patients with pleural effusions, the position of the trachea should always be ascertained because it indicates the relationship between the pleural pressures in the two hemithoraces.

The percussion note over a pleural effusion is dull or flat. The dullness is maximum at the lung bases where the thickness of the fluid is the greatest. As mentioned earlier, however, the percussion note may not be duller if only a thin rim of fluid is present. Light percussion is better than heavy percussion for identifying small amounts of pleural fluid. If the dullness to percussion shifts as the position of the patient is changed, one can be almost certain that free pleural fluid is present.

Auscultation over the pleural fluid characteristically reveals decreased or absent breath sounds. Near the superior border of the fluid, however, breath sounds may be accentuated. This phenomenon has been attributed to increased conductance of breath sounds through the partially atelectatic lung beneath the fluid (7). This accentuation of breath sounds does not mean that an associated parenchymal infiltrate is present. Auscultation may also reveal a pleural rub. Pleural rubs are characterized by coarse, creaking, leathery sounds most commonly heard during the latter part of inspiration and the early part of expiration, to give a to-and-fro pattern of sound. Pleural rubs, caused by the rubbing together of the roughened pleural surfaces during respiration, are often associated with local pain on breathing that subsides with breath-holding. Pleural rubs often appear as pleural effusions diminish in size either spontaneously or as a result of treatment. The rub appears because the pleural fluid is no longer present between the roughened pleural surfaces.

Obviously, the chest is not the only structure that should be examined when evaluating a patient with pleural effusion; hints as to the origin of the effusion are often present elsewhere. The effusion is probably due to congestive heart failure if the patient has cardiomegaly, neck vein distension, or peripheral edema. Signs of joint disease or subcutaneous nodules suggest that the pleural effusion is due to rheumatoid disease or lupus erythematosus. An enlarged, nontender nodular liver or the presence of hypertrophic osteoarthropathy suggests metastatic disease, as do breast masses or the absence of a breast. Abdominal tenderness suggests a subdiaphragmatic process, whereas tense ascites suggests cirrhosis. Lymphadenopathy suggests lymphoma, metastatic disease, or sarcoidosis.

SEPARATION OF TRANSUDATIVE FROM EXUDATIVE EFFUSIONS

The accumulation of clinically detectable quantities of pleural fluid is distinctly abnormal. A diagnostic thoracentesis (see Chapter 23) should be attempted whenever the thickness of pleural fluid on the decubitus radiograph is greater than 10 mm or whenever loculated pleural fluid is demonstrated with ultrasound unless the patient has typical congestive heart failure. A properly performed diagnostic thoracentesis takes less than 10 minutes and should cause no more morbidity than a venipuncture. The information available from examination of the pleural fluid is invaluable.

Pleural effusions have classically been divided into transudates and exudates (8). A transudative pleural effusion develops when the systemic factors influencing the formation or absorption of pleural fluid are altered so that pleural fluid accumulates. The pleural fluid is a transudate. The fluid may originate in the lung, the pleura, or the peritoneal cavity

(9). The permeability of the capillaries to proteins is normal in the area where the fluid is formed. Examples of conditions producing transudative pleural effusions are left ventricular failure producing increased pulmonary interstitial fluid and a resulting pleural effusion, ascites due to cirrhosis with movement of fluid through the diaphragm, and decreased serum oncotic pressure with hypoproteinemia. In contrast, an exudative pleural effusion develops when the pleural surfaces or the capillaries in the location where the fluid originates are altered such that fluid accumulates. The pleural fluid is an exudate. The two most common causes of exudative pleural effusions are increased permeability of the capillaries in the lung to protein, as with parapneumonic effusions, and decreased lymphatic clearance of the fluid from the pleural space, as in some types of malignant disease (see Chapter 3).

The first question to answer in assessing a patient with a pleural effusion is whether that effusion is a transudate or an exudate. If the effusion is a transudate, no further diagnostic procedures are necessary, and therapy is directed to the underlying congestive heart failure, cirrhosis, or nephrosis. Alternately, if the effusion proves to be an exudate, a more extensive diagnostic investigation is indicated to delineate the cause of the effusion.

For many years, a pleural fluid protein level of 3.0 g/dl was used to separate transudates from exudates, with exudative pleural effusions characterized by a protein level above 3.0 g/dl (10, 11). Use of this one simple test led to the misclassification of approximately 10% of pleural effusions, however (10–12). My colleagues and I subsequently demonstrated that with the use of simultaneously obtained serum and pleural fluid protein and lactic acid dehydrogenase (LDH) values, 99% of pleural effusions could be correctly classified as either transudates or exudates (12). Exudative pleural effusions meet at least one of the following criteria, whereas transudative pleural effusions meet none: (Light's criteria)

1. Pleural fluid protein divided by serum protein greater than 0.5
2. Pleural fluid LDH divided by serum LDH greater than 0.6

3. Pleural fluid LDH greater than two-thirds the upper limit of normal for the serum LDH.

In recent years, other researchers have proposed new tests to differentiate transudates and exudates. Two reports (13, 14) indicated that transudates tend to have a pleural fluid cholesterol level below 60 mg/dl, whereas most exudative pleural effusions have cholesterol levels that exceed this value. Another report (15) demonstrated that transudates had a gradient between the serum and the pleural fluid for albumin that exceeded 1.2 g/100 ml while exudates had a gradient that was more than 1.2 g/100 ml. Lastly, another report (16) concluded that a value of 0.6 for the pleural fluid-to-serum bilirubin effectively separates transudates and exudates with exudates having the higher values.

Two subsequent reports (17, 18) have compared Light's criteria with the other proposed tests and have concluded that Light's criteria best separates exudates and transudates. In the study of Romero and associates (17) of 297 patients including 44 transudates and 253 exudates, Light's criteria were superior to the cholesterol in making the distinction. In this study with Light's criteria, 98% of the exudates and 77% of the transudates were correctly classified (17). In a subsequent study of 393 patients from South Africa (18) including 123 with transudates and 270 with exudates, Light's criteria were found to be superior to the serum-effusion albumin gradient, the effusion cholesterol concentration, and the pleural fluid:serum bilirubin ratio (18). Again in this study, Light's criteria identified 98% of the exudates correctly, but were less accurate in identifying transudates (18).

In summary, it appears that Light's criteria remain the best biochemical means by which pleural effusions can be classified as transudates or exudates. If it is thought that the patient has a transudative pleural effusion clinically, but Light's exudative criteria are met, then it is reasonable to measure the serum-pleural fluid albumin gradient. If this is above 1.2 g/dl, then the patient in all probability has a transudative pleural effusion (18). Use of the serum-pleural fluid albumin gradient alone will result in the misclassification of many exudates as transudates (18).

Specific Gravity

The specific gravity of the pleural fluid as measured with a hydrometer was used in the past to separate transudates from exudates (8), because it was a simple and rapid method of estimating the protein content of the fluid. A specific gravity of 1.015 corresponds to a protein content of 3.0 g/dl, and this value was used to separate transudates from exudates (19). At the present time, refractometers are usually used to estimate the specific gravity of pleural fluid. Unfortunately, the scale on the commercially available refractometers is calibrated for the specific gravity of urine rather than pleural fluid. A reading of 1.020 on the urine specific gravity scale corresponds to a pleural fluid protein level of 3.0 g/dl. However, there is a scale on the same refractometer for protein levels, which is valid for pleural fluid. Since the only reason to measure specific gravity is to estimate the protein level, the pleural fluid specific gravity measurement is extraneous and confusing and should no longer be ordered (20). A rapid estimate of the pleural fluid protein content can be obtained at the patient's bedside with the protein scale on the refractometer, however (20).

Other Characteristics of Transudates

Most transudates are clear, straw-colored, nonviscid, and odorless. Approximately 15% have red cell counts above 10,000/mm^3, however, so the discovery of blood-tinged pleural fluid does not mean that the fluid is not a transudate. Because red blood cells contain a large amount of LDH, one might suppose that the LDH level in a blood-tinged or bloody transudative pleural effusion would be so elevated that it would meet the criteria for an exudative pleural effusion. Such does not appear to be the case, however. The LDH isoenzyme present in red blood cells is LDH-1, and in one study of 23 patients with bloody pleural effusions (pleural fluid red cell counts greater than 100,000/mm^3), the fraction of LDH-1 in the pleural fluid was not much increased (21).

The pleural fluid white blood cell count of most transudates is less than 1000/mm^3, but about 20% have white blood cell counts that exceed 1000/mm^3 (22). Pleural fluid white blood cell counts above 10,000/mm^3 are rare with transudative pleural effusions. The differential white cell count in transudative pleural effusions may be dominated by polymorphonuclear leukocytes, small lymphocytes, or other mononuclear cells. In a series of 47 transudative effusions, 6 (13%) had more than 50% polymorphonuclear leukocytes, whereas 16 (34%) had predominantly small lymphocytes and 22 (47%) had predominantly other mononuclear cells (22). The pleural fluid glucose level is similar to the serum glucose level, but the pleural fluid amylase level is low (23). The pleural fluid pH with transudative pleural effusions is higher than the simultaneously obtained blood pH (24), probably because of active transport of bicarbonate from the blood into the pleural space (25).

GENERAL TESTS FOR DIFFERENTIATING CAUSES OF EXUDATES

Appearance of Fluid

The gross appearance of the pleural fluid frequently yields useful diagnostic information. The color, turbidity, viscosity, and odor should be described. Most transudative and many exudative pleural effusions are clear, straw-colored, nonviscid, and odorless. Any deviations should be noted and investigated.

A reddish color indicates that blood is present, and a brownish tinge indicates that the blood has been present for a prolonged period. If the pleural fluid is blood-tinged, the pleural fluid red blood cell count is between 5,000 and 10,000/mm^3. If the pleural fluid appears grossly bloody, a hematocrit should be obtained to determine whether the patient has a hemothorax (see Chapter 20).

Turbid pleural fluid can occur from either increased cellular content or increased lipid content. These two entities can be differentiated if the pleural fluid is centrifuged and the supernatant is examined. If turbidity remains after centrifugation, it is in all probability due to increased lipid content, and the fluid should be sent for lipid analysis (see the discussion later in this chapter). Alternately, if the supernatant is clear, the original turbidity was due to increased numbers of cells or other debris. The discovery of pleural fluid that looks like chocolate sauce or anchovy paste is suggestive of amebiasis with a hepatopleural fistula (26).

This appearance is due to the presence of a mixture of blood, cytolyzed liver tissue, and small solid particles of liver parenchyma that have resisted dissolution.

A clear or bloody viscous fluid is suggestive of malignant mesothelioma; the high viscosity is secondary to an elevated pleural fluid hyaluronic acid level (27). Of course, the fluid from a long-standing pyothorax is also viscid because of the large amounts of cells and debris in the fluid.

The odor of all pleural fluids should be noted. One can immediately establish two diagnoses by smelling the pleural fluid. A feculent odor indicates that the patient has an anaerobic infection of his pleural space. If the pleural fluid smells like urine, the patient probably has a urinothorax.

Red Blood Cell Count

Only 5,000 to 10,000 red blood cells/mm^3 need be present to impart a red color to pleural fluid. If a pleural effusion has a total volume of 500 ml and the red cell count in the peripheral blood is 5,000,000/mm^3, a leak of only 1 ml blood into the pleural space will result in a blood-tinged pleural effusion. It is probably for this reason that the presence of blood-tinged or serosanguineous pleural fluid has little diagnostic significance. Over 15% of transudative and over 40% of all types of exudative pleural fluids are blood-tinged (22); that is, they have pleural fluid red cell counts between 5,000 and 100,000/mm^3.

Occasionally, pleural fluid obtained by diagnostic thoracentesis appears bloody. In such cases one can assume that the red cell count in the pleural fluid is above 100,000/mm^3. One should obtain a hematocrit on such pleural fluids to document the amount of blood in the pleural fluid. If the hematocrit of the pleural fluid is greater than 50% of the peripheral hematocrit, a hemothorax is present, and one should consider inserting chest tubes (see Chapter 20). Usually, the hematocrit of bloody pleural fluid is much lower than one would expect from its gross appearance.

The presence of bloody pleural fluid suggests one of three diagnoses, namely, malignant disease, trauma, or pulmonary embolization. In a series of 22 bloody pleural effusions

Table 4.1. Etiology of 25 Effusions Containing More Than 10,000 WBC/mm³

Diagnosis	Number with >10,000 WBC/mm³	Total Number of Effusions	Percentage having >10,000 WBC/mm³
Parapneumonic effusion	13	26	50
Malignant disease	3	43	7
Pulmonary embolization	3	8	37
Tuberculosis	2	14	14
Pancreatitis	2	5	40
Postmyocardial infarction syndrome	1	3	33
Systemic lupus erythematosus	1	1	100

that I observed on medical wards, 12 were due to malignant disease, 5 to pulmonary embolization, 2 to trauma, 2 to pneumonia, and 1 was a transudative effusion secondary to cirrhosis (22). The traumatic origin of the pleural effusion may not be obvious, particularly when the patient is on a medical ward. The patient may have broken a rib while coughing or suffered trauma during an episode of inebriation that is not remembered.

Pleural fluid red blood cell counts are usually done with an automated Coulter counter. In our experience, the red blood cell counts of pleural fluid reported by this method are virtually meaningless. Frequently, red cell counts above 30,000/mm³ are reported when the pleural fluid is clear and yellow and the red blood cell count should be less than 5,000/mm³. It is unclear why the pleural fluid red cell counts are so inaccurate. It may be that the Coulter counter is calibrated for much higher red blood cell counts or that debris in the pleural fluid is mistaken for red blood cells by the machine. In view of the inaccuracies of the automated counts, more reliance should be placed on the gross description of the pleural fluid. If the pleural fluid is grossly bloody, then a hematocrit should be obtained on the pleural fluid to quantitate the amount of blood.

At times, it is unclear whether blood in the pleural fluid resulted from or was present prior to the thoracentesis. If the blood is a result of the thoracentesis, the degree of red discoloration of the fluid should not be uniform throughout the course of aspiration. Examination of the fluid microscopically may also be useful. If the red blood cells were present before the thoracentesis, the macrophages in the pleural fluid usually contain hemoglobin inclusions. If there are no plate-

lets present, the blood is not the result of a traumatic thoracentesis (28). Creation of the red blood cells in the pleural fluid rarely occurs because the osmotic pressure of the pleural fluid is similar to that of serum.

White Blood Cell Count

The pleural fluid white blood count is of limited diagnostic use. Most transudates have white cell counts below 1,000/mm³, whereas most exudates have white cell counts above 1,000/mm³ (12). Pleural fluid white blood cell counts above 10,000/mm³ are most commonly seen with parapneumonic effusions, but are also seen with many other diseases (22), as shown in Table 4.1. I have seen pleural fluid white blood cell counts above 50,000/mm³ with both pancreatic disease and pulmonary embolization. With grossly purulent pleural fluid, the pleural fluid white blood cell count is frequently much lower than one would anticipate because debris rather than cells accounts for much of the turbidity.

Differential White Cell Count

Examination of a Wright stain of pleural fluid is one of the most informative tests on pleural fluid. Because the pleural fluid white blood cell count is frequently less than 5000/mm³, it is useful to concentrate the cells before staining. This procedure is easily accomplished by centrifuging about 10 ml fluid and then resuspending the button of cells in about 0.5 ml supernatant. After thorough mixing, slides are made similarly to those for examining peripheral blood and are stained in the usual way. Occasionally, large amounts of fibrinogen adhere to the cells. In such cases, resuspension in saline solution, followed by centrifugation, is indicated in order to evaluate cellular morphologic features.

Although most laboratories divide pleural fluid white cells into polymorphonuclear leukocytes and mononuclear cells, I prefer to divide them into three categories: polymorphonuclear leukocytes, small lymphocytes, and other mononuclear cells, because of the diagnostic significance of small lymphocytes (see "Lymphocytes," later in this chapter). The polymorphonuclear leukocytes include neutrophils, eosinophils, and basophils, whereas the other mononuclear cells include mesothelial cells, macrophages, plasma cells, and malignant cells. Excellent color plates demonstrating the morphologic and staining characteristics of the different cells in pleural effusions are contained in the monograph by Spriggs and Boddington (29).

Neutrophils

Because neutrophils are the cellular component of the acute inflammatory response, they predominate in pleural fluid resulting from acute inflammation such as occurs with pneumonia, pancreatitis, pulmonary embolization, subphrenic abscess, and early tuberculosis. Although over 10% of transudative pleural effusions contain predominantly neutrophils, pleural fluid neutrophilia in transudates has no clinical significance (22). The significance of neutrophils in an exudative pleural effusion is that they indicate acute inflammation of the pleural surface.

Interleukin 8 (IL-8) appears to be one of the primary chemotaxins for neutrophils in the pleural space (30, 31). The number of neutrophils in pleural fluid is correlated with the IL-8 level and empyemas have the highest levels of IL-8. The addition of IL-8 neutralizing serum decreases the chemotactic activity for neutrophils in empyema fluids (31). The cellular source of IL-8 is unknown (30).

Examination of the pleural fluid neutrophils in patients with parapneumonic effusions is useful in identifying those that are infected. If pleural infection is present, the neutrophils undergo a characteristic degeneration. The nucleus becomes blurred and no longer is stained purple. The cytoplasm shows toxic granulation initially. Subsequently, the neutro-

philic granules become indistinct and then are lost. Finally, only a smear cell remains (29).

Eosinophils

Most clinicians feel that significant numbers of eosinophils (more than 10%) in pleural fluid should be a clue to the origin of the pleural effusion. In most instances, however, the pleural fluid eosinophilia is due to either air or blood in the pleural space and therefore does not contribute any diagnostic information in these situations. Charcot-Leyden crystals (32), as well as Curschmann's spirals (33), are occasionally found in the pleural fluid of patients with pleural eosinophilia. Their presence appears to have no diagnostic significance.

In the past few years the mechanisms responsible for pleural fluid eosinophilia have been somewhat clarified. Pleural fluid from patients with eosinophilic pleural effusions stimulates bone marrow cells to form colonies of eosinophils (34, 35). In addition, when eosinophils are incubated in the presence of eosinophilic pleural fluid, their survival is prolonged (34). Peripheral blood from patients with eosinophilic pleural effusions does not stimulate the bone marrow to form eosinophil colonies and does not prolong survival of eosinophils. The factor responsible for the increased colony forming activity and the increased survival appears to be interleukin 5 (IL-5) (34, 35), although IL-3 and granulocyte/macrophage colony-stimulating factor (GM-CSF) may also play a role (34). The source of the IL-5 appears to be the CD4[+] lymphocyte in the pleural fluid (35), but the eosinophils in the pleural fluid may themselves also produce IL-5 (34). The source of the eosinophils in eosinophilic pleural effusions appears to be the bone marrow; no progenitor cells are present in the pleural space. It is not known what stimulates the CD4[+] lymphocytes to produce the IL-5. However, it probably results from another cytokine since the intrapleural injection of IL-2 into malignant pleural effusions results in an eosinophilic pleural effusion with a high level of IL-5 (36). There are factors other than IL-5 that recruit eosinophils to the pleural space. Antibodies to IL-5 will eliminate the eosinophilic influx to an allergen but not to endotoxin in the mouse (37).

The most common cause of pleural fluid eosinophilia is air in the pleural space. In a series of 127 cases with more than 20% eosinophils in the pleural fluid, 81 (64%) were thought to have pleural fluid eosinophilia secondary to air in the pleural space (29). In a review of 343 pleural effusions with greater than 10% eosinophils, 95 (28%) had air in the pleural space (38). It is likely that the pleural fluid eosinophilia in many of the other patients in this series was also due to the introduction of air into the pleural space during a prior thoracentesis. On numerous occasions over the past two decades, I have seen patients who had no pleural fluid eosinophilia at the initial thoracentesis, but who had many eosinophils at a subsequent thoracentesis. In each case, a small pneumothorax resulted from the initial thoracentesis. The mechanism responsible for the pleural fluid eosinophilia in response to air in the pleural space is unknown but is probably related to the cytokines as outlined above. When patients with spontaneous pneumothorax undergo thoracotomy, a reactive eosinophilic pleuritis frequently exists in the resected parietal pleura (39).

The second most common cause of pleural fluid eosinophilia is blood in the pleural space. Following traumatic hemothorax, pleural fluid eosinophils do not usually become numerous until the second week (29). There is frequently an associated peripheral blood eosinophilia that does not disappear until the pleural effusion is completely resolved (40). The pleural effusions associated with pulmonary embolization are frequently bloody and contain numerous eosinophils. Bloody pleural fluids due to malignant disease are not usually characterized by eosinophilia (22, 29). In a study conducted by my colleagues and myself of bloody pleural effusions, none of the 11 cases of malignant pleural effusions with pleural fluid red cell counts greater than 100,000/mm^3 had more than 10% eosinophils (22).

If neither air nor blood is present in the pleural space, several unusual diagnoses should be considered. Pleural eosinophilia is common in patients with asbestos-related pleural effusions. In a review of eosinophilic pleural effusions (38), 15 of 29 (52%) of asbestos pleural effusions had more than 10% eosinophils in the pleural fluid. The pleural effusions second-ary to drug reactions are frequently eosinophilic. Offending drugs include dantrolene, bromocriptine, and nitrofurantoin (see Chapter 17). Pleural effusions secondary to parasitic diseases such as paragonimiasis (41), hydatid disease (42), amebiasis (29), or ascariasis (29) frequently contain a large percentage of eosinophils. Lastly, the pleural effusion associated with the Churg-Strauss syndrome is eosinophilic (43).

If none of the foregoing rare diseases is causing the pleural effusion, the following statements are pertinent to patients with eosinophilic pleural effusions. If the patient has pneumonia and pleural effusion, the presence of pleural fluid eosinophilia is a good prognostic sign because such an effusion rarely becomes infected. If the patient has not had a previous thoracentesis or pneumothorax, it is unlikely that he has tuberculosis (29, 38). It is also unlikely that he has a malignant disease unless he has Hodgkin's disease (29, 38). The origin of approximately 25% of eosinophilic effusions is not established, and these effusions resolve spontaneously. Indeed, no etiology was established for 35% of 343 eosinophilic pleural effusions in the review of Adelman and coworkers (38). I believe that most of these undiagnosed eosinophilic pleural effusions are due to viral infections or occult pulmonary emboli.

Basophils

Basophilic pleural effusions are distinctly uncommon. I have not seen a pleural effusion that contained more than 2% basophils. A few basophils are usually present in pleural effusions with eosinophils. Basophil counts over 10% are most common with leukemic pleural involvement (29).

Lymphocytes

The discovery that more than 50% of the white blood cells in an exudative pleural effusion are small lymphocytes is important diagnostically because it means that the patient probably has a malignant disease or tuberculosis. In two series (22, 44) 96 of 211 exudative pleural effusions had more than 50% small lymphocytes. Of these 96 effusions, 90 (94%) were due to tuberculosis or malignant disease.

Because these diseases can be diagnosed with pleural biopsy, the presence of predominantly small lymphocytes in an exudative pleural effusion is usually an indication for such a biopsy. When the foregoing series are analyzed, almost all the effusions secondary to tuberculosis (43 of 46), but only two-thirds of the effusions secondary to malignant disease (47 of 70) had predominantly small lymphocytes. Approximately one-third of transudative pleural effusions (22) contain predominantly small lymphocytes, and lymphocytosis in these effusions is not an indication for pleural biopsy.

Several papers have assessed the diagnostic utility of separating the pleural lymphocytes into T and B lymphocytes (45–48). In general, this separation has not been useful. With most disease states, the pleural fluid contains a higher percentage of T lymphocytes ($\sim 70\%$), a lower percentage of B lymphocytes ($\sim 10\%$), and a higher percentage of null cells ($\sim 20\%$), than the corresponding peripheral blood (45, 46). The partitioning of lymphocytes may be useful, however, when chronic lymphatic leukemia or lymphoma is suspected. In a report of 4 such patients, all had more than 80% B lymphocytes in their pleural fluid (47).

The recent development of monoclonal antibodies has permitted a further subdivision of T lymphocytes. In comparison to peripheral blood, in pleural fluid the ratio of the helper/inducer cells (OKT4$^+$) to the suppressor/cytotoxic cells (OKT8$^+$) is higher regardless of the etiology of the pleural effusion (49–51). Therefore, this subdivision is not useful diagnostically. Natural killer (NK) cells are lymphocytes derived from an unimmunized host that lyse certain tumor cell lines and virus-infected cells. In general, the percentage of T lymphocytes in pleural fluid that is identified as NK cells by either the Leu 7 or Leu 11 monoclonal antibody is much lower than in the peripheral blood, whether the patient has tuberculosis or malignancy (51, 52). However, there is a discrepancy between the number of NK positive cells and the NK activity of the cells when patients with tuberculosis are compared to patients with malignancy. Although the number of NK cells is comparable in the two populations, there is much more NK activity in the tuberculous pleural effusions (52). The

explanation for the functional difference remains in doubt.

Mesothelial Cells

These cells line the pleural cavities. They frequently become dislodged from the pleural surfaces and are present in the small amount of normal pleural fluid (53). These cells are usually 12 to 30 µm in diameter, but multinucleated forms may have diameters up to 75 µm. Their cytoplasm is light blue (Fig. 4.1A) and often contains a few vacuoles. The nucleus is large (9–22 µm) and stains purplish with a uniform appearance. The nucleus usually contains 1 to 3 bright blue nucleoli (29).

Mesothelial cells are significant for two different reasons. First, their presence or absence is often useful diagnostically because these cells are uncommon in tuberculous effusions. Spriggs and Boddington analyzed 65 tuberculous effusions and found that only 1 effusion had more than a single mesothelial cell per 1000 cells (29). My colleagues and I have confirmed the paucity of mesothelial cells in tuberculous pleural effusions (22), as have Yam (44) and Hurwitz and associates (54). The lack of mesothelial cells is not diagnostic of tuberculosis, however. It simply indicates that the pleural surfaces have become extensively involved by the disease process so that the mesothelial cells cannot enter the pleural space. The absence of mesothelial cells is common with complicated parapneumonic effusions and with other conditions in which the pleura becomes coated with fibrin. It is also common with malignant effusions after sclerosing agents have been injected to effect a pleurodesis. Second, mesothelial cells, particularly in their activated form, may be confused with malignant cells. Frequently, an experienced pathologist is required to make the differentiation. Immunohistochemistry is useful in making this distinction (see discussion later in this chapter).

Macrophages

Macrophages by definition are cells that store vital dyes. It appears that the origin of the pleural fluid macrophages can be either the circulating monocyte or the mesothelial cells (55). Macrophages vary in diameter from

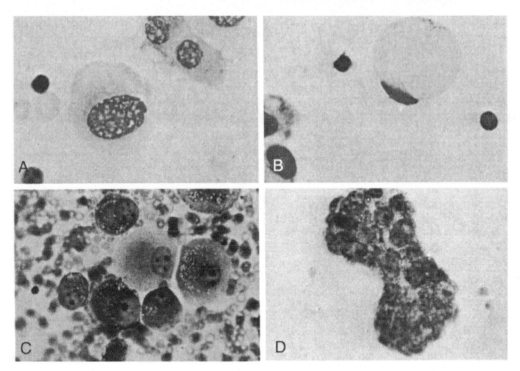

Figure 4.1A. Mesothelial cell. Note that the mesothelial cell is large in comparison to the lymphocyte and has light blue cytoplasm and light blue nucleoli of varying shapes and sizes. **B.** Signet-ring cell. This macrophage, which has engorged itself with pleural debris, is not a malignant cell. **C.** Malignant cells. Several large cells are similar, but vary in size. Note the large, dark nucleoli, which are so different from the nucleoli in the mesothelial cell. **D.** Clump of malignant cells from the pleural fluid of a patient with metastatic adenocarcinoma.

15 to 50 μm and have irregular nuclei. Their cytoplasm is gray, cloudy, and full of vacuoles. At times, the macrophage may become engorged with debris, to take on the appearance of a "signet-ring" cell with the nucleus flattened against the side of the cell (Fig. 4.1*B*). It is important to realize that these are not malignant cells. During phagocytosis, macrophages may engulf polymorphonuclear leukocytes or red blood cells. These cells may be evident within the macrophage in various stages of digestion. If red cells have been ingested, the iron pigment is retained as dark blue or brown staining material (29). In general, the presence of macrophages in pleural fluid is of limited diagnostic use. It is important not to confuse macrophages with mesothelial cells because macrophages are sometimes present in tuberculous pleural effusions (29).

Plasma Cells

These cells are of the lymphoid series and produce immunoglobulins. Morphologically, they are larger than small lymphocytes and have an eccentric nucleus and deeply staining basophilic cytoplasm with a clear area at the cell center (Golgi zone) (29). Mature forms have well-defined nuclear chromatin blocks. The presence of many plasma cells in the pleural fluid suggests multiple myeloma. Smaller numbers of plasma cells are not of any particular diagnostic importance. In a series of 16 effusions with more than 5% plasma cells, 4 were due to malignant disease, 3 to tuberculosis, 3 to congestive heart failure, 3 to pulmonary embolization, 2 to pneumonia, 1 to sepsis, and 2 were of undetermined origin (29).

Protein Measurements

The pleural fluid protein levels are generally higher in exudative pleural effusions than in transudative pleural effusions, and this observation serves as a basis for separating transudates from exudates (see the foregoing discussion on this differentiation in this chapter). Pleural fluid protein levels are not useful in separating the various types of exudative effu-

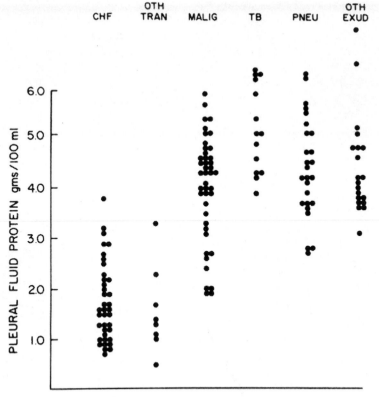

Figure 4.2.   Pleural fluid protein levels in effusion secondary to congestive heart failure (CHF), other transudates (OTH TRAN), malignant disease (MALIG), tuberculosis (TB), pneumonia (PNEU), and other exudates (OTH EXUD). Each point represents one pleural fluid. Note that the distribution of protein levels for all categories of exudative pleural effusions is similar. (From Light RW, MacGregor MI, Luchsinger PC, Ball WC: Pleural effusions: the diagnostic separation of transudates and exudates. Ann Intern Med 1972;77:507–513.)

sions, however, because the protein level in most exudates is elevated to a comparable degree (Fig. 4.2). At times, a pleural fluid meets the exudative criteria with its LDH, but not with its protein level. Such exudative pleural effusions are almost always parapneumonic effusions or are secondary to malignant pleural disease (12).

Simultaneous electrophoretic studies of serum and pleural fluid demonstrate that the pattern in the pleural fluid is essentially an image of that in the serum, except proportionately more albumin is present in the pleural fluid (56, 57). Along the same lines, the ratio of the pleural fluid to the serum IgG, IgA, and IgM is always below unity and appears to have no diagnostic value (1, 58). The ratio of the concentration of these proteins is inversely related to their molecular weight (58). The one immunoglobulin measurement that may be diagnostically useful is IgE. Yokogawa and coworkers measured the pleural fluid and serum IgE levels in 5 patients with paragonimiasis (59). In all 5 patients, the pleural fluid IgE level was above 4000 IU and exceeded the serum level. A subsequent report, however, measured the pleural fluid and serum IgE levels in 7 patients with eosinophilic pleural effusions and 7 with noneosinophilic pleural effusions. The pleural fluid levels and the ratio of the pleural fluid/serum IgE concentration were comparable in the two groups and it was concluded that pleural fluid IgE was the result of passive diffusion from the serum (60). None of the patients in this latter series, however, had paragonimiasis.

Glucose Measurement

Measurement of the pleural fluid glucose level is useful in the differential diagnosis of exudative pleural effusions because a low pleural fluid glucose level (less than 60 mg/dl) indicates that the patient probably has one of four disorders, namely, tuberculosis, malignant disease, rheumatoid disease, or parapneumonic effusion. Other rare causes of a low glucose pleural effusion include paragonimiasis, hemothorax, the Churg-Strauss syndrome and occasionally lupus pleuritis. The pleural fluid glucose level of all transudates and of most exudates parallels that of the serum. In my experience, it is not necessary to obtain pleural fluid glucose levels with the patient fasting or to take the serum glucose level into consideration when evaluating the pleural fluid glucose level.

The pleural fluid glucose level is reduced in some patients with tuberculous pleuritis. Indeed, early reports indicated that low pleural fluid glucose levels were seen only with tuberculous pleural effusions (61, 62). Subsequent studies (23, 63–65), however, revealed that low pleural fluid glucose levels also occurred with malignant and rheumatoid disease and parapneumonic effusion. The distribution of pleural fluid glucose levels for tuberculous and malignant pleural effusions is in fact similar (23). The majority of patients with tuberculous pleuritis have a pleural fluid glucose level above 80 mg/dl (23). Accordingly, a low pleural fluid glucose level is compatible with the diagnosis of tuberculous pleuritis, but it is not necessary for the diagnosis.

Approximately 15 to 25% of patients with malignant pleural effusions have pleural fluid glucose levels below 60 mg/dl (23, 63, 66) and the level may be less than 10 mg/dl. Patients with malignant pleural effusions and a low glucose level have a greater tumor burden in their pleural space than do those with normal pleural fluid glucose levels. In one report of 77 patients with malignant pleural effusion who underwent thoracoscopic examination (66) the extent of the tumor at thoracoscopy was significantly higher in those 16 patients in whom the pleural fluid glucose was less than 60 mg/dl. In addition, those patients with a low pleural fluid glucose are more likely to have positive pleural fluid cytology, are more likely to have a positive pleural biopsy (67), are less likely to have a good result from chemical pleurodesis (66, 68), and have a shortened life expectancy (68, 69).

Pleural effusions due to rheumatoid disease (see Chapter 14) classically have a low pleural fluid glucose level. Carr and Power first reported that rheumatoid pleural effusions had a low pleural fluid glucose level (64). In a subsequent review of 76 cases of rheumatoid pleural effusions (70), 42% had pleural fluid glucose levels below 10 mg/dl, and 78% had levels below 30 mg/dl. The explanation for the low pleural fluid glucose level in this condition appears to be a selective block to the entry of glucose into the pleural effusion (71). The pleural fluid glucose level in effusions secondary to lupus erythematosus is usually normal. In one report of 9 patients, the pleural fluid glucose level exceeded 80 mg/dl in all (72). In a subsequent report (73), the pleural fluid glucose level was below 50 mg/dl in 2 of 14 (14%) of patients with lupus pleuritis.

The pleural fluid glucose level can also be low with parapneumonic effusion (65, 74). If the pleural fluid is thick and purulent, the pleural fluid glucose level is frequently close to zero (65). Even in more serous fluid, the glucose level may be reduced. The more the pleural fluid glucose level is reduced, the more likely one is dealing with a complicated parapneumonic pleural effusion. Tube thoracostomy should be instituted in patients with a parapneumonic effusion if the glucose level is below 40 mg/dl (see Chapter 9) (74).

Amylase Determination

Pleural fluid amylase determinations are useful in the differential diagnosis of exudative pleural effusions because a pleural fluid amylase level above the upper normal limits for serum indicates that the patient has one of three problems: pancreatic disease, malignant tumor, or esophageal rupture (23). Approximately 10% of patients with inflammatory pancreatic disease have an accompanying pleural effusion (75). In such persons, the pleural fluid amylase level is usually raised well above the normal upper limits for serum and is also higher than the simultaneously sampled serum (23, 75). On rare occasions, the pleural fluid amylase is normal at the time of the original thoracentesis, only to become elevated at the time of a subsequent thoracentesis. In some patients with acute pancreatitis with pleural effusion, the chest symptoms of pleuritic chest pain and dyspnea may overshadow the abdominal symptoms. In such instances, an elevated pleural fluid amylase level may be the first hint of a pancreatic problem (23).

Patients with chronic pancreatic disease may also present with a pleural effusion with a high amylase content (76). The effusion results when a sinus tract connects the pancreatic pseudocyst and the pleural space. The patients typically appear chronically ill without abdominal symptoms and look like they have cancer. If a pleural fluid amylase level is not measured, the correct diagnosis may never be established.

The pleural fluid amylase level is elevated in approximately 10% of malignant pleural effusions (23, 77). The serum amylase level is also elevated in about 50% of patients with malignant pleural effusions and an elevated pleural fluid amylase. The pleural fluid amylase level in malignant pleural effusions is usually only minimally to moderately elevated, in contrast to the marked elevations with pancreatitis or esophageal rupture. The primary site of the tumor in patients with neoplastic pleural effusions and elevated pleural fluid amylase levels is usually not the pancreas (23, 77). Because the amylase in malignant pleural effusions is of the salivary type (78), amylase isoenzyme determinations are useful in distinguishing between malignant and pancreas-related pleural effusions.

The pleural fluid amylase level is also elevated with esophageal rupture (23, 79). The origin of the amylase with esophageal rupture has been shown to be the salivary gland rather than the pancreas (80). With the tear in the esophagus, the swallowed saliva with its high amylase content passes into the pleural space. Because the early diagnosis of esophageal perforation is imperative, owing to the high mortality rate without rapid operative intervention, the pleural fluid amylase determination should be made promptly when this diagnosis is suspected. In animal experiments, the pleural fluid amylase concentration is elevated within 2 hours of esophageal rupture (81).

Lactic Acid Dehydrogenase (LDH) Measurement

The pleural fluid LDH level is used to separate transudates from exudates (see the discussion earlier in this chapter). Most patients who meet the criteria for exudative pleural effusions with LDH but not with protein levels have either parapneumonic effusions or malignant pleural disease. Although initial reports suggested that the pleural fluid LDH level was increased only in patients with malignant pleural disease (82), subsequent reports demonstrated that the pleural fluid LDH was elevated in most exudative effusions regardless of origin (Fig. 4.3), and therefore, this determination is of no use in the differential diagnosis of exudative pleural effusions (12).

The level of the pleural fluid LDH is a reliable indicator of the degree of pleural inflammation; the higher the LDH, the more inflamed the pleural surfaces. Serial measurement of the pleural fluid LDH levels are informative when one is dealing with a patient with an undiagnosed pleural effusion. If with repeated thoracenteses, the pleural fluid LDH level becomes progressively higher, the degree of inflammation in the pleural space is increasing and one should be aggressive in pursuing a diagnosis. Alternatively, if the pleural fluid LDH level decreases with time, the process is resolving and one need not be as aggressive in the approach to the patient.

When bloody pleural fluid is obtained, one might wonder whether the LDH measurement would be useful since red blood cells contain large amounts of LDH. The presence of blood in the pleural fluid, however, usually does not adversely affect the measurement of the LDH. In one study, LDH isoenzyme analysis was performed on 12 pleural fluids that had contained more than 100,000 erythrocytes/mm^3. In only one effusion was the LDH-1 more than 5% above that in the serum, and the total pleural fluid LDH in that effusion was only 107 (21).

Even though the total pleural fluid LDH level is not useful in distinguishing among

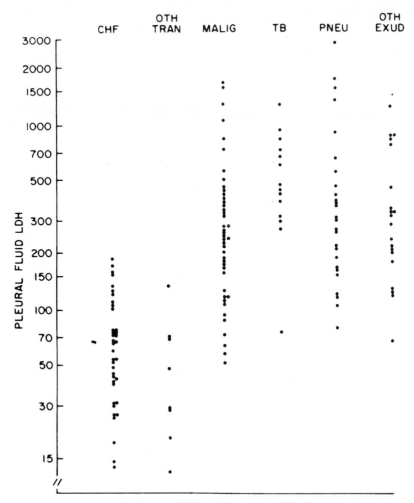

Figure 4.3. Pleural fluid lactic dehydrogenase (LDH) levels. See the legend of Figure 4.2 for explanation of abbreviations. Note the similar distributions of the LDH levels for all categories of exudative pleural effusions. (From Light RW, MacGregor MI, Luchsinger PC, Ball WC: Pleural effusions: the diagnostic separation of transudates and exudates. Ann Intern Med 1972;77:507–513.)

various exudative pleural effusions, one might suppose that LDH isoenzymes would be useful in the differentiation. Two studies have shown that LDH isoenzymes have limited value in the differential diagnosis of exudative pleural effusions, however (21, 83). All benign effusions with elevated pleural fluid LDH levels and most malignant effusions are characterized by a higher percentage of LDH-4 and LDH-5 in the pleural fluid than in the corresponding serum (21). The increased amounts of LDH-4 and LDH-5 are thought to arise from the inflammatory white blood cells in the pleural effusion (21). Approximately one-third of malignant pleural effusions have a different pleural fluid LDH isoenzyme pattern, which is characterized by large amounts (more than 35%) of LDH-2 and less LDH-4 and LDH-5. None of 31 benign exudates in 1 series had more than 35% LDH-2 (21). No relationship exists between the histologic type of the malignant pleural disease and the pleural fluid LDH-isoenzyme pattern (22). At present, the only situation in which we obtain LDH isoenzyme analysis of pleural fluid is when there is a bloody pleural effusion in a patient who clinically is thought to have a transudative pleural effusion. If the LDH is in the exudative range and the protein is in the transudative range, the demonstration that the majority of the pleural LDH is LDH-1 indicates that the increase in the LDH is due to the blood.

pH and Pco₂ Measurement

Measurement of the pleural fluid pH and P_{CO_2} is useful in the differential diagnosis of exudative pleural effusions. If the pleural fluid pH is less than 7.20, it means that the patient has 1 of 10 conditions: (*a*) complicated parapneumonic effusion, (*b*) esophageal rupture, (*c*) rheumatoid pleuritis, (*d*) tuberculous pleuritis, (*e*) malignant pleural disease, (*f*) hemothorax, (*g*) systemic acidosis, (*h*) paragonimiasis, (*i*) lupus pleuritis, or (*j*) urinothorax.

The pleural fluid pH is obviously influenced by the arterial pH. With transudative pleural effusions, the pleural fluid pH is usually higher than the simultaneous blood pH (24), presumably because of active transport of bicarbonate from the blood into the pleural space (25). If a low pleural fluid pH is discovered, the arterial pH should be checked to ensure that the patient does not have systemic acidosis. With certain exudative effusions, the pleural fluid pH falls substantially below that of the arterial pH. The explanation for the relative pleural fluid acidosis is as follows. The relationship between the pleural fluid pH and the blood pH depends upon the extent to which the blood and pleural fluid P_{CO_2} and bicarbonate are in equilibrium. In conditions associated with pleural fluid acidosis, lactic acid accumulates in the pleural fluid (84, 85), presumably from anaerobic glycolysis in the pleural fluid or tissues. The hydrogen ions associated with the lactic acid combine with bicarbonate to form water and carbon dioxide. Accordingly, the pleural fluid P_{CO_2} increases and the pH decreases. Because the addition of 1 mEq fixed acid to 1 L pleural fluid results in an increase of 33 mm Hg in the P_{CO_2} but in a decrease of only 1 mEq in the bicarbonate concentration (86), pleural fluid acidosis is characterized by a P_{CO_2} that is increased proportionately more than the bicarbonate is reduced (24, 84).

The increased pleural fluid P_{CO_2} could result from either an increased production of CO_2 or a decreased diffusion of CO_2 from the pleural fluid to blood or a combination of these factors. It is my belief that limited diffusion of CO_2 out of the pleural space is the predominant mechanism. In Figure 4.4*A*, it can be seen that changes in the arterial P_{CO_2} of a patient with a malignant pleural effusion and mild pleural fluid acidosis were not associated with changes in the pleural fluid P_{CO_2}. Similarly, in a second patient, the administration of bicarbonate with an increase in the arterial pH from 7.40 to 7.59 did not change the pleural fluid pH or bicarbonate level (Fig. 4.4*B*). When pleural fluids are incubated at 37°C in vitro, no correlation exists between the rate of acid accumulation in vitro and the pleural fluid pH in vivo (86, 87), with the possible exception of patients with complicated parapneumonic effusions in whom the rate of acid accumulation is high (87).

When the pleural fluid pH is used as a diagnostic test, it must be measured with the same care as arterial pH. The fluid should be collected anaerobically in a heparinized syringe (see Chapter 23). It should be placed in ice for transfer to the laboratory because of spontaneous acid generation by the fluid. Pleural fluid maintained at 0°C has a constant pH for at least 12 hours (86). If frank pus is obtained at thoracentesis, one should not submit it for pH determination because the thick, purulent fluid may clog the blood gas machine, and laboratory personnel may hesitate to analyze subsequent pleural fluids.

In general, pleural fluids with a low pH also have low glucose and high LDH levels (84). If the laboratory reports a low pH with normal glucose and low LDH levels, the pH measurement is probably in error. In like manner, a low glucose level with a normal pH and a low LDH is probably a laboratory error. The only reason to measure the pleural fluid P_{CO_2} is to verify the pleural fluid pH because a low pleural fluid pH is almost always associated with a high P_{CO_2} (24, 84). The pleural fluid P_{CO_2} adds nothing diagnostically.

The pleural fluid pH is most useful in determining whether chest tubes should be inserted in parapneumonic effusions (see Chapter 9). If the pleural fluid pH is below 7.00, the patient invariably has a complicated parapneumonic effusion, and tube thoracostomy should be instituted. If the pleural fluid pH is above 7.20, the patient will probably not require chest tubes, whereas if the pleural fluid pH is between 7.00 and 7.20, the patient may or

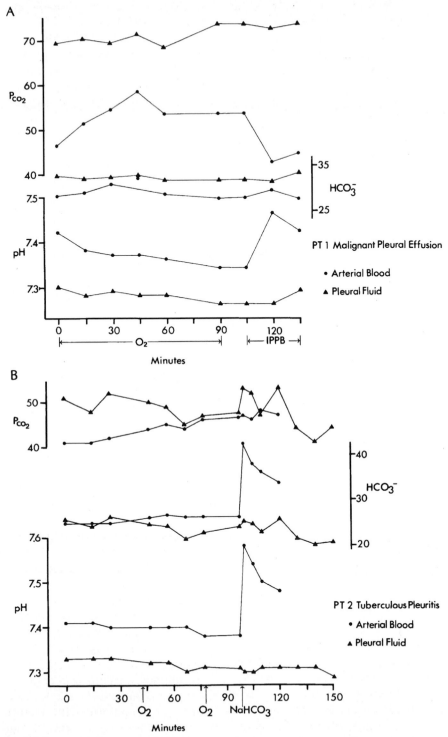

Figure 4.4. Relationship between pleural fluid and arterial pH, P_{CO_2} and HCO_3^-. **A.** Patient with a malignant pleural effusion in whom the administration of supplemental oxygen resulted in an increase in the Pa_{CO_2} from 46 to 58. Note that no concomitant change is seen in the pleural fluid P_{CO_2}. **B.** Patient with a slightly acidic pleural fluid. The administration of bicarbonate raised the arterial pH from 7.40 to 7.59, but had no influence on the pleural fluid pH.

may not require tube thoracostomy (74). If the patient has an infection with *Proteus* organisms, the pleural fluid pH may be elevated because these organisms produce ammonia by their urea-splitting ability, which can increase the pH (88). In patients with parapneumonic effusions, the pleural fluid pH may fall before the pleural fluid glucose level becomes depressed (74, 89).

The pleural fluid pH is also decreased with esophageal rupture (79, 90). In fact, Dye and Laforet (90) concluded that a pleural fluid pH of less than 6.0 was highly suggestive of esophageal rupture. These workers attributed the low pleural fluid pH to the reflux of gastric acid through the rent in the esophagus into the pleural space. Subsequent studies in rabbits (91), however, have demonstrated that the pleural fluid pH becomes just as acidic after esophageal rupture if the esophagogastric junction is ligated. It appears the low pleural fluid pH is due to infection in the pleural space rather than to acid reflux. Over the past few years, we have seen several patients with pleural infection without esophageal rupture in whom the pleural fluid pH was below 6.0. In summary, esophageal rupture is associated with a low pleural fluid pH because of the concomitant pleural infection and not acid reflux. A pleural fluid pH below 6.0 is not diagnostic of esophageal rupture.

Patients with pleural effusions secondary to both malignant disease and tuberculosis may have a low pleural fluid pH (24, 84, 92). When my colleagues and I wrote our first paper on pleural fluid pH (24), we concluded that the pleural fluid pH was useful in distinguishing tuberculous from malignant pleural effusions; a pleural fluid pH below 7.30 was suggestive of tuberculosis, whereas a pleural fluid pH above 7.40 was suggestive of malignant disease. Subsequent studies by others (85, 92, 93), however, and my own observations have not supported this conclusion. At present, I consider the pleural fluid pH valueless in distinguishing tuberculous from malignant pleural effusions. The pleural fluid pH does provide information about malignant pleural effusions since patients with a low pleural fluid pH have a shorter life expectancy and are less likely to have a favorable response to pleurodesis (93, 94).

The pleural fluid pH is almost always less than 7.20 with rheumatoid pleural effusions (72). The pleural fluid pH with lupus pleuritis is usually above 7.35 (72), but occasionally is less than 7.20 (73). The pleural fluid pH tends to be low with both paragonimiasis (41) and the Churg-Strauss syndrome (43) and these are the only two conditions where a low pleural fluid pH is associated with pleural eosinophilia. Another situation in which the pleural fluid pH may be decreased is with a large hemothorax (24). The metabolism of the many red blood cells in this condition, in conjunction with the atelectatic underlying lung, is the probable explanation for the decreased pH. Finally, the pleural fluid pH may be reduced with urinothorax (95). This is the only situation in which a transudative pleural fluid has a low pH without concomitant systemic acidosis.

TESTS FOR DIAGNOSING PLEURAL MALIGNANCY

Cytologic Examination of Pleural Fluid

Cytologic examination of pleural fluid is one of the most informative laboratory procedures in the diagnosis of pleural effusions because with it a definitive diagnosis can be made in over 50% of patients with malignant disease involving the pleura. Malignant cells have several characteristics that differentiate them from other cells in the pleural fluid (29). Malignant cells in a given pleural effusion are recognizably similar and are different from any nonmalignant cells in pleural fluid (Fig. 4.1C). With their similar characteristics, however, a marked variation in size and shape is seen, so that one cell may have many times the diameter of its twin.

Frequently, malignant cells are large. The nuclei of malignant cells may exceed 50 μm in diameter, in contrast with mesothelial cell nuclei, which rarely exceed 20 μm in diameter. Small lymphocytes, by comparison, have a diameter of about 10 μm. The nucleoli of malignant cells are often large, exceeding 5 μm in diameter, whereas the nucleoli of nonmalignant cells in pleural fluid usually do not exceed 3 μm. Malignant cells have a high nucleocytoplasmic ratio. Indeed the nuclear size of the cells in pleural effusions has been used diagnostically. Marchevsky and associates performed a computer-assisted morphometric study of 48 pleural fluids including 20 benign fluids, 8 mesotheliomas, and 20 carcinomas (96). If the mean nuclear diameter exceeded 10.5 μm or the mean nuclear diameter exceeded 9.3 μm and the mean nuclear diameter divided by the cytoplasmic diameter exceeded 0.74, the patient had a malignant pleural effusion. This morphologic analysis was not able to separate carcinomas from mesotheliomas.

There are, however, cytologic characteristics that tend to be different for mesothelioma and from adenocarcinomas. Stevens and coworkers (97) compared the cytologic characteristics of 44 cases of malignant mesothelioma and 46 cases of metastatic adenocarcinomas. They concluded that the following five features separate malignant mesothelioma from adenocarcinoma with better than 95% accuracy. Mesotheliomas tend to have true papillary aggregation, multinucleation with atypia and cell-to-cell apposition, while adenocarcinomas tend to have acinus-like structures and balloonlike vacuolation (97).

Malignant cells sometimes aggregate, and large balls or clumps of cells are characteristic of adenocarcinoma (Fig. 4.1D). Although aggregates of 20 or more benign mesothelial cells occasionally occur, the bizarre, large, vacuolated cells with adenocarcinoma allow for a differentiation between these entities. Small numbers of mitotic figures frequently occur in benign effusions, and accordingly, the presence of such figures is not indicative of malignant disease. Both malignant cells and macrophages may have vacuolation.

The accuracy of the cytologic diagnosis of malignant pleural effusions has been reported to be anywhere between 40 and 87% (98–100). Several factors influence the percentages in the various reports. First, in many patients with proven malignant disease and pleural effusion, the effusion is not related to malignant involvement of the pleura, but rather is secondary to other factors such as congestive heart failure, pulmonary emboli, pneumonia, lymphatic blockade, or hypoproteinemia. In such patients, one cannot expect the pleural fluid cytologic test result to be positive. For example, it is unusual for the results of pleural fluid cytologic tests to be positive in patients with squamous cell carcinoma (22, 29, 101), because the pleural effusions are usually due to bronchial obstruction or lymphatic blockade. Second, the frequency of positive cytologic results depends upon the tumor type. For example, with lymphoma, the cytologic examination was positive in 75% of patients with diffuse histiocytic lymphoma, but in only 25% of patients with Hodgkin's disease in one series (102). The cytologic test is more frequently positive with adenocarcinomas than with sarcomas (101). Third, the accuracy depends on the way in which the specimens are examined. If both cell blocks and smears are prepared and examined, the percentage of positive diagnoses will be greater than if only one method is used (103). Fourth, the more separate specimens submitted for cytologic examination, the higher the percentage of positive reports (22, 102). In my own experience in patients with proved malignant disease involving the pleural space, the initial pleural fluid cytologic examination is positive in about 60% of patients, and if 3 separate specimens are submitted, nearly 80% of the patients will have positive results (22). The third specimen frequently contains fresher cells that allow the diagnosis to be made. Fifth, the incidence of positive diagnoses is obviously dependent upon the skill of the cytologist.

In summary, when 3 separate pleural fluid specimens from a patient with malignant pleural disease are submitted to an experienced cytologist, one should expect a positive diagnosis in about 80% of patients. Because it is important to prevent the pleural fluid specimen from clotting, about 0.5 ml heparin should be added to the syringe during a diagnostic thoracentesis (see Chapter 23). If a larger volume of pleural fluid is obtained during a therapeutic thoracentesis for submission to a cytologist, additional heparin should be added. From the examination of the exfoliated cancer cells, it is usually possible to classify the neoplasm accurately into its histologic type such as adenocarcinoma. Only occasionally is it possible to suggest with confidence the primary site of the neoplasm (101).

Electron Microscopic Examination

Several reports have discussed the use of either transmission electron microscopy (104–106) or scanning electron microscopy (107) in the diagnosis of malignant pleural effusions. Electron microscopy has its greatest utility in differentiating metastatic adenocarcinoma from mesotheliomas. The ultrastructural features of mesotheliomas are so characteristic as to be almost diagnostic. These characteristics include the absence of microvillus core rootlets, glycocalyceal bodies, and secretory granules; the presence of intracellular desmosomes, junctional complexes, and intracytoplasmic lumina; and characteristic microvilli. The appearance of the microvilli is the most important diagnostic feature. With adenocarcinoma they are less abundant and are usually short and stubby, while with mesothelioma they are numerous and are characteristically long and thin (106, 107).

Despite much progress in the identification of malignant cells in pleural fluid and the distinction of adenocarcinomas from mesotheliomas, in many cases morphologic analysis does not provide a definitive answer. Over the past decade much research has been devoted toward the development of tests that would better make this distinction. The newer tests evaluated have included histochemical studies, immunohistochemical studies, studies of lectin binding, and flow cytometry.

Histochemical Studies

The two primary histochemical tests used to separate mesotheliomas from adenocarcinomas are the Alcian blue stain and the periodic acid-Schiff stain after diastase digestion (PAS-D). The Alcian blue stain detects the acid mucins characteristic of mesothelioma (108). In one study the Alcian blue stain was positive in 14 of 29 (47%) of mesotheliomas (108), but in none of 44 patients with adenocarcinoma. The PAS-D stain detects neutral mucins, which are diagnostic of adenocarcinomas. In one recent study the PAS-D stain was positive in 27

of 44 (61%) patients with adenocarcinoma, but in no patients with mesothelioma (108). In summary, if the cells stain positive with PAS-D, the patient in all probability has an adenocarcinoma. If the cells stain positive with Alcian blue, the patient in all probability has a mesothelioma. If the cells stain positive with neither, no conclusion can be made.

Immunohistochemical Studies

With the development of the necessary technology for monoclonal antibodies (MAb), numerous papers have been published in the past ten years that have assessed the diagnostic utility of MAb in the diagnosis of pleural malignancy. The basis for this approach is the thought that there are antigens that are unique for benign mesothelial cells, adenocarcinoma cells, and malignant mesothelioma cells. If monoclonal antibodies are developed against these specific antigens, then positive identification of these cells can be made when tissue samples or cytologic preparations are incubated with the antibody and then counterstained with immunoalkaline phosphatase or some similar method. The antibodies that have shown the most promise include the following: anti-carcinoembryonic antigen (CEA), B72.3, Leu-M1, BER-EP4, EMA, MFG, antikeratin, CA-125, vimentin, and thrombomodulin.

There have been several studies which have compared the usefulness of the different antibodies in distinguishing the three different cells (109–111). The antibodies that have done the best in the majority of the comparison studies are CEA, B72.3, Leu-M1, and EMA. Interestingly, all of these tend to be positive for adenocarcinoma and negative for malignant mesothelioma and benign mesothelial proliferation. Therefore, they are of limited use in the distinction of benign mesothelial cells from malignant mesothelial cells. Each of these is positive in 50–80% of adenocarcinomas and each is on rare occasions positive with mesotheliomas.

In view of the above, a panel of monoclonal antibodies should be assessed when immunohistochemistry is used to differentiate adenocarcinoma and mesothelioma. The utility of using such a panel was shown in a study by Brown and coworkers (111) who evaluated the usefulness of the monoclonal antibodies in a series of 103 adenocarcinomas and 34 mesotheliomas. They found that the three most useful antibodies were CEA, B72.3, and Leu-M1. If the specimen were positive for all three, the specificity for adenocarcinoma was 100% and the sensitivity was 70%. If the specimen were positive with 2 or 3 of the antibodies, the sensitivity increased to 97%, but there was one false positive. If the specimen were positive with only 1 of the three antibodies, then two of the patients had adenocarcinoma and two of the patients had mesothelioma. If the specimen were positive for none of the antigens, then the specificity for mesothelioma was 99% and the sensitivity was 91%. However, it must be emphasized that the benign mesothelial cells will also be negative for these antigens.

In summary, many articles have been devoted to the immunohistochemical differentiation of metastatic adenocarcinoma from mesothelioma from benign mesothelial cells. There are not good antibodies for positively identifying malignant mesothelioma or for distinguishing malignant mesothelioma from benign mesothelial proliferation. Nevertheless, immunohistochemical tests using a panel of antibodies are very useful in making the diagnosis of adenocarcinoma. Moreover, if it is known that the patient has a malignancy, the demonstration of positive immunohistochemistry with two of the following three antibodies, CEA, B72.3 and Leu-M1, virtually establishes the diagnosis of adenocarcinoma. If none of the three tests is positive, the patient in all probability has mesothelioma.

The are some additional points that need to be made about the immunohistochemical tests. For some of the antibodies, the pattern of the staining is very important. It is therefore very important to have an experienced immunohistochemist performing the tests. There are new antibodies being evaluated continuously and hopefully within the near future, antibodies will be developed that are specific for malignant mesothelioma and benign mesothelial cells. Up until this time, the immunohisto-

chemical tests are not useful in identifying the origin of the tumor.

It appears that immunohistochemistry is quite useful in establishing the diagnosis of a lymphomatous pleural effusion. Guzman and coworkers performed immunocytochemical analysis with the peroxidase-antiperoxidase adhesive slide assay for detection of cell surface antigens using a broad panel of monoclonal antibodies in nine patients with pleural lymphoma (112). They were able to clearly recognize 6 cases of B cell lymphoma, one case of Hodgkin's disease, and one case of hairy cell leukemia (112).

A role for immunohistochemical tests in establishing the diagnosis of squamous cell carcinoma or small cell carcinoma involving the pleura remains to be demonstrated.

Immunohistochemical tests on cell blocks of pleural fluid are available from Smith Kline Beecham Clinical Laboratories (Philadelphia, PA) at a cost of $75 per antibody.

Cancer-Associated Antigens

Another approach to the diagnosis of malignant pleural diseases has been to measure the pleural fluid levels of the cancer-associated antigens CA 15-3 (113) and carbohydrate antigen 19-9 (CA 19-9) (114) using monoclonal antibodies. CA 15-3 is composed of two different antigenic determinants recognized by murine monoclonal antibodies (115D8 and DF3). CA 19-9 has been described as an antigen detected by a monoclonal antibody specific for cells of human carcinoma of the colon. When the levels of these two antigens are compared in tuberculous and malignant pleural effusions, the overlap between the two groups is substantial and accordingly these measurements do not appear to be useful diagnostically (113, 114). In like manner the measurement of tumor-associated trypsin inhibitor in the pleural fluid is not useful diagnostically (115).

Enolase is a glycolytic enzyme that is found in extracts of neuroendocrine tumors including small cell lung carcinoma. Pleural effusions due to small cell lung carcinoma tend to have higher levels of enolase than do effusions due to non small cell lung carcinoma or tuberculosis, but again the overlap is such that the measurement of the enolase levels do not appear to be useful in the differential diagnosis of pleural disease (116).

Oncogenes

The development of cancer is a multistep process in which multiple genetic alterations must occur. The transforming genes are collectively called oncogenes. The oncogenes may be related to viruses, environmental carcinogens, or spontaneous mutations. Since the oncogenes are associated with the development of malignancy, one might hypothesize that patients with pleural malignancy would have cells in their pleural fluid containing oncogenes. There have been at least two different studies testing this hypothesis. Tawfik and Coleman (117) reported that benign and malignant effusions did not differ significantly in their expression of the c-myc oncogene. Athanassiadou and coworkers (118) reported that although 21 of 24 malignant effusions (87%) were positive for the c-Ha-ras oncogene, the diagnostic usefulness of the test was limited since 6 of 16 benign effusions (37%) also tested positive.

Carcinoembryonic Antigen (CEA)

Several papers have concluded that measurement of the CEA levels in pleural fluid is useful in establishing the diagnosis of malignant pleural effusions (114, 119–122). Rittgers and associates reported that 34% of 70 malignant pleural effusions had CEA levels above 12 ng/ml (119), whereas only 1% of 101 benign effusions had CEA levels this high. Vladutiu and coworkers reported that 39% of 37 patients with malignant pleural effusion had CEA levels above 10 ng/ml (120), while only 1 of 21 patients with benign disease exceeded this level. Tamura and colleagues (122) reported that 33 of 66 (50%) patients with a malignant pleural effusion had a pleural fluid CEA level above 10 ng/ml, whereas none of 39 patients with benign disease had pleural fluid CEA levels above this value. Pleural fluid CEA levels above 10 are not diagnostic of malignant pleural effusion. McKenna and associates (121) reported 1 patient with tuberculous pleuritis with a pleural fluid CEA level of 53 ng/ml. In

another report (123) pleural fluid CEA levels exceeded 15 ng/ml in 4 of 9 benign exudates, including one value of 245 ng/ml. In view of the foregoing, it appears that a pleural fluid CEA level above 10 ng/ml is highly suggestive, but not diagnostic, of a malignant pleural effusion. When the CEA levels are elevated, cytology of the pleural fluid is usually positive. In one study of patients with malignancy and a pleural effusion with negative cytology, the CEA exceeded 20 ng/ml in only 5 of 26 (19%) (1). At the present time, routine pleural fluid CEA determinations are not indicated. Cytology, immunohistochemical staining, and pleural biopsy provide a more definite answer.

Hyaluronic Acid

Pleural fluid from patients with mesotheliomas is sometimes abnormally viscid. The increased viscosity in such fluids is due to the presence of increased amounts of hyaluronate, which was previously called hyaluronic acid. Rasmussen and Faber examined the diagnostic usefulness of pleural fluid hyaluronic acid levels in 202 exudates including 19 malignant mesotheliomas (27). These investigators found that 7 of 19 pleural fluids (37%) from patients with malignant mesotheliomas had hyaluronate concentrations above 1 mg/ml, whereas none of the other pleural fluids had hyaluronate levels above 0.8 mg/ml. More recently, Nurminen and coworkers (124) assayed the levels of hyaluronate in 1039 pleural effusions including 50 from patients with mesothelioma. They reported that when a cutoff level of 75 mg/L was used, the assay specificity for malignant mesothelioma was 100% and the sensitivity was 56%. Two more recent papers (125, 126) have reported that the mean levels of hyaluronate are comparable in patients with mesothelioma and metastatic adenocarcinoma. The explanation for the discrepant results appears to be methodologic (127). The measurements of Nurminen were obtained with high pressure liquid chromatography (HPLC) while those of the other two groups were by radioimmunoassay. Unfortunately, the only commercially available measurement in the United States of which I am aware is a radioimmunoassay (Specialty Laboratories, San Diego, CA, Smith Kline Beecham Clinical Laboratories, Philadelphia, PA). Until the results with this assay are verified, it cannot be recommended on a routine basis.

Lectin Binding

Lectins are a class of glycoproteins of non-immune origin that bind specifically to carbohydrate groups found ubiquitously in various biologic products. Kawai and coworkers investigated lectin binding in 23 pleural mesotheliomas, 6 effusions with reactive mesothelial cells, and 28 well-differentiated pulmonary adenocarcinomas (128). In this study some of the lectins were much more likely to bind to adenocarcinomas than to reactive mesothelial cells or mesothelioma cells. These workers could not find significant differences in lectin binding between mesotheliomas and reactive mesothelial cells. Additional research in this area may well demonstrate that studies of lectin binding are useful diagnostically. At the present time, such studies should be considered experimental.

Flow Cytometry

Flow cytometry provides a method for the rapid quantitative measurement of nuclear DNA. It has been proposed as a suitable tool for differentiating between benign and malignant cells as most malignant tumor cells possess an abnormal number of chromosomes (aneuploidy), and consequently an abnormal DNA content (DNA aneuploidy) (129). However, a substantial percentage of metastatic adenocarcinomas and most malignant mesotheliomas are diploid via flow cytometry (130, 131). Accordingly, the routine use of flow cytometry to quantitate nuclear DNA levels for the differentiation of benign and malignant effusions cannot be recommended.

Flow cytometry can also be used to rapidly and specifically define the surface markers of lymphocytes (132) using immunocytometry. Accordingly, the cell lineage (T or B cells) and the clonality of a population of lymphocytes can be determined. These techniques can therefore be used to establish the diagnosis of pleural lymphomas and are recommended in lymphocytic pleural effusions on which the diagnosis of lymphoma is a consideration (132).

Chromosomal Analysis

Abnormalities undoubtedly exist in the chromosome number and structure in some patients with malignant pleural effusions (133, 134). Malignant cells have more chromosomes and marker chromosomes, which are chromosomes with structural abnormalities (translocation, deletion, acentric, dicentric, inversion, isochromosome, or ring) (133). It remains to be demonstrated that there is a place for chromosomal analysis in the routine examination of pleural fluid.

TESTS FOR DIAGNOSING PLEURAL TUBERCULOSIS

Adenosine Deaminase (ADA) Measurement

Measurement of the adenosine deaminase (ADA) level in pleural fluid is diagnostically useful because ADA levels tend to be higher in tuberculous pleural effusions than in other exudates (114, 135–138). ADA is the enzyme that catalyzes the conversion of adenosine to inosine. In one of the early reports the ADA levels were evaluated in the pleural fluid of 221 patients. The pleural fluid ADA level exceeded 70 U/L in 33 of 46 (72%) of patients with tuberculous pleuritis. In contrast, none of 173 pleural fluids from patients with other diagnoses had levels this high. Moreover, all 48 pleural fluids from patients with TB had ADA levels above 45 U/L while only 5 of the 173 (3%) other pleural fluids had ADA levels above 45 U/L (136). Fontan Bueso and colleagues reported similar results in a group of 138 pleural effusions including 61 due to TB and 42 due to malignancy (137).

More recently Valdés and associates (138) reported their results on 405 pleural fluids, including 91 due to tuberculosis, 110 due to malignancy, 58 due to pneumonia, 10 due to empyema, 88 transudates and 48 miscellaneous. Their results are very similar to those of previous workers with the exception that empyemas also had very high ADA levels (Fig. 4.5). Measurement of the ratio of the pleural fluid to the serum ADA is much less useful diagnostically (138).

From the foregoing three series (136–138), it appears that a pleural fluid ADA level above

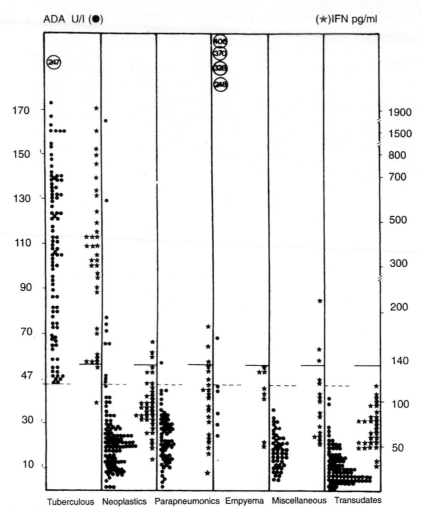

Figure 4.5. Pleural fluid ADA and interferon gamma levels in 430 cases. (From Valdes L, San Jose E, Alvarez D, Sarandeses A, Pose A, Chomon B, Alvarez-Dobano JM, Salgueiro M, Rodriguez Suarez JR: Diagnosis of tuberculous pleurisy using the biologic parameters adenosine deaminase, lysozyme, and interferon gamma. Chest 1993;103:458–465.)

70 U/L is highly suggestive of tuberculous pleuritis, while a pleural fluid ADA level below 40 U/L virtually rules out this diagnosis. Some caution must be used in relying on ADA levels exclusively to establish the diagnosis of tuberculous pleuritis. If the patient is immunocompromised and has tuberculous pleuritis, the pleural fluid ADA level may be below 40 U/L (139). Patients with rheumatoid pleuritis frequently have ADA levels that exceed 70 U/L as do patients with empyema (138, 140). High pleural fluid ADA levels have also been reported with a very small percent of other neoplasms (141). It appears that separation of the molecular forms of ADA by polyacrylamide

gel electrophoresis may be diagnostically useful. Ungerer and Grobler performed this analysis on pleural fluid from 30 patients with tuberculosis and 10 other exudates with high (greater than 60 U/L) pleural fluid ADA levels (141). They identified two ADA forms, a small form and a large form. Without exception, the tuberculous effusions had only the large form. All the other effusions contained both forms with the small form being predominant.

Essentially all the reports from Europe and South Africa have been very positive in finding that the pleural fluid ADA level is useful diagnostically. Interestingly, reports from Asia have been much less positive (114, 122, 142) with much lower mean levels of ADA being reported from Asia. It is unclear whether the differences in the results are due to ethnic differences or methodologic differences.

In view of the foregoing, it is recommended that facilities in which a sizable percentage of the cases of pleural effusions are due to tuberculosis develop the faculty to perform ADA assays on pleural fluid. An ADA level above 70 U/L in a patient who does not have an empyema or rheumatoid arthritis is essentially diagnostic of tuberculous pleuritis. Unfortunately, to my knowledge, there is no place in the United States where ADA levels can be obtained commercially.

Gamma Interferon

There have been several reports in the past few years that have demonstrated that pleural fluids from patients with tuberculous pleuritis tend to have higher levels of gamma interferon than do other types of exudates (113, 142–145). Pleural fluid gamma interferon levels from the 145 patients reported by Valdés and associates are shown in Figure 4.5. As can be seen from this figure, 26 of 35 patients (74%) with tuberculous pleurisy had gamma interferon levels above 200 pg/ml, while only 1 effusion of 110 other effusions that were not empyemas had gamma interferon levels that exceeded this.

Gamma interferon is produced by the $CD4^+$ lymphocytes from patients with tuberculous pleuritis (144). The production of gamma interferon appears to be a useful defense mechanism. Interferon gamma enhances poly myristate acetate (PMA)-induced hydrogen peroxide production in macrophages, facilitating elimination of intracellular parasites. This lymphokine also inhibits mycobacterial growth in human monocytes (144).

In view of the above, it appears that measurement of the gamma interferon level is very useful in the diagnosis of tuberculous pleuritis. One must be careful in interpreting the results from a given laboratory, however, because different laboratories report their results in different units. Unfortunately, as with ADA, there is no commercial laboratory in the United States that measures gamma interferon levels in pleural fluid.

Lysozyme Measurement

The level of lysozyme in the pleural fluid tends to be higher in the pleural fluid from patients with tuberculous pleuritis than in other types of exudates (137, 138, 146, 147). Lysozyme is a bacteriolytic protein with low molecular weight distributed extensively in organic fluids. In general the lysozyme levels in tuberculous pleural effusions are greater than those in malignant pleural effusions, but there is so much overlap that the pleural fluid levels themselves are not particularly useful diagnostically. There was one report that suggested that the ratio of the pleural fluid to the serum lysozyme level was useful in separating the two diseases (147). Verea Hernando and colleagues (147) reported results for 54 patients with tuberculous pleural effusions and 35 patients with malignant pleural effusions. All the patients with tuberculosis had a ratio above 1:2, whereas only 1 of the 35 patients (3%) with malignant pleural effusions had ratios above 1:2. A recent study by Valdés and associates (138) did not duplicate these good results; nearly one-third of the patients with tuberculous pleuritis had a lysozyme ratio less than 1:1 and many other exudates had ratios that exceeded this value. In this latter paper both the gamma interferon and the ADA were superior to the lysozyme ratio in differentiating tuberculous from nontuberculous exudates (138). At the present time the routine measurement of pleural fluid lysozyme to help in establishing the diagnosis of pleural tuberculosis cannot be recommended.

Tuberculous Antigens and Their Antibodies

In recent years the possibility of establishing the diagnosis of tuberculous pleuritis by the demonstration of tuberculous antigens or specific antibodies against tuberculous proteins in the pleural fluid has been investigated. Two reports have evaluated the diagnostic utility of measuring the levels of different tuberculous antigens in the pleural fluid (148, 149). Although the mean levels of tuberculous antigens were higher in the pleural fluid of patients with tuberculous pleuritis than in the pleural fluid of other patients, there was so much overlap, that the test was of little diagnostic use. In a similar vein there have been at least six separate reports (150–155), which have indicated that patients with tuberculous pleural effusions tend to have higher levels of specific antituberculous antibodies in their pleural fluid than do patients with other types of exudative effusions. The source of the antibodies, however, is apparently the serum rather than local antibody production in the pleural space (152). Accordingly it is unlikely that measurement of the antituberculous antibodies in the pleural fluid will add anything diagnostically to measurement of the antituberculous antibodies in the serum (152).

IMMUNOLOGIC STUDIES

Because nearly 5% of patients with rheumatoid arthritis (RA) (156) and 50% of patients with systemic lupus erythematosus (SLE) (157) have pleural effusions sometime during the course of their disease, and because such effusions may be manifest before the underlying disease is obvious (72, 156), it is important to consider these diagnostic possibilities in patients with exudative pleural effusions of undetermined origin. Numerous papers have assessed the diagnostic utility of various immunologic measurements of the pleural fluid in establishing these diagnoses.

Rheumatoid Factor (RF)

Berger and Seckler (158) first reported that RF was elevated in the pleural fluid of patients with rheumatoid pleuritis. Subsequently, Levine and coworkers (159) studied pleural fluid RF levels in 65 patients with pleural effusions and found that 41% of patients with bacterial pneumonia and 20% of patients with carcinoma had pleural fluid RF titers equal to or greater than 1:160. In 7 of the 65 fluids, the pleural fluid RF titers were greater than the serum titers, but the pleural fluid titer was greater than 1:640 in only 1 of the patients. These workers concluded that the RF titers in pleural fluid were not useful diagnostically. Halla and coworkers (72), however, found that the pleural fluid RF was elevated in 11 of 11 seropositive patients with rheumatoid pleural effusions. In each patient, the pleural fluid RF titer was equal to or greater than 1:320 and was equal to or greater than that in the serum.

In view of the last-mentioned study, I recommend that RF titers be determined in pleural fluid when the diagnosis of rheumatoid pleuritis is considered. The demonstration of a pleural fluid RF titer equal to or greater than 1:320 and equal to or greater than the serum titer is strong evidence that the patient has a rheumatoid pleural effusion.

Antinuclear Antibodies

Measurement of the antinuclear antibody (ANA) levels in pleural fluid appears to be the best test for establishing the diagnosis of lupus pleuritis. In one study the serum and pleural fluid ANA levels were measured in 13 patients with lupus pleuritis (73). In 11 of 13 patients the pleural fluid ANA titer was equal to or greater than 1:160 and in 9 of 13 patients the pleural fluid to serum ANA ratio was equal to or greater than 1.0. In contrast, the pleural fluid to serum ANA ratio was less than 1.0 in 4 patients who had SLE, but pleural effusions due to other etiologies. The pleural fluid ANA titers were negative in 67 patients with pleural effusions of other etiologies (73). An earlier report measured ANA levels in 100 consecutive pleural fluids and found ANA only in the pleural fluid of patients with lupus pleuritis (160). Patients who are suspected of having systemic lupus erythematosus should have the ANA levels in their pleural fluid measured.

LE Cells

The demonstration of LE cells in a pleural effusion was thought to be diagnostic of lupus pleuritis (73). LE cells are formed when polymorphonuclear leukocytes ingest extracellular nuclear material, to form a polymorphonuclear leukocyte with a large inclusion of nuclear material. Most pleural effusions secondary to SLE contain LE cells (73). With the development of better immunologic tests for SLE, LE preparations are being done less and less frequently. Testing of the pleural fluid for LE cells is not recommended unless the laboratory is proficient in this test.

RA Cells

Granular white cells containing cytoplasmic inclusions can be found in the synovial fluid of many patients with rheumatoid arthritis. These cells are called RA cells only when liberation of RF from the cell can be demonstrated. RA cells have been demonstrated in the pleural fluid of patients with rheumatoid pleuritis (161). Because many pleural fluids contain many white blood cells with cytoplasmic inclusions, because the demonstration of the liberation of RF is time-consuming, and because the diagnosis of rheumatoid pleuritis can usually be established by other means, I do not recommend searching for RA cells in pleural fluid.

Complement Levels

Most patients with pleural effusions secondary to either SLE or RA have reduced pleural fluid complement (Fig. 4.6), whether whole complement (CH_{50}) (162, 163), C3 (72, 164), or C4 (72, 162) is measured. The measurement of pleural fluid complement does not absolutely separate patients with SLE or RA from patients with other exudative pleural effusions, as shown in Figure 4.6, regardless of whether CH_{50}, C3, or C4 is measured. Nevertheless, a CH_{50} level below 10 U/ml (162) or a

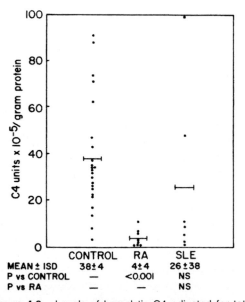

C4 level below 10×10^{-5} U/g protein (72) is seen with most patients with either RA or SLE and rarely with other diseases. Since the ANA levels and the RF titers appear to be more specific and more sensitive at identifying individuals with pleural effusions due to RA or SLE, it is recommended that pleural fluid complement levels not be routinely obtained.

Immune Complexes

Patients with pleural effusions secondary to RA or SLE also have higher pleural fluid levels of immune complexes than patients with effusions due to other causes (72, 164, 165). The separation of pleural effusions secondary to SLE and RA from other exudative pleural effusions is less distinct when pleural fluid immune complex levels are used than when pleural fluid complement is used, because a substantial percentage of other exudative pleural effusions have elevated pleural fluid immune complex levels (72, 164). The presence of pleural fluid immune complexes also depends on the assay system (72). Patients with SLE have higher levels of immune complexes when the assay is performed with the C1q component of complement or the Raji cell assay than with monoclonal rheumatoid factor. With RA, the level of immune complexes in the pleural fluid is higher than that in the simultaneous serum, whereas in other disease states, the serum level of immune complexes is higher (72). Because measurement of the immune complex level appears to add no information to that obtained from measuring complement levels, it is recommended that pleural fluid immune complex determinations be performed only in research situations.

LIPID STUDIES

Pleural fluid is occasionally milky or opalescent. This opalescence is sometimes mistakenly attributed to myriad white blood cells in the pleural fluid, and the patient is treated for an empyema. This mistake is not made if the supernatant of the centrifuged pleural fluid is examined. In empyema, the supernatant is clear, whereas in a chylous or chyliform effusion, the supernatant remains cloudy or milky. Some pleural fluids with high lipid content also contain numerous red blood cells, and their color is accordingly red or brown. The

Figure 4.6. Levels of hemolytic C4 adjusted for total protein in control, rheumatoid arthritis (RA), and systemic lupus erythematosus (SLE) pleural fluids. Note that the pleural fluid from the patients with RA and SLE has lower levels of hemolytic C4. (From Halla JT, Schrohenloher RE, Volanakis JE: Immune complexes and other laboratory features of pleural effusions. Ann Intern Med 1980;92:748–752.)

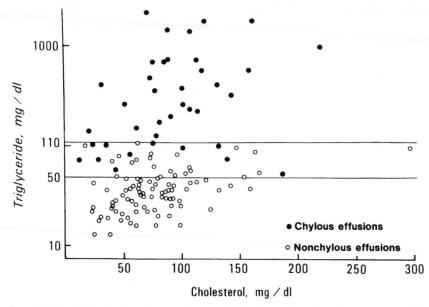

Figure 4.7. Scattergram of cholesterol and triglyceride values in pleural fluid. *Solid dots* represent patients whose effusions contained chylomicrons and were considered chylous. *Open circles* represent patients without chylomicrons whose effusions were considered nonchylous. All patients with triglyceride levels above 110 mg/dl had chylous effusions, whereas no patient with triglyceride levels below 50 mg/dl had a chylous effusion. (From Staats BA, Ellefson RD, Budahn LL, et al: The lipoprotein profile of chylous and nonchylous pleural effusions. Mayo Clin Proc 1980;55:700–704.)

supernatants of all pleural fluids should be examined for turbidity. Lipid studies of the pleural fluid should be ordered when turbidity persists in the supernatant.

The persistent cloudiness of these pleural fluids after centrifugation is due to their high lipid content, which can result from one of two mechanisms. First, the lymphatic duct may be disrupted so that chyle accumulates in the pleural space. The patient is then said to have a chylothorax, and the pleural effusion is called a chylous pleural effusion. Second, large amounts of cholesterol or lecithin-globulin complexes can accumulate for unknown reasons in the pleural fluid. The patient is then said to have a pseudochylothorax and a chyliform pleural effusion. Although some authors have separated pseudochylothoraces into chyliform pleural effusions, characterized by high lecithin-globulin levels, and pseudochylous effusions, characterized by the presence of cholesterol crystals (166, 167), I see no advantage to making this differentiation. It is important to distinguish chylous pleural effusions from chyliform pleural effusions because only the first indicates disruption of the thoracic duct.

The diagnosis of chylothorax is best made by measuring the triglyceride levels in the pleural fluid. If the pleural fluid triglyceride level exceeds 110 mg/dl, the patient probably has a chylothorax; if the triglyceride level is below 50 mg/dl, the patient does not have a chylothorax (Fig. 4.7). If the triglyceride level is between 50 and 110 mg/dl, the patient may or may not have a chylothorax (168). When the diagnosis is uncertain, lipoprotein analysis of the fluid should be ordered. The demonstration of chylomicrons in the pleural fluid with lipoprotein analysis is diagnostic of chylothorax (168, 169). Most patients with chylothoraces and pleural fluid triglyceride levels below 110 mg/ml are malnourished. Patients with chyliform pleural effusions often have pleural fluid triglyceride levels above 250 mg/dl (170), but their clinical picture of a long-standing pleural effusion with thickened pleura is easily differentiated from that of an acute pleural effusion with normal pleural surfaces, as seen with a chylous effusion. If any doubt exists, lipoprotein analysis of the pleural fluid should be performed.

Other studies useful for diagnosing turbid pleural fluids are the total lipid content, the cholesterol content, and microscopic examination of the sediment. Most pleural effusions that are cloudy on account of high lipid levels have a total fat content greater than 400 mg/dl (171). The cholesterol levels in the pleural fluid are elevated in high-lipid pleural effusions due to high numbers of cholesterol crystals or lecithin-globulin complexes (167), but cholesterol levels may also be elevated in chylous pleural effusions (168), as demonstrated in Figure 4.7. When the turbidity is due to high numbers of cholesterol crystals, examination of the pleural fluid sediment reveals the cholesterol crystals, which are large, rhombic or polyhedric crystals, as illustrated in Figure 21.1.

MICROBIOLOGIC STUDIES ON PLEURAL FLUID

Cultures

Pleural fluid from patients with undiagnosed exudative pleural effusions should be cultured for bacteria (both aerobically and anaerobically), mycobacteria, and fungi. For aerobic and anaerobic bacterial cultures, we prefer to inoculate blood culture media right at the bedside. For mycobacterial cultures, use of a BACTEC system with bedside inoculation provides higher yields and faster results than do conventional methods. In one study, the median time for the BACTEC cultures to become positive was 18 days (range 3–40) while the median time for conventional cultures was 33.5 days (range 21–48) (172). A Gram stain of the fluid should also be obtained. Routine smears for mycobacteria are not indicated because they are almost always negative, unless the patient has a tuberculous empyema.

Countercurrent Immunoelectrophoresis (CIE)

The goal with CIE is to identify bacterial antigens in pleural fluid and thus to establish a presumptive bacteriologic diagnosis in patients with parapneumonic pleural effusions. CIE depends upon the interaction of an antigen with a negative charge and a specific antibody with a positive charge in an electrical field to form a distinct precipitin line (173, 174). The advantage of CIE over bacterial cultures is that results are available within hours rather than days, so that appropriate antibiotics can be administered sooner. CIE is most useful in the diagnosis of pleural effusions in children, in whom most pleural effusions are due to bacterial infections with *Streptococcus pneumoniae*, *Staphylococcus aureus*, or *Haemophilus influenzae*. These are the 3 bacteria for which antigens are available to perform CIE studies. In a series of 87 pediatric patients with pleural effusions (173), pleural fluid cultures were positive for 1 of these 3 bacteria in 34 patients, and CIE correctly identified the offending organisms in 33 (97%). In about 25% of those patients, the Gram stain of the pleural fluid was negative. In an additional 23 patients, CIE identified antigens in the pleural fluid when the pleural fluid cultures were negative (173).

Another advantage of CIE is it remains positive for several days after antibiotic therapy is initiated (173, 174). To my knowledge, examination of pleural fluid with CIE has not been performed on a large series of adult patients with pleural effusion. The disadvantage of CIE in the adult patient with a complicated parapneumonic effusion is that many such effusions are due to anaerobic bacteria (74), and antigens for all the anaerobic organisms are not yet available for routine use. Certainly, if CIE is readily available, it should be performed on the pleural fluid from patients with an acute febrile illness and pleural effusion.

Direct Gas-Liquid Chromatography

Most anaerobic bacteria produce volatile fatty acids. Demonstration of such fatty acids by direct gas-liquid chromatography of the pleural fluid has been proposed as a means to establish the diagnosis of anaerobic pleural infections. In one report, pleural fluids from 52 patients including 14 with anaerobic infections were analyzed with direct gas-liquid chromatography (175). Multiple volatile fatty acids or succinic acid were present in 13 of the 14 (93%) of the fluids from patients with anaerobic infections. Succinic acid was the major product in 10 patients, and 9 of them had infections due to *Bacteroides*. In contrast, pleural fluid from other patients did not contain multiple volatile fatty acids or succinic acid (175). Direct gas-liquid chromatography is a difficult and expensive procedure, however, and it requires specially trained technicians. The resources required for gas-liquid chromatography are probably better spent in upgrading anaerobic culture techniques.

MISCELLANEOUS TESTS ON PLEURAL FLUID

Cytokines

Cytokines are soluble peptides secreted by cells that affect the behavior of either the same or other nearby cells through nonenzymatic means. Often they are glycopeptides, and typically they exert their effects at very low concentrations in the picomolar to nanomolar range. Within this broad heading are a number of subclasses, including polypeptide growth factors, interleukins, interferons, and colony stimulating factors.

In recent years, much research has been devoted toward understanding the role of these peptides. It is not surprising, therefore, that there have been numerous reports assessing the diagnostic utility of the levels of different cytokines in the pleural fluid. In general, with the exception of gamma interferon, the diagnostic usefulness of cytokine levels in pleural fluid remains to be demonstrated. Nevertheless, I have elected to include a brief discussion of the more commonly studied cytokines because their study has provided clues about the pathogenesis and resolution of pleural injury.

Interleukin-1 (IL-1)

IL-1 has an essential role in T-cell activation. The primary sources of IL-1 are blood monocytes and tissue macrophages. When the IL-1 levels were compared in 20 malignant pleural effusions and 20 tuberculous pleural effusions, the tuberculous pleural effusions were found to have significantly higher mean levels, but there was a lot of overlap between the two groups (145).

Interleukin-2 (IL-2)

IL-2 plays a crucial role in the mediation of the immune response. It induces and maintains the proliferation of T lymphocytes following mitogen or antigen activation and it also induces production of cytotoxic lymphocytes, natural killer cells, and lymphokine-activated killer cells. As with IL-1, the pleural fluid levels of IL-2 are higher with tuberculous pleuritis than with malignant pleural effusion, but there is much overlap (145). One of the first events with T-cell activation is the synthesis and surface expression of a receptor of IL-2 (IL-2R) along with the release of a shorter soluble form of IL-2R. The median levels of the soluble IL-2R are higher in tuberculous effusions than in malignant pleural effusions than in parapneumonic pleural effusions than in transudative pleural effusions, but again there is substantial overlap (176).

Interleukin-3 (IL-3)

IL-3 induces the proliferation of eosinophils in vitro and also prolongs their survival. In patients with eosinophilic pleural effusions, IL-3 appears to help promote the eosinophil proliferation and also prolongs the survival of eosinophils. It appears, however, that IL-3 is less important than IL-5 in promoting these two activities in patients with eosinophilic pleural effusions. Blocking antibodies to IL-5 neutralize more of these activities than do blocking antibodies to IL-3 (34). IL-3 is not detectable in eosinophilic pleural effusions (35).

Interleukin-5 (IL-5)

IL-5 also induces the proliferation of eosinophils in vitro and prolongs their survival. Pleural fluid IL-5 levels are elevated in patients with posttraumatic eosinophilic pleural effusions (35). The pleural fluid from such individuals acts as a stimulus for eosinophil colony formation and this stimulatory capability is largely blocked by specific antibodies toward IL-5. In like manner eosinophilic pleural fluid will enhance the survival of eosinophils and this capability is largely blocked by specific antibodies toward IL-5. It therefore appears that IL-5 is one of the primary factors responsible for eosinophilic pleural effusions (34, 35).

Interleukin-6 (IL-6)

IL-6 plays a pivotal role in inflammatory responses such as the induction of acute phase proteins and the synthesis of immunoglobulins. It has been shown (177) that the mean IL-6 levels are much higher in exudates than in transudates and that tuberculous effusions contain significantly higher levels of IL-6 than do malignant pleural effusions. Since the IL-6 levels are significantly higher in the pleural fluid than they are in the serum, IL-6 is probably produced in the pleural space (177).

Interleukin-8 (IL-8)

IL-8 is a powerful neutrophil chemotaxin that contributes to the influx of neutrophils into the pleural space (30, 31, 178). IL-8 levels are most elevated in the pleural fluid from patients with empyema (30, 31, 178). There is a significant correlation between the numbers of neutrophils in empyema fluid and the level of IL-8 in the fluid (30, 31). Neutrophil chemotactic activity is correlated with IL-8 activity and the majority of the neutrophil chemotactic activity in pleural fluid is neutralized with anti-IL-8 antibodies (30).

Monocyte Chemotactic Peptide

Monocyte chemotactic peptide-1 (MCP-1) is a cytokine that is chemotactic for monocytes. Antony and coworkers (31) have shown that the pleural fluid levels of MCP-1 are higher in patients with malignant pleural effusions and tuberculous pleural effusions than they are in patients with parapneumonic effusions or congestive heart failure. There is a correlation between the number of monocytes and the pleural fluid MCP-1 levels in patients with malignant pleural effusions. Specific neutralizing antibodies to MCP-1 eliminate approximately 70% of the monocyte chemotactic activity (31).

Fibrinogen and Fibrin Degradation Products (FDP)

The fibrinogen levels in pleural fluid are low in comparison to those in plasma (56, 179, 180). Glauser and colleagues were unable to detect fibrinogen in 15 of 23 effusions (179), including all 4 that were loculated, whereas Widstrom and coworkers were unable to detect fibrinogen in 18 of 20 pleural fluids (180). The results indicate that pleural fluid fibrinogen levels are not useful diagnostically and should not be measured. Although an early report suggested that elevated levels of FDP were indicative of a malignant pleural effusion (181), subsequent reports have revealed that the pleural fluid FDP levels are elevated with all exudative pleural effusions (180, 182), and they are therefore of no diagnostic use.

In certain conditions involving the pleura, e.g., parapneumonic effusions, loculations may develop in the pleural space. The loculations are due to fibrin membranes. One might hypothesize that the development of the loculations would depend upon the balance between the procoagulant and the fibrinolytic activity in the pleural space. Idell and coworkers (183) measured the procoagulant and fibrinolytic activity in 36 pleural fluids including 21 due to malignancy, 3 due to empyema, 8 due to congestive heart failure, and 4 due to pneumonia. They found that procoagulant activity was present in some of the exudates, but its presence did not necessarily correlate with loculation and its level did not serve to differentiate the different exudates. The transudates had no procoagulant active. Fibrinolytic activity was absent in all the exudates while 5 of the 8 transudates had fibrinolytic activity (183). In view of the above measurement of the procoagulant activity in pleural fluids does not appear to be useful either diagnostically or prognostically.

Other Proteins

Numerous studies have evaluated the diagnostic usefulness of measuring other proteins in the pleural fluid including mucoproteins (57), fibronectin (184), acid glycosaminoglycans (mucopolysaccharides) (185), β_2-microglobulins (120), and α-fetoprotein (120). The pleural fluid levels of these proteins are not useful in the differential diagnosis of exudative pleural effusions.

Other Enzyme Determinations

Many other enzymes, including aldolase (186), glutamic-oxaloacetic transaminase, glutamic-pyruvic transaminase (186), phosphohexose isomerase (186), malic dehydrogenase (186), isocitric dehydrogenase (186), glutathione reductase (186), alkaline phosphatase (187), angiotensin-converting enzyme (188), and transketolase, have been measured in the pleural fluid and have been found to give no useful diagnostic information. One report suggested that elevation of the acid phosphatase level in the pleural fluid was diagnostic of metastatic prostatic carcinoma (189), but a second report indicated that approximately 10% of all pleural effusions have acid phosphatase levels above the upper normal limit for serum and higher than in the corresponding serum (190).

INVASIVE SURGICAL PROCEDURES

Pleural Biopsy

Needle biopsy of the pleura (see Chapter 23) is useful in establishing the diagnosis of malignant or tuberculous pleural effusions. Therefore, if one of these diagnoses is suspected, this procedure should be undertaken. If the patient has a transudative effusion or if the effusion is known to be due to pneumonia, pulmonary embolus, pancreatitis, or collagen vascular disease, no reason exists to perform the pleural biopsy. In fact, a pleural biopsy is contraindicated if the patient has a complicated parapneumonic effusion because of the likely development of subcutaneous abscesses at the biopsy site (191).

With tuberculous pleuritis, the initial needle biopsy is positive for granulomas in 50 to 80% of patients (192–195). If the initial biopsy is nondiagnostic and the patient has tuberculous pleuritis, a second biopsy will be diagnostic 10 to 40% of the time (191, 195, 196). The demonstration of granulomas on the pleural biopsy is virtually diagnostic of tuberculous pleuritis; caseous necrosis or acid-fast bacilli need not be demonstrated. On rare occasions, however, fungus diseases, sarcoidosis, and rheumatoid pleuritis can produce granulomatous pleuritis (197) and these possibilities should be kept in mind when granulomatous pleuritis is discovered. When tuberculous pleuritis is suspected, it is useful to culture a portion of the pleural biopsy specimen for mycobacteria. In a series of 21 patients with tuberculous pleuritis (193), cultures of 16 of 21 pleural biopsy specimens (76%) were positive for tuberculosis, and 5 of the specimens did not reveal granulomas on microscopic examination. In this particular series of 21 patients, the first pleural biopsy was diagnostic for tuberculosis in 20 of 21 (95%) of the patients by microscopic examination or by culture.

Needle biopsy of the pleura is also useful in establishing the diagnosis of malignant pleural effusion. The incidence of positive pleural biopsies ranges from 39 to 75% (100, 191, 192, 195, 196, 198, 199). In general, cytologic examination of the pleural fluid establishes the diagnosis more frequently than pleural biopsy, but because a pleural biopsy is sometimes positive when the cytologic test is negative or inconclusive (198, 199), both procedures are recommended when a malignant pleural effusion is suspected and the initial cytology is negative.

When no pleural fluid is present but the pleura is thickened, needle biopsy of the pleura can still be used to establish the diagnosis of tuberculosis or malignant disease. Levine and Cugell, who performed needle biopsies of the pleura in 45 patients who had pleural thickening without any free pleural fluid, were able to establish the diagnosis of malignant disease in 13 and tuberculosis in 3 of these patients, to give an overall diagnostic yield of 36% (196).

Thoracoscopy

Thoracoscopy (see Chapter 25), also called pleuroscopy, is useful diagnostically in patients in whom the origin of a pleural effusion remains unclear after routine fluid analysis and needle biopsy of the pleura. With the advent of video-assisted thoracic surgery (VATS), there has been renewed interest in the use of thoracoscopy for the diagnosis of pleural disease. The visibility of the entire thoracic cavity obtained with VATS compares favorably with that obtained by direct view through a limited axillary, inframammary, or lateral thoracotomy (200). For VATS general anesthesia is recommended (200).

Thoracoscopy is an excellent means by which malignant disease of the pleural can be established. Recently two separate studies, each with 102 patients, were published that reported diagnostic yields of 93% (201) and 80% (202). However, when these two studies are examined in detail, one finds that the only diagnosis that was definitely established is malignancy. When the above two studies are combined, the diagnosis of malignancy was established in 99 of 117 patients (85%), with malignancy including 51 of 56 (91%) with mesothelioma.

Where is the rightful place of pleuroscopy in the management of the patient with an undiagnosed pleural effusion? Pleuroscopic examination is best at diagnosing malignant pleural effusions, but what is the hurry to establish this diagnosis? No definitive treatment exists for most malignant pleural effusions, and this diagnosis can usually be established by pleural fluid cytologic study, immunohistochemical tests, or pleural biopsy. Thoracoscopy is recommended for the patient with an undiagnosed pleural effusion in whom the diagnosis of malignancy is strongly suspected, and in whom at least two pleural fluid cytologies and one needle biopsy of the pleura have been negative. When one does thoracoscopy for diagnostic purposes, it is important to be prepared to perform a procedure to create a pleurodesis at the time of surgery. Our preferred method is the insufflation of 2 to 5 grams of talc. Thoracoscopy is also excellent for managing patients with complex pneumothoraces (see Chapter 19) and for breaking down loculations in patients with complicated parapneumonic effusions (see Chapter 9).

Bronchoscopy

In patients with pleural effusions and other abnormalities on their chest radiographs such as infiltrates, masses, or atelectasis, bronchoscopic examination is useful in establishing the cause of the parenchymal disease and, accordingly, of the pleural effusion. Chang and Perng (203) performed fiberoptic bronchoscopy in 59 patients who had concurrent pulmonary lesions and were able to establish a diagnosis in 43 (73%). If no parenchymal lesion is apparent on the routine chest radiographs, CT scan of the chest should be obtained. If there is a parenchymal lesion, bronchoscopy should then be performed with special attention directed toward the abnormal area.

Bronchoscopy should also be performed if the patient has hemoptysis. In the series of Chang and Perng (203), bronchoscopy yielded a diagnosis in 47 of 58 patients (81%) with hemoptysis and pleural effusion. If the patient has neither a parenchymal abnormality nor hemoptysis, but has a pleural effusion occupying more than three-fourths of the hemithorax, there is substantial yield from bronchoscopy. Bronchoscopy established the diagnosis in 7 of 18 such patients in one series (204).

Bronchoscopy is probably not indicated for the patient with a pleural effusion and no parenchymal abnormality, hemoptysis, and less than a massive effusion. In one series, the bronchoscopy was diagnostic in only 1 of 48 (2%) such patients (204). Similarly bronchoscopy is rarely diagnostic in the patient with a cytologically positive pleural effusion and no parenchymal abnormality. In one series of 17 such patients (205), the bronchoscopy was diagnostic in only 2 (12%).

Open Pleural Biopsy

Open thoracotomy with direct biopsy of the pleura has been supplanted by video-assisted thoracoscopy in many institutions. The main indication for open pleural biopsy (or for thoracoscopy) is progressive undiagnosed pleural disease. If both procedures are available, thoracoscopy is usually preferred because it is associated with less morbidity.

It should be emphasized that open pleural biopsy does not always provide a diagnosis in a patient with an undiagnosed pleural effusion. Douglass and associates (206) reported that thoracotomy failed to provide a specific diagnosis for 7 of 21 patients with pleural effusion. The group at the Mayo Clinic reviewed their experience with open pleural biopsy for undiagnosed pleural effusion between 1962 and 1972 and reported that during this time period no diagnosis was established in 51 such patients (207). In 31 of the patients (61%) there was no recurrence of the pleural effusion, and no cause ever became apparent. However, 13 of the patients were eventually proven to have malignant disease (6 patients with lymphoma, 4 patients with mesothelioma, and 3 with other malignancy).

Lung Scans and Pulmonary Arteriograms

It is estimated that over 150,000 cases of pleural effusions secondary to pulmonary emboli occur annually in the United States (see Chapter 14). Because the pleural effusion with pulmonary embolization can be either a transudate or an exudate, it is recommended that the diagnosis of pulmonary embolization be considered in every patient with a pleural effusion.

Accordingly, I recommend a perfusion lung scan for all patients with pleural effusions in whom the origin of the effusion is not evident after the initial evaluation, including a diagnostic thoracentesis. The interpretation of the perfusion lung scan is difficult in patients with pleural fluid (208). Obviously, areas of the hemithorax occupied by the pleural fluid receive no perfusion. With large effusions, perfusion to the entire ipsilateral lung may be attenuated because of reflex vasoconstriction on the ipsilateral side. In addition, if perfusion scans are obtained in a recumbent patient, the fluid can gravitate into the fissure to produce large perfusion defects (see Fig. 14.1). If the ventilation lung scan is subsequently performed with the patient erect, areas of gross mismatching of the ventilation and perfusion may be seen, owing merely to the presence of the pleural fluid.

In a patient without parenchymal infiltrates, the diagnosis of pulmonary embolization is suggested if mismatches of ventilation and perfusion occupy more than 75% of the volume of a lung segment or if more than 1 area of mismatching occupies 25 to 75% of the volume of a single segment (209). In a patient with a parenchymal infiltrate, a larger defect on the perfusion scan than on the ventilation scan suggests pulmonary emboli. If the perfusion and ventilation scans are equivocal, evidence for deep venous thrombosis should be sought, or a pulmonary arteriogram should be obtained.

REFERENCES

1. Marel M, Štastny B, Melínová L, Svandová E, Light RW: Diagnosis of pleural effusions—experience with clinical studies 1986-1990. Chest 1995, in press.
2. Anthonisen NR, Martin RR: Regional lung function in pleural effusion. Am Rev Respir Dis 1977;116: 201-207.
3. Light RW, Stansbury DW, Brown SE: The relationship between pleural pressures and changes in pulmonary function after therapeutic thoracentesis. Am Rev Respir Dis 1986;133:658-661.
4. Vaska K, Wann LS, Sagar K, Klopfenstein HS: Pleural effusion as a cause of right ventricular diastolic collapse. Circulation 1992;86:609-617.
5. Brandstetter RD, Cohen RP: Hypoxemia after thoracentesis. A predictable and treatable condition. JAMA 1979;242:1060-1061.
6. Pavlin J, Cheney FW Jr: Unilateral pulmonary edema in rabbits after re-expansion of collapsed lung. J Appl Physiol 1979;46:31-35.
7. Bernstein A, White FZ: Unusual physical findings in pleural effusion: intrathoracic manometric studies. Ann Intern Med 1952;37:733-738.
8. Paddock FK: The diagnostic significance of serous fluids in disease. N Engl J Med 1940;223:1010-1015.
9. Broaddus VC, Light RW: What is the origin of pleural transudates and exudates? (Editorial) Chest 1992;102:658.
10. Leuallen EC, Carr DT: Pleural effusion, a statistical study of 436 patients. N Engl J Med 1955;252:79-83.
11. Carr DT, Power MH: Clinical value of measurements of concentration of protein in pleural fluid. N Engl J Med 1958;259:926-927.
12. Light RW, MacGregor MI, Luchsinger PC, Ball WC: Pleural effusions: the diagnostic separation of transudates and exudates. Ann Intern Med 1972;77: 507-513.
13. Hamm H, Brohan U, Bohmer R, Missmahl HP: Cholesterol in pleural effusions: a diagnostic aid. Chest 1987;92:296-302.
14. Valdes L, Pose A, Suarez J, Gonzalez-Juanatey JR, Sarandeses A, San Jose E, Alvarez Dobana JM, Salgueiro M, Rodriguez Sudrez JR: Cholesterol: A useful parameter for distinguishing between pleural exudates and transudates. Chest 1991;99:1097-1102.
15. Roth BJ, O'Meara TF, Cragun WH: The serum-effusion albumin gradient in the evaluation of pleural effusions. Chest 1990;98:546-549.
16. Meisel S, Shamiss A, Thaler M, Nussinovitch N, Rosenthal T: Pleural fluid to serum bilirubin concentration ratio for the separation of transudates from exudates. Chest 1990;98:141-144.
17. Romero S, Candela A, Martin C, Hernandez L, Trigo C, Gil J: Evaluation of different criteria for the separation of pleural transudates from exudates. Chest 1993;104:399-404.
18. Burgess LJ, Maritz FJ, Taljaard FFJ: Comparative analysis of the biochemical parameters used to distinguish between pleural transudates and exudates. Chest 1995, in press.
19. Paddock FK: The relationship between the specific gravity and the protein content in human serous effusions. Am J Med Sci 1941;201:569-574.
20. Light RW: Falsely high refractometric readings for the specific gravity of pleural fluid. Chest 1979;76: 300-301.
21. Light RW, Ball WC: Lactate dehydrogenase isoenzymes in pleural effusions. Am Rev Respir Dis 1973;108:660-664.
22. Light RW, Erozan YS, Ball WC: Cells in pleural fluid: their value in differential diagnosis. Arch Intern Med 1973;132:854-860.
23. Light RW, Ball WC: Glucose and amylase in pleural effusions. JAMA 1973;225:257-260.

24. Light RW, MacGregor MI, Ball WC Jr, Luchsinger PC: Diagnostic significance of pleural fluid pH and PCO_2. Chest 1973;64:591–596.

25. Rolf LL, Travis DM: Pleural fluid-plasma bicarbonate gradients in oxygen-toxic and normal rats. Am J Physiol 1973;224:857–861.

26. Lyche KD, Jensen WA, Kirsch CM, Yenokida GG, Maltz GS, Knauer CM: Pleuropulmonary manifestations of hepatic amebiasis. West J Med 1990;153:275–278.

27. Rasmussen KN, Faber V: Hyaluronic acid in 247 pleural fluids. Scand J Respir Dis 1967;48:366–371.

28. Judson MA, Lazarchick J, Sahn SA: Pleural fluid platelets: can they help identify traumatic thoracenteses? Am J Respir Crit Care Med 1994;149:A1104.

29. Spriggs AI, Boddington MM: The Cytology of Effusions. 2nd ed. New York: Grune & Stratton, 1968.

30. Broaddus VC, Hebert CA, Vitangcol RV, Hoeffel JM, Bernstein MS, Boylan AM: Interleukin-8 is a major neutrophil chemotactic factor in pleural liquid of patients with empyema. Am Rev Respir Dis 1992;146:825–830.

31. Antony VB, Godbey SW, Kunkel SL, Hott JW, Hartman D, Burdick MD, Strieter M: Recruitment of inflammatory cells to the pleural space. Chemotactic cytokines, IL-8, and monocyte chemotactic peptide-1 in human pleural fluids. J Immunol 1993;151:7216–7223.

32. Naylor B, Novak PM: Charcot-Leyden crystals in pleural fluids. Acta Cytol 1985;29:781–784.

33. Wahl RW: Curschmann's spirals in pleural and peritoneal fluids. Report of 12 cases. Acta Cytol 1986;30:147–151.

34. Nakamura Y, Ozaki T, Kamei T, Kawaji K, Banno K, Miki S, Fujisawa K, Yasuoka S, Ogura T: Factors that stimulate the proliferation and survival of eosinophils in eosinophilic pleural effusion: relationship to granulocyte/macrophage colony-stimulating factor, interleukin-5, and interleukin-3. Am J Respir Cell Mol Biol 1993;8:605–611.

35. Schandene L, Namias B, Crusiaux A, Lybin M, Devos R, Velu T, Capel P, Bellens R, Goldman M: IL-5 in post-traumatic eosinophilic pleural effusion. Clin Exper Immunol 1993;93:115–119.

36. Nakamura Y, Ozaki T, Yanagawa H, Yasuoka S, Ogura T: Eosinophil colony-stimulating factor induced by administration of interleukin-2 into the pleural cavity of patients with malignant pleurisy. Am J Respir Cell Mol Biol 1990;3:291–300.

37. Bozza PT, Castro-Faria-Neto HC, Penido C, Larangeira AP, Silva PM, Martins MA, Cordeiro RS: IL-5 accounts for the mouse pleural eosinophil accumulation triggered by antigen but not by LPS. Immunopharmacology 1994;27:131–136.

38. Adelman M, Albelda SM, Gottlieb J, Haponik EF: Diagnostic utility of pleural fluid eosinophilia. Am J Med 1984;77:915–920.

39. Askin FB, McCann BG, Kuhn C: Reactive eosinophilic pleuritis. Arch Pathol Lab Med 1977;101:187–191.

40. Maltais F, Laberge F, Cormier Y: Blood hypereosinophilia in the course of posttraumatic pleural effusion. Chest 1990;98:348–351.

41. Johnson RJ, Johnson JR: Paragonimiasis in Indochinese refugees: Roentgenographic findings with clinical correlations. Am Rev Respir Dis 1983;128:534–538.

42. Yacoubian HD: Thoracic problems associated with hydatid cyst of the dome of the liver. Surgery 1976;79:544–548.

43. Erzurum SE, Underwood GA, Hamilos DL, Waldron JA: Pleural effusion in Churg-Strauss syndrome. Chest 1989;95:1357–1359.

44. Yam LT: Diagnostic significance of lymphocytes in pleural effusions. Ann Intern Med 1967;66:972–982.

45. Pettersson T, Klockans M, Hellström P-E, et al: T and B lymphocytes in pleural effusions. Chest 1978;73:49–51.

46. Potrykus AM, Steinmann G, Stein E, Mertelsmann R: T- and B-cell responses in patients with malignant pleural effusions. Br J Cancer 1981;43:471–477.

47. Domagala W, Emeson EE, Kos LG: T and B lymphocyte enumeration in the diagnosis of lymphocyte-rich pleural fluids. Acta Cytol 1981;25:108–110.

48. Moisan T, Chandrasekhar AJ, Robinson J, et al: Distribution of lymphocyte subpopulations in patients with exudative pleural effusions. Am Rev Respir Dis 1978;117:507–511.

49. Kockman S, Bernard J, Lavaud F, et al: T-lymphocyte subsets in pleural fluids: discrimination according to traditional and monoclonal antibody-defined markers. Eur J Respir Dis 1984;65:586–591.

50. Lucivero G, Pierucci G, Bonomo L: Lymphocyte subsets in peripheral blood and pleural fluid. Eur Respir J 1988;1:337–340.

51. Guzman J, Bross KJ, Wurtemberger G, Costabel U: Immunocytology in malignant pleural mesothelioma: expression of tumor markers and distribution of lymphocyte subsets. Chest 1989;95:590–595.

52. Okubo Y, Nakata M, Kuroiwa Y, et al: NK cells in carcinomatous and tuberculous pleurisy: phenotypic and functional analyses of NK cells in peripheral blood and pleural effusions. Chest 1987;92:500–504.

53. Miserocchi G, Agostoni E: Contents of the pleural space. J Appl Physiol 1971;30:208–213.

54. Hurwitz S, Leiman G, Shapiro C: Mesothelial cells in pleural fluid: TB or not TB? S Afr Med J 1980;57:937–939.

55. Antony VB, Sahn SA, Antony AC, Repine JE: Bacillus Calmette-Guerin-stimulated neutrophils release chemotaxins for monocytes in rabbit pleural space in vitro. J Clin Invest 1985;76:1514–1521.

56. Luetscher JA Jr: Electrophoretic analysis of the proteins of plasma and serous effusions. J Clin Invest 1941;20:99–106.

57. Zinneman HH, Johnson JJ, Lyon RH: Proteins and mucoproteins in pleural effusions. Amer Rev Tuberc Pulmon Dis 1957;76:247–255.

58. Telvi L, Jaybert F, Eyquem A, et al: Study of immunoglobulins in pleura and pleural effusions. Thorax 1979;34:389–392.

59. Yokogawa M, Kojima S, Araki K, et al: Immunoglobulin E: raised levels in sera and pleural exudates of

patients with paragonimiasis. Am J Trop Med Hyg 1976:25:581-586.

60. Nash DR, Wallace RJ Jr: Immunoglobulin E and other immunoglobulins in patients with eosinophilic pleural effusions. J Lab Clin Med 1985;106: 512-516.

61. Calnan WL, Winfield BJO, Crowley MF, Bloom A: Diagnostic value of the glucose content of serous pleural effusions. Br Med J 1951;1:1239-1240.

62. Barber LM, Mazzadi L, Deakins DO, et al: Glucose level in pleural fluid as a diagnostic aid. Dis Chest 1957;31:680-681.

63. Berger HW, Maher G: Decreased glucose concentration in malignant pleural effusions. Am Rev Respir Dis 1971;103:427-429.

64. Carr DT, Power MH: Pleural fluid glucose with special reference to its concentration in rheumatoid pleurisy with effusion. Dis Chest 1960;37:321-324.

65. Vianna NJ: Nontuberculous bacterial empyema in patients with and without underlying diseases. JAMA 1971;215:69-75.

66. Rodriguez-Panadero F, Lopez Mejias J: Low glucose and pH levels in malignant pleural effusions. Am Rev Respir Dis 1989;139:663-667.

67. Sahn SA, Good JT Jr: Pleural fluid pH in malignant effusions. Ann Intern Med 1988;108:345-349.

68. Sanchez-Armengol A, Rodriguez-Panadero F: Survival and talc pleurodesis in metastatic pleural carcinoma, revisited. Report of 125 cases. Chest 1993;104:1482-1485.

69. Rodriguez-Panadero F, Lopez-Mejias J: Survival time of patients with pleural metastatic carcinoma predicted by glucose and pH studies. Chest 1989;95: 320-324.

70. Lillington GA, Carr DT, Mayne JG: Rheumatoid pleurisy with effusion. Arch Intern Med 1971;128: 764-768.

71. Dodson WH, Hollingsworth JW: Pleural effusion in rheumatoid arthritis. N Engl J Med 1966;275:1337-1342.

72. Halla JT, Schrohenloher RE, Volanakis JE: Immune complexes and other laboratory features of pleural effusions. Ann Intern Med 1980;92:748-752.

73. Good JT Jr, King TE, Antony VB, Sahn SA: Lupus pleuritis: clinical features and pleural fluid characteristics with special reference to pleural fluid antinuclear antibodies. Chest 1983;84:714-718.

74. Light RW, Girard WM, Jenkinson SG, George RB: Parapneumonic effusions. Am J Med 1980;69:507-511.

75. Kaye MD: Pleuropulmonary complications of pancreatitis. Thorax 1968;23:297-306.

76. Rockey DC, Cello JP: Pancreaticopleural fistula. Report of 7 cases and review of the literature. Medicine 1990;69:332-344.

77. Ende N: Studies of amylase activity in pleural effusions and ascites. Cancer 1960;13:283-287.

78. Kramer MR, Cepero RJ, Pitchenik AE: High amylase in neoplasm-related pleural effusion. Ann Intern Med 1989;110:567-569.

79. Abbott OA, Mansour KA, Logan WC, et al: Atraumatic so-called "spontaneous" rupture of the esophagus. J Thorac Cardiovasc Surg 1970;59:67-83.

80. Sherr HP, Light RW, Merson MH, et al: Origin of pleural fluid amylase in esophageal rupture. Ann Intern Med 1972;76:985-986.

81. Maulitz RM, Good JT Jr, Kaplan RL, et al: The pleuropulmonary consequences of esophageal rupture: an experimental model. Am Rev Respir Dis 1979;120:363-367.

82. Wroblewski F, Wroblewski R: The clinical significance of lactic dehydrogenase activity of serous effusions. Ann Intern Med 1958;48:813-822.

83. Raabo E, Rasmussen KN, Terkildsen TC: A study of the isoenzymes of lactic dehydrogenase in pleural effusions. Scand J Respir Dis 1966;47:150-156.

84. Potts DE, Willcox MA, Good JT Jr, et al: The acidosis of low-glucose pleural effusions. Am Rev Respir Dis 1978;117:665-671.

85. Chavalittamrong B, Angsusingha K, Tuchinda M, et al: Diagnostic significance of pH, lactic acid dehydrogenase, lactate and glucose in pleural fluid. Respiration 1979;38:112-120.

86. Light RW, Luchsinger P: Metabolic activity of pleural fluid. J Appl Physiol 1973;34:97-101.

87. Taryle DA, Good JT Jr, Sahn SA: Acid generation by pleural fluids: possible role in the determination of pleural fluid pH. J Lab Clin Med 1979;93:1041-1046.

88. Pine JR, Hollman JL: Elevated pleural fluid pH in *Proteus mirabilis* empyema. Chest 1983;84:109-111.

89. Potts DE, Levin DC, Sahn SA: Pleural fluid pH in parapneumonic effusions. Chest 1976;70:328-331.

90. Dye RA, Laforet EG: Esophageal rupture: diagnosis by pleural fluid pH. Chest 1974;66:454-456.

91. Good JT Jr, Taryle DA, Sahn SA: The pathogenesis of the low pleural fluid pH in esophageal rupture. Am Rev Respir Dis 1983;127:702-704.

92. Good JT Jr, Taryle DA, Maulitz RM, et al: The diagnostic value of pleural fluid pH. Chest 1980;78: 55-59.

93. Rodriguez-Panadero F, Lopez-Mejias L: Survival time of patients with pleural metastatic carcinoma predicted by glucose and pH studies. Chest 1989;95: 320-324.

94. Sahn SA, Good JT Jr: Pleural fluid pH in malignant effusions. Ann Intern Med 1988;108:345-349.

95. Miller KS, Wooten S, Sahn SA: Urinothorax: a cause of low pH transudative pleural effusions. Am J Med 1988;85:448-449.

96. Marchevsky AM, Hauptman E, Gil J, Watson C: Computerized interactive morphometry as an aid in the diagnosis of pleural effusions. Acta Cytol 1987; 31:131-136.

97. Stevens MW, Leong AS, Fazzalari NL, Dowling KD, Henderson DW: Cytopathology of malignant mesothelioma: a stepwise logistic regression analysis. Diag Cytopath 1992;8:333-342.

98. Jarvi OH, Kunnas RJ, Laitio MT, Tyrkko JES: The accuracy and significance of cytologic cancer diagnosis of pleural effusions. Acta Cytol 1972;16:152-157.

99. Grunze H: The comparative diagnostic accuracy, efficiency and specificity of cytologic techniques used in the diagnosis of malignant neoplasm in serous effusions of the pleural and pericardial cavities. Acta Cytol 1964;8:150-164.

100. Bueno CE, Clemente G, Castro BC, Martin LM, Ramos SR, Panizo AG, Glez-Rio JM: Cytologic and bacteriologic analysis of fluid and pleural biopsy specimens with Cope's needle. Arch Intern Med 1990;150:1190-1194.

101. Naylor B, Schmidt RW: The case for exfoliative cytology of serous effusions. Lancet 1964;1:711-712.

102. Melamed MR: The cytological presentation of malignant lymphomas and related diseases in effusions. Cancer 1963;16:413-431.

103. Dekker A, Bupp PA: Cytology of serous effusions. An investigation into the usefulness of cell blocks versus smears. Am J Clin Pathol 1978;70:855-860.

104. Gondos B, McIntosh KM, Renston RH, King EB: Application of electron microscopy in the definitive diagnosis of effusions. Acta Cytol 1978;22:297-304.

105. Warhol MJ, Hickey WF, Corson JM: Malignant mesothelioma. Ultrastructural distinction from adenocarcinoma. Am J Surg Pathol 1982;6:307-314.

106. Coleman M, Henderson DW, Mukherjee TM: The ultrastructural pathology of malignant pleural mesothelioma. Pathol Ann 1989;24:303-353.

107. Jandik WR, Landas SK, Bray CK, Lager DJ: Scanning electron microscopic distinction of pleural mesotheliomas from adenocarcinomas. Modern Path 1993;6:761-764.

108. Warnock ML, Stoloff A, Thor A: Differentiation of adenocarcinoma of the lung from mesothelioma. Periodic acid-Schiff, monoclonal antibodies B72.3, and Leu M1. Am J Pathol 1988;133:30-38.

109. Wirth PR, Legier J, Wright GL Jr: Immunohistochemical evaluation of seven monoclonal antibodies for differentiation of pleural mesothelioma from lung adenocarcinoma. Cancer 1991;67:655-662.

110. Frisman DM, McCarthy WF, Schleiff P, Buckner SB, Nocito JD Jr, O'Leary TJ.: Immunocytochemistry in the differential diagnosis of effusions: use of logistic regression to select a panel of antibodies to distinguish adenocarcinomas from mesothelial proliferations. Modern Path 1993;6:179-184.

111. Brown RW, Clark GM, Tandon AK, Allred DC: Multiple-marker immunohistochemical phenotypes distinguishing malignant pleural mesothelioma from pulmonary adenocarcinoma. Human Path 1993;24:347-354.

112. Guzman J, Bross KJ, Costabel U: Malignant lymphoma in pleural effusions: an immunocytochemical cell surface analysis. Diag Cytopath 1991;7:113-118.

113. Shimokata K, Totani Y, Nakanishi K, et al: Diagnostic value of cancer antigen 15-3 (CA15-3) detected by monoclonal antibodies (115D8 and DF3) in exudative pleural effusions. Eur Respir J 1988;1:341-344.

114. Niwa Y, Kishimoto H, Shimokata K: Carcinomatous and tuberculous pleural effusion. Comparison of tumor markers. Chest 1985;87:351-355.

115. Klockars M, Pettersson T, Froseth B, Selroos O, Stenman U-H: Concentration of tumor-associated trypsin inhibitor (TATI) in pleural effusions. Chest 1990;98:1159-1164.

116. Shimokata K, Niwa Y, Yamamoto M, Sasou H, Morishita M: Pleural fluid neuron-specific enolase. Chest 1989;95:602-603.

117. Tawfik MS, Coleman DV: C-myc expression in exfoliated cells in serous effusions. Cytopath 1991;2:83-92.

118. Athanassiadou PP, Veneti SZ, Kyrkou KA, Athanassiades PH: Detection of c-Ha-ras oncogene expression in pleural and peritoneal smear effusions by in situ hybridization. Cancer Detect Prevent 1993;17:585-590.

119. Rittgers RA, Loewenstein MS, Feinerman AE, et al: Carcinoembryonic antigen levels in benign and malignant pleural effusions. Ann Intern Med 1978;88:631-634.

120. Vladutiu AO, Brason FW, Adler RH: Differential diagnosis of pleural effusions: clinical usefulness of cell marker quantitation. Chest 1981;79:297-301.

121. McKenna JM, Chandrasekhar AJ, Henkin RE: Diagnostic value of carcinoembryonic antigen in exudative pleural effusions. Chest 1980;78:587-590.

122. Tamura S, Nishigaki T, Moriwaki Y, et al: Tumor markers in pleural effusion diagnosis. Cancer 1988;61:298-302.

123. Stanford CF, Neville AM, Laurence DJR: Concurrent assays of plasma and pleural-effusion levels of carcinoembryonic antigen in the diagnosis of pulmonary disease. Lancet 1978;3:53.

124. Nurminen M, Dejmek A, Martensson G, Thylen A, Hjerpe A: Clinical utility of liquid-chromatographic analysis of effusions for hyaluronate content. Clin Chem 1994;40:777-780.

125. Hillerdal G, Lindqvist U, Engström-Laurent A: Hyaluronan in pleural effusions and in serum. Cancer 1991;67:2410-2414.

126. Pettersson T, Froseth B, Riska H, Klockars M: Concentration of hyaluronic acid in pleural fluid as a diagnostic aid for malignant mesothelioma. Chest 1988;94:1037-1039.

127. Martensson G, Thylen A, Lindquist U, Hjerpe A: The sensitivity of hyaluronan analysis of pleural fluid from patients with malignant mesothelioma and a comparison of different methods. Cancer 1994;73:1406-1410.

128. Kawai T, Greenberg SD, Truong LD, et al: Differences in lectin binding of malignant pleural mesothelioma and adenocarcinoma of the lung. Am J Pathol 1988;130:401-410.

129. Croonen AM, van der Valk P, Herman CJ, Lindeman J: Cytology, immunopathology and flow cytometry in the diagnosis of pleural and peritoneal effusion. Lab Invest 1988;58:725-732.

130. Rijken A, Dekker A, Taylor S, Hoffman P, Blank M, Krause JR: Diagnostic value of DNA analysis in effusions by flow cytometry and image analysis. A prospective study on 102 patients as compared with cytologic examination. Am J Clin Pathol 1991; 95:6-12.

131. Pinto MM: DNA analysis of malignant effusions. Comparison with cytologic diagnosis and carcinoembryonic antigen content. Analytic Quant Cytol Histol 1992;14:222-226.

132. Moriarty AT, Wiersema L, Snyder W, Kotylo PK, McCloskey DW: Immunophenotyping of cytologic specimens by flow cytometry. Diag Cytopath 1993; 9:252-258.

133. Dewald G, Dines DE, Weiland LH, Gordon H: Usefulness of chromosome examination in the diagnosis of malignant pleural effusions. N Engl J Med 1976;295:1494-1500.

134. Korsgaard R: Chromosome analysis of malignant human effusions in vivo. Scand J Respir Dis 1979; 105(suppl):1-100.

135. Piras MA, Gakis C, Budroni M, Andreoni G: Adenosine deaminase activity in pleural effusions: an aid to differential diagnosis. Br Med J 1978;4:1751-1752.

136. Ocana IM, Martinez-Vazquez JM, Seguna RM, et al: Adenosine deaminase in pleural fluids. Chest 1983; 84:51-53.

137. Fontan Bueso J, Verea H, Perez J, et al: Diagnostic value of simultaneous determination of pleural adenosine deaminase and pleural lysozyme/serum lysozyme ratio in pleural effusion. Chest 1988;93:303-307.

138. Valdes L, San Jose E, Alvarez D, Sarandeses A, Pose A, Chomon B, Alvarez-Dobano JM, Salgueiro M, Rodriguez Suarez JR: Diagnosis of tuberculous pleurisy using the biologic parameters adenosine deaminase, lysozyme, and interferon gamma. Chest 1993; 103:458-465.

139. Hsu WH, Chiang CD, Huang PL: Diagnostic value of pleural adenosine deaminase in tuberculous effusions of immunocompromised hosts. J Formosan Med Assoc 1993;92:668-670.

140. Ocana I, Ribera E, Martinez-Vazquez JM, et al: Adenosine deaminase activity in rheumatoid pleural effusion. Ann Rheum Dis 1988;47:394-397.

141. Ungerer JP, Grobler SM: Molecular forms of adenosine deaminase in pleural effusions. Enzyme 1988; 40:7-13.

142. Aoki Y, Katoh O, Nakanishi Y, Kuroki S, Yamada H: A comparison study of IFN-gamma, ADA, and CA125 as the diagnostic parameters in tuberculous pleuritis. Resp Med 1994;88:139-143.

143. Ribera E, Ocana I, Martinez-Vazquez JM, et al: High level of interferon gamma in tuberculous pleural effusion. Chest 1988;93:308-311.

144. Barnes PF, Mistry SD, Cooper CL, Pirmez C, Rea TH, Modlin RL: Compartmentalization of a CD4+ T lymphocyte subpopulation in tuberculous pleuritis. J Immunol 1989;142:1114-1119.

145. Shimokata K, Saka H, Murate T, Hasegawa Y, Hasegawa T: Cytokine content in pleural effusion. Chest 1991;99:1103-1107.

146. Asseo PP, Tracopoulos GD, Kotsovoulou-Fouskak V: Lysozyme (muramidase) in pleural effusions and serum. Am J Clin Pathol 1982;78:763-767.

147. Verea Hernando HRA, Masa Jimenez JF, Dominguez Juncal L, et al: Meaning and diagnostic value of determining the lysozyme level of pleural fluid. Chest 1987;91:342-345.

148. Baig MME, Pettengell KE, Simgee AE, et al: Diagnosis of tuberculosis by detection of mycobacterial antigens in pleural effusions and ascites. S Afr Med J 1986;69:101-102.

149. Yew WW, Chan CY, Kwan SY, Cheung SW, French GL: Diagnosis of tuberculous pleural effusion by the detection of tuberculostearic acid in pleural aspirates. Chest 1991;100:1261-1263.

150. Banchuin N, Pumprueg U, Pimolpan V, et al: Anti-PPD IgG responses in tuberculous pleurisy. J Med Assoc Thai 1987;70:321-325.

151. Dhand R, Gangul NK, Vaishnavi C, et al: False-positive reactions with enzyme-linked immunosorbent assay of Mycobacterium tuberculosis antigens in pleural fluid. J Med Microbiol 1988;26:241-243.

152. Levy H, Wayne LG, Anderson BE, et al: Antimycobacterial antibody levels in pleural fluid reflect passive diffusion from serum. Chest 1989;92:1855.

153. Caminero JA, Rodriguez de Castro F, Carrillo T, Diaz F, Rodriguez Bermejo JC, Cabrera P: Diagnosis of pleural tuberculosis by detection of specific IgG anti-antigen 60 in serum and pleural fluid. Respiration 1993;60:58-62.

154. Van Vooren JP, Farber CM, De Bruyn J, Yernault JC: Antimycobacterial antibodies in pleural effusions. Chest 1990;97:88-90.

155. Murate T, Mizoguchi K, Amano H, Shimokata K, Matsuda T: Antipurified-Protein-Derivative antibody in tuberculous pleural effusions. Chest 1990;97:670-673.

156. Walker WC, Wright V: Rheumatoid pleuritis. Ann Rheum Dis 1967;26:467-474.

157. Winslow WA, Ploss LN, Loitman B: Pleuritis in systemic lupus erythematosus: its importance as an early manifestation in diagnosis. Ann Intern Med 1958;49:70-88.

158. Berger HW, Seckler SG: Pleural and pericardial effusions in rheumatoid disease. Ann Intern Med 1966;64:1291-1297.

159. Levine H, Szanto M, Grieble HG, et al: Rheumatoid factor in non-rheumatoid pleural effusions. Ann Intern Med 1968;69:487-492.

160. Leechawengwong M, Berger HW, Sukumaran M: Diagnostic significance of antinuclear antibodies in pleural effusion. Mt Sinai J Med 1979;46:137-139.

161. Carmichael DS, Golding DN: Rheumatoid pleural effusion with "RA cells" in the pleural fluid. Br Med J 1967;1:814.

162. Hunder GG, McDuffie FC, Hepper NGG: Pleural fluid complement in systemic lupus erythematosus

and rheumatoid arthritis. Ann Intern Med 1972;76: 357-362.

163. Glovsky MM, Louie JS, Pitts WH Jr, Alenty A: Reduction of pleural fluid complement activity in patients with systemic lupus erythematosus and rheumatoid arthritis. Clin Immunol Immunopathol 1976;6:31-41.

164. Andrews BS, Arora NS, Shadforth MF, et al: The role of immune complexes in the pathogenesis of pleural effusions. Am Rev Respir Dis 1981;124:115-120.

165. Hunder GG, McDuffie FC, Huston KA, et al: Pleural fluid complement, complement conversion, and immune complexes in immunologic and nonimmunologic diseases. J Lab Clin Med 1977;90:971-980.

166. Bruneau R, Rubin P: The management of pleural effusions and chylothorax in lymphoma. Radiology 1965;85:1085-1092.

167. Hughes RL, Mintzer RA, Hidvegi DF, et al: The management of chylothorax. Chest 1979;76:212-218.

168. Staats BA, Ellefson RD, Budahn LL, et al: The lipoprotein profile of chylous and nonchylous pleural effusions. Mayo Clin Proc 1980;55:700-704.

169. Seriff NS, Cohen ML, Samuel P, Schulster PL: Chylothorax: diagnosis by lipoprotein electrophoresis of serum and pleural fluid. Thorax 1977;32:98-100.

170. Coe JE, Aikawa JK: Cholesterol pleural effusion. Arch Intern Med 1961;108:763-774.

171. Roy PH, Carr DT, Payne WS: The problem of chylothorax. Mayo Clin Proc 1967;42:457-467.

172. Maartens G, Bateman ED: Tuberculous pleural effusions: increased culture yield with bedside inoculation of pleural fluid and poor diagnostic value of adenosine deaminase. Thorax 1991;46:96-99.

173. Lampe RM, Chottipitayasunondh T, Sunakorn P: Detection of bacterial antigen in pleural fluid by counterimmunoelectrophoresis. J Pediatr 1976;88: 557-560.

174. Coonrod JD, Wilson HD: Etiologic diagnosis of intrapleural empyema by counterimmunoelectrophoresis. Am Rev Respir Dis 1976;113:637-641.

175. Thadephalli H, Gangopadhyay PK: Rapid diagnosis of anaerobic empyema by direct gas-liquid chromatography of pleural fluid. Chest 1980;77:507-513.

176. Chang SC, Hsu YT, Chen YC, Lin CY: Usefulness of soluble interleukin 2 receptor in differentiating tuberculous and carcinomatous pleural effusions. Arch Intern Med 1994;154:1097-1101.

177. Yokoyama A, Maruyama M, Ito M, Kohno N, Hiwada K, Yano S: Interleukin 6 activity in pleural effusion. Chest 1992;102:1055-1059.

178. Miller EJ, Idell S: Interleukin-8: an important neutrophil chemotaxin in some cases of exudative pleural effusions. Exp Lung Res 1993;19:589-601.

179. Glauser FL, Otis PT, Levine RI, Smith WR: In vitro pleural fluid clottability and fibrinogen content. Chest 1975;68:205-208.

180. Widstrom O, Kockum C, Nilsson BS: Fibrinogen, fibrin(ogen) degradation products and fibrinopeptide A in pleural effusions. Scand J Respir Dis 1978;59:210-215.

181. Astedt B, Adielsson G, Mattsson W: Fibrin/fibrinogen degradation products in pleural exudate. Lancet 1976;2:414.

182. Raja OG, Casson IF: Fibrinogen degradation products in pleural effusions. Br J Dis Chest 1980;74: 164-168.

183. Idell S, Girard W, Koenig KB, McLarty J, Fair DS: Abnormalities of pathways of fibrin turnover in the human pleural space. Am Rev Respir Dis 1991;144: 187-194.

184. Delpuech P, Desch G, Fructus F: Fibronectin is unsuitable as a tumor marker in pleural effusions. Clin Chem 1989;35:166-168.

185. Arai H, Endo M, Yokosawa A, et al: On acid glycosaminoglycans (mucopolysaccharides) in pleural effusion. Am Rev Respir Dis 1975;111:37-42.

186. Brauer MJ, West M, Zimmerman HJ: Comparison of glycolytic and oxidative enzyme and transaminase values in benign and malignant effusions with those in serums. Cancer 1963;16:533-541.

187. Feldstein AM, Samachson J, Spencer H: Levels of calcium, phosphorus, alkaline phosphatase and protein in effusion fluid and serum in man. Am J Med 1963;35:530-535.

188. Bedrossian CWM, Stein DA, Miller WC, Woo J: Levels of angiotensin-converting enzyme in pleural effusion. Arch Pathol Lab Med 1981;105:345-346.

189. Veran P, Moigneteau C, Lasausse G, et al: Les phosphatases des épanchements pleuraux de diverses natures. Leur intérêt dans le cancer de la prostate. J Fr Med Chir Thorac 1965;19:621-643.

190. Migueres J, Jover A, Abou P: Valeur théorique et pratique de certains dosages enzymatiques au cours des épanchements pleuraux (amylase, phosphatases, lacticodeshydrogenase). A propos de 129 observations. J Fr Med Chir Thorac 1969;23:443-458.

191. Scerbo J, Keltz H, Stone DJ: A prospective study of closed pleural biopsies. JAMA 1971;218:377-380.

192. Mestitz P, Purves MJ, Pollard AC: Pleural biopsy in the diagnosis of pleural effusion. Lancet 1958;2: 1349-1353.

193. Levine H, Metzger W, Lacera D, Kay L: Diagnosis of tuberculous pleurisy by culture of pleural biopsy specimen. Arch Intern Med 1970;126:269-271.

194. Poppius H, Kokkola K: Diagnosis and differential diagnosis in tuberculous pleurisy. Scand J Respir Dis 1968;63(suppl):105-110.

195. Von Hoff DD, LiVolsi V: Diagnostic reliability of needle biopsy of the parietal pleura. Am J Clin Pathol 1975;64:200-203.

196. Levine H, Cugell DW: Blunt-end needle biopsy of pleura and rib. Arch Intern Med 1971;109:516-525.

197. Nelson O, Light RW: Granulomatous pleuritis secondary to blastomycosis. Chest 1977;71:433-434.

198. Salyer WR, Eggleston JC, Erozan YS: Efficacy of pleural needle biopsy and pleural fluid cytopathol-

ogy in the diagnosis of malignant neoplasm involving the pleura. Chest 1975;67:536–539.

199. Frist B, Kahan AV, Koss LG: Comparison of the diagnostic values of biopsies of the pleura and cytologic evaluation of pleural fluids. Am J Clin Pathol 1979;72:48–51.

200. Landreneau RJ, Hazelrigg SR, Mack MJ, Keenan RJ, Ferson PF: Video-assisted thoracic surgery for pulmonary and pleural disease. In: Shields TW, ed. General Thoracic Surgery. Malvern, PA: Williams & Wilkins, 1994;4:508–528.

201. Menzies R, Charbonneau M: Thoracoscopy for the diagnosis of pleural disease. Ann Intern Med 1991; 114:271–276.

202. Hucker J, Bhatnagar NK, al-Jilaihawi AN, Forrester-Wood CP: Thoracoscopy in the diagnosis and management of recurrent pleural effusions. Ann Thorac Surg 1991;52:1145–1147.

203. Chang S-C, Perng RP: The role of fiberoptic bronchoscopy in evaluating the causes of pleural effusions. Arch Intern Med 1989;149:855–857.

204. Poe RH, Levy PC, Israel RH, Ortiz CR, Kallay MC: Use of fiberoptic bronchoscopy in the diagnosis of bronchogenic carcinoma. A study in patients with idiopathic pleural effusions. Chest 1994;105:1663–1667.

205. Feinsilver SH, Barrows AA, Braman SS: Fiberoptic bronchoscopy and pleural effusion of unknown origin. Chest 1986;90:514–515.

206. Douglass BE, Carr DT, Bernatz PE: Diagnostic thoracotomy in the study of "idiopathic" pleural effusion. Am Rev Tuberc 1956;954–957.

207. Ryan CJ, Rodgers RF, Unni KK, Hepper NC: The outcome of patients with pleural effusion of indeterminate cause at thoracotomy. Mayo Clin Proc 1981;56:145–149.

208. Baum S, Vincent NR, Lyons KP, et al: Atlas of Nuclear Medicine Imaging. New York: Appleton-Century-Crofts, 1981.

209. Biello DR, Mattar AG, McKnight RC, Siegel BA: Ventilation-perfusion studies in suspected pulmonary embolism. AJR 1979;133:1033–1037.

CHAPTER 5
Approach to the Patient

Whenever a patient with an abnormal chest radiograph is evaluated, the possibility of a pleural effusion should be considered. Increased densities on the chest radiograph are frequently attributed to parenchymal infiltrates when they actually represent pleural fluid. Most patients with pleural effusions have blunting of the posterior costophrenic sulcus on the lateral chest radiograph. If this angle is blunted, bilateral decubitus chest radiographs should be obtained to ascertain whether free pleural fluid is present (see Chapter 3). This chapter provides a guide to the approach to a patient with an undiagnosed pleural effusion. The management of patients with pleural effusions due to specific diseases is discussed in the chapters on those diseases.

FREQUENCIES OF VARIOUS DIAGNOSES

Pleural effusions can occur as complications of many different diseases (Table 5.1). The vigor with which various diagnoses are pursued depends on the likelihood that the individual has that particular disease. Table 5.2 shows the approximate annual incidence for the most common causes of pleural effusions. These data are rough estimates of the incidence of the various types of pleural effusions. A recent epidemiologic study from the Czech Republic found that the four leading causes of pleural effusions in order were congestive heart failure, malignancy, pneumonia, and pulmonary embolism (1). Congestive heart failure and cirrhosis cause almost all transudative pleural effusions, whereas malignant disease, pneumonia, and pulmonary embolization are the three main causes of exudative pleural effusions.

SEPARATION OF EXUDATES FROM TRANSUDATES

If free pleural fluid is demonstrated on the decubitus film, one should consider performing a diagnostic thoracentesis (Fig. 5.1). It has been my experience that diagnostic thoracentesis is difficult if the thickness of the fluid on the decubitus radiograph is less than 10 mm. If the thickness of the fluid is greater than 10 mm, however, consideration should be given to performing a diagnostic thoracentesis (see Chapter 23). If the patient has obvious congestive heart failure, I perform a diagnostic thoracentesis if any of the following three conditions are met: (a) the effusions are not bilateral and comparably sized; (b) the patient has pleuritic chest pain; or (c) the patient is febrile. Otherwise, treatment of the congestive heart failure is initiated. If the pleural effusions do not rapidly disappear, I then perform a diagnostic thoracentesis several days later. It must be remembered, however, that the characteristics of the pleural fluid may occasionally change from those of a transudate to those of an exudate with diuresis. Chakko and coworkers (2) treated 9 patients with congestive heart failure for a mean of 6 days and found that in 3 of the 9 patients a pleural fluid that was a transudate initially developed the characteristics of an exudate with diuresis. We performed a similar study (3) on 12 patients in whom the repeat thoracentesis was performed 12 to 48 hours after diuresis was initiated and found that in only 1 patient had the characteristics of the pleural fluid become exudative.

One of the main purposes of the diagnostic thoracentesis is to determine whether the patient has a transudative or an exudative pleural effusion. This distinction is made by analysis of the levels of protein and lactic acid dehydrogenase (LDH) in the pleural fluid and in the serum (4). If none of the criteria in Figure 5.1 is met, then the patient has a transudative pleural effusion. Therefore, the pleural surfaces can be ignored while the congestive heart failure, cirrhosis, or nephrosis, for example, is treated. Alternately, if any of the three criteria in Figure 5.1 are met, the patient has an exudative pleural effusion, that is, a pleural effusion resulting from local

Table 5.1   Differential Diagnoses of Pleural Effusion

Transudative Pleural Effusions
  Congestive heart failure
  Cirrhosis
  Nephrotic syndrome
  Superior vena caval obstruction
  Fontan procedure
  Urinothorax
  Peritoneal dialysis
  Glomerulonephritis
  Myxedema
  Pulmonary emboli
  Sarcoidosis
Exudative Pleural Effusions
  Neoplastic disease
    Metastatic disease
    Mesothelioma
  Infectious diseases
    Bacterial infections
    Tuberculosis
    Fungal infections
    Parasitic infections
    Viral infections
  Pulmonary embolization
  Gastrointestinal disease
    Pancreatic disease
    Subphrenic abscess
    Intrahepatic abscess
    Intrasplenic abscess
    Esophageal perforation
    After abdominal surgery
    Diaphragmatic hernia
    Endoscopic variceal sclerosis
    After liver transplant
  Collagen vascular diseases
    Rheumatoid pleuritis
    Systemic lupus erythematosus

Drug-induced lupus
Immunoblastic lymphadenopathy
Sjögren's syndrome
Familial Mediterranean fever
Churg-Strauss syndrome
Wegener's granulomatosis
Drug-induced pleural disease
  Nitrofurantoin
  Dantrolene
  Methysergide
  Bromocriptine
  Amiodarone
  Procarbazine
  Methotrexate
Miscellaneous diseases and conditions
  Asbestos exposure
  Postpericardiectomy or postmyocardial infarction
    syndrome
  Meigs' syndrome
  Yellow nail syndrome
  Sarcoidosis
  Pericardial disease
  After coronary artery bypass surgery
  After lung transplant
  Fetal pleural effusion
  Uremia
  Trapped lung
  Radiation therapy
  Ovarian hyperstimulation syndrome
  Postpartum pleural effusion
  Amyloidosis
  Electrical burns
  Iatrogenic injury
Hemothorax
Chylothorax

Table 5.2   Approximate Annual Incidence of Various Types of Pleural Effusions in the United States

Congestive heart failure	500,000
Pneumonia (bacterial)	300,000
Malignant disease	200,000
Lung	60,000
Breast	50,000
Lymphoma	40,000
Other	50,000
Pulmonary embolization	150,000
Viral disease	100,000
Cirrhosis with ascites	50,000
Gastrointestinal disease	25,000
Collagen vascular disease	6,000
Tuberculosis	2,500
Asbestos exposure	2,000
Mesothelioma	1,500

disease where the fluid originated, and further investigation should be directed toward the genesis of the local disease.

If there is a significant likelihood that the patient has a transudative pleural effusion, the most cost-effective use of the laboratory is to only obtain the protein and LDH levels of the pleural fluid at the initial diagnostic thoracentesis. Pleural fluid can be set aside for other tests if the fluid proves to be an exudate. Peterman and Speicher (5) reviewed the charts of 83 patients whose pleural fluid was a transudate by protein and LDH levels during a 1-year period. They found that 725 additional studies were performed on these 83 pleural fluids. Only 9 of the 725 studies yielded a positive result, and the positive result was eventually proven to be false in 7 of the 9 studies. If no tests other than the protein and LDH had been obtained in these 83 patients, there would have been a mean cost savings of $185 per patient.

In recent years several alternatives to the protein and LDH have been proposed to separate transudative and exudative pleural effusions. These have included a pleural fluid cholesterol level of 60 mg/dl (6, 7), a gradient between the serum and pleural albumin that exceeds 1.2 gm/100 ml (8), and a pleural fluid:serum bilirubin level of 0:6 (9). However, when these tests are compared directly with Light's criteria (10, 11), Light's criteria appear to be the most accurate. The primary problem is that Light's criteria incorrectly identify some transudates due to congestive heart failure as exudates (11). If a patient has congestive heart failure and the exudative criteria of Light are met, the serum-to-pleural fluid albumin gradient should be evaluated. If this exceeds 1.2 gm/dl, the patient probably has a transudative pleural effusion (11).

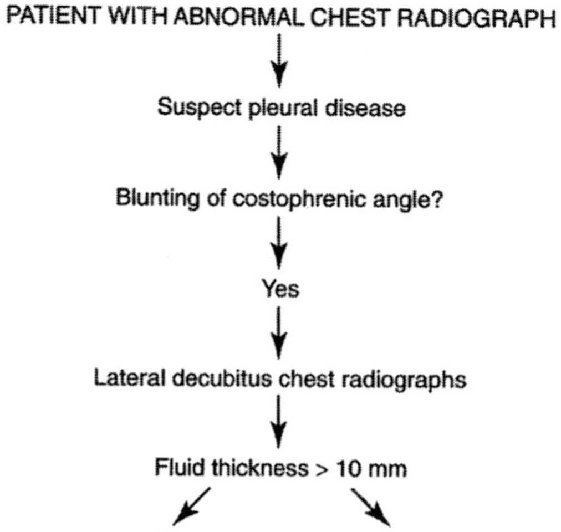

DIFFERENTIATING AMONG VARIOUS EXUDATIVE PLEURAL EFFUSIONS

In order to differentiate among the various causes of exudative pleural effusions, one should initially examine the gross appearance of the fluid, the pleural fluid differential cell count and cytologic test, the pleural fluid glucose, amylase, and LDH levels, and the pleural fluid pH measurement. Other tests can then be ordered on an individual basis.

Although each patient with an exudative pleural effusion should be assessed individually, the flow diagrams in Figures 5.2 through 5.4 are rough guides for evaluating such a patient.

Appearance of Pleural Fluid

The gross appearance of the pleural fluid should always be noted and evaluated as outlined in Figure 5.2. If the pleural fluid appears bloody, a hematocrit should be obtained on the fluid. The hematocrit is frequently much lower than one would expect from the appearance of the pleural fluid. The blood in the pleural fluid is not significant if the pleural fluid hematocrit is less than 1% (12). If the pleural fluid hematocrit is greater than 1%, the patient most likely has malignant pleural disease, a pulmonary embolus, or a traumatically induced pleural effusion (12). If the hematocrit is greater than 50% of that of the peripheral blood, the patient has a hemothorax, and one should consider performing a tube thoracostomy (see Chapter 20).

If the pleural fluid is turbid or milky or if it is bloody, the supernatant of the pleural fluid should be examined to see whether it is cloudy. If the pleural fluid was turbid when originally withdrawn, but the turbidity clears with centrifugation, the turbidity was due to cells or debris in the pleural fluid. If the turbidity persists after centrifugation, the patient probably has a chylothorax or a pseudochylothorax (see Chapter 21). These two entities can be differentiated by the pa-

PATIENT WITH ABNORMAL CHEST RADIOGRAPH

↓

Suspect pleural disease

↓

Blunting of costophrenic angle?

↓

Yes

↓

Lateral decubitus chest radiographs

↓

Fluid thickness > 10 mm

Yes → Diagnostic thoracentesis

No → Observe

Any of the following met?
PF/serum protein > 0.5
PF/serum LDH > 0.6
PF LDH > 2/3 upper normal serum limit

Yes → Exudate → Appearance of pleural fluid
Amylase and glucose of pleural fluid
Cytology and differential cell count of pleural fluid
(Figs. 5.2–5.4)

No → Transudate → Treat CHF, cirrhosis, or nephrosis

Figure 5.1. Algorithm for separating transudative from exudative pleural effusions.

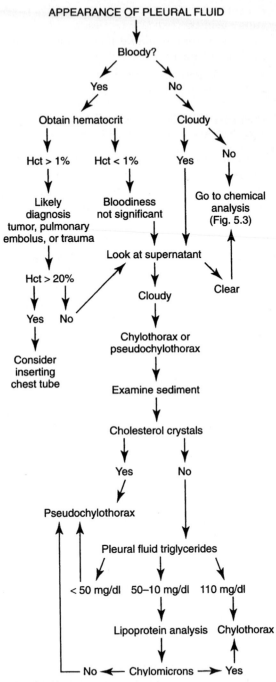

APPEARANCE OF PLEURAL FLUID

Bloody?

Yes — No

Obtain hematocrit — Cloudy

Hct > 1% — Hct < 1% — Yes — No

Likely diagnosis tumor, pulmonary embolus, or trauma — Bloodiness not significant — Go to chemical analysis (Fig. 5.3)

Hct > 20% — Look at supernatant

Yes — No — Cloudy — Clear

Consider inserting chest tube

Chylothorax or pseudochylothorax

Examine sediment

Cholesterol crystals

Yes — No

Pseudochylothorax

Pleural fluid triglycerides

< 50 mg/dl — 50–10 mg/dl — 110 mg/dl

Lipoprotein analysis — Chylothorax

No ← Chylomicrons → Yes

Figure 5.2. Algorithm for evaluating appearance of pleural fluid.

tient's history, examination of the sediment for cholesterol crystals, and lipid analysis of the supernatant (Fig. 5.2). Pseudochylothoraces usually occur when the pleural effusion has been present for many years. Cholesterol crystals may be found in the sediment, and

high levels of triglycerides are not usually present in the pleural fluid. In contrast, chylothoraces are more acute, do not contain cholesterol crystals, and are characterized by high levels of triglycerides. The management of a patient with a chylothorax or a pseudochylothorax is discussed in Chapter 21.

Pleural Fluid Amylase and Glucose Measurements

In the differential diagnosis of exudative pleural effusions, one should first measure the pleural fluid amylase and glucose levels, because if the amylase is elevated or the glucose is reduced, the spectrum of diagnostic possibilities is dramatically reduced. An elevated pleural fluid amylase level is only seen in pancreatic pleural effusions, esophageal perforation, and malignant pleural effusions (13). These three conditions are easily differentiated, and their management is discussed in Chapters 7 and 15.

The demonstration of a reduced pleural fluid glucose level (less than 60 mg/dl) is useful because it indicates that the patient probably has one of four conditions: parapneumonic effusion, tuberculous pleuritis, malignant pleural effusion, or rheumatoid pleural effusion (13). Other rare causes of a low glucose pleural effusion include paragonimiasis, hemothorax, the Churg-Strauss syndrome, urinothorax, and occasionally lupus pleuritis. A flow diagram for diagnosing patients with low pleural fluid glucose is shown in Figure 5.3. Most patients with a reduced pleural fluid glucose level also have a reduced pleural fluid pH and an increased pleural fluid LDH level. Laboratory errors in the performance of one of these three tests should be suspected when these relationships are not maintained.

Patients with either parapneumonic effusions or tuberculous pleuritis may have an acute illness characterized by fever, cough, pleuritic chest pain, and a low pleural fluid glucose level. Patients with parapneumonic effusions usually have radiologically evident parenchymal infiltrates, whereas those with tuberculous pleuritis usually have no infiltrates. The differential cell count on the pleural fluid is also useful in making the differentiation because most patients with parapneumonic effusions have predominantly polymorphonuclear leukocytes in their pleural fluid, but most patients with tuberculous pleuritis have predominantly lymphocytes.

Patients with subacute or chronic symptoms and a low pleural fluid glucose level may have malignant pleural disease, rheumatoid disease, or tuberculosis, or even a chronic bacterial infection. The diagnosis of rheumatoid pleuritis (see Chapter 17) is usually easy. The differentiation among tuberculosis, malignant disease, and chronic bacterial infection may be more difficult. The pleural biopsy and cytologic examination, however, are usually positive in the patient with tuberculosis or malignant disease and a low pleural fluid glucose level. If a definite diagnosis is not obtained after two pleural fluid cytologies and one needle biopsy of the pleura, the next diagnostic procedure should be thoracoscopy.

Other Diagnostic Tests

In patients with exudative pleural effusions and normal levels of pleural fluid glucose and amylase, one must first consider the pleural fluid cytologic examination (Fig. 5.4). If this test is positive, the diagnosis of malignant pleural disease is established, and the patient can be managed as outlined in Chapter 7. Immunohistochemical tests are also useful in establishing the diagnosis of a malignant pleural effusion and differentiating adenocarcinoma from mesothelioma (see Chapter 4). If

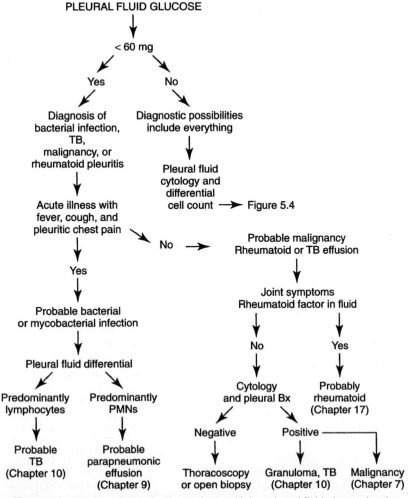

Figure 5.3. Algorithm for evaluating patients with low pleural fluid glucose levels.

the pleural fluid cytologic test is negative, the differential cell count of the pleural fluid should be examined. When polymorphonuclear leukocytes predominate in the pleural fluid, an acute process is affecting the pleural surfaces, and the chest radiograph should be evaluated for parenchymal infiltrates. The presence of an infiltrate indicates that the patient probably has parapneumonic effusion, pulmonary embolus, or bronchogenic carcinoma. The diagnosis of a parapneumonic effusion is likely if purulent sputum is present. When purulent sputum or peripheral leukocytosis is not seen, the patient should have a lung scan to rule out pulmonary embolus. In the event of a negative lung scan, a bronchoscopy with transbronchial biopsy should be performed to determine the cause of the parenchymal infiltrate. A pleural biopsy with repeated pleural fluid cytologic studies should also be done. If after all these studies the diagnosis is still not clear, video-assisted thoracoscopy (Chapter 25)

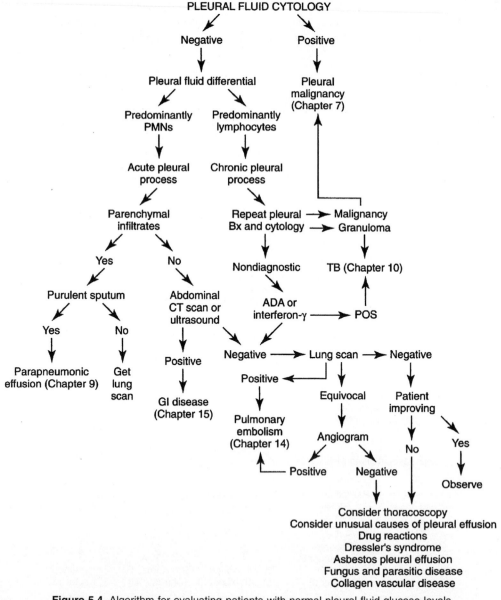

Figure 5.4. Algorithm for evaluating patients with normal pleural fluid glucose levels.

should be performed if the infiltrate is worsening or the effusion is increasing in size.

The patient with an exudative pleural effusion with predominantly polymorphonuclear leukocytes and without parenchymal infiltrates most likely has pulmonary embolus, viral infection, gastrointestinal disease, asbestos pleural effusion, malignant pleural disease, or acute tuberculous pleuritis. Accordingly, a lung scan and a CT scan or an ultrasonic examination of the abdomen should be obtained, and a careful history should be taken for asbestos exposure. If these tests are nondiagnostic and a second thoracentesis reveals predominantly mononuclear cells with a lower pleural fluid LDH than on the original thoracentesis, the patient probably has a viral infection and can be observed. The diagnosis of tuberculous pleuritis must be excluded, however (see Chapter 10).

The patient with an exudative pleural effusion with predominantly mononuclear cells in the pleural fluid has a chronic process involving the pleural space. Malignant disease, pulmonary embolization, and tuberculosis are the three most common causes of this picture. An elevated level of adenosine deaminase (ADA) activity (more than 70 IU/L) or interferon-γ in the pleural fluid essentially establishes the diagnosis of tuberculous pleuritis (see Chapter 4). If these tests are not diagnostic of tuberculosis, the patient should be subjected to a needle biopsy of the pleura in conjunction with a repeat pleural fluid cytology. The pleural biopsy specimen should be cultured for mycobacteria, and the patient should have a purified protein derivative (PPD) skin test. If the PPD is positive the patient should be treated for tuberculosis (see Chapter 10). If these tests are nondiagnostic, a lung scan should be obtained to rule out pulmonary embolization. If an infiltrate is present on the chest radiograph, bronchoscopic examination with transbronchial lung biopsy should also be performed.

Unusual Exudative Effusions

In many patients, no definite diagnosis is established when the diagnostic tests outlined in the previous section have been completed. In such cases, more unusual causes of

pleural effusion should be considered. Every patient with an undiagnosed pleural effusion should have a lung scan to rule out pulmonary embolization. In the patient with predominantly polymorphonuclear leukocytes persisting in the pleural fluid and without parenchymal infiltrates, the diagnosis of intrahepatic or subphrenic abscess should be pursued. Patients should be carefully questioned regarding asbestos exposure or the ingestion of drugs that produce a pleural effusion either directly (see Chapter 17) or by drug-induced lupus (see Table 16.1). A history of a recent (within 12 months) myocardial infarction or a cardiac operation suggests Dressler's syndrome (see Chapter 18). An elevated creatinine level implicates uremia, whereas yellow nails or lymphedema suggests the yellow nail syndrome (see Chapter 18). A chronic pleural effusion with negative pleural pressures during thoracentesis indicate a trapped lung (see Chapter 18).

Undiagnosed Pleural Effusion

If no diagnosis has been obtained after an initial diagnostic thoracentesis, a repeat diagnostic thoracentesis with pleural biopsy, and a perfusion lung scan, how aggressive should one be in pursuing a diagnosis? Poe and co-workers (14) followed 143 patients seen at a community teaching hospital in New York for 12 to 72 months after the initial pleural biopsy was nondiagnostic. Thirty of the 143 patients (21%) were eventually shown to have malignant disease (29 patients) or tuberculosis (1 patient). In all 29 patients who had malignant disease, the neoplasm was strongly suspected by clinical criteria such as weight loss, constitutional symptoms, or a history of a previous cancer. Leslie and Kinasewitz (15) reported similar findings in 53 patients with nonspecific pleuritis on the pleural biopsy specimen. None of their 53 patients had evidence of either granulomatous infection or intrapleural malignancy during a mean follow-up period of 33 months.

With the results of the foregoing two series in mind, my approach to the patient with an undiagnosed pleural effusion after the initial diagnostic thoracentesis, a repeat diagnostic thoracentesis with pleural biopsy, and a negative perfusion lung scan, is as follows. This approach is in part based on the knowledge that the diagnosis that one is most likely to establish is malignant disease, and virtually all patients with pleural malignancy are incurable. Moreover, if a pleural malignancy is present, the diagnosis will soon become apparent, and the delay in diagnosis probably is of little consequence to the patient.

One must rule out the diagnosis of tuberculous pleuritis (see Chapter 10). If the PPD is positive, I will treat the patient with two antituberculous drugs for 6 months. If the PPD is negative, I will repeat the PPD in 6 weeks. If it has converted at this time, I will then treat the patient for tuberculosis. I will also treat the patient for tuberculosis if the pleural fluid ADA is above 70 IU/L or if the pleural fluid interferon-γ levels are markedly elevated.

If the patient appears to be improving clinically, my approach is conservative. I am guided by the patient's symptoms, chest x-ray findings, and the level of LDH in the pleural fluid. If the patient's symptoms are decreasing and if the chest x-ray is improving, I am content to observe the patient. One parameter to follow is the level of LDH in the pleural fluid, because it accurately reflects the level of inflammation in the pleural space. If with successive thoracenteses the pleural fluid LDH decreases, then the process is resolving.

If the patient is not doing well clinically, a more aggressive approach may be indicated. Increases in the patient's symptoms, the amount of fluid on the chest x-ray, or the level of LDH in the pleural fluid are indications that there is progression of the process in the pleural space. Another indication for an aggressive approach is the patient who is desperate to have the cause of his pleural disease defined. The three alternatives to be considered are a repeat needle biopsy of the pleura, thoracoscopy, or an open thoracotomy. In general the next procedure of choice is video-assisted thoracoscopy. Thoracoscopy is particularly good at establishing the diagnosis of malignancy, including mesothelioma. Alternately, a thoracotomy with open pleural biopsy can be performed. In my opinion, thoracoscopy is preferred because there is at least equal visualization and less morbidity than with the thoracotomy.

REFERENCES

1. Marel M, Arustova M, Stasny B, Light RW: Incidence of pleural effusion in a well-defined region: epidemiologic study in central Bohemia. Chest 1993;104:1486–1489.
2. Chakko SC, Caldwell SH, Sforza PP: Treatment of congestive heart failure: its effect on pleural fluid chemistry. Chest 1989;95:978–982.
3. Shinto RA, Light RW: The Effects of Diuresis upon the Characteristics of Pleural Fluid in Patients with Congestive Heart Failure. Am J Med 1990;88:230–233.
4. Light RW, MacGregor MI, Luchsinger PC, Ball WC: Pleural effusions: the diagnostic separation of transudates and exudates. Ann Intern Med 1972;77:507–513.
5. Peterman TA, Speicher CE: Evaluating pleural effusion: a two-stage laboratory approach. JAMA 1984;252:1051–1053.
6. Hamm H, Brohan U, Bohmer R, Missmahl HP: Cholesterol in pleural effusions: a diagnostic aid. Chest 1987;92:296–302.
7. Valdes L, Pose A, Suarez J, Gonzalez-Juanatey JR, Sarandeses A, San Jose E, Alvarez Dobana JM, Salgueiro M, Rodriguez Sudrez JR: Cholesterol: A useful parameter for distinguishing between pleural exudates and transudates. Chest 1991;99:1097–1102.
8. Roth BJ, O'Meara TF, Cragun WH: The serum-effusion albumin gradient in the evaluation of pleural effusions. Chest 1990;98:546–549.
9. Meisel S, Shamiss A, Thaler M, Nussinovitch N, Rosenthal T: Pleural fluid to serum bilirubin concentration ratio for the separation of transudates from exudates. Chest 1990;98:141–144.
10. Romero S, Candela A, Martin C, Hernandez L, Trigo C, Gil J: Evaluation of different criteria for the separation of pleural transudates from exudates. Chest 1993;104:399–404.
11. Burgess LJ, Maritz FJ, Taljaard FFJ: Comparative analysis of the biochemical parameters used to distinguish between pleural transudates and exudates. Chest 1995, in press.
12. Light RW, Erozan YS, Ball WC: Cells in pleural fluid: their value in differential diagnosis. Arch Intern Med 1973;132:854–860.
13. Light RW, Ball WC: Glucose and amylase in pleural effusions. JAMA 1973;225:257–260.
14. Poe RH, Israel RM, Utell MJ, et al: Sensitivity, specificity, and predictive values of closed pleural biopsy. Arch Intern Med 1984;144:325–328.
15. Leslie WK, Kinasewitz GT: Clinical characteristics of the patient with nonspecific pleuritis. Chest 1988;94:603–608.

CHAPTER 6

Transudative Pleural Effusions

Transudative pleural effusions occur when the systemic factors influencing the formation and absorption of pleural fluids are altered so that pleural fluid accumulates. In this chapter, the various causes of transudative pleural effusions are discussed.

CONGESTIVE HEART FAILURE

Congestive heart failure is probably the most common cause of pleural effusion. The reason for the low incidence of pleural effusions secondary to heart failure in most studies is that researchers interested in pleural effusions usually do not see most patients with pleural effusions of this origin. In a recent epidemiological study from the Czech Republic, congestive heart failure was the most common cause of pleural effusion (1). The incidence of pleural effusions in congestive heart failure is high. Logue and colleagues (2) reported that 58% of 114 patients with left ventricular failure had pleural effusions. Race and associates (3) reviewed the autopsies at the Mayo Clinic between 1948 and 1953 of 402 patients who had had congestive heart failure during life. The researchers found that 290 of the patients (72%) had pleural effusions with volumes greater than 250 ml. Of the patients with pleural effusions, 88% had bilateral pleural effusions, whereas 8% and 4% had unilateral right- and left-sided effusions, respectively (3).

Pathophysiology

In recent years concepts of pleural fluid formation and resorption in patients with heart failure have undergone significant modifications. In the past, it was believed that the pleural fluid that accumulated in patients with congestive heart failure was due to increased pressure in the capillaries in the visceral or the parietal pleura. These increased pressures were thought to result in an increased entry of fluid into the pleural space from the parietal pleura and a decreased removal of fluid through the visceral pleura according to Starling's equation.

The current theories on pleural fluid formation and resorption give us a different entry pathway and a different exit pathway for pleural fluid in patients with congestive heart failure. It appears that the majority of the fluid that enters the pleural space in patients with congestive heart failure comes from the alveolar capillaries rather than the pleural capillaries (4). When the pressure in the pulmonary capillaries is elevated, increased amounts of fluid enter the interstitial spaces of the lung. The increased fluid in the interstitial spaces results in an increased interstitial pressure in the subpleural interstitial spaces (5). The fluid then moves from the pulmonary interstitial spaces across the visceral pleura into the pleural space. There appears to be relatively little resistance to fluid movement from the pulmonary interstitial spaces across the visceral pleura (4). In sheep with pulmonary edema from volume overloading, approximately 25% of the pulmonary edema fluid exits the lung through the visceral pleura (6).

Presently, it is believed that almost all fluid exits the pleural space through the lymphatics in the parietal pleura rather than by passively diffusing across the visceral pleura (see Chapter 2). Pleural fluid accumulates in patients with congestive heart failure when the rate of entry of fluid into the pleural space exceeds the capability of the lymphatics in the parietal pleura to remove the fluid. In normal sheep, the capacity of the lymphatics to remove fluid is approximately 0.28 ml/kg/hour (7). If there is elevated pressure in the systemic veins, the lymphatic clearance is decreased (8).

In the clinical situation, it appears that the accumulation of pleural fluid in patients with congestive heart failure is related more to left ventricular failure than to right ventricular failure. Wiener-Kronish and associates (9) prospectively evaluated 37 patients admitted to a coronary care unit with congestive heart failure secondary to ischemic heart disease or to cardiomyopathy. They found that 19 patients had a pleural effusion and the mean wedge pressure in the patients with effusion (24.1 ± 1.3 mm Hg) was significantly higher than this pressure in those without effusion (17.2 ± 1.5 mm Hg). There also was a greater likelihood of finding pleural effusions if severe rather than mild pulmonary edema was found roentgenographically. In a subsequent study (10), these same researchers were unable to demonstrate any pleural effusions in 27 patients with chronic pulmonary hypertension or chronically elevated right atrial pressures.

In summary, it appears that pleural fluid accumulates in patients with congestive heart failure when they have left ventricular failure. The high pressures in the pulmonary capillaries lead to increased amounts of fluid in the interstitial spaces. The fluid in the interstitial spaces enters the pleural space through the highly permeable visceral pleura. Fluid accumulates when the entry of fluid overwhelms the capacity of the lymphatics in the parietal pleura to remove the fluid. Some fluid may enter the pleural space from the capillaries in either pleural surface. Elevation of the systemic venous pressure may decrease the lymphatic clearance from the pleural space.

Clinical Manifestations

Pleural effusions due to congestive heart failure are usually associated with other manifestations of that disease. The patient often has a history of increasing dyspnea on exertion, increasing peripheral edema, and orthopnea or paroxysmal nocturnal dyspnea. The dyspnea is frequently out of proportion to the size of the effusion. Physical examination usually reveals signs of both right-sided heart failure with distended neck veins and peripheral edema and left-sided heart failure with rales and an S3 ventricular gallop as well as signs of the pleural effusion(s).

The chest radiograph almost always reveals cardiomegaly and usually bilateral pleural effusions. Congestive heart failure is by far the most common cause of bilateral pleural effusions, but if cardiomegaly is not present, an alternate explanation should be sought. In a series (11) of 78 patients with bilateral pleural effusions but a normal-sized heart, only 3 (4%) were due to congestive heart failure. Although in the past it was thought that pleural effusions due to congestive heart failure were commonly unilateral on the right or at least were much larger on the right side, such does not appear to be the case. In the autopsy series of Race and colleagues (3), 88% of the patients studied had bilateral pleural effusions. Moreover, the mean volume of pleural fluid in the right pleural space (1084 ml) was only slightly greater than the mean volume of pleural fluid in the left pleural space (913 ml). In this series, 35 patients had unilateral pleural effusions, and of these 35 patients, 16 (46%) had either pulmonary embolism or pneumonia (3). When two series (12, 13) comprising 124 patients are combined, 100 patients (81%) had bilateral pleural effusions, 15 (12%) had unilateral right-sided effusions, and 9 (7%) had unilateral left-sided effusions. Therefore, the presence of a unilateral pleural effusion or of bilateral pleural effusions of disparate size is an indication to search for other causes of the effusion.

Diagnosis

The diagnosis of pleural effusions secondary to congestive heart failure comes readily to mind every time a patient is seen with congestive heart failure. One must be careful to avoid the trap of ascribing the pleural effusion to congestive heart failure when it has another cause. In the series of Race and coworkers (3), over 25% of the patients with congestive heart failure and pleural effusions had either pulmonary emboli or pneumonia at autopsy. Certainly if the patient is febrile, has pleural effusions that are greatly disparate in size, has a unilateral pleural effusion, has pleuritic chest pain, or does not have cardiomegaly, a diagnostic thoracentesis should be performed.

If the patient has cardiomegaly and bilateral pleural effusions, is afebrile and does not have pleuritic chest pain, we initiate treatment of the congestive heart failure and observe the patient to see if the pleural fluid is resorbed. If the effusions do not disappear within a few days, we then perform a diagnostic thoracentesis. One problem with this approach is that with diuresis the characteristics of the pleural fluid may change from those of a transudate to those of an exudate. Chakko and coworkers (14) treated 9 patients with congestive heart failure for a mean of 6 days and found that in 3 of the 9 patients a pleural fluid that was a transudate initially developed the characteristics of an exudate. We performed a similar study (15) on 12 patients in whom the repeat thoracentesis was performed 12 to 48 hours after diuresis was initiated and found that in only 1 patient had the characteristics of the pleural fluid become exudative. In those patients whose pleural fluid developed exudative characteristics the protein ratio was 0.62 or less, the LDH ratio was less than 1.00 and the LDH level was less than 250 U/L.

The pleural fluid from a patient with congestive heart failure is typically a transudate with a ratio of pleural fluid to serum protein below 0.5, a ratio of pleural fluid to serum LDH under 0.6, and an absolute pleural fluid LDH level below two-thirds the upper limit of normal for serum (16). If the foregoing criteria are satisfied in a patient with congestive heart failure, the patient has a transudative pleural effusion that can be ascribed to the congestive heart failure, and no further diagnostic studies are indicated. Such transudative pleural effusions may be blood-tinged, and the pleural fluid differential cell count may reveal predominantly polymorphonuclear leukocytes, small lymphocytes, or other mononuclear cells (17). If the foregoing criteria are not satisfied but congestive heart failure appears to be the likely explanation for the pleural effusion, the pleural fluid to serum albumin gradient should be examined. If this gradient is greater than 1.2 gm/dl, the pleural effusion in all probability is due to the congestive heart failure and additional diagnostic studies are not indicated (18). If the protein and LDH criteria are not met and the albumin gradient is less than 1.2 gm/dl, the pleural effusion is not due to the heart failure. Rather, the patient has an exudative pleural effusion, and further diagnostic tests such as pleural fluid cytologic study, lung scans, and pleural biopsy should be performed.

Treatment

The preferred treatment of pleural effusion secondary to heart failure is with digitalis, diuretics, and afterload reduction. When the heart failure is successfully managed, the pleural effusion disappears. Occasionally, large pleural effusions cause patients to be initially dyspneic. The removal of 500 to 1000 ml pleural fluid from such persons may rapidly relieve the symptoms.

Patients with large pleural effusions and refractory heart failure sometimes receive symptomatic relief from therapeutic thoracentesis. In such patients, pleurodesis with a sclerosing agent may be considered. Spicer and Fisher (18) reported symptomatic relief lasting at least 8 months in a patient following pleurodesis with silver nitrate. In the past 12 years, I have attempted pleurodesis with tetracycline or a tetracycline derivative in 8 such patients. In 5 patients, pleurodesis brought about several months of symptomatic relief. At the present time we recommend minocycline or doxycycline at a dose of 5 mg/kg or 5 g of talc in a slurry (19) as the sclerosing agent in this situation. Bleomycin is not recommended in this situation since it is not an effective agent in the rabbit model with normal pleura (20).

An alternative approach is to use a pleuroperitoneal shunt. The shunt consists of two catheters connected with a valved pump chamber. The two one-way valves in the pump chamber are positioned such that fluid can only flow from the pleural space to the peritoneal cavity through the pump chamber. Since the pleural pressure is almost always more negative than the peritoneal pressure, the pumping chamber must be used to move fluid from the pleural cavity to the peritoneal cavity. Little and coworkers reported that 2 patients with refractory pleural effusions secondary to congestive heart failure were managed successfully with the pleuroperitoneal shunt (21).

HEPATIC HYDROTHORAX

Pleural effusions occur occasionally as a complication of hepatic cirrhosis. Pleural effusions usually occur only when ascitic fluid is present. Lieberman and associates (22) reviewed 330 patients with cirrhosis and ascites and found that 18 (5.5%) had pleural effusions; Johnston and Loo found that 6% of 200 patients with cirrhosis had pleural effusions. In the second series, none of the 54 patients with cirrhosis without ascites had a pleural effusion (23). In some patients the ascites is not clinically evident, but it can almost always be demonstrated with ultrasonography (24). The pleural effusion in patients with cirrhosis and ascites is usually right-sided (67%), but occasionally is left-sided (16%) or bilateral (16%) (22, 23).

Pathophysiology

Patients with cirrhosis frequently have decreased plasma oncotic pressure (23), and from Figure 2.1 one might hypothesize that the pleural effusions arise because of it. Indeed, in the experimental animal, the induction of decreased plasma oncotic pressure leads to the accumulation of pleural fluid (25). This mechanism does not appear to be the predominant cause of pleural effusions in patients with cirrhosis and ascites, however. Rather, the pleural effusions appear to be produced by movement of the ascitic fluid from the peritoneal cavity into the pleural cavity.

Johnston and Loo (23) demonstrated that after the intraperitoneal injection of India ink, cells in the pleural fluid contained many carbon particles, whereas cells in the peripheral blood contained none. In addition, after the intravenous injection of radiolabeled albumin, the albumin first appeared in the peritoneal fluid and then in the pleural fluid. Following the intraperitoneal injection of radiolabeled albumin, the concentration of the labeled protein was greater in the pleural fluid than in the plasma; after intrapleural injection, the labeled protein appeared in the plasma before it appeared in the peritoneal fluid (23). Because no air entered the pleural space following the intraperitoneal injection of carbon dioxide in 1 patient, these researchers concluded that the pleural effusion arose from the transfer of ascitic fluid from the peritoneal to the pleural space by the lymphatic vessels. This conclusion appears to have been incorrect. Datta and colleagues (26) injected radiolabeled human serum albumin into the peritoneal cavity of a patient with ascites and a large pleural effusion. They were able to demonstrate that when the labeled protein was picked up into the lymphatic system in the diaphragm, it flowed into normal mediastinal lymphatic channels and from them into the subclavian vein. It did not enter the pleural space.

Studies by Lieberman and colleagues (22) suggest that fluid passes directly from the peritoneal to the pleural cavity through pores in the diaphragm. These researchers introduced 500 to 1000 ml air into the peritoneal cavity of 5 patients with cirrhosis, ascites, and pleural effusions. In all 5 patients, a pneumothorax developed 1 to 48 hours after the induction of the pneumoperitoneum. Thoracoscopic examination was performed in 3 other patients after the induction of the pneumoperitoneum, and in 1 of these patients, air bubbles were seen coming through an otherwise undetectable diaphragmatic defect (22). At postmortem examination, diaphragmatic defects were demonstrated in 2 of the patients (22). More recently Mouroux and coworkers (27) were able to visualize the defects in 4 patients during thoracoscopy.

From the foregoing studies, it is evident that the pleural fluid in these patients originates from the ascitic fluid. It is probable that the fluid passes directly into the pleural space through defects in the diaphragm. In the patient with tense ascites and increased intraabdominal pressure, the diaphragm may be stretched, causing microscopic defects. The increased hydrostatic pressure in the ascitic fluid results in a one-way transfer of fluid from the peritoneal to the pleural cavity. In some patients, transfer of ascitic fluid across the diaphragm by the lymphatic vessels may be important in the production of the pleural effusion. My experience with the placement of chest tubes in such patients leads me to believe that the direct movement of fluid is the dominant mechanism. In order to control the symptoms from large hydrothoraces in several patients with cirrhosis and ascites, I have performed tube thoracostomy followed by the injection of a sclerosing agent. In each instance, the placement of the chest tube was

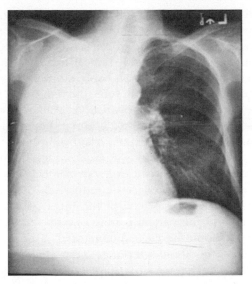

Figure 6.1. Posteroanterior chest radiograph demonstrating a large right pleural effusion. This patient with massive ascites suddenly developed shortness of breath. A previous chest radiograph (see Figure 3.4) had suggested a subpulmonic pleural effusion.

followed by rapid (within minutes) diminution in the amount of ascites.

Clinical Manifestations

Patients with pleural effusions from cirrhosis and ascites have clinical pictures dominated by the cirrhosis and ascites. At times, these patients develop acute dyspnea in association with large pleural effusions. Although the pleural effusions may be small to moderate in size, frequently they are large and occupy the entire hemithorax (Fig. 6.1). The large effusions probably occur because the diaphragmatic defect permits fluid to flow from the peritoneal into the pleural cavity until the pleural pressure approaches the peritoneal pressure. Indeed, the pleural pressures in patients with pleural effusions secondary to ascites are higher than in patients with other transudative pleural effusions (28).

Diagnosis

The diagnosis of pleural effusion secondary to cirrhosis and ascites is usually easy. Both a paracentesis and a thoracentesis should be performed to ascertain that the ascites and pleural fluid are compatible with the diagnosis and do not have high polymorphonuclear cell counts. The pleural fluid protein level is usually higher than the ascitic fluid protein level (22), but is still below 3.0 g/dl, and the pleural fluid LDH is low. The pleural fluid is occasionally blood-tinged or is frankly bloody, but such findings have no significance and are probably due to the patient's poor coagulation status. The differential cell count may reveal predominantly polymorphonuclear leukocytes, small lymphocytes, or other mononuclear cells. Amylase levels should be determined and cytologic examination should be performed on both fluid specimens to rule out pancreatic ascites or malignant disease.

In patients with cirrhosis, ascites and pleural effusion, it is important to be aware of the possibility of spontaneous bacterial empyema, which is somewhat analogous to the spontaneous bacterial peritonitis that occurs in these patients (29). If the pleural fluid polymorphonuclear cell count exceeds 500 cells/mm^3, the diagnosis of spontaneous bacterial empyema is strongly suggested (29). Xiol and coworkers (29) reported on 11 episodes of spontaneous bacterial empyemas in 8 patients. All but one of the patients had concomitant spontaneous bacterial peritonitis. The organism most commonly responsible for the spontaneous bacterial empyema is *Escherichia coli* (29).

Patients with spontaneous bacterial empyema should be treated with appropriate antibiotics, but it does not appear that tube thoracostomy is necessary (29).

Treatment

The management of pleural effusions associated with cirrhosis and ascites should be directed toward treatment of the ascites because the hydrothorax is an extension of the peritoneal fluid. The patient should be put on a low salt diet, and diuretics should be administered. The best diuretic therapy appears to be the combination of furosemide and spironolactone. The initial starting dose is 40 mg furosemide and 100 mg spironolactone. This combination appears to have the optimal ratio for the two diuretics. The doses can be increased up to 160 mg furosemide and 400 mg spironolactone daily (30). Serial therapeutic thoracenteses are not indicated because the pleural fluid rapidly reaccumulates. In addition, serial thoracenteses further deplete the patient's body protein. If the pleural fluid has a protein level of 2.5 g/dl, a therapeutic thoracentesis of 2000 ml will remove 50 g protein.

Certain patients are refractory to salt restriction and diuretics and remain symptomatic from the presence of the large pleural effusion. In such patients there are four alternatives: (*a*) tube thoracostomy followed by the injection of a sclerosing agent such as talc to effect a pleurodesis, (*b*) implantation of a peritoneal-to-venous shunt device, (*c*) thoracoscopy with the insufflation of talc, or (*d*) thoracotomy with surgical repair of the diaphragmatic leak.

Falchuk and coworkers (31) reported the successful control of a hydrothorax in 2 patients after a pleurodesis was effected by the intrapleural injection of tetracycline. The chest radiograph of a patient we treated successfully with tetracycline is shown in Figure 6.2. Tube thoracostomy with pleural sclerosis can be dangerous to the patient. Runyon and coworkers (32) reported 2 patients in whom chest tube placement led to massive protein and

electrolyte depletion and death. These authors concluded that chest tube insertion is relatively contraindicated in the patient with hepatic hydrothorax, and surgical repair of the diaphragmatic leak is probably the preferable mode of treatment. If tube thoracostomy is performed in a patient with a large amount of ascites, it is important to observe the patient carefully after the tube has been inserted because the amount of ascites rapidly decreases and may lead to hypovolemia. Therefore, if this procedure is performed, the patient should be placed in the intensive care unit, and the patient's urine output and vital signs should be closely monitored. If the patient's condition deteriorates, the chest tube should be temporarily clamped to allow equilibration, and one should consider administering fluids and salt-free albumin intravenously.

Although implantation of a peritoneojugular shunt might at first glance appear to be a good alternative in the management of hepatic hydrothorax, shunts frequently do not control the pleural effusion. The explanation for the ineffectiveness of the shunt has to do with the pressure differences among the peritoneal cavity, the pleural space, and the systemic veins. Because the pleural pressure is less than the central venous pressure, fluid will preferentially move to the pleural space rather than to the central veins (33).

Thoracoscopy may have a role in the management of patients with hepatic hydrothorax. Vargas and coworkers (34) have recently reported that the insufflation of 2 g of talc at the time of thoracoscopy controlled the pleural effusion in 5 of 6 patients with cirrhosis and ascites. The 6th patient had a recurrence of the effusion shortly after the insufflation, but after a second insufflation had no subsequent recurrence. Mouroux and associates (27) have recently reported that thoracoscopy with the application of biological glue to the diaphragmatic defects controlled hepatic hydrothorax in 4 of 4 patients. Since these researchers administered talc concomitantly with the biological glue, the relative roles of the two agents in preventing the reaccumulation of the pleural fluid are unclear.

The most aggressive approach in the management of hepatic hydrothorax is to perform a thoracotomy, repair the diaphragmatic de-

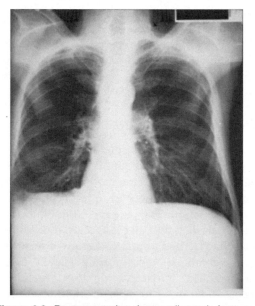

Figure 6.2. Posteroanterior chest radiograph from patient with the massive hepatic hydrothorax in Figure 6.1 after a pleurodesis was effected by the intrapleural injection of tetracycline. At the time this radiograph was obtained, the patient had tense ascites and peripheral edema; however, the patient has had no recurrence of his pleural effusion during 8 months of follow-up.

fects, and abrade the pleural surface in an attempt to effect a pleurodesis (24). This aggressive approach carries a significant risk to the patient with severe underlying medical problems. Fluid balance may also be a problem following surgery. In 1 patient the initial postoperative chest tube output was 14 L/day (24).

PLEURAL EFFUSION AS A COMPLICATION OF PERCUTANEOUS TRANSHEPATIC CORONARY VEIN OCCLUSION

Patients with bleeding esophageal varices are sometimes managed by injecting Gelfoam or other materials transhepatically into the coronary vein, in the hope that the injected material will lodge in the esophageal veins and will stop the bleeding. To perform this procedure, the liver is entered through the diaphragm (35). In at least 1 patient, a large pleural effusion requiring tube thoracostomy developed following this procedure (35). On several occasions I have observed that pleural fluid rapidly accumulates after this procedure in patients who had ascites before the procedure. I hypothesize that the pleural effusion arose because the iatrogenic diaphragmatic defect allowed the ascitic fluid to flow into the pleural space. Pleural effusions may also appear by the same mechanism after percutaneous transhepatic cholangiography.

PERITONEAL DIALYSIS

During the past 15 years, there has been an increasing use of continuous ambulatory peritoneal dialysis (CAPD) in the treatment of chronic renal failure. Pleural effusions can result from CAPD due to the movement of the dialysate from the peritoneal cavity into the pleural cavity via a mechanism similar to that with cirrhosis and ascites. Nomoto and coworkers (36) reviewed 3195 patients on CAPD from 161 medical centers in Japan. They reported that 1.6% developed this complication secondary to movement of the dialysate from the peritoneal cavity through the diaphragm into the pleural space (36). The effusion developed within 30 days of initiating the dialysis in 50% of the patients, but 18% had been on dialysis for more than a year before the effu-

sion developed (36). The pleural effusion is right-sided about 90% of the time, but can be bilateral or left-sided (36). Pleural effusions can also develop as a complication of acute peritoneal dialysis (37).

The diagnosis of a pleural effusion secondary to peritoneal dialysis is usually very easy. The pleural fluid in these patients is characterized by a glucose level intermediate between that of the dialysate and the serum, a protein level below 1.0 g/dl, and a low LDH.

When a patient on peritoneal dialysis develops a pleural effusion, the dialysis usually must be stopped. If further peritoneal dialysis is deemed appropriate, there are two approaches. First, a tube thoracostomy can be performed with instillation of a sclerosing agent such as a tetracycline derivative or talc (38). If this approach is taken, small-volume peritoneal dialysis can be performed for 10 to 14 days during which the pleurodesis is done (38). The second approach is an attempt to close the pleuroperitoneal communication surgically. At the time of thoracotomy, two to three liters of dialysate are rapidly run into the peritoneal cavity and the diaphragm is inspected for seepage through holes or blisters. Sites of leakage are repaired using nonabsorbable sutures reinforced with Teflon felt patches (39).

OTHER CAUSES OF TRANSUDATIVE PLEURAL EFFUSIONS

Nephrotic Syndrome

Pleural effusion is common in patients with the nephrotic syndrome. In a study of 52 patients (40), 21% had pleural effusions. With the nephrotic syndrome, the pleural effusions are usually bilateral and are frequently infrapulmonary in location (40). Pleural effusions arise because the decreased plasma oncotic pressure upsets the normal equilibrium, as shown in Figure 2.1.

The diagnosis of pleural effusion secondary to the nephrotic syndrome is not difficult in the typical clinical situation. A diagnostic thoracentesis should be performed to ascertain that the pleural fluid is indeed a transudate. One should always consider the possibility of pulmonary emboli in patients with the nephrotic syndrome and pleural effusion. In one series of 36 patients with the nephrotic syndrome, 22% had pulmonary emboli (41). In addition, the nephrotic syndrome may be due to or complicated by renal vein thrombosis, and in such instances, the incidence of pulmonary emboli is high (41). A lung scan should be obtained in all patients with the nephrotic syndrome and pleural effusion. If the lung scan is equivocal, evidence for deep venous thrombosis should be sought with venograms, impedance plethysmograms, or a pulmonary arteriogram.

The treatment of the pleural effusion associated with the nephrotic syndrome should be aimed at decreasing the protein loss in the urine in order to increase the plasma protein. This is best accomplished by administering angiotensin-converting enzyme inhibitors, lowering the protein content of the diet, and using nonsteroidal antiinflammatory agents cautiously (42). Serial therapeutic thoracenteses should not be performed because they only further deplete the protein stores. In selected individuals who are symptomatic from the pleural effusion, one should consider a pleurodesis with a sclerosing agent such as talc.

Superior Vena Caval Obstruction

In sheep, elevation of the pressure in the superior vena cava will lead to the accumulation of pleural fluid. Allen and coworkers (8) demonstrated that once the pressure in the superior vena cava was elevated above 15 mm Hg, pleural fluid accumulated. The higher the pressure in the superior vena cava, the greater the fluid accumulation. The fluid was transudative in that the ratio of the pleural fluid to serum protein was less than 0.5. These workers attributed the pleural fluid formation to either lymph leakage out of the lymphatics that pass through the chest or obstruction of lung and/or chest lymphatics with subsequent leakage of interstitial fluid into the pleural space.

In the clinical situation most patients that have superior vena caval obstruction do not have a pleural effusion. If such a patient has a pleural effusion, one should try to exclude other causes such as malignant disease involving the pleura. In neonates, however, superior vena caval thrombosis is associated with the development of bilateral pleural effusions. Dhande and colleagues (43) reported a series

of 5 babies who developed superior vena caval obstruction as a complication of the use of central venous catheters. The effusions occurred 7 to 19 days after the initial placement or change of a central venous catheter. All required repeated thoracenteses to remove pleural fluid that accumulated at a rate of up to 200 ml/kg/day. The fluid was a clear transudate (protein level 1.2 to 2.2 g/dl), but became chylous when feedings were given. These workers attributed the pleural fluid accumulation to obstruction of thoracic lymph flow into the venous system.

Fontan Procedure

With the Fontan procedure the right ventricle is bypassed by an anastomosis between the superior vena cava, the right atrium, or the inferior vena cava and the pulmonary artery (44). The procedure is typically performed for tricuspid atresia or univentricular heart. Pleural effusion appears to be a significant problem after the Fontan procedure. The development of the effusions postoperatively in these patients is probably related to the increased systemic venous pressure. It is unclear, however, whether increased pleural fluid transudation from the parietal pleura, decreased lymphatic clearance from the pleural space, or lymphatic leakage into the pleural space is responsible for the large accumulations of pleural fluid. Zellers and associates (45) analyzed pleural fluid formation after this procedure on 46 patients. They reported that the median amount of pleural drainage was 3220 ml with a range of 155 to 31,000 ml. Most of the patients had pleural drainage from both sides. The mean duration of the pleural fluid drainage was 14 days. The intrapleural administration of tetracycline at the end of the surgical procedure had no effect on the amount or the duration of the fluid drainage (45). In patients who have markedly prolonged pleural fluid drainage, consideration should be given to the implantation of a pleuroperitoneal shunt (46).

Urinothorax

Pleural effusion can develop when there is retroperitoneal urinary leakage secondary to urinary obstruction, trauma, retroperitoneal inflammatory or malignant processes, failed nephrostomy, or kidney biopsy (47, 48). Such a pleural fluid accumulation is called a urinothorax. This is a rare cause of pleural effusions; only 21 cases had been reported by 1986 (48). The pleural effusion tends to develop within hours after the precipitating event and dissipates rapidly once the obstruction is relieved. It is believed that the urine moves retroperitoneally into the pleural space.

The diagnosis is usually easy if it is considered. The pleural fluid looks and smells like urine and has the biochemical characteristics of a transudate. Confirmation of the diagnosis can be obtained with simultaneous measurements of the pleural fluid and creatinine levels. Only with urinothorax is the pleural fluid creatinine greater than the serum creatinine (49). The pleural fluid with a urinothorax at times has a low pH (50) or a low glucose level (49), both uncommon features with a transudative pleural effusion.

Glomerulonephritis

Patients with acute glomerulonephritis frequently have pleural effusions. In a series of 76 children, 42 (55%) had pleural effusions (51). The pleural effusions are transudative and are probably due to increased intravascular pressures because most patients have cardiomegaly or peripheral edema in addition to the pleural effusions.

Myxedema

Pleural effusions occasionally occur as a complication of myxedema. In one review of 128 patients with hypothyroidism from the Massachusetts General Hospital and the Medical University of South Carolina, pleural effusion occurred in 28 patients, but the pleural effusion was felt to be due to the hypothyroidism in only 6 patients (52). In 1 of these 6 patients the pleural effusion was felt to be secondary to a myxedematous pericardial effusion, while in the other five there was no evidence of pericardial disease. When the pleural effusion occurs simultaneously with a pericardial effusion, the pleural fluid is usually a transudate (53). The isolated pleural effusion secondary to hypothyroidism can be either an exudate or a transudate (52). The diagnosis is one of exclusion in a patient with hypothyroid-

ism. The obvious treatment for pleural effusions associated with myxedema is thyroid replacement.

Meigs' Syndrome

Although the pleural fluid associated with Meigs' syndrome (benign ovarian tumors with ascites and pleural effusion) is often considered a transudate (54), the pleural fluid protein levels are usually above 3.5 g/dl, (55, 56) and therefore the effusions are exudates. Accordingly, this syndrome is further discussed in Chapter 18.

Pulmonary Embolus

About 20% of the pleural effusions that occur with pulmonary embolization are transudates. This condition is discussed in detail in Chapter 14.

Sarcoidosis

This condition is occasionally accompanied by a transudative rather than an exudative pleural effusion (see Chapter 18).

REFERENCES

1. Marel M, Stastny B, Light RW: Incidence of pleural effusion in the Central Bohemia Region. Chest 1993; 104:1486–1489.
2. Logue RB, Rogers JV Jr, Gay BB Jr: Subtle roentgenographic signs of left heart failure. Am Heart J 1963; 65:464–473.
3. Race GA, Scheifley CH, Edwards JE: Hydrothorax in congestive heart failure. Am J Med 1957;22:83–89.
4. Wiener-Kronish JP, Broaddus VC: Interrelationship of pleural and pulmonary interstitial liquid. Annu Rev Physiol 1993;55:209–226.
5. Bhattacharya J, Gropper MA, Staub NC: Interstitial fluid pressure gradient measured by micropuncture in excised dog lung. J Appl Physiol 1984;56:271–277.
6. Broaddus VC, Wiener-Kronish JP, Staub NC: Clearance of lung edema into the pleural space of volume-loaded anesthetized sheep. J Appl Physiol 1990;68; 2623–2630.
7. Broaddus VC, Wiener-Kronish JP, Berthiauma Y, Staub NC: Removal of pleural liquid and protein by lymphatics in awake sheep. J Appl Physiol 1988;64: 384–390.
8. Allen SJ, Laine GA, Drake RE, Gabel JC: Superior vena caval pressure elevation causes pleural effusion formation in sheep. Am J Physiol 1988;255(3 Pt 2):H492–H495.
9. Wiener-Kronish JP, Goldstein R, Matthay RA, et al: Relationship of pleural effusions to pulmonary hemo-

dynamics in patients with congestive heart failure. Am Rev Respir Dis 1985;132:1253-1256.

10. Wiener-Kronish JP, Goldstein R, Matthay RA, et al: Lack of association of pleural effusion with chronic pulmonary arterial and right atrial hypertension. Chest 1987;92:967-970.

11. Rabin CB, Blackman NS: Bilateral pleural effusion: its significance in association with a heart of normal size. J Mt Sinai Hosp 1957;24:45-63.

12. Peterman TA, Brothers SK: Pleural effusions in congestive heart failure and in pericardial disease. N Engl J Med 1983;309:313.

13. Weiss JM, Spodick DH: Laterality of pleural effusions in chronic congestive heart failure. Am J Cardiology 1984;53:951.

14. Chakko SC, Caldwell SH, Sforza PP: Treatment of congestive heart failure: its effect on pleural fluid chemistry. Chest 1989;95:978-982.

15. Shinto RA, Light RW: The effects of diuresis upon the characteristics of pleural fluid in patients with congestive heart failure. Am J Med 1990;88:230-233.

16. Light RW, MacGregor MI, Luchsinger PC, Ball WC: Pleural effusions: the diagnostic separation of transudates and exudates. Ann Intern Med 1972;77:507-513.

17. Light RW, Erozan YS, Ball WC: Cells in pleural fluid: their value in differential diagnosis. Arch Intern Med 1973;132:854-860.

18. Spicer AJ, Fisher JA: Recurring pleural effusion in congestive heart failure treated by pleurodesis. J Ir Med Assoc 1969;62:177-178.

19. Webb WR, Ozmen V, Moulder PV, Shabahang B, Breaux J: Iodized talc pleurodesis for the treatment of pleural effusions. J Thorac Cardiovasc Surg 1992;103:881-885.

20. Vargas FS, Wang N-S, Lee HM, Gruer SE, Sassoon CSH, Light RW: Effectiveness of bleomycin in comparison to tetracycline as pleural sclerosing agent in rabbits. Chest 1993;104:1582-1584.

21. Little AG, Kodowaki MH, Ferguson MK, Staszek VM, Skinner DB: Pleuro-peritoneal shunting. Alternative therapy for pleural effusions. Ann Surg 1988;208:443-450.

22. Lieberman FL, Hidemura R, Peters RL, Reynolds TB: Pathogenesis and treatment of hydrothorax complicating cirrhosis with ascites. Ann Intern Med 1966;64:341-351.

23. Johnston RF, Loo RV: Hepatic hydrothorax: studies to determine the source of the fluid and report of thirteen cases. Ann Intern Med 1964;61:385-401.

24. Rubinstein D, McInnes IE, Dudley FJ: Hepatic hydrothorax in the absence of clinical ascites: diagnosis and management. Gastroenterology 1985;88:188-191.

25. Mellins RB, Levine OR, Fishman AP: Effect of systemic and pulmonary venous hypertension on pleural and pericardial fluid accumulation. J Appl Physiol 1970;29:564-569.

26. Datta N, Mishkin FS, Vasinrapee P, Niden AH: Radionuclide demonstration of peritoneal-pleural communication as a cause for pleural fluid. JAMA 1984;252:210.

27. Mouroux J, Hebuterne X, Perrin C, Venissac N, Benchimol D, Rampal P, Richelme H: Treatment of pleural effusion of cirrhotic origin by videothoracoscopy. Brit J Surg 1994;81:546-547.

28. Light RW, Jenkinson SG, Minh V, George RB: Observations on pleural pressures as fluid is withdrawn during thoracentesis. Am Rev Respir Dis 1980;121:799-804.

29. Xiol X, Castellote J, Baliellas C, Ariza J, Gimenez Roca A, Guardiola J, Casais L: Spontaneous bacterial empyema in cirrhotic patients: analysis of eleven cases. Hepatology 1990;11:365-370.

30. Runyon BA: Care of patients with ascites. N Engl J Med 1994;330:337-342.

31. Falchuk KR, Jacoby I, Colucci WS, Rybak ME: Tetracycline-induced pleural symphysis for recurrent hydrothorax complicating cirrhosis. Gastroenterology 1977;72:319-321.

32. Runyon BA, Greenblatt M, Ming RHC: Hepatic hydrothorax is a relative contraindication to chest tube insertion. Am J Gastroenterol 1986;81:566-567.

33. Ikard RW, Sawyers JL: Persistent hepatic hydrothorax after peritoneojugular shunt. Arch Surg 1980;115:1125-1127.

34. Vargas FS, Milanez JR, Filomeno LT, Fernandez A, Jatene A, Light RW: Intrapleural talc for the prevention of recurrence in benign or undiagnosed pleural effusion. Chest 1994;106:1771-1775.

35. Widrich WC, Johnson WC, Robbins AH, Nabseth DC: Esophagogastric variceal hemorrhage: its treatment by percutaneous transhepatic coronary vein occlusion. Arch Surg 1978;113:1331-1338.

36. Nomoto Y, Suga T, Nakajima K, Sakai H, Osawa G, Ota K, Kawaguchi Y, et al: Acute hydrothorax in continuous ambulatory peritoneal dialysis—A collaborative study of 161 centers. Am J Nephrol 1989;9:363-367.

37. Rudnick MR, Coyle JF, Beck LH, McCurdy DK: Acute massive hydrothorax complicating peritoneal dialysis, report of 2 cases and a review of the literature. Clin Nephrol 1979;12:38-44.

38. Chow CC, Sung JY, Cheung CK, et al: Massive hydrothorax in continuous ambulatory peritoneal dialysis: diagnosis, management and review of the literature. NZ Med J 1988;27:475-477.

39. Allen SM, Matthews HR: Surgical treatment of massive hydrothorax complicating continuous ambulatory peritoneal dialysis. Clin Nephrol 1991;36:299-301.

40. Cavina C, Vichi G: Radiological aspects of pleural effusions in medical nephropathy in children. Ann Radiol Diagn 1958;31:163-202.

41. Llach F, Arieff AI, Massry SG: Renal vein thrombosis and nephrotic syndrome: a prospective study of 36 adult patients. Ann Intern Med 1975;83:8-14.

42. Palmer BF: Southwestern internal medicine conference: nephrotic edema—pathogenesis and treatment. Am J Med Sci 1993;306:53-67.

43. Dhande V, Kattwinkel J, Alford B: Recurrent bilateral pleural effusions secondary to superior vena cava

obstruction as a complication of central venous catheterization. Pediatrics 1983;72:109–113.

44. Laks H, Milliken JC, Perloff JK, et al: Experience with the Fontan procedure. J Thorac Cardiovasc Surg 1984;88:939–951.

45. Zellers TM, Driscoll DJ, Humes RA, Feldt RH, Puga FJ, Danielson GK: Glenn shunt: effect on pleural drainage after modified Fontan operation. J Thorac Cardiovasc Surg 1989;98:725–729.

46. Sade RM, Wiles HB: Pleuroperitoneal shunt for persistent pleural drainage after Fontan procedure. J Thorac Cardiovasc Surg 1990;100:621–623.

47. Belie JA, Milan D: Pleural effusion secondary to ureteral obstruction. Urology 1979;14:27–29.

48. Sulcate JR: Urinothorax: report of 4 cases and review of the literature. J Urol 1986;135:805–808.

49. Stark D, Shades J, Baron RL, Koch D: Biochemical features of urinothorax. Arch Intern Med 1982;142:1509–1511.

50. Miller KS, Wooden S, San SA: Urinothorax: a cause of low pH transudative pleural effusions. Am J Med 1988;85:448–449.

51. Kirkpatrick JA Jr, Fleisher DS: The roentgen appearance of the chest in acute glomerulonephritis in children. J Pediatr 1964;64:492–498.

52. Gottehrer A, Roa J, Stanford GG, Chernow B, Sahn SA: Hypothyroidism and pleural effusions. Chest 1990;98:1130–1132.

53. Smolar EN, Rubin JE, Avramides A, Carter AC: Cardiac tamponade in primary myxedema and review of the literature. Am J Med Sci 1976;272:345–352.

54. Lowell JR: Pleural Effusions. A Comprehensive Review. Baltimore: University Park Press, 1977.

55. Neustadt JE, Levy RC: Hemorrhagic pleural effusion in Meigs' syndrome. JAMA 1968;204:179–180.

56. Solomon S, Farber SJ, Caruso LJ: Fibromyomata of the uterus with hemothorax. Meigs' syndrome? Arch Intern Med 1971;127:307–309.

CHAPTER 7
Malignant Pleural Effusions

INCIDENCE

Malignant disease involving the pleura is the second leading cause of exudative pleural effusions after parapneumonic effusions. Because many of the parapneumonic effusions are small and are not subjected to thoracentesis, malignancy is probably the leading cause of exudative effusions subjected to thoracentesis. In our series from Baltimore, 42% of 102 exudative pleural effusions were due to malignant disease (1). In a recent epidemiologic study from the Czech Republic, malignancy accounted for 24% of all the pleural effusions (2).

Carcinoma of the lung and breast and lymphomas account for approximately 75% of malignant pleural effusions (Table 7.1). Metastatic ovarian carcinoma is the fourth leading cause of malignant pleural effusions, whereas sarcomas, particularly melanoma, account for a small percentage of malignant pleural effusions. No other single tumor accounts for more than 1% of malignant pleural effusions. In about 6% of patients with malignant pleural effusions, the primary tumor is not identified (3, 4).

Lung Cancer

In most series, lung cancer is the leading cause of malignant pleural effusion (5). When patients with lung cancer are first evaluated, about 15% have a pleural effusion (6). During the course of this disease, however, at least 50% of patients with disseminated lung cancer develop a pleural effusion. Pleural effusions occur with all the cell types of lung carcinoma, but appear to be most frequent with adenocarcinoma (5, 7). The incidence of pleural effusions in patients with small cell lung carcinoma is about 10% (8).

Breast Carcinoma

The second leading cause of malignant pleural effusion is metastatic breast carcinoma.

Fracchia and colleagues (9) reviewed 601 patients with disseminated breast carcinoma and found that 48% had pleural effusions. The effusions were large enough to warrant therapeutic intervention in 48% of the patients. Goldsmith and coworkers (10) reviewed the autopsies of 365 patients who had died of disseminated breast carcinoma and reported that 46% had pleural effusions. Pleural effusions were more common with lymphangitic spread (63%) than without lymphangitic spread (41%) (10). In this series, the pleural effusions were on the same side as the primary breast carcinoma in 58% of these patients, on the opposite side in 26%, and on both sides in 16% (10). In a second series, the effusion was ipsilateral in 70%, contralateral in 20%, and bilateral in 10% (11). With breast carcinoma, the mean interval between the development of the primary tumor and the appearance of the pleural effusion is about 2 years (12), but this interval can be as long as 20 years (13).

Lymphomas

Lymphomas, including Hodgkin's disease, are the third leading cause of malignant pleural effusions. Vieta and Craver (14) reviewed radiographs of 335 patients with Hodgkin's disease and reported that 16% had pleural effusions. Autopsy on 51 of the 335 cases revealed that 39% had pleural effusions, 29% had involvement of the parietal pleura, and 74% had mediastinal or hilar lymph node involvement (14). These same authors (14) reviewed the radiographs of 239 patients with non-Hodgkin's lymphoma and reported that 17% had pleural effusions. In 55 autopsies, 38% had pleural fluid, 30% had involvement of the parietal pleura, and 65% had mediastinal or hilar lymph node involvement. Vieta and Craver (14) also reported that 12% of 158 patients with lymphatic leukemia and 4% of 52 patients with myelogenous leukemia had pleural effusions. Parietal pleural involvement was uncommon at autopsy with leukemia, how-

Table 7.1.   Causes of Malignant Pleural Effusions In Two Different Series

Tumor	Spriggs and Boddington[a]		Anderson[b]	
	n	%	n	%
Lung carcinoma	275	43	32	24
Breast carcinoma	157	25	35	26
Lymphoma and leukemia	52	8	34	26
Ovarian carcinoma	27	4	9	7
Sarcoma (including melanoma)	13	2	5	4
Uterine and cervical carcinoma	6	1	3	2
Stomach carcinoma	18	3	1	1
Colon carcinoma	9	1	0	0
Pancreatic carcinoma	7	1	0	0
Bladder carcinoma	7	1	0	0
Other carcinoma	23	4	6	4
Primary unknown	40	6	8	6
	634		133	

[a]Data from Spriggs AI, Boddington MM: The Cytology of Effusions. 2nd ed. New York: Grune & Stratton, 1968.
[b]Data from Anderson CB, Philpott GW, Ferguson TB: The treatment of malignant pleural effusions. Cancer 1974; 33:916–922.

ever. Patients with Hodgkin's disease who have pleural effusions almost invariably have intrathoracic lymph node involvement, frequently without microscopic pleural involvement (15). Most patients with lymphoma or leukemia do not have pleural effusions when their disease is first diagnosed. The median time between diagnosis of the malignancy and the development of the pleural effusion in this group is slightly under 2 years (16). There has been, however, a recent series where during a 7-year period 19 patients with non-Hodgkin's lymphoma presented with pleural effusion (17). The pleural effusion associated with lymphoma is frequently a chylothorax (18).

PATHOPHYSIOLOGIC FEATURES

A malignant tumor can directly or indirectly lead to a pleural effusion in several different ways (Table 7.2). In some patients with pleural metastases, the presence of these metastases increases the permeability of the pleural surfaces so that more fluid enters the pleural space than can be removed. Indeed, in the series of Leckie and Tothill (19), a patient with bronchogenic carcinoma had the second highest amount of protein entering the pleural space of the 40 patients studied. This mechanism, however, is probably not the predominant cause of pleural effusions in malignant disease. In both bronchogenic carcinoma and other metastatic carcinomas of the pleura, the mean amount of protein entering the pleural

Table 7.2.   Mechanisms by which Malignant Disease Leads to Pleural Effusions

Direct Result
  Pleural metastases with increased permeability
  Pleural metastases with obstruction of pleural
    lymphatic vessels
  Mediastinal lymph node involvement with
    decreased pleural lymphatic drainage
  Thoracic duct interruption (chylothorax)
  Bronchial obstruction (decreased pleural
    pressures)
  Pericardial involvement
Indirect Result
  Hypoproteinemia
  Postobstructive pneumonitis
  Pulmonary embolism
  Postradiation therapy

space is similar to that seen with congestive heart failure (19).

Decreased clearance of fluid from the pleural space is probably the mechanism responsible for the pleural effusions in the majority of cases. Leckie and Tothill (19) reported that the mean amount of protein leaving the pleural space in patients with malignant pleural effusions was less than that leaving the pleural space with tuberculosis, pulmonary embolism, or congestive heart failure. This decreased lymphatic drainage can occur through two separate mechanisms. First, because the fluid leaves the pleural space through stomas in the lymphatic vessels in the parietal pleura (20), metastases to the parietal pleura that obstruct these stomas can decrease fluid clearance. Second, the lymphatic vessels of the parietal pleura drain mainly through the mediastinal lymph nodes. Therefore, neoplastic involvement of the mediastinal lymph nodes can decrease the lymphatic clearance of the pleural space.

Malignant tumors can also produce pleural effusions by obstructing the thoracic duct, in which case the resulting pleural effusion is a chylothorax. In fact, the majority of chylothoraces that are not traumatic in origin are secondary to neoplastic involvement of the thoracic duct. Lymphomas are responsible for 75% of chylothoraces secondary to malignant disease (see Chapter 21).

Another mechanism by which malignant tumors produce pleural effusion is through bronchial obstruction. When a neoplasm obstructs the mainstem bronchus or a lobar bronchus, the lung distal to the obstruction becomes atelectatic. Therefore, the remaining lung has to overexpand or the ipsilateral hemithorax has to contract to compensate for the loss of volume of the atelectatic lung. These events result in a more negative pleural pressure, and it is easy to see from Figure 2.1 that such a negative pleural pressure causes pleural fluid to accumulate. My associates and I studied a patient with obstruction of the bronchus intermedius in whom the pleural pressure dropped from -12 to -48 cm H_2O as 200 ml pleural fluid were removed (21).

Pericardial involvement is frequent with metastatic malignant diseases. When a pericardial effusion is caused by such involvement and hydrostatic pressures become elevated in the systemic and pulmonary circulation, transudative pleural effusions may result.

Not all pleural effusions in patients with malignant disease are related to intrathoracic involvement by the neoplasm. Many patients with malignant disease are malnourished with hypoproteinemia, and this disorder can lead to the formation of transudative pleural effusions (see Chapter 6). Pulmonary infection distal to a partially or totally occluded bronchus may produce a parapneumonic effusion (see Chapter 9). The incidence of pulmonary embolization is higher in patients with malignant disease, and emboli can cause pleural effusions (see Chapter 14). Patients with intrathoracic neoplasms frequently receive radiotherapy to their chests, and this treatment can also result in pleural effusions (see Chapter 18) as can some types of chemotherapy (see Chapter 17).

Autopsy Studies

The most detailed autopsy series on pleural involvement in malignant disease are those of Meyer (22) and Rodriguez-Panadero and co-workers (23). It appears that pleural metastases with bronchogenic carcinoma are usually due to pulmonary arterial emboli to the ipsilateral pleura. Virtually all patients with metastatic pleural involvement from lung carcinoma have involvement of the visceral pleura (22, 23). In the series of Rodriguez-Panadero and associates, pulmonary vascular invasion by the tumor was found in 19 of the 24 cases (23). Parietal pleural metastases result from direct extension from the visceral pleura (22, 23).

In patients with nonbronchogenic carcinoma, the visceral pleura is almost always involved also. Involvement of the parietal pleura again appears to result from direct extension from the visceral pleura (22, 23). The origin of these metastases is controversial. Meyer attributed them to tertiary spread from secondary hepatic tumors (22). In his series of 23 patients with pleural metastases, 19 (83%) had hepatic metastases. In the series of Rodriguez-Panadero and coworkers, however, hepatic metastases could only be demonstrated in 71% of the patients and they attributed the visceral pleural metastases to blood-borne metastases from the primary (23). The latter explanation appears more plausible to me. The presence of pleural metastases does indicate systemic dissemination of the disease and renders the patient incurable with surgery alone.

Not all patients with pleural metastases have pleural effusions. In Meyer's series, only 60% of patients with pleural metastases had pleural effusion (22). In Rodriguez-Pandero's study only 30 of 55 patients (55%) with metastatic disease to the pleura had pleural effusion (23). Meyer found that the presence of a pleural effusion was more closely related to neoplastic invasion of the mediastinal lymph nodes than to the extent of pleural involvement by nodular metastases (22). He concluded that the pleural effusions secondary to intrathoracic malignant disease are usually due to lymphatic obstruction (22).

CLINICAL MANIFESTATIONS

The most common symptom reported by patients with malignant pleural effusions is dyspnea, which occurs in more than 50% (7). Symptoms attributable to the tumor itself are also frequent. In one series, weight loss occurred in 32%, malaise in 21%, and anorexia in 14% of patients (7). When patients with malignant pleural effusions are compared to those with benign pleural effusions, patients with malignant pleural effusions are more likely to have dull chest pain (34% versus 11%) while patients with benign disease are more likely to have pleuritic chest pain (51% versus 24%) (24). Temperature elevations are significantly more common in patients with benign disease (73%) than in patients with malignant disease (37%) (24).

Chest Radiographs

The size of a malignant pleural effusion varies from a few milliliters to several liters, with the fluid occupying the entire hemithorax and shifting the mediastinum to the contralateral side. Malignant disease is the most common cause of a massive pleural effusion and accounted for 31 of 46 (67%) of effusions occupying an entire hemithorax in one series (25).

Almost all patients with pleural effusions secondary to bronchogenic carcinoma have radiographically demonstrable pulmonary abnormalities in addition to the effusion. A therapeutic thoracentesis at times must be done before the pulmonary abnormality is evident. Although almost all patients with pleural effusions secondary to lymphoma have mediastinal lymph node involvement at autopsy, this involvement is not always evident in chest radiographs (14). In a series of 22 patients with chylothorax due to lymphoma, only 5 patients (23%) had hilar or mediastinal adenopathy demonstrable on routine chest radiographs (26). In another series, however, 71% of 21 patients with pleural effusions secondary to lymphoma had visible mediastinal lymph node involvement on chest radiographs (27).

In a third series of 19 patients with non-Hodgkin's lymphoma, only 4 patients had mediastinal lymphadenopathy (17). The chest radiographs of patients with pleural effusions due to malignant tumors other than lung carcinoma or lymphoma often reveal only a pleural effusion. In a series of 105 patients with pleural effusion due to breast carcinoma (13), only 9% had radiographically evident pulmonary metastases.

In certain instances the chest computed tomography (CT) scan is useful in patients with malignant pleural effusion. O'Donovan and Eng (28) reviewed the CT findings in 86 patients with documented malignant effusions. They reported the following incidences of concurrent abnormalities: pericardial effusion 3%, pericardial thickening 14%, mediastinal adenopathy 43%, chest wall involvement 12%, lymphangitic carcinoma 7%, and suspicious lung masses, nodules, or infiltrates 53%.

Pleural Fluid

The pleural fluid from a malignant pleural effusion is an exudate (29). The ratio of the pleural fluid to the serum protein level is less than 0.5 in about 20% of malignant pleural effusions (7, 29), but the lactic acid dehydrogenase (LDH) ratio exceeds 0.60 or the absolute pleural fluid LDH meets exudative criteria in this 20% (29). Most pleural effusions that meet exudative criteria by the LDH level but not by the protein level are malignant pleural effusions (29).

The presence of grossly bloody pleural fluid (red blood cell count greater than 100,000/mm^3) suggests malignant pleural disease. In our series of 22 such effusions, my colleagues and I reported that 12 (55%) of the bloody pleural effusions were due to malignant disease (1). A pleural effusion that is not bloody is still likely to be malignant since nearly 50% of malignant pleural effusions have pleural fluid red blood cell counts under 10,000/mm^3, however (1). The pleural fluid white blood cell count with malignant pleural effusion is variable, with the usual count between 1,000 and 10,000/mm^3 (1). The predominant cells in the pleural fluid differential white cell count of these effusions are lymphocytes in about 45%, other mononuclear cells in about 40%, and polymorphonuclear leukocytes in about 15% (1). Pleural fluid eosinophilia is uncommon in malignant pleural effusions.

The pleural fluid glucose level is reduced to below 60 mg/dl in approximately 15 to 20% of malignant pleural effusions (7, 30, 31). A low pleural fluid glucose in association with a malignant pleural effusion indicates that the patient has a high tumor burden in his pleural space. Rodriguez-Panadero and Lopez-Mejias (31) performed thoracoscopy on 77 patients with a malignant pleural effusion and found that the extent of the tumor was significantly greater in those with a low pleural fluid glucose. Cytology and pleural biopsy are more likely to be positive in patients with low-glucose pleural effusions (31). Because of the large tumor burden, patients with a low pleural fluid glucose level have a poor prognosis. In one series (32), the mean survival time of those with a pleural fluid glucose below 60 mg/dl was 1.4 months, compared to a mean survival time of 5.9 months in patients with pleural fluid glucose levels above 60 mg/dl. It appears that the low glucose levels with malignant pleural effusion are due to impaired glucose transfer from blood to pleural fluid (33). Increased glucose utilization by the pleural tumor probably also plays a role in producing the low pleural fluid glucose.

Approximately one-third of patients with malignant pleural effusions have a pleural fluid pH below 7.30 (31, 34, 35). Patients with a low pleural fluid pH also tend to have a low pleural glucose (31, 35). As one might anticipate, they have a greater tumor burden, are more likely to have positive pleural fluid cytology and pleural biopsy, and have a shorter survival than individuals with malignant pleural effusions and a pH level above 7.30 (31, 35). The pathogenesis of the low pH with malignant pleural effusions appears to be due to the combination of acid production by the pleural fluid or the pleura and a block to the movement of carbon dioxide out of the pleural space (33).

Approximately 10% of patients with malignant pleural effusions have an elevated pleural fluid amylase level (30, 36). Usually, the primary tumor is not in the pancreas in these patients (30, 36). Analysis of the amylase isoenzymes has demonstrated that the amylase in malignant effusions is the salivary rather than the pancreatic isoenzyme (37), and therefore amylase isoenzyme analysis can be used to differentiate pancreatic effusions from malignant effusions.

DIAGNOSIS

The diagnosis of a malignant pleural effusion is established by demonstrating malignant cells in the pleural fluid or in the pleura itself. In most cases, this is done by cytologic examination of the pleural fluid, needle biopsy of the pleura, or thoracoscopy.

Cytologic Examination

The characteristics of malignant cells in pleural fluid are described in Chapter 4. The percentage of cases in which cytologic study of the pleural fluid establishes the diagnosis of a malignant pleural effusion ranges from 40 to 87% (38–42). The reasons for this variability in the diagnostic yield with cytologic study are discussed in Chapter 4. When three separate pleural fluid specimens from a patient with malignant pleural disease are submitted to an experienced cytologist, one should expect a positive diagnosis in about 80% of patients. The incidence of positive results depends on the primary tumor. Positive results are uncommon with squamous cell carcinoma because the pleural effusions are usually due to bronchial obstruction or lymphatic blockade (1, 3, 43). With lymphoma, the cytologic test is positive in only 10 to 25% (17, 44). By cytologic examination, the neoplasm can usually be classified into a histologic type such as adenocarcinoma, but the primary site of the tumor cannot usually be identified (43).

Immunohistochemical Tests

The use of monoclonal antibodies directed against various antigens appears to be useful in distinguishing malignant from benign pleural effusions (45–47). Metastatic adenocarcinomas tend to stain positive with anti-CEA, anti-B72.3, and anti-Leu M1, whereas reactive mesothelial cells or malignant mesothelial cells do not stain positive with any of these monoclonal antibodies (see Chapter 4. Over 95% of adenocarcinomas will stain positive for at least two of the above three antigens while almost no mesotheliomas stain positive for more than one (47). The technology with these monoclonal antibodies is likely to improve rapidly, and it is recommended that all laboratories who deal with significant numbers of pleural fluids develop the capability to perform these immunohistochemical tests.

Tumor Markers in Pleural Fluid

The tumor marker most commonly measured in pleural fluid is carcinoembryonic antigen (CEA). Approximately 30–40% of patients with malignant pleural effusions have pleural fluid CEA levels that exceed 10 ng/ml and only a rare benign effusion has levels that exceed this value (48, 49). However, since most patients with an elevated CEA level also have positive pleural fluid cytology (24), the performance of this measurement is not routinely recommended. Other tumor markers that have been evaluated include CA 15-3 (50), CA 19-9 (51), neuron-specific enolase (52) and sialyl state-specific mouse embryonic antigen (SSEA-1) (53). For all these markers, malignant effusions tend to have higher levels than benign effusions, but there is sufficient overlap that the tests are not generally useful diagnostically.

Pleural Biopsy

The incidence of positive pleural biopsies in patients with malignant pleural effusions ranges from 39 to 75% (41, 54, 55). In general, cytologic study of the pleural fluid establishes the diagnosis more frequently than pleural biopsy. Because the pleural biopsy is sometimes positive when the cytologic examination is negative or inconclusive (41, 42, 56, 57) both procedures are recommended when a malignant pleural effusion is suspected. Pleural biopsy has a lower diagnostic yield than pleural fluid cytologic examination because, in about 50% of patients with malignant pleural disease, the costal parietal pleura is not involved (58).

Thoracoscopy or Open Thoracotomy

In many patients with exudative pleural effusions, no diagnosis is reached after an extensive workup including two or more pleural biopsies and pleural fluid cytologic examinations, and lung scans. The following approach to such patients is recommended. If the patient has a positive skin test to purified protein derivative (PPD), the patient should be treated for tuberculosis. Obviously if the patient does not improve with antituberculous therapy, a more invasive procedure should be performed. If the patient has a negative PPD, a CT scan of the chest should be obtained to delineate whether there are parenchymal abnormalities or findings suggestive of mesothelioma. If parenchymal abnormalities are present, a bronchoscopy should be performed. If the CT scan suggests mesothelioma, then thoracoscopy should be performed to establish this diagnosis.

If the CT scan shows nothing other than the pleural effusion, the approach to the patient should be governed by the clinical picture. If there is nothing in the patient's history to suggest carcinoma and if the patient's symptoms are improving, then it is probably best to observe the patient for several weeks as only a small percentage of these patients have malignant pleural disease (59). Alternatively, if the symptoms of the patient are worsening or if there is something in the clinical picture that suggests malignancy, the patient should undergo thoracoscopy. If facilities for thoracoscopy are not available, an alternative approach is to do a thoracotomy with open biopsy of the pleura.

Mesothelioma?

The possibility of a malignant mesothelioma (see Chapter 8) should be considered whenever a patient's pleural fluid cytologic study or pleural biopsy suggests metastatic adenocarcinoma, because the epithelial form of malignant mesothelioma is frequently misinterpreted as adenocarcinoma on cytologic examination or pleural biopsy (60). If no primary tumor is evident, a CT scan of the thorax should be obtained. If the CT scan suggests mesothelioma, one should consider thoracoscopy or exploratory thoracotomy for staging and possible radical pleuropneumonectomy (see Chapter 8).

Electron microscopy is very useful in differentiating metastatic adenocarcinoma from mesothelioma. The appearance of the microvilli is the most important diagnostic feature. With mesothelioma, the microvilli are characteristically numerous, long, and thin while with metastatic adenocarcinoma they are less abundant and are short and stubby (61, 62). As discussed above, immunohistochemical tests are also very effective in differentiating mesothelioma from metastatic adenocarcinoma.

Histochemical tests are also useful in distinguishing metastatic carcinoma from mesothelioma. If staining remains positive with periodic acid-Schiff (PAS) after diastase digestion, the patient has metastatic carcinoma (63). If the cells or tissue stain positive with Alcian blue (which detects acid mucins), the patient has mesothelioma. If neither stain is positive, no conclusion can be made with histochemistry (63).

Lipid Analysis

The possibility of a chylothorax should be considered in every patient with malignant disease and a pleural effusion. If a chylothorax is present, the mediastinal lymph nodes are probably involved, and the treatment of choice is radiation to the mediastinum or chemotherapy. The supernatant of the pleural fluid from patients with malignant pleural effusions should be examined. If the supernatant is turbid, a chylothorax should be suspected, and the triglyceride level in the pleural fluid should be determined. If the pleural fluid triglyceride level exceeds 110 mg/dl, the patient probably has a chylothorax; if the level is below 50 mg/dl, the patient does not have a chylothorax (18). If the level is between 50 and 110 mg/dl, lipoprotein electrophoresis should be performed (18) (see Chapter 21).

Other Diagnostic Tests

Numerous papers have recommended various diagnostic tests such as flow cytometry, chromosomal analysis of pleural fluid cells, or LDH isoenzymes in the diagnosis of malignant pleural effusions. These various tests are discussed in Chapter 4. In general, they are not recommended. Flow cytometry with immunophenotyping is useful in making the diagnosis of lymphoma (17).

Unknown Primary

Most patients who are diagnosed with a malignant pleural effusion already are known to have a malignancy. However, if the patient presents with a malignant pleural effusion, where is its likely origin? A recent article reviewed 18 patients whose first evidence of cancer was a malignant pleural effusion (64). The mean survival of these 18 patients was 9.6 months. The primary tumors were as follows: lung cancer 12, mesothelioma 2, ovarian carcinoma 2, and unknown 2. None were from a breast cancer.

Patients with a malignant pleural effusion and an unknown primary tumor should have a CT of the chest and abdomen. If pulmonary parenchymal abnormalities are discovered, then a bronchoscopy is indicated with special attention to the area of abnormality. If there are no parenchymal abnormalities, then bronchoscopy will probably be nondiagnostic (65). Masses in the abdomen should be evaluated. If the patient has symptoms referable to a specific organ, that organ should be evaluated. If the patient is female, mammography and a careful pelvic examination should be performed. If the foregoing sequence of tests does not identify the site of the primary tumor, it is recommended that further tests not be undertaken.

TREATMENT

A simplified algorithm for the management of patients with malignant pleural effusion is given in Figure 7.1. The initial step is to identify the location of the primary lesion. Frequently the location of the primary is already known when the pleural effusion is first identified. If the primary is unknown, then the procedures outlined in the previous paragraph should be followed.

Only a rare patient with a primary bronchogenic carcinoma and a pleural effusion should be considered to be a surgical candidate. If the pleural fluid cytology is positive, the patient has disseminated disease and is not an operative candidate. If the pleural fluid cytology is negative, consideration should be given to performing curative surgery. Decker and coworkers (66) reviewed 68 patients meeting these criteria who underwent mediastinoscopic examination or exploratory thoracotomy. These investigators found that 4 patients (6%) had surgically resectable lesions,

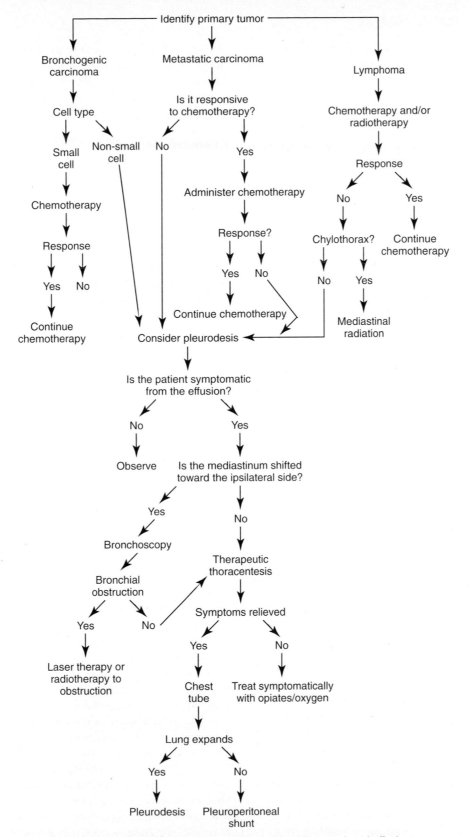

Figure 7.1. Algorithm for managing patients with malignant pleural effusions.

and these 4 all remained free of disease for at least 3 years (66). In such patients, a CT scan of the chest should be obtained to evaluate the mediastinal lymph nodes. If the CT scan demonstrates lymph node enlargement, a mediastinoscopy should be performed. If the CT scan demonstrates no lymph node enlargement, consideration should be given to an exploratory thoracotomy if the patient has no other contraindication to curative resection.

Systemic Chemotherapy

The main reason to identify the primary tumor is to decide whether systemic chemotherapy is indicated. The presence of a malignant pleural effusion usually indicates disseminated tumor, at least for nonbronchogenic carcinoma (22). Therefore, the only hope for cure or prolonged palliation is with systemic chemotherapy. Fentiman and coworkers (13) reported that pleural effusions were controlled in 7 of 22 patients (32%) with metastatic breast carcinoma who were given systemic chemotherapy, whereas Jones and coworkers (67) reported positive responses in 6 of 8 patients (75%) given systemic chemotherapy. Livingston and coworkers (68) reported that 36% of 53 patients with small cell lung carcinoma had complete disappearance of their pleural effusions with chemotherapy. The median survival of patients with small cell lung carcinoma with limited disease and a pleural effusion is 13.9 months, compared to a median survival of 18.3 months if no pleural effusion is present (69). In addition, pleural effusions in lymphomas respond to chemotherapy (26).

In patients undergoing systemic chemotherapy, pleural effusions should be aspirated before chemotherapy is given because the antineoplastic drugs may accumulate in the pleural space and lead to increased systemic toxicity (8).

Mediastinal Radiation

When a patient with a malignant pleural effusion has a chylothorax, the thoracic duct is involved by the neoplastic process. It is therefore logical to administer radiotherapy to the mediastinum in such patients who have tumor types against which primary chemotherapy is not effective. In one series, mediastinal radiation resulted in adequate control of the chylothorax for the remainder of the patient's life in 68% of those with lymphomas and in 50% of those with metastatic carcinoma (70).

Chemical Pleurodesis

Chemical pleurodesis should be considered in patients with malignant pleural effusions who are not candidates for systemic chemotherapy and who do not have a chylothorax. This procedure should also be considered in those who have failed systemic chemotherapy or mediastinal radiotherapy. When managing such a patient, the first question to answer is whether the patient is symptomatic from the effusion. The only symptom likely to be relieved with pleurodesis is dyspnea. If the patient does not have symptoms attributable to the pleural effusion, it does not make sense to insert a chest tube and to attempt a pleurodesis just to make the chest radiograph look better. In a similar vein, if the patient is moribund from disseminated tumor, he should not be tortured for the last few days of his life with chest tubes. If a patient's quality of life is diminished by dyspnea and he has a life expectancy of more than a few weeks, however, one should consider pleurodesis. This local therapy probably does not improve the duration of the patient's life, but can improve the quality of life.

Before a pleurodesis is attempted, the position of the mediastinum on the chest radiograph should be evaluated, because its position tells much about the pleural pressure on the side of the effusion. If the mediastinum is shifted toward the side of the effusion (Fig. 7.2), the pleural pressure is more negative on the side of the effusion. Pleurodesis is then unlikely to be successful because the ipsilateral lung is unable to expand. In such patients, a bronchoscopic examination should be performed to assess the patency of the major bronchi. If neoplastic obstruction of the bronchi is discovered, radiotherapy or laser therapy should be given in an attempt to relieve the bronchial obstruction. If no obstructing lesion is found, the lung is probably encased by the tumor, and a pleurectomy (discussed later in this chapter) should be considered.

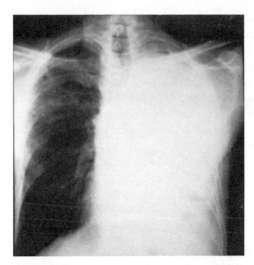

Figure 7.2. Posteroanterior chest radiograph from a patient with a malignant pleural effusion. Note that the mediastinum is shifted toward the side of the effusion.

If the mediastinum is in midline position or has shifted to the contralateral side (Fig. 7.3), then a therapeutic thoracentesis should be performed. The purpose of this procedure is to determine whether it relieves the dyspnea of the patient. Only those patients who experience significant symptomatic improvement from this thoracentesis should be considered to be candidates for chemical pleurodesis. If over 1000 ml pleural fluid are removed during this procedure, pleural pressures should be monitored (21).

If the patient experiences symptomatic improvement after a therapeutic thoracentesis, a tube thoracostomy should be performed. A chest tube with additional holes cut in the side is inserted in the midaxillary line through the seventh or eighth intercostal space (see Chapter 24). The chest tube is connected to a water-sealed drainage system, and the effusion is allowed to drain (71). Negative pressure should not be applied to the chest tube in this situation because the combination of a chronic pleural effusion and the application of negative pleural pressure can cause reexpansion pulmonary edema (see Chapter 19). If successful reexpansion of the lung cannot be accomplished with tube thoracostomy, as shown in Figure 7.3B, sclerosing agents should not be injected into the pleural space. Their injection can only thicken the visceral pleura and allow even less lung expansion. If the lung does not expand with tube thoracostomy, consideration should be given to implanting a pleuroperitoneal shunt (discussed later in this chapter) particularly if the mediastinum is shifted away from the side of the effusion (Fig. 7.3A). If the patient is in excellent condition, pleurectomy can be considered (discussed later in this chapter).

If the pleural fluid glucose is less than 60 mg/dl or if the pleural fluid pH is less than 7.30, pleurodesis is less likely to be successful (35, 72). In one large series in which pleurodesis was attempted with talc insufflation during thoracoscopy, pleurodesis failed in 6 of 14 patients (43%) if the pH was below 7.20, compared with 8 of 92 patients (9%) if the pleural fluid pH was above 7.20 (72). Comparable findings have been reported when the pleurodesis was attempted with intrapleural tetracycline (35). It is recommended that pleurodesis be attempted in patients who have malignant pleural effusions with a low pH if they are good candidates since more than 50% of those with a low pleural fluid pH will be successfully managed with chemical pleurodesis.

Choice of Sclerosing Agent

Originally, antineoplastic agents such as nitrogen mustard (73) or radioisotopes (74) were injected into the pleural space in the hope that these agents would kill the tumor cells and control the pleural effusion. It was subsequently shown that the injection of these agents often controlled the pleural effusion when tumor cells persisted, and that the effectiveness of intrapleural therapy was related more to the creation of a pleurodesis preventing reaccumulation of the pleural fluid than to any antineoplastic effect of the agent administered (75, 76). The effectiveness of intracavitary nitrogen mustard (4) is much greater when the instillation of this agent is combined with tube thoracostomy.

Subsequent to the demonstration of the importance of the chemical pleuritis in controlling pleural effusions, nonspecific irritants such as quinacrine (77), talc (78), and tetracycline (79) were combined with tube thoracostomy in an attempt to control malignant effusions. At the time that the previous edition of this book was written, tetracycline was considered the agent of choice. Since the last edition, parenteral tetracycline has become unavailable due to more stringent manufacturing requirements. Subsequently there have been many publications advocating various sclerosants. The four agents that are presently most commonly recommended are talc, either insufflated or as a slurry; the tetracycline derivatives minocycline and doxycycline, the antineoplastic bleomycin, and *Corynebacterium parvum*. A brief discussion of these four categories of agents follows.

Talc.   Insufflated talc was first used in 1935 by Bethune (80) to produce a pleurodesis. Subsequent studies have shown that insufflated talc is very effective for creating a pleurodesis. In dogs the intrapleural insufflation of talc is more effective at producing a pleurodesis than are tetracycline, yttrium-aluminum garnet laser, or argon beam electro-

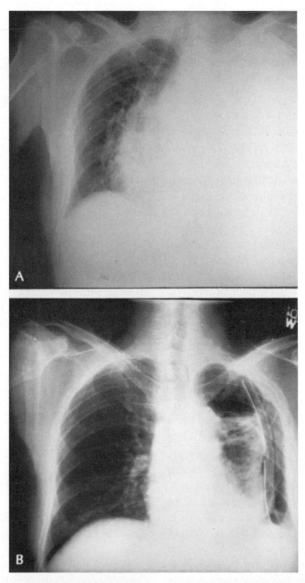

Figure 7.3A. Posteroanterior chest radiograph from a patient with a malignant pleural effusion. Note that the mediastinum is shifted away from the side with the pleural effusion. **B.** Posteroanterior chest radiograph from same patient after insertion of a chest tube into the left pleural space. Note that the left lung is not well-expanded. Accordingly, a sclerosing agent should not be injected into the pleural space.

coagulation, and is comparable to mechanical abrasion (81). Insufflated talc is also very effective at creating a pleurodesis in patients with malignant pleural effusion. Aelony and coworkers (82) reported that 2.5 g aerosolized talc effectively controlled 23 of 28 (82%) of malignant pleural effusions. Hartman and associates (83) reported that the intrapleural insufflation of 3 to 6 g aerosolized talc controlled malignant pleural effusions in 37 of 39 (95%) patients for 90 days. The side effects of talc insufflation are relatively minor (82, 83). The primary disadvantage of insufflated talc is that the insufflation must be done in conjunction with thoracoscopy or thoracotomy.

It appears that talc in a slurry is also very effective in producing a pleurodesis. The preparation is called a slurry because the talc does not dissolve in the saline, but rather is suspended in the solution. In the rabbit, the intrapleural administration of 400 mg/kg talc produces a pleurodesis that is comparable to that produced with 35 mg/kg tetracycline (84). The intrapleural administration of talc slurry in rabbits is not associated with the development of fibrothorax or hemothorax (84) as is the intrapleural administration of the tetracycline derivatives (85). The intrapleural administration of talc slurry effectively controls malignant pleural effusions. Adler and Sayek (78) treated 44 hemithoraces with malignant pleural effusion with 10 g talc in 250 ml saline and reported control of the effusion in 41 (93%). Webb and coworkers (86) reported a 100% success rate in 28 patients with malignant effusions who were given 5 g talc and 3 g thymol iodine in 50 ml saline. Miller and Unger reported complete control of the effusion in 7 of 8 patients (87). Most recently Kennedy and coworkers (88) reported that 10 g talc mixed in 150 to 250 ml normal saline solution effectively controlled 38 of 47 (81%) of malignant pleural effusions.

It appears that the intrapleural administration of talc is associated with relatively few side effects. One possible significant side effect is the development of respiratory failure. The intrapleural administration of talc has been reported to cause acute pneumonitis (89) and the adult respiratory distress syndrome (90). Both of these reports involved only patients that had received talc in a slurry, and in

retrospect we speculate that the patients possibly had reexpansion pulmonary edema rather than an adverse reaction to talc. In the recent series reported by Kennedy and coworkers (88), 5 of 58 patients (9%) had respiratory failure associated with the talc slurry pleurodesis. In 2 of the patients the respiratory failure was not thought to be due to the talc. A third patient received simultaneous bilateral talc instillation that was followed by the development of fever, bilateral infiltrates, and hypoxemic respiratory failure requiring intubation and mechanical ventilation. The other 2 patients developed increasing hypoxia, but recovered without requiring mechanical ventilation. There were no episodes of respiratory failure reported in the other three series (79, 86, 91) with a total of 88 patients who used talc in a slurry. Further studies are necessary to document the incidence of respiratory failure following talc in a slurry and to document whether the incidence is different than with other compounds. Similar problems have been reported after the intrapleural administration of bleomycin (92).

Tetracycline Derivatives. During the 1980s tetracycline was probably the agent most commonly used for creating a pleurodesis. Tetracycline 35 mg/kg is effective in creating a pleurodesis in rabbits (93). Tetracycline is also effective in treating malignant pleural effusions. Sherman and coworkers (94) reported that tetracycline 1500 mg effectively controlled 94.4% of 108 malignant pleural effusions. In a recent review of 11 reports involving 359 patients, the success rate with tetracycline was 67% (95).

Parenteral tetracycline is no longer available in the United States, although it remains available in some countries, such as Germany (96). Accordingly the tetracycline derivatives minocycline and doxycycline have been evaluated. In the rabbit, minocycline 7 mg/kg produces pleurodesis that is comparable to that produced by tetracycline 35 mg/kg (85). One disturbing aspect of the intrapleural administration of tetracycline derivatives in animals is that it is associated with a high incidence of hemothorax, which is frequently fatal (85). Such hemothoraces are not seen after talc administration (84). The significance of these hemothoraces is unclear since they have not been reported in humans to my knowledge.

Doxycycline and minocycline are effective at producing pleurodesis in patients with malignant pleural effusion. When three reports (97–99) with a total of 62 patients are combined, there was complete initial control of the effusion in 47 (76%). There has also been one report in which the administration of minocycline 300 mg controlled 6 of 7 malignant pleural effusions (100). The degree of chest pain with the tetracycline derivatives appears to be comparable to that with tetracycline itself (98).

Bleomycin and Mitoxantrone.   Bleomycin is another agent that has become popular recently as a sclerosing agent for malignant pleural effusions. The popularity of bleomycin is due in part to a controlled study by Ruckdeschel and associates comparing the results with 60 units of bleomycin and 1000 mg tetracycline (101) in 44 patients. The rate of success with bleomycin at 30 days (64%) was significantly better than that with tetracycline (33%). It should be noted that less than an optimal dose of tetracycline was used in this study and the rate of success with tetracycline was much less than that generally reported.

Overall, it appears that bleomycin is less effective than talc or the tetracycline derivatives in producing a pleurodesis. In a review of 8 reports with a total of 199 patients using bleomycin to treat malignant pleural effusions, the overall success rate was only 54% (95). In the rabbit model, bleomycin is ineffective in producing a pleurodesis (102). Lastly, bleomycin is much more expensive (~$1000) than the tetracycline derivatives or talc. Therefore, it cannot be recommended.

Another antineoplastic agent that has shown some promise as a pleural sclerosant is mitoxantrone. A recent paper found that mitoxantrone was comparable to bleomycin in controlling malignant pleural effusions (103). One advantage of mitoxantrone over bleomycin is that mitoxantrone binds to cell membranes and therefore is likely to remain in the pleural space longer (104). There have been limited clinical studies that have addressed the effectiveness of intrapleural mitoxantrone as a treatment for malignant pleural effusion. Maiche and coworkers (103) treated 15 pa-

tients with 30 mg mitoxantrone in 30 ml saline and reported that the effusion was controlled in 10 (67%). Kelly and associates (105) administered 20 mg/m^2 to 15 patients with metastatic sarcoma and reported that complete resolution of the effusion was achieved in 76% of the patients. Groth and associates (106) treated 54 patients with 30 mg mitoxantrone and reported that 71% of the patients had complete disappearance of the effusion for 2 months. In the animal model, the intrapleural administration of high doses of mitoxantrone produces a pleurodesis, but there is much cardiotoxicity (107). Interestingly, the intrapleural injection of mitoxantrone leads to proportionately more inflammation than does the intrapleural injection of tetracycline derivatives or talc (107). At the present time, mitoxantrone is not recommended as a sclerosing agent because it is no more effective than talc or the tetracycline derivatives and it has more toxicity (107).

Other antineoplastic agents such as cisplatin, doxorubicin, etoposide, fluorouracil, and mitomycin C have been evaluated for the treatment of pleural effusions and the response rates have been less than 50% for almost all (95). Therefore, their use cannot be recommended.

Corynebacterium parvum.   Over the last decade there have been several articles advocating the use of intrapleural *C. parvum* for the control of malignant pleural effusions (108–111). *C. parvum* is an anaerobic Gram-positive bacterium showing remarkable immunostimulating and cytotoxic effects. One advantage of *C. parvum* use is that it can be injected directly into the pleural space, and no chest tube is necessary. The usual dose is 7 mg of dried, killed *C. parvum*. When nine reports involving a total of 169 patients are combined, the success rate with *C. parvum* was 76%, which compares favorably with the tetracycline derivatives but is slightly inferior to talc (95). *C. parvum* injected intrapleurally is ineffective in the rabbit model (112) and *C. parvum* is not available in the United States.

Agent of Choice.   Based upon the above information, the following recommendations for the selection of an agent for pleurodesis in patients with malignant pleural effusions are made. If a patient has a malignant pleural effusion diagnosed during thoracoscopy or at thoracotomy, insufflated talc is the agent of choice. If a patient has a malignant pleural effusion diagnosed less invasively, then 5 g talc in a slurry is probably the treatment of choice. A reasonable alternative is doxycycline 500 mg or 7 mg *C. parvum* if it is available. Bleomycin is not recommended because overall it is less effective and it is more expensive.

Intrapleural Injection of Sclerosing Agent

The recommended procedure for the intrapleural injection of a sclerosing agent is as follows. Unless *C. parvum* is being used, tube thoracostomy should be performed. The first decision that must be made is what size of chest tubes to use. It appears that large tubes are not necessary. Walsh and associates (113) reported that they successfully managed 10 of 11 patients (91%) with 9F catheters inserted percutaneously. Groth et al. reported that they managed 100 patients with 16F to 20F catheters (106).

Once the chest tube has been inserted, how long should one wait before injecting the sclerosing agent? It is important to make certain that the underlying lung has fully expanded before the injection is made. If the underlying lung has not expanded, then the injection of a sclerosing agent will only lead to additional thickening of the visceral pleura, which will further compromise the function of the underlying lung. Some authors have advocated that the sclerosing agent not be injected until the drainage from the chest tube is less than 150 ml/day (101). However, a recent study lends no support to this practice. Villanueva and coworkers (114) randomly assigned patients to a group in which tetracycline was not instilled until the drainage was less than 150 ml/day and a group in which tetracycline was instilled as soon as the lung had reexpanded. The rate of success was the same in each group (80%), but the duration of the chest tubes was much less in the latter group (2 days) than in the former group (7 days). In view of this study, it is recommended that the sclerosant be injected as soon as the lung has reexpanded.

If talc is used as the sclerosing agent, how should it be prepared? It is important to obtain asbestos-free talc to minimize the risk of carcinogenicity. Elaborate procedures, which include sterilization by gamma irradiation, have been proposed (115), but it appears that the talc can be adequately sterilized in an autoclave with dry heat for 6 hours at 270°F (116). The sterilized talc is put into a syringe with 50 ml saline. Then right before the injection, the syringe is agitated to disperse the suspended talc.

Because the injection of the tetracycline produces an intense pleuritis that can be very painful, some authors (117, 118) have suggested that the patient should be given a local anesthetic, such as lidocaine hydrochloride, intrapleurally. There are no controlled studies evaluating the efficacy of intrapleural lidocaine. Since talc in a slurry appears to be less painful than the tetracycline derivatives, intrapleural lidocaine is no longer recommended. Systemic analgesia with agents such as 10 mg morphine sulfate parenterally is recommended.

After the sclerosant is injected, the tube is flushed with an additional 100–200 ml saline solution. The chest tube is then clamped for about 2 hours. Although in the past it has been recommended that the patient be moved into different positions so that the sclerosant contacts all the pleural surfaces, this does not appear to be necessary. In animals the dispersal of radioisotopes injected intrapleurally is similar whether the animals are rotated or not (119). In humans the dispersal of the injected radioisotopes is similar whether or not the patients are rotated (120). Rotation did not have a statistically significant effect on the results of pleurodesis in one randomized study with tetracycline derivatives (121). The rate of success with rotation was 73.7% while the rate of success with no rotation was 61.9% (121). Rotation through the different positions is still recommended if the patient has any air in the pleural space.

After these 2 hours, the chest tube is unclamped and negative pressure (−15 to −20 cm H_2O) is applied to the chest tube. Suction is maintained for at least 24 hours and until the pleural drainage is less than 150 ml/day. The keys to the success of this procedure are the pleuritis produced by the sclerosant and the approximation of the visceral and the parietal pleura by the chest tubes so that a pleural symphysis can occur. There appears to be no advantage if the sclerosant is injected twice. In

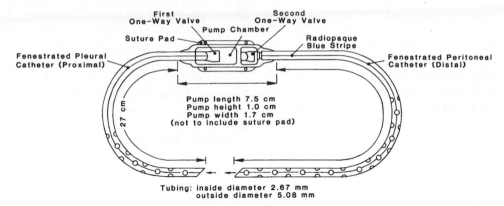

First One-Way Valve
Second One-Way Valve
Pump Chamber
Suture Pad
Radiopaque Blue Stripe
Fenestrated Pleural Catheter (Proximal)
Fenestrated Peritoneal Catheter (Distal)

Pump length 7.5 cm
Pump height 1.0 cm
Pump width 1.7 cm
(not to include suture pad)

27 cm

Tubing: inside diameter 2.67 mm
outside diameter 5.08 mm

Figure 7.4. Diagram of the Denver Pleuro-Peritoneal Shunt, which consists of a fenestrated pleural catheter, a flexible pump chamber containing two one-way valves, and a fenestrated peritoneal catheter. The one-way valves open at a positive pressure of about 1 cm H_2O.

one study (122), 25 patients received one injection of tetracycline, 20 mg/kg, and 25 patients received instillations of tetracycline, 20 mg/kg, on 2 consecutive days. Effusions recurred in 4 patients in each group (122).

Alternatives to Pleurodesis

If the patient is not a good candidate for chemical pleurodesis, there are several options available that include symptomatic treatment, the implantation of a pleuroperitoneal shunt, serial thoracentesis, pleurectomy, and pleural radiotherapy.

Symptomatic Treatment

The two primary symptoms associated with a malignant pleural effusion are chest pain and shortness of breath. If the patient has chest pain, sufficient analgesics should be given to control the pain. There is no reason to worry about narcotic addiction since the life expectancy of the patient is so short.

If the primary symptom is dyspnea, the patient should be given opiates and/or oxygen. Both opiates and oxygen will relieve the dyspnea. The disadvantage of opiates is that their administration can be associated with an increase in the $PaCO_2$, which in turn will lead to a decrease in the PaO_2. The disadvantage of oxygen is that it is very expensive and is not very portable. Opiates are probably underused in the treatment of dyspnea associated with pleural effusions.

Pleuroperitoneal Shunt

An alternative approach to the management of patients with malignant pleural effusions is the placement of a pleuroperitoneal shunt (123–126), which is marketed commercially by Denver Biomaterials, Evergreen, CO. This device consists of two catheters connected with a valved pump chamber (Fig. 7.4). The two one-way valves in the pump chamber are positioned such that fluid can only flow from the pleural space to the pump chamber to the peritoneal cavity. These valves open at a positive pressure of about 1 cm H_2O. Because the pleural pressure is almost always more negative than the peritoneal pressure, the pumping chamber must be used to move fluid from the pleural cavity to the peritoneal cavity. The capacity of the pump chamber is approximately 1.5 ml. When the pump chamber is compressed, fluid is forced from the chamber into the peritoneal cavity. Then when the pump chamber is released, negative pressure created in the pump chamber draws fluid from the pleural cavity to the pump chamber.

Little and associates (124) reported their experience with the insertion of these shunts into 29 patients, of whom 22 had malignant pleural disease. Eight of the patients had had chest tube placement previously with attempted sclerosis with tetracycline. In most instances, shunt implantation was performed in the operating room, using general anesthesia, but in 4 patients, local anesthesia was used. The pump chamber is placed in a subcutaneous pocket caudad to a skin incision in the lateral part of the inframammary crease and fixed to the tissues with sutures through the sewing holes in the base of the pump chamber. Because the chamber does not lie directly beneath the incision, pump compression does not traumatize the incision and is therefore less painful. The pleural catheter is inserted at the lateral and superior aspect of the incision with a Seldinger-type introducer kit. The abdominal catheter is tunneled subcutaneously across the costal margin and inserted, via a 3-cm skin incision, into the peritoneal cavity through a small incision in the peritoneum. Pump compression by physicians and nurses is initiated in the recovery room and is then started by the patient or the patient's family on the first postoperative day. Within 3 days of shunt placement, pump compression usually causes no discomfort. Most patients are ready for discharge from the hospital within 48 hours of the operation. Selected patients can have the procedure performed on an outpatient basis.

Little and associates (124) reported excellent results in their 29 patients. Three patients never pumped on their shunts; one obese patient was unable to localize the pump chamber, a 90-year-old man suffering from senility was simply unable to comply, and one patient developed a cancer phobia and refused to touch her shunt. Two patients died shortly after implantation from disseminated malignant disease. Excellent results were obtained in 20 of the remaining 24 patients. The 14 patients with malignant effusions had a median survival of 4 months, and there were no instances of peritoneal tumor seeding. In 5 patients the shunts became occluded by fibrinous debris between 3 weeks and 2 months after the operation. Replacement was uneventful in all five instances.

Since these original reports (123, 124) there have been several additional reports (125–128). In these latter four studies, a total of 84 patients with malignancy were treated and 76 had failed pleurodesis or had a trapped lung. Alleviation of dyspnea and control of the effusion was obtained in more than 90% of the patients. These results are particularly impressive when one realizes that more than 90% of the patients in these four series had failed previous therapy. The primary complication with the pleuroperitoneal shunt is that in about 15%, the shunt becomes occluded and has to be replaced.

What should be the place of the pleuroperitoneal shunt in the management of patients with malignant pleural effusions? The shunt should certainly be used in the patient in whom the lung does not expand after tube thoracostomy. It is also recommended that the shunt be used in any patient who fails pleurodesis.

There are no studies comparing the efficacy of the shunt and chemical pleurodesis. The advantages of the shunt include the following: (a) the total hospitalization time is less than with chemical pleurodesis; (b) the amount of pain is probably less than with pleurodesis; (c) the procedure can be done on an outpatient basis; and (d) the patient may benefit psychologically from using the pump when he is dyspneic. The disadvantages of the shunt include the following: (a) the shunt becomes obstructed in some patients; (b) insertion frequently requires general anesthesia; and (c) the patient must use the pump daily.

At the present time I have no strong preference for either chemical pleurodesis or implantation of the shunt. Controlled studies are necessary to determine the relative advantages and disadvantages cf each procedure. I have been surprised that the shunt has not become more widely used for the primary treatment of malignant pleural effusions over the past few years.

Pleurectomy

In carefully selected individuals, pleurectomy can be of use in controlling malignant pleural effusions. Pleurectomy may be attempted in two different situations (129). The first is in the patient who undergoes a diagnostic thoracotomy for an undiagnosed pleural effusion. If malignant disease is found, an immediate parietal pleurectomy is useful to prevent recurrence of the effusion (129). Parietal pleurectomy consists of stripping all the parietal pleura from the rib cage and the mediastinum. The second situation is in the symptomatic patient with a persistent pleural effusion and trapping of the ipsilateral lung so that the injection of sclerosing agents is contraindicated. The surgical procedure involves decortication of the trapped lung in conjunction with parietal pleurectomy. Pleurectomy controls the pleural effusion in over 90% of cases (129). It is a substantial operation with a mortality rate of about 10%, however (129). A pleurectomy combined with decortication is recommended only in a patient who is symptomatic from the pleural effusion, who is in good overall condition, and whose primary tumor either is under control or is progressing slowly. I have yet to see such a patient, but an occasional patient with breast carcinoma meets these criteria.

Thoracentesis

In the past, many patients with malignant pleural effusions were managed with repeated therapeutic thoracenteses for symptomatic relief. This regimen has several drawbacks. After therapeutic thoracentesis, malignant pleural effusions reaccumulate rapidly, usually within 1–3 days (4). Repeated thoracenteses lead to protein depletion; the removal of 2000 ml pleural fluid containing 4.0 g/dl protein deprives the patient of 80 g protein. The patient has to visit the physician frequently for the procedure. In addition, repeated thoracenteses often lead to loculation of the pleural fluid that makes subsequent pleurodesis difficult (4). In view of these disadvantages, serial therapeutic thoracentesis should only be performed in moribund patients in whom the procedure offers symptomatic relief.

An alternative to serial therapeutic thoracentesis is the placement of a catheter in the pleural space. Robinson and associates (130) recently reported a series of 9 patients who had an indwelling Tenckhoff catheter placed in the pleural space. The Tenckhoff catheter is made of translucent silicone rubber tubing. A felt cuff comes attached to the catheter and is positioned just within the skin exit site. The catheter is equipped with a plastic occluding device, which may be opened to drain the fluid. The fluid is drained whenever the patient becomes symptomatic. In the series of Robinson all patients reported excellent palliation. The mean volume of drainage was 477 ml/24 hours. The serum protein level de-

creased slightly from 6.5 to 6.2 g/dl during the treatment period. Local wound cellulitis developed at 3 of the 12 catheter exit sites, but this resolved with oral antibiotic therapy. No pleural space infection developed (130). This mode of therapy appears to be an alterative to pleuroperitoneal shunting. The disadvantage is that the patient may lose protein from the repeated fluid removal, but this may not be important clinically.

Pleural Radiotherapy

The role of mediastinal radiotherapy in treating the patient with malignant disease and a chylothorax is well established, as discussed earlier, but the role of radiotherapy to the pleura itself in the management of malignant effusions is not yet defined. Strober and colleagues reported that malignant pleural effusions were controlled in 7 of 10 patients to whom they administered super-voltage therapy using a moving strip technique (131). Until additional studies are completed, however, the rightful place of pleural radiotherapy in the management of malignant pleural effusions remains to be determined.

Experimental Treatments

There are several different approaches that have been tested in a research setting that show promise for the treatment of patients with malignant pleural effusions. All the following treatments should be regarded as experimental.

There have been at least three reports (132–134) evaluating the efficacy of OK-432, an immune modulator purified from the SU strain of *Streptococcus pyogenes*. The usual regimen involves the placement of a pigtail catheter in the pleural space and weekly injections of OK-432 until the effusion ceases to reaccumulate. In one study of 26 patients the mean number of OK-432 injections was 1.9 (132). OK-432 can control the pleural effusion in approximately 75% of patients, but its administration is associated with significant side effects (132). In one series of 26 patients, fever above 38°C occurred in 20, chills in 4, chest pain in 2, dyspnea in 3, and no toxicity in 5 (132).

Attempts have been made to increase the effectiveness of chemotherapeutic agents by attaching them to particles that would remain in the pleural space for a longer period. Hagiwara and associates (135) tried adsorbing mitomycin C to activated carbon particles. The acute toxicity of the activated carbon particles with the mitomycin C is about 20% that of mitomycin C solutions alone. These workers treated 17 patients with malignant pleural effusions in this manner and reported that 12 responded completely (135). There were significant side effects, however, in that 80% developed general fatigue and loss of appetite, 53% developed fever above 38°C, 47% developed thrombocytopenia, and 35% developed leukopenia. The number of side effects probably preclude this regimen for generalized use, but the general approach of using activated carbon to keep the sclerosing agent in the pleural space deserves further attention. In a similar manner Ike and associates (136) used microspheres containing adriamycin and reported that the effusions were controlled in 6 of 7 patients and there were no systemic symptoms.

Four separate reports (137–140) have assessed the value of intrapleural interferon in the management of malignant pleural effusions. The intrapleural administration of interferon results in a decreased number of malignant cells and an increased number of lymphocytes, neutrophils, and monocytes in the pleural fluid (137, 139). However, since the complete response rate was less than 50% in two of the reports (138, 140), it appears unlikely that this agent will ever achieve a prominent role in the management of malignant pleural effusions.

Liu and coworkers (141) assessed the therapeutic efficacy of the intrapleural transfer of autologous or allogeneic lymphokine-activated killer (LAK) cells, which had been cultured in vitro with recombinant interleukin-2 (IL-2). Each patient received one injection of LAK cells and recombinant IL-2 intrapleurally daily for the 10 days prior and the 10 days following the LAK cell administration. When autologous cells were used, the pleural effusion completely disappeared in 31 of 45 patients (68.8%). When allogeneic LAK cells were used, the pleural effusion completely disappeared in 40 of 76 patients (52.6%). Yasumoto and colleagues (142) have reported similar results in a much smaller group of patients. These studies show that modulation of the immune response intrapleurally can result in control of malignant pleural effusions. Practically, however, since this procedure is so much more time consuming and expensive than pleurodesis with talc or a tetracycline derivative, it must be simplified if it is going to be widely used.

Pectasides and coworkers (143) administered tumor-associated monoclonal antibodies radiolabeled with iodine-131 to 10 patients with malignant pleural effusions. In 7 of the patients, the effusions were completely controlled after one injection. There was no toxicity with the regimen. The disadvantages of this approach are that it is expensive and the patient must remain in the hospital until the radioactivity dissipates.

There has been one case report (144) advocating the use of the trimidyne Nd:YAG Optilase laser for control of a malignant pleural effusion. Obviously, this approach much be considered experimental until its efficacy and safety have been evaluated in controlled studies.

PROGNOSIS

The prognosis of patients with malignant pleural effusions is not good, although it obviously varies according to the histologic features of the tumor. In the series from 1977 of Chernow and Sahn (7), which reviewed all patients with positive pleural fluid cytology or pleural biopsy in a given hospital, the mean survival was 3.1 ± 0.5 months after diagnosis of the malignant pleural effusion, with a 54% mortality rate within 1 month and an 84% mortality by 6 months. The mean survival was only 2.2 months in patients with lung cancer, whereas it was 7.3 months in patients with breast carcinoma. In a more recent series (72) the mean survival was 4.3 months with non-small cell lung carcinoma, 3.7 months with small cell lung cancer, 7.4 months with breast carcinoma, 5 months with gastrointestinal cancer, and 9.4 months with ovarian carcinoma. In another series of 105 malignant pleural effusions secondary to breast carcinoma (13), the mean survival was 15.7 months, with about 20% of the patients living 3 years after the onset of the pleural effusion.

The prognosis of patients is worse if the pleural fluid glucose level is below 60 mg/dl or the pleural fluid pH is below 7.30. Sanchez-Armengol and Rodriguez-Panadero (72) reviewed their experience with 119 patients who had the diagnosis of malignant pleural effusion made during thoracoscopy. They reported that the mean survival was 1.9 months in 14 patients with a low pleural fluid glucose level and a low pleural fluid pH compared to 5.7 months in the remaining patients. Sahn and Good (35) reported that the mean survival of 20 patients with a pleural fluid pH below 7.30 was 2.1 months, compared with a mean survival of 9.8 months in 40 patients with a normal pleural fluid pH. When patients with specific tumor types were analyzed, those with a low pleural fluid pH or glucose level always tended to have a poorer prognosis.

REFERENCES

1. Light RW, Erozan YS, Ball WC: Cells in pleural fluid: their value in differential diagnosis. Arch Intern Med 1973;132:854–860.
2. Marel M, Arustova M, Stasny B, Light RW: Incidence of pleural effusion in a well-defined region: epidemiologic study in central Bohemia. Chest 1993;104:1486–1489.
3. Spriggs AI, Boddington MM: The Cytology of Effusions. 2nd ed. New York: Grune & Stratton, 1968.
4. Anderson CB, Philpott GW, Ferguson TB: The treatment of malignant pleural effusions. Cancer 1974;33:916–922.
5. Johnston WW: The malignant pleural effusion: a review of cytopathologic diagnoses of 584 specimens from 472 consecutive patients. Cancer 1985;56:905–909.
6. Cohen S, Hossain S: Primary carcinoma of the lung: a review of 417 histologically proved cases. Dis Chest 1966;49:67–73.
7. Chernow B, Sahn SA: Carcinomatous involvement of the pleura. Am J Med 1977;63:695–702.
8. Herrstedt J, Clementsen P, Hansen OP: Increased myelosuppression during cytostatic treatment and pleural effusion in patients with small cell lung cancer. Eur J Cancer 1992;28A:1070–1073.
9. Fracchia AA, Knapper WH, Carey JT, Farrow JH: Intrapleural chemotherapy for effusion from metastatic breast carcinoma. Cancer 1970;26:626–629.
10. Goldsmith HS, Bailey HD, Callahan EL, Beattie EJ Jr: Pulmonary lymphangitic metastases from breast carcinoma. Arch Surg 1967;94:483–488.
11. Banerjee AK, Willetts I, Robertson JF, Blamey RW: Pleural effusion in breast cancer: a review of the Nottingham experience. Europ J Surg Oncol 1994;20:33–36.
12. Raju RN, Kardinal CG: Pleural effusion in breast carcinoma: analysis of 122 cases. Cancer 1981;48:2524–2527.
13. Fentiman IS, Millis R, Sexton S, Hayward JL: Pleural effusion in breast cancer: a review of 105 cases. Cancer 1981;47:2087–2092.
14. Vieta JO, Craver LF: Intrathoracic manifestations of the lymphomatoid diseases. Radiology 1941;37:138–158.
15. Stolberg HO, Patt NL, MacEwen KF, et al: Hodgkin's disease of the lung: roentgenologic-pathologic correlation. AJR 1964;92:96–115.
16. van de Molengraft FJ, Vooijs GP: The interval between the diagnosis of malignancy and the development of effusions, with reference to the role of cytologic diagnosis. Acta Cytol 1988;32:183–187.
17. Celikoglu F, Teirstein AS, Krellenstein DJ, Strauchen JA: Pleural effusion in non-Hodgkin's lymphoma. Chest 1992;101:1357–1360.
18. Staats BA, Ellefson RD, Budahn LL, et al: The lipoprotein profile of chylous and nonchylous pleural effusions. Mayo Clin Proc 1980;55:700–704.
19. Leckie WJH, Tothill P: Albumin turnover in pleural effusions. Clin Sci 1965;29:339–352.
20. Wang NS: The preformed stomas connecting the pleural cavity and the lymphatics in the parietal pleura. Am Rev Respir Dis 1975;111:12–20.
21. Light RW, Jenkinson SG, Minh V, George RB: Observations on pleural pressures as fluid is withdrawn during thoracentesis. Am Rev Respir Dis 1980;121:799–804.
22. Meyer PC: Metastatic carcinoma of the pleura. Thorax 1966;21:427–433.
23. Rodriguez-Panadero F, Borderas Naranjo F, Lopez Mejias J: Pleural metastatic tumours and effusions. Frequency and pathogenic mechanisms in a postmortem series. Eur Respir J 1989;2:366–369.
24. Marel M, Štastny B, Melínová L, Svandová E, Light RW: Diagnosis of pleural effusions—experience with clinical studies 1986–1990. Chest 1995, in press.
25. Maher GG, Berger HW: Massive pleural effusion: malignant and nonmalignant causes in 46 patients. Am Rev Respir Dis 1972;105:458–460.
26. Weick JK, Kiely JM, Harrison EG Jr, et al: Pleural effusion in lymphoma. Cancer 1973;31:848–853.
27. Bruneau R, Rubin P: The management of pleural effusions and chylothorax in lymphoma. Radiology 1965;85:1085–1092.
28. O'Donovan PB, Eng P: Pleural changes in malignant pleural effusions: appearance on computed tomography. Cleve Clin J Med 1994;61:127–131.
29. Light RW, MacGregor MI, Luchsinger PC, Ball WC: Pleural effusions: the diagnostic separation of transudates and exudates. Ann Intern Med 1972;77:507–513.
30. Light RW, Ball WC: Glucose and amylase in pleural effusions. JAMA 1973;225:257–260.
31. Rodriguez-Panadero F, Lopez-Mejias J: Low glucose and pH levels in malignant pleural effusions. Am Rev Respir Dis 1989;139:663–667.

32. Rodriguez-Panadero F, Lopez-Mejias J: Survival time of patients with pleural metastatic carcinoma predicted by glucose and pH studies. Chest 1989;95: 320-324.

33. Good JT Jr, Taryle DA, Sahn SA: The pathogenesis of low glucose, low pH malignant effusions. Am Rev Respir Dis 1985;131:737-741.

34. Light RW, MacGregor MI, Ball WC Jr, Luchsinger PC: Diagnostic significance of pleural fluid pH and P_{CO_2}. Chest 1973;64:591-596.

35. Sahn SA, Good JT Jr: Pleural fluid pH in malignant effusions. Ann Intern Med 1988;108:345-349.

36. Ende N: Studies of amylase activity in pleural effusions and ascites. Cancer 1960;13:283-287.

37. Kramer MR, Saidana MJ, Cepero RJ, Pitchenik AE: High amylase levels in neoplasm-related pleural effusion. Ann Intern Med 1989;110:567-569.

38. Jarvi OH, Kunnas RJ, Laitio MT, Tyrkko JES: The accuracy and significance of cytologic cancer diagnosis of pleural effusions. Acta Cytol 1972;16:152-157.

39. Grunze H: The comparative diagnostic accuracy, efficiency and specificity of cytologic techniques used in the diagnosis of malignant neoplasm in serous effusions of the pleural and pericardial cavities. Acta Cytol 1964;8:150-164.

40. Dekker A, Bupp PA: Cytology of serous effusions. An investigation into the usefulness of cell blocks versus smears. Am J Clin Pathol 1978;70:855-860.

41. Prakash URS, Reiman HM: Comparison of needle biopsy with cytologic analysis for the evaluation of pleural effusion: analysis of 414 cases. Mayo Clin Proc 1985;60:158-164.

42. Bueno CE, Clemente G, Castro BC, Martin LM, Ramos SR, Panizo AG, Glez-Rio JM: Cytologic and bacteriologic analysis of fluid and pleural biopsy specimens with Cope's needle. Arch Intern Med 1990;150:1190-1194.

43. Naylor B, Schmidt RW: The case for exfoliative cytology of serous effusions. Lancet 1964;1:711-712.

44. Melamed MR: The cytological presentation of malignant lymphomas and related diseases in effusions. Cancer 1963;16:413-431.

45. Wirth PR, Legier J, Wright GL Jr: Immunohistochemical evaluation of seven monoclonal antibodies for differentiation of pleural mesothelioma from lung adenocarcinoma. Cancer 1991;67:655-662.

46. Frisman DM, McCarthy WF, Schleiff P, Buckner SB, Nocito JD Jr, O'Leary TJ: Immunocytochemistry in the differential diagnosis of effusions: use of logistic regression to select a panel of antibodies to distinguish adenocarcinomas from mesothelial proliferations. Modern Path 1993;6:179-184.

47. Brown RW, Clark GM, Tandon AK, Allred DC: Multiple-marker immunohistochemical phenotypes distinguishing malignant pleural mesothelioma from pulmonary adenocarcinoma. Human Path 1993;24: 347-354.

48. Rittgers RA, Loewenstein MS, Feinerman AE, et al: Carcinoembryonic antigen levels in benign and malignant pleural effusions. Ann Intern Med 1978; 88:631-634.

49. Tamura S, Nishigaki T, Moriwaki Y, et al: Tumor markers in pleural effusion diagnosis. Cancer 1988; 61:298-302.

50. Shimokata K, Totani Y, Nakanishi K, et al: Diagnostic value of cancer antigen 15-3 (CA15-3) detected by monoclonal antibodies (115D8 and DF3) in exudative pleural effusions. Eur Respir J 1988;1: 341-344.

51. Niwa Y, Kishimoto H, Shimokata K: Carcinomatous and tuberculous pleural effusion. Comparison of tumor markers. Chest 1985;87:351-355.

52. Shimokata K, Niwa Y, Yamamoto M, Sasou H, Morishita M: Pleural fluid neuron-specific enolase. Chest 1989;95:602-603.

53. Iguchi H, Hara N, Miyazaki K, Ohtsu Y, Sonoda F, Ohta M: Elevation of sialyl stage-specific mouse embryonic antigen levels in pleural effusion in patients with adenocarcinoma of the lung. Cancer 1989;63:1327-1330.

54. Scerbo J, Keltz H, Stone DJ: A prospective study of closed pleural biopsies. JAMA 1971;218:377-380.

55. Von Hoff DD, LiVolsi V: Diagnostic reliability of needle biopsy of the parietal pleura. Am J Clin Pathol 1975;64:200-203.

56. Salyer WR, Eggleston JC, Erozan YS: Efficacy of pleural needle biopsy and pleural fluid cytopathology in the diagnosis of malignant neoplasm involving the pleura. Chest 1975;67:536-539.

57. Frist B, Kahan AV, Koss LG: Comparisons of the diagnostic values of biopsies of the pleura and cytologic evaluation of pleural fluids. Am J Clin Pathol 1979;72:48-51.

58. Canto A, Rivas J, Saumench J, et al: Points to consider when choosing a biopsy method in cases of pleurisy of unknown origin. Chest 1983;84:176-179.

59. Poe RH, Israel RH, Utell MJ, et al: Sensitivity, specificity, and predictive values of closed pleural biopsy. Arch Intern Med 1984;144:325-328.

60. Antman KH: Clinical presentation and natural history of benign and malignant mesothelioma. Semin Oncol 1981;8:313-320.

61. Coleman M, Henderson DW, Mukherjee TM: The ultrastructural pathology of malignant pleural mesothelioma. Pathol Ann 1989;24:303-353.

62. Jandik WR, Landas SK, Bray CK, Lager DJ: Scanning electron microscopic distinction of pleural mesotheliomas from adenocarcinomas. Modern Path 1993; 6:761-764.

63. Warnock ML, Stoloff A, Thor A: Differentiation of adenocarcinoma of the lung from mesothelioma: periodic acid-Schiff, monoclonal antibodies B72.3, and Leu M1. Am J Pathol 1988;133:30-38.

64. Monte SA, Ehya H, Lang WR: Positive effusion cytology as the initial presentation of malignancy. Acta Cytol 1987;31:448-452.

65. Feinsilver SH, Barrows AA, Braman SS: Fiberoptic bronchoscopy and pleural effusion of unknown origin. Chest 1986;90:514-515.

66. Decker DA, Dines DE, Payne WS, et al: The significance of a cytologically negative pleural effusion in bronchogenic carcinoma. Chest 1978;74:640-642.

67. Jones SE, Durie BGM, Salmon SE: Combination chemotherapy with Adriamycin and cyclophosphamide for advanced breast cancer. Cancer 1975;36:90-97.

68. Livingston RB, McCracken JD, Trauth CJ, Chen T: Isolated pleural effusion in small cell lung carcinoma: favorable prognosis. Chest 1982;81:208-211.

69. Albain KS, Crowley JJ, LeBlanc M, Livingston RB: Determinants of improved outcome in small-cell lung cancer: an analysis of the 2,580-patient Southwest Oncology Group data base. J Clin Oncol 1990;8:1563-1574.

70. Roy PH, Carr DT, Payne WS: The problem of chylothorax. Mayo Clin Proc 1967;42:457-467.

71. Leininger BJ, Barker WL, Langston HT: A simplified method for management of malignant pleural effusion. J Thorac Cardiovasc Surg 1969;58:758-763.

72. Sanchez-Armengol A, Rodriguez-Panadero F: Survival and talc pleurodesis in metastatic pleural carcinoma, revisited. Report of 125 cases. Chest 1993;104:1482-1485.

73. Weisberger AS, Levine B, Storaasli JP: Use of nitrogen mustard in treatment of serous effusions of neoplastic origin. JAMA 1955;159:1704-1706.

74. Ariel IM, Oropeza R, Pack GT: Intracavitary administration of radioactive isotopes in the control of effusions due to cancer. Cancer 1966;19:1096-1101.

75. Austin EH, Flye MW: The treatment of recurrent malignant pleural effusion. Ann Thorac Surg 1979;28:190-203.

76. Izbicki R, Weyhing BT, Baker L, et al: Pleural effusion in cancer patients: a prospective randomized study of pleural drainage with the addition of radio-active phosphorous to the pleural space vs. pleural drainage alone. Cancer 1975;36:1511-1518.

77. Dollinger MR, Krakoff IH, Karnofsky DA: Quinacrine (Atabrine) in the treatment of neoplastic effusions. Ann Intern Med 1967;66:249-257.

78. Adler RH, Sayek I: Treatment of malignant pleural effusion: a method using tube thoracostomy and talc. Ann Thorac Surg 1976;22:8-15.

79. Rubinson RM, Bolooki H: Intrapleural tetracycline for control of malignant pleural effusion: a preliminary report. South Med J 1972;65:847-849.

80. Bethune N: Pleural poudrage: new technique for deliberate production of pleural adhesions as preliminary to lobectomy. J Thorac Cardiovasc Surg 1935;4:251-261.

81. Bresticker MA, Oba J, LoCicero J 3d, Greene R: Optimal pleurodesis: a comparison study. Ann Thorac Surg 1993;55:364-366.

82. Aelony Y, King R, Boutin C: Thoracoscopy talc poudrage for chronic recurrent pleural effusions. Ann Intern Med 1991;115:778-782.

83. Hartman DL, Gaither JM, Kesler KA, Mylet DM, Brown JW, Mathur PN: Comparison of insufflated talc under thoracoscopic guidance with standard tetracycline and bleomycin pleurodesis for control of malignant pleural effusions. Cardiovasc Surg 1993;105:743-748.

84. Light RW, Vargas FS, Sassoon CSH, Gruer SE, Wang NS: Induction of a pleurodesis by the intrapleural injection of talc slurry in rabbits. Chest 1993;104:161S.

85. Light RW, Wang NS, Sassoon CSH, Gruer SE, Vargas FS: Comparison of the effectiveness of tetracycline and minocycline as pleural sclerosing agents in rabbits. Chest 1994;106:577-582.

86. Webb WR, Ozmen V, Moulder PV, Shabahang B, Breaux J: Iodized talc pleurodesis for the treatment of pleural effusions. J Thorac Cardiovasc Surg 1992;103:881-886.

87. Miller WC, Unger KM: Talc slurry for pleurodesis. (LTE) Chest 1994;107:1906-1907.

88. Kennedy L, Rusch VW, Strange C, Ginsberg RJ, Sahn SA: Pleurodesis using talc slurry. Chest 1994;106:342-346.

89. Bouchama A, Chastre J, Gaudichet A, et al: Acute pneumonitis with bilateral effusion after talc pleurodesis. Chest 1984;86:795-797.

90. Rinaldo JE, Owens GR, Rogers RM: Adult respiratory distress syndrome following intrapleural instillation of talc. J Thorac Cardiovasc Surg 1983;85:523-526.

91. Sorensen PG, Svendsen TL, Enk B: Treatment of malignant pleural effusion with drainage, with and without instillation of talc. Eur J Respir Dis 1984;65:131-135.

92. Audu PB, Sing RF, Mette SA, Fallahnejhad M: Fatal diffuse alveolar injury following use of intrapleural bleomycin. Chest 1993;103:1638.

93. Sahn SA, Good JT: The effect of common sclerosing agents on the rabbit pleural space. Am Rev Respir Dis 1981;124:65-67.

94. Sherman S, Grady KJ, Seidmen JC: Clinical experience with tetracycline pleurodesis of malignant pleural effusions. South Med J 1987;80:716-719.

95. Walker-Renard PB, Vaughan LM, Sahn SA: Chemical pleurodesis for malignant pleural effusion. Ann Intern Med 1994;120:56-64.

96. Costabel U: Adieu, Tetracycline Pleurodesis (but not in Germany). Chest 1993;103:984.

97. Robinson LA, Fleming WH, Galbraith TA: Intrapleural doxycycline control of malignant pleural effusions. Ann Thorac Surg 1993;55:1115-1121.

98. Heffner JE, Standerfer RJ, Torstveit J, Unruh L: Clinical efficacy of doxycycline for pleurodesis. Chest 1994;105:1743-1747.

99. Mansson T: Treatment of malignant pleural effusion with doxycycline. Scand J Infect Dis Suppl 1988;53:29-34.

100. Hatta T, Tsubuota N, Yoshimura M, Yanagawa M: Effect of intrapleural administration of minocycline on postoperative air leakage and malignant pleural effusion. Kyobu Geka 1990;43:283-286.

101. Ruckdeschel JC, Moores D, Lee JY, Einhorn LH, Mandelbaum I, Koeller J, et al: Intrapleural therapy for malignant pleural effusions. A randomized com-

parison of bleomycin and tetracycline. Chest 1991;
100:1528–1535.

102. Vargas FS, Wang NS, Despars JA, Gruer SE, Sassoon C, Light RW: Effectiveness of bleomycin in comparison to tetracycline as pleural sclerosing agent in rabbits. Chest 1993;104:1582–1584.

103. Maiche AG, Virkkunen P, Kontkanen T, Moykkynen K, Porkka K: Bleomycin and mitoxantrone in the treatment of malignant pleural effusions. Am J Clin Oncol 1993;16:50–53.

104. Alberts DS, Surwit EA, Peng Y-M, McCloskey T, Rivest R, Graham V, McDonald L, Roe D: Phase I clinical and pharmacokinetic study of mitoxantrone given to patients by intraperitoneal administration. Cancer Res 1988;48:5874–5877.

105. Kelly J, Holmes EC, Rosen G: Mitoxantrone for malignant pleural effusion due to metastatic sarcoma. Surg Oncol 1993;2:299–301.

106. Groth G, Gatzemeier U, Haubingen K, Heckmayr M, Magnussen H, Neuhauss R, Pavel JV: Intrapleural palliative treatment of malignant pleural effusions with mitoxantrone versus placebo (pleural tube alone). Ann Oncol 1991;2:213–215.

107. Light RW, Gruer SE, Wang NS, Teixeira LR, Silva LMMF, Vargas FS: Acute and chronic pleuropulmonary changes induced by intrapleural mitoxantrone in rabbits. Am J Respir Crit Care Med 1994;149:A973.

108. Feletti R, Ravazzoni C: Intrapleural *Corynebacterium parvum* for malignant pleural effusions. Thorax 1983;38:22–24.

109. Leahy BC, Honeybourne D, Brear SG, et al: Treatment of malignant pleural effusions with intrapleural *Corynebacterium parvum* or tetracycline. Eur J Respir Dis 1985;66:50–54.

110. Hillerdal G, Kiviloog J, Nou E, Steinholtz L: *Corynebacterium parvum* in malignant pleural effusion: a randomized prospective study. Eur J Respir Dis 1986;69:204–206.

111. Casali A, Gionfra T, Rinaldi M, et al: Treatment of malignant pleural effusions with intracavitary *Corynebacterium parvum*. Cancer 1988;62:806–811.

112. Vargas FS, Cukier A, Teixeira LR, Terra-Filho M, Light RW: Effectiveness of *Corynebacterium parvum* as pleural sclerosing agent in rabbits. Am J Respir Crit Care Med 1994;149:A972.

113. Walsh FW, Alberts WM, Solomon DA, Goldman AL: Malignant pleural effusions: pleurodesis using a small-bore percutaneous catheter. South Med J 1989;82:963–965.

114. Villanueva AG, Gray AW Jr, Shahian DM, Williamson WA, Beamis JF Jr: Efficacy of short term versus long term tube thoracostomy drainage before tetracycline pleurodesis in the treatment of malignant pleural effusions. Thorax 1994;49:23–25.

115. Bubik JS: Preparation of sterile talc for treatment of pleural effusion [letter]. AM J Hospit Pharm 1992; 49:562–563.

116. Aelony Y: Talc sterilization for thoracoscopic talc poudrage. Am J Respir Crit Care Med 1994;149: 512A.

117. Wallach HW: Intrapleural therapy with tetracycline and lidocaine for malignant pleural effusions. Chest 1978;73:246.

118. Sherman S, Ravikrishnan KP, Patel AS, et al: Optimum anesthesia with intrapleural lidocaine during chemical pleurodesis with tetracycline. Chest 1988; 93:533–536.

119. Vargas FS, Teixeira LR, Coelho IJC, Braga GA, Terra-Filho M, Light RW: Distribution of pleural injectate: effect of volume of injectate and animal rotation. Chest 1994;106:1246–1249.

120. Lorch DG, Gordon L, Wooten S, et al: Effect of patient positioning on distribution of tetracycline in the pleural space during pleurodesis. Chest 1988;93:527–529.

121. Dryzer SR, Allen ML, Strange C, Sahn SA: A comparison of rotation and nonrotation in tetracycline pleurodesis. Chest 1993;104:1763–1766.

122. Landvater L, Hix WR, Mills M, et al: Malignant pleural effusion treated by tetracycline sclerotherapy: a comparison of single vs repeated instillation. Chest 1988;93:1196–1198.

123. Cimochowski GE, Joyner LR, Fardin R, et al: Pleuroperitoneal shunting for recalcitrant pleural effusion. J Thorac Cardiovasc Surg 1986;92:866–870.

124. Little AG, Kadowaki MH, Ferguson MK, et al: Pleuroperitoneal shunting: alternative therapy for pleural effusions. Ann Surg 1988;208:443–450.

125. Tzeng E, Ferguson MK: Predicting failure following shunting of pleural effusions. Chest 1990;98:890–893.

126. Lee KA, Harvey JC, Reich H, Beattie EJ: Management of malignant pleural effusions with pleuroperitoneal shunting. J Am College Surg 1994;178:586–588.

127. Tsang V, Fernando HC, Goldstraw P: Pleuroperitoneal shunt for recurrent malignant pleural effusion. Thorax 1990;45:369–372.

128. Ponn RB, Blancaflor J, D'Agostino RS, Kiernan ME, Toole AL, Stern H: Pleuroperitoneal shunting for intractable pleural effusions. Ann Thorac Surg 1991; 51:605–609.

129. Martini N, Bains MS, Beattie EJ Jr: Indications for pleurectomy in malignant effusion. Cancer 1975;35: 734–738.

130. Robinson RD, Fullerton DA, Albert JD, Sorensen J, Johnston MR: Use of pleural Tenckhoff catheter to palliate malignant pleural effusion. Ann Thorac Surg 1994;57:286–288.

131. Strober SJ, Klotz E, Kuperman A, Ghossein NA: Malignant pleural disease: a radiotherapeutic approach to the problem. JAMA 1973;226:296–299.

132. Luh KT, Yang PC, Kuo SH, Chang DB, Yu CJ, Lee LN: Comparison of OK-432 and mitomycin C pleurodesis for malignant pleural effusion caused by lung cancer. A randomized trial. Cancer 1992;69: 674–679.

133. Kan N, Kodama H, Hori T, Takenaka A, Yasumura T, Kato H, Ogawa H, Mukaihara S, Kudo T, Ohsumi K, et al: Intrapleural adaptive immunotherapy for breast cancer patients with cytologically-confirmed malignant pleural effusions: an analysis of 67 pa-

tients in Kyoto and Shiga Prefecture, Japan. Breast Can Res Treat 1993;27:203–210.

134. Chao TY, Hwang WS: Treating carcinomatous pleural effusion by intrapleural injection of OK-432 in patients with non-small-cell lung cancer. Chung Hua I Hsueh Tsa Chih (Taipei) 1993;52:229–234.

135. Hagiwara A, et al: Chemotherapy for carcinomatous peritonitis and pleuritis with MMC-CH, mitomycin C absorbed on activated carbon particles: clinical trials. Cancer 1987;59:245–251.

136. Ike O, Shimizu Y, Hitomi S, Wada R, Ikada Y: Treatment of malignant pleural effusions with doxorubicin hydrochloride containing poly(L-lactic acid) microspheres. Chest 1991;99:911–915.

137. Jereb B, Us-Krasovec M, Cervek J, Soos E: Intrapleural application of human leukocyte interferon (LHI) in breast cancer patients with ipsilateral pleural carcinomatosis. J Interferon Res 1987;7:357–363.

138. Rosso R, Rimoldi R, Salvati F, et al: Intrapleural natural beta interferon in the treatment of malignant pleural effusions. Oncology 1988;45:253–256.

139. Tercelj-Zorman M, Mermolja M, Jereb M, et al: Human leukocyte interferon alpha (HLI-alpha) for treatment of pleural effusion caused by non small cell lung cancer. A pilot study. Acta Oncol 1991; 963–965.

140. Bhatia A, Rice TW, McLain D, Herzog P, Budd GT, Murthy S, Kirby TJ, Bukowski RM: A phase I trial of intrapleural recombinant human interferon alpha (rHuIFN alpha 2b) in patients with malignant pleural effusions. J Cancer Res Clin Oncol 1994;120:169–172.

141. Liu X, Li D, Zhang C, Ba D, Liu J, Wan T, Li Z, Jin Y, He Y: Treatment of 121 patients with malignant effusion due to advanced lung cancer by intrapleural transfer of autologous or allogeneic LAK cells combined with rIL-2. Chinese Med Sci J 1993;8:186–189.

142. Yasumoto K, Mivazaki K, Nagishma A, et al: Induction of lymphokine-activated killer cells by intrapleural instillations of recombinant interleukin-2 in patients with malignant pleurisy due to lung cancer. Cancer Res 1987;47:2184–2187.

143. Pectasides D, Stewart S, Courtenay-Luck N, et al: Antibody-guided irradiation of malignant pleural and pericardial effusions. Br J Cancer 1986;53:727–732.

144. Jensen MO, Matthees DJ, Antonenko D: Laser thoracoscopy for pleural effusion. Am Surg 1992;58:667–669.

CHAPTER 8

Malignant and Benign Mesotheliomas

MALIGNANT MESOTHELIOMAS

Malignant mesotheliomas are thought to arise from the mesothelial cells that line the pleural cavities. Individuals with a history of exposure to asbestos have a much greater risk of developing these neoplasms. Malignant mesothelioma, with its dismal prognosis, should be differentiated from the benign mesothelioma with its excellent prognosis, discussed later in this chapter. About 20% of mesotheliomas arise in the peritoneal cavity (1), but only pleural mesotheliomas are discussed in this chapter.

Incidence

The current annual incidence of malignant mesotheliomas is approximately 11.4/1,000,000 in males and 2.8/1,000,000 in females in the United States (1). Thus, about 2,000 cases of malignant mesothelioma can be expected annually in the United States. The incidence of mesothelioma approximately doubled between 1975 to 1979 and 1980 to 1984 (1). That the incidence of mesothelioma is increasing is to be expected because asbestos use became widespread only in the last 60 years (2). The incidence of malignant mesothelioma is much higher in asbestos workers. Between January 1, 1967 and December 31, 1976, there were 2,271 deaths among 17,800 asbestos insulation workers, and 2.8% of the deaths were due to pleural mesothelioma (3).

Etiologic Factors

The occurrence of mesothelioma in many persons is certainly related to previous exposure to asbestos. Asbestos is a fibrous silicate of various chemical types. The main types of asbestos are chrysotile and the amphiboles, which include crocidolite, amosite, tremolite, actinolite, and anthophyllite. The different types of asbestos vary in their ability to induce mesothelioma (4). Fibers with the greatest length-to-diameter ratio are the most carcinogenic (4). Chrysotile accounts for about 90% of the commercial asbestos, but probably is related to the development of mesothelioma only when the level of exposure is high (5). It appears that the lack of the association between malignancy and chrysotile exposure is due to the fact that it is cleared from the lungs in a matter of weeks, while the amphiboles are only cleared in a matter of decades (5). Crocidolite and amosite are the most carcinogenic amphiboles. Tremolite is a potent inducer of mesothelioma when the fibers have a high length-to-diameter ratio, such as occurs in some areas of Greece (6), but the tremolite that contaminates chrysotile ore has a short length and appears to be a low-grade mesothelial carcinogen (6). No case of mesothelioma has been reported to date among Finnish miners exposed to anthophyllite asbestos, although there is a high incidence of pleural calcification as a result of this exposure.

Epidemiologic studies have implicated asbestos in the pathogenesis of malignant mesothelioma. The percentage of patients with mesothelioma who have a history of occupational exposure to asbestos ranges from 10% in a series from the Mayo Clinic (7) to 70% in New England, England, and South Africa (8), where shipyards or asbestos mines are located. The risk of developing mesothelioma from asbestos exposure appears to be higher in manufacturing industries than in mining and milling. Because asbestos is found in a variety of industrial products, including insulation, roofing and ceiling tiles, brake linings, and numerous small appliances, many individuals are unaware of their exposure to this substance.

Further evidence implicating asbestos as an etiologic agent in mesotheliomas comes from animal studies. The intrapleural injection of any of the different types of asbestos (including chrysotile) results in the production of mesotheliomas in 8 to 66% of animals, depending upon the dose. These mesotheliomas are histologically identical to the human tumor (9, 10).

The interval between the first exposure to asbestos and the emergence of the tumor is usually 20 to 40 years (11). Mesotheliomas have developed in children, however, and the parents of some of these children worked with asbestos (12). In contrast to the other manifestations of asbestosis such as parenchymal fibrosis or pleural plaques, no close relationship exists between the degree and duration of asbestos exposure and the development of mesotheliomas (12).

An interesting paper on the epidemiology of mesotheliomas is that of Baris and colleagues, who studied the population of Karain, a small village in Turkey (13). In this particular village, with a population under 600, about 1% of the population dies each year of malignant mesothelioma. Villagers are usually aged 40 to 60 when the mesotheliomas develop. Asbestos does not occur in the local soil or rocks, nor is it handled in the village. The atmosphere at Karain contains increased amounts of erionite, however, a mineral of the zeolite family and the major contributor to the Karain clouds. This report suggests that the inhalation of airborne respirable fibers other than asbestos can be associated with the subsequent development of pleural mesotheliomas (13). Indeed, when erionite fibers are administered intrapleurally to rats, they are two orders of magnitude more carcinogenic than crocidolite (14).

There are probably other factors related to the development of pleural mesothelioma. Antman and associates (15) reported that mesothelioma developed in proximity to a field of therapeutic radiation administered 10 to 31 years previously in 4 patients. Roviaro and coworkers (16) reviewed 35 cases of pleural mesothelioma and found that 3 of the patients had calcified posttuberculous fibrothorax.

At times the asbestos exposure may not be obvious. In one report (17), 5 cases of mesothelioma developed in a Native American pueblo of approximately 2000 persons. Epidemiologic investigation revealed that asbestos mats were used to insulate work tables against the intense heat of brazing torches and molten metal in the preparation of silver jewelry. In addition, the villagers scrubbed leather with cakes of asbestos to make their leggings and moccasins a brilliant white.

Pathologic Features

Malignant mesotheliomas in the earliest stages appear grossly as multiple white or gray granules, nodules, or flakes on normal or opaque visceral or parietal pleura (18). As the tumor progresses, the pleural surface becomes progressively thicker and nodular in appearance. The growing tumor extends in all directions to form a continuous layer encasing the lung and leading to contraction of the involved hemothorax. In advanced cases, the diaphragm, liver, pericardium, heart, contralateral pleura, and other mediastinal structures may be involved. At autopsy, hematogenously disseminated metastases are present in about 50% of patients. In contrast to other sarcomas, however, the hematogenous metastases are usually clinically silent, and death generally results from complications arising from the primary lesion (8).

Microscopically, malignant mesotheliomas are characterized by marked structural variation within a single tumor or among different tumors with a similar gross appearance (18). Histologically, malignant mesotheliomas are classified as epithelial, mesenchymal, or mixed tumors (19). The neoplastic cells of the epithelial form may show various epithelial arrangements such as papillary, tubular, tubulopapillary, cordlike, and sheetlike patterns (19). The epithelial cells may take various shapes, but most commonly are cuboidal and uniform in size with vesicular nuclei. The mesenchymal (fibrous) form resembles a spindle cell sarcoma in that the cells are spindle-shaped with a parallel arrangement, and have ovoid or elongated nuclei with well-developed nucleoli (19). The mixed form reveals features of both the epithelial and mesenchymal forms.

The frequency of the three main histologic types varies in different series. In a compilation of 819 cases from the literature, 50% were epithelial, 34% were mixed, and 16% were mesenchymal (20). The more separate biopsies obtained, the more likely for the tumor to be classified as mixed. In one series of 44 mesotheliomas, careful review of the pathologic material led the authors to classify all 44 as mixed tumors (21).

Electron microscopic study of mesotheliomas reveals abundant long, slender microvilli and prominent desmosomes; with metastatic adenocarcinoma, the microvilli are short and blunt (8). In addition, malignant mesotheliomas have a different distribution of intracellular organelles than metastatic carcinomas (19).

Clinical Manifestations

Two-thirds of patients with malignant mesothelioma are between the ages of 40 and 70 years (8, 22), and many have a history of exposure to asbestos 20 or more years in the past. Most patients initially experience the insidious onset of chest pain or shortness of breath (4). Patients usually have had symptoms for several months before they see a physician (4). The chest pain is usually nonpleuritic and is frequently referred to the upper abdomen or shoulder because of diaphragmatic involvement. As the disease progresses, the patients lose weight and develop a dry, hacking cough and progressive dyspnea. Some patients have irregular episodes of low-grade fever (22). Occasionally, the presenting sign is either intermittent hypoglycemia or hypertrophic pulmonary osteoarthropathy (8), but these disorders are much more common with benign mesothelioma.

Radiographic Manifestations

The chest radiograph (Fig. 8.1) reveals a pleural effusion in about 75% of patients (23). This effusion is frequently large, occupying 50% or more of the hemithorax and obscuring the pleural tumor. In about one-third of patients, pleural plaques are evident in the opposite hemithorax (24). With progression of the disease, the tumor encases the ipsilateral lung and thereby produces a mediastinal shift to the side of the effusion and results in a loculated pleural effusion. In the late stages of the disease, the chest radiograph may show mediastinal widening, enlargement of the cardiac shadow due to infiltration of the pericardium, and destruction of the ribs or soft tissue masses (11).

Because routine chest radiographs often underestimate the extent of the disease, chest computed tomography (CT) scans are invaluable in delineating the extent of the disease (23-25). Chest CT scans should be obtained in all patients in whom a malignant mesothelioma is considered (Fig. 8.1C). The CT scan reveals that the pleura is thickened, with an irregular, often nodular internal margin that serves to distinguish this tumor from other types of pleural thickening. These changes are most pronounced at the base of the lung. The CT scan usually reveals marked thickening of the major fissure due to a combination of fibrosis, tumor, and associated fluid. The fissure may also appear nodular because of tumor infiltration (24). At times, pleural thickening is seen predominantly along the mediastinum. In such cases, the pulmonary margin is irregular, and separate nodules representing either metastases or lymph node infiltration may be seen in the juxtamediastinal tissue.

The volume of the hemithorax with malignant mesothelioma is quite varied. If the patient has a pleural effusion with pleural thickening and decreased volume of the ipsilateral hemithorax, it is very suggestive of mesothelioma. In one series, the volume of the hemithorax was reduced in 42% of 50 cases of mesothelioma (23). It should be emphasized, however, that contralateral mediastinal shift is seen in about 15% of cases and this is usually due to a large effusion (23).

The CT scan is also useful in demonstrating disease beyond the pleura and thereby is quite useful in staging the disease. It often reveals intrapulmonary nodules that are not apparent on the standard chest radiograph (24). The CT scan may reveal chest wall invasion, diaphragmatic invasion, or extension of the tumor to the liver or retroperitoneal space. CT scans are not without their problems with mesothelioma; it is often very difficult to distinguish pleural disease alone from associated pericardial disease, and extensive pleural disease often envelops and obscures the nodal anatomy in the hilar and middle mediastinal nodal groups (23).

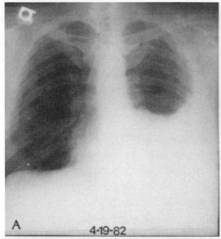

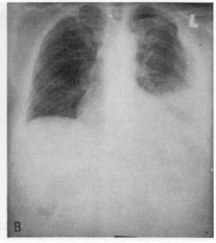

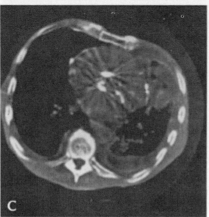

Figure 8.1. Malignant mesothelioma. **A.** Posteroanterior chest radiograph demonstrating left pleural effusion and thickening of the pleura over the upper left lung. **B.** Posteroanterior chest radiograph from the same patient after therapeutic thoracentesis revealing a small left lung and marked pleural thickening. **C.** CT scan of chest demonstrating shrunken left hemithorax and shift of the mediastinum toward the left. Pericardial calcifications due to previous asbestos exposure are also present.

Pleural Fluid

The pleural fluid with mesotheliomas is yellow in about 50% of patients and serosanguineous in the remainder. This fluid is exudative. In approximately one-third of patients, the pleural fluid glucose is below 50 mg/dl and the pleural fluid pH is below 7.20 (26). Patients with a low pleural fluid pH or low pleural fluid glucose levels tend to have a poorer prognosis (26). The pleural fluid generally is cellular and contains a mixture of normal mesothelial cells, differentiated and undifferentiated malignant mesothelial cells, and varying numbers of lymphocytes and polymorphonuclear leukocytes (27).

At times, the pleural fluid of patients with malignant mesothelioma is viscid, owing to the presence of large amounts of hyaluronate, which was previously called hyaluronic acid. Nurminen and coworkers (28) assessed the diagnostic utility of hyaluronate levels by as-saying the levels in 1039 pleural fluids, including 50 from mesothelioma. They found that with a cutoff of 75 mg/L for hyaluronate, the assay specificity for malignant mesothelioma was 100% and the sensitivity was 56% (28). It should be noted that another study (29) demonstrated that the hyaluronate measurements were much less useful. It appears that the poor results in the latter study are probably attributable to procedural mistakes (30). The results by Nurminen (28) were obtained by high performance liquid chromatography (HPLC), and this assay is not generally available in the United States.

Diagnosis

The diagnosis of malignant mesothelioma should be considered in all patients with exudative pleural effusions. The suspicion of mesothelioma should be higher in middle-aged or older patients with persistent chest pain or shortness of breath, particularly if there is a history of asbestos exposure. The chest CT scan is frequently suggestive of the diagnosis. Although a diagnosis of malignancy can be established by cytologic smears or needle biopsies of the pleura, these procedures usually cannot distinguish between a metastatic adenocarcinoma and a mesothelioma. In one series (31) 80 patients with mesothelioma had pleural fluid cytology. In 20 patients (25%), cytologic examination of the pleural fluid established that the patient had malignant disease, but in none could the diagnosis of mesothelioma be established definitely with only cytology. There are, however, certain cytological features that assist in making this differentiation. One report (32) compared the cytological features of 44 cases of malignant mesothelioma and 46 cases of metastatic adenocarcinomas and concluded that the following five features separate malignant mesothelioma from adenocarcinoma with better than 95.4% accuracy. Mesotheliomas tend to have true papillary aggregation, multinucleation with atypia, and cell-to-cell apposition, while adenocarcinomas tend to have acinuslike structures and balloonlike vacuolation (32). Needle biopsy of the pleura is usually not diagnostic of mesothelioma. In one report (31) the needle biopsy was diagnostic of mesothelioma in only 18 of 84 cases (21%).

Accordingly, more invasive procedures are necessary to provide a larger tissue sample so that a definitive diagnosis can be made. If the patient has skin deposits, these should be biopsied. However, usually the diagnosis must be made with thoracoscopy or open biopsy. The diagnosis of mesothelioma is made about 90% of the time with thoracoscopy. When two recent series (33, 34) are combined, the diagnosis was established in 51 of the 56 (90%) patients. These results are similar to those with thoracotomy and open biopsy (22). Thoracoscopy is therefore the procedure of choice because its diagnostic yield is similar to that of open thoracotomy, but the procedure is less invasive (35).

Since malignant mesothelioma often infiltrates needle tracts, thoracotomy scars, and chest tube drainage sites (36) it has been suggested that one should avoid performing such procedures in patients with suspected mesothelioma (36). The occurrence of such skin deposits, however, appears to have little clinical consequence because they are not painful and cause no other morbidity (31). Accordingly I am not hesitant to perform such procedures when they are clinically indicated in patients suspected of having malignant mesothelioma.

Over the past 2 decades, three new techniques have been developed that improve the accuracy in diagnosing mesothelioma. These three techniques are histochemical staining with periodic acid-Schiff stain, immunoperoxidase studies with monoclonal antibodies, and electron microscopy. In order to obtain these special studies, biopsy specimens should be immediately fixed in neutral buffered formalin, and a small piece should be fixed in glutaraldehyde for electron microscopy.

The differentiation of the epithelial variety of malignant mesothelioma from the more common metastatic adenocarcinoma is frequently difficult. The periodic acid-Schiff stain is probably the single most reliable histochemical method available to distinguish mesotheliomas from adenocarcinomas. The presence of strongly positive vacuoles after diastase digestion effectively establishes the diagnosis of adenocarcinoma, although not all adenocarcinomas have this staining characteristic. In addition, most mesotheliomas contain large amounts of hyaluronate that stain positively with colloidal iron or Alcian blue stains. To be unequivocally positive, absence or attenuation of blue staining after pretreatment of a serial section with bovine testicular hyaluronidase overnight is required (37).

The value of pleural fluid cytologic examination in establishing the diagnosis of malignant mesothelioma is limited by the subtle differences between benign and malignant mesothelial cells. However, immunohistochemical studies on cell blocks from pleural fluid are useful in distinguishing mesothelioma from adenocarcinoma (38–40) (see Chapter 4). When one desires to make this distinction, immunohistochemical tests should be performed with carcinoembryonic antigen (CEA), B72.3, and Leu M1. If two or three of the tests are positive, the patient in all probability has adenocarcinoma. If none of the tests are positive, the patient in all probability has mesothelioma. It should be noted that with benign mesothelial cells, the tests will also be negative. Immunohistochemical studies are recommended if there is any doubt as to whether the patient has adenocarcinoma or mesothelioma.

Electron microscopy is also useful in distinguishing mesotheliomas from metastatic adenocarcinomas. The ultrastructural features of mesotheliomas are so characteristic as to be almost diagnostic. These characteristics include the absence of microvillus core rootlets, glycocalyceal bodies and secretory granules, the presence of intracellular desmosomes, junctional complexes, and intracytoplasmic lumina and characteristic microvilli. The appearance of the microvilli is the most important diagnostically; in mesothelioma they are numerous and are characteristically long and thin, whereas in adenocarcinoma they are typically much less frequent and are usually short and stubby (41, 42). In one study (42), the mean length:diameter ratio for the mesotheliomas with scanning electron microscopy was 19.7:1 (range 13.7–23.5:1) while that for adenocarcinomas was 2.5:1 (range 1.3–4.1). Scanning electron microscopy can be used when glutaraldehyde-fixed, plastic-embedded tissue is not available for transmission electron microscopy (42).

Flow cytometry does not appear to be particularly useful in establishing the diagnosis of malignant mesothelioma. Burmer and coworkers (43) performed flow cytometry on 46 cases of malignant pleural mesothelioma and 31 nonmesothelioma malignancies of the pleural space. They reported that 65% of the mesotheliomas were diploid in DNA content, with intermediate-to-low proliferative rates. In contrast, 85% of the nonmesothelial malignant neoplasms were aneuploid.

Management and Prognosis

In general, the prognosis of patients with malignant mesothelioma is dismal. The median survival time is about 7 months after diagnosis (22, 44). Survival is related to the stage of the disease (Table 8.1) at the time of diagnosis, with median survivals of 13 months, 9 months, and 2 months for stage I, II, and III disease, respectively (45). Patients with the epithelial variant have a longer median survival rate (46).

Table 8.1. Pathologic Staging of Diffuse Malignant Mesothelioma of the Pleura

Stage	Manifestation
I	Tumor confined within the capsule of the parietal pleura, i.e., involving only the ipsilateral pleura, lung, pericardium, and diaphragm
II	Tumor involving chest wall or mediastinal structures; possible lymph node involvement inside the chest
III	Tumor penetrating diaphragm to involve the peritoneum; contralateral pleural involvement; lymph node involvement outside the chest
IV	Distant bloodborne metastases

Modified from Butchart EG, Ashcroft T, Barnsley WC, Holden MP: The role of surgery in diffuse malignant mesothelioma of the pleura. Semin Oncol 1981;8:321–328. By permission of Grune & Stratton.

Survival varies inversely with age, with the longest survival occurring in the youngest age group (44). Survival is also poorer in patients with regional lymph node involvement. In one series, the 5-year survival rate was 45% in patients with the epithelial variant and negative mediastinal lymph nodes who underwent radical surgery followed by chemotherapy and radiotherapy. Patients with an aneuploid pattern on flow cytometry also have a worse prognosis (47). The prognosis is better in women than it is in men (44). Hematogenously disseminated metastases can be documented at autopsy in approximately 50% of patients, but death is usually from respiratory failure rather than from complications of the metastases (48).

Staging

When a patient is suspected of having a mesothelioma, the extent of the disease should be staged because the stage of the disease dictates the therapeutic approach. The staging scheme proposed by Butchart and coworkers (49) is shown in Table 8.1. In recent years there have been other staging systems proposed, namely, those by Chahinian (50) and the Union Internationale Contre le Cancer (UICC) (51). The latter two systems are based on the tumor-node-metastasis (TMN) categories. In order to stage the disease, the following studies are required: a barium swallow to assess esophageal involvement; a bronchoscopic examination to assess involvement of the tracheobronchial tree; a chest CT scan to assess mediastinal or chest wall involvement; brain, liver, and bone scans to look for distant metastases, and possibly, a pneumoperitoneogram to look for diaphragmatic penetration (49).

Equally important is the characterization of the tumor microscopically. The epithelial mesothelioma has a better prognosis than the mesenchymal mesothelioma (46). It is also likely that the responses to chemotherapy and to radiotherapy may depend on the microscopic characteristics of the tumor. Therefore, it is important to characterize malignant mesotheliomas carefully microscopically so that the optimal therapy for this tumor can be developed.

No satisfactory treatment exists for malignant mesothelioma. There are no controlled studies demonstrating that any treatment is effective in prolonging survival. It is unclear whether any of the available treatments prolong life. Law and coworkers (52) compared the survival rates in 64 untreated patients and 52 treated patients seen at the Brompton and the Royal Marsden Hospitals between 1971 and 1980. The two groups of patients had comparable clinical conditions at the time of presentation. Whether or not the patient received treatment depended on the attending physician; some treated all patients while others managed all patients symptomatically. The survival curves for the 64 untreated patients and the 12 patients who received radiotherapy, the 28 patients who received decortication, and the 12 patients who received chemotherapy, were virtually identical. The median survival was about 18 months; 10% of patients survived more than 4 years, including 7 of the 64 (11%) of the untreated patients (52). These results indicate that controlled cooperative studies are needed to assess the effectiveness of the various treatment modalities proposed for malignant mesothelioma.

Surgical Treatment

Surgical management appears to be the only form of therapy that offers the patient any hope for cure. Butchart and coworkers (49) operated on 29 patients with malignant mesothelioma between 1959 and 1972 and re-

ported that 2 patients (7%) were alive, without evidence of recurrence, 3.5 and 6 years after operation. The surgical resections performed by this group were extensive, with removal of the pleura, lung, lymph nodes, ipsilateral pericardium, and diaphragm. The in-hospital postoperative mortality rate was 31%. These workers concluded that radical pleuropneumonectomy was only indicated for patients under the age of 60 who are fit and who have stage I tumors of the epithelial type.

DaValle and colleagues (53) performed extrapleural pneumonectomies in 33 patients with malignant mesothelioma. Their operative mortality rate was 9%, and serious postoperative complications occurred in 24% of the patients. Five of their 33 patients lived more than 3 years, but 3 of these patients subsequently died of mesothelioma.

Sugarbaker and colleagues (46) recently reported their results for 52 patients who underwent an extrapleural pneumonectomy followed by chemotherapy and radiotherapy. They only operated on patients who were Butchart stage I preoperatively after CT scan and magnetic resonance imaging (MRI) of the mediastinum. They operated on 32 patients with the epithelial-type tumor and these patients had 1-, 2-, and 3-year survival rates of 77%, 50%, and 42%, respectively. If the patients had negative mediastinal lymph nodes at surgery, the 5-year survival rate was 45%. In contrast the 20 patients with the sarcomatous or mixed-cell type had 1- and 2-year survival rates of 45% and 7.5%, and none lived longer than 25 months. It is unclear the role that chemotherapy and radiotherapy played in this series.

Based upon the above series, it is recommended that patients in relatively good health who have stage I disease of the epithelial type be subjected to this radical surgery. However, it should be recognized that this is only a small fraction of the patients with mesothelioma (54).

Other researchers have recommended that only pleurectomies be performed (22, 55). Wanebo and colleagues (55) performed pleurectomies on 33 patients with malignant mesothelioma of whom 17 had the epithelial variant and 16 the mesenchymal variant. Four of the 17 patients with the epithelial variant

(23%), and 3 of the 16 patients with the mesenchymal type (19%) were disease-free at 17 to 69 months postoperatively. These authors followed their surgical procedures with high-dose radiotherapy or systemic chemotherapy because tumor was left behind when pneumonectomies were not performed. The regimens of chemotherapy and radiotherapy were not consistent, and therefore their roles in combination with resection remain to be defined. The large advantage that this surgery has over the extrapleural pneumonectomy is that it has a much lower associated morbidity and mortality (22). However, it appears less likely to cure the patient since tumor is left behind.

Controlled studies are needed to compare the extrapleural pneumonectomy with the pleurectomy with no surgery.

Chemotherapy

The role of chemotherapy in the treatment of malignant mesothelioma remains to be defined. No chemotherapy trials have stratified patients according to histologic form or stage of the disease. Moreover, until recently, most patients with mesothelioma did not have objective parameters to follow, in that the extent of the disease could not be gauged accurately from the chest radiographs. The availability of CT scan of the chest has corrected this deficiency, however.

Doxorubicin (adriamycin) appears to be the most active single agent against mesothelioma (56). In a series of 36 patients, 16 patients (44%) had some regression of their tumor after doxorubicin administration, and an additional 4 patients (11%) had stabilization of their disease (56). As single agents, alkylating drugs (cyclophosphamide, mechlorethamine, melphalan), 5-fluorouracil, and procarbazine all appear to be effective in some cases of malignant mesothelioma (57).

Combination chemotherapy with or without radiotherapy and/or surgery has also been tried for malignant mesothelioma, but no strong evidence suggests that a combined regimen is more effective than symptomatic therapy (57–59). Cooperative studies in which the tumors are carefully staged and classified histologically are needed to determine the optimal chemotherapeutic regimen for malignant mesothelioma. Until such studies are completed, it is recommended that patients with inoperable mesotheliomas be carefully staged and treated with doxorubicin alone until progression of the disease is evident. At that time, the more toxic multiple-drug regimens should be considered.

Radiotherapy

The results with radiotherapy in the treatment of malignant mesothelioma have been disappointing. External radiotherapy does not control mesotheliomas locally and is associated with severe toxicity in the underlying lung (60). It is not recommended at the present time. There may be a place for internal radiation therapy in the management of malignant mesothelioma (57). In one report from the Memorial Sloan-Kettering Cancer Center, 33 patients were treated with the implantation of permanent radioactive iodine-125 sources in residual tumor. This report concluded that the local radiotherapy improved the length of survival (57).

Palliative Therapy

Shortness of breath and chest pain are the two most troublesome symptoms in patients with malignant mesothelioma. The shortness of breath can be due either to the presence of a large pleural effusion or to invasion of the lung or mediastinum by the tumor. If the patient is breathless and has a pleural effusion, a therapeutic thoracentesis should be performed. If the shortness of breath is relieved by the thoracentesis, a pleurodesis should be attempted (31), or a pleuroperitoneal shunt inserted. Details concerning both these procedures are delineated in Chapter 7. If the shortness of breath is not relieved by the thoracentesis, then oxygen or opiates should be prescribed.

The other main symptom in patients with malignant mesothelioma is chest pain, frequently caused by tumor invasion of the chest wall. In such persons, local palliative radiotherapy may relieve the symptoms (11), but frequently, the response is minimal or nonexistent (31, 36). More often, strong analgesics must be administered to control the pain.

Another troublesome symptom in approximately one-third of patients is intermittent fever and sweating (31). Law and coworkers (31) reported that the administration of prednisolone was of some benefit in alleviating the fever and sweating and usually improved the appetite and the well-being of the patient.

BENIGN FIBROUS MESOTHELIOMAS

Benign fibrous mesotheliomas are localized pleural tumors with a good prognosis, in contrast to malignant mesotheliomas. These tumors are uncommon, but over a 25-year period, 52 cases were seen at the Mayo Clinic (61). Most patients with benign fibrous mesothelioma have no history of asbestos exposure (61, 62).

Pathologic Features

Grossly benign fibrous mesotheliomas appear as firm, encapsulated yellow tumors, which may be vascular with prominent veins over their external surfaces (63). About 70% of benign fibrous mesotheliomas arise from the visceral pleura, whereas 30% arise from the parietal pleura. At times, these tumors invade the lung and chest wall locally (64). Benign fibrous mesotheliomas are characterized histologically by uniform, elongated spindle cells and varied amounts of collagen and reticulum fibers in bundles of many sizes (61). The cell of origin of this tumor is not yet known; some believe that the tumor arises from the multipotential subpleural fibroblasts (62, 65), whereas others believe that the tumor arises from the mesothelial cell (64). An absolute distinction between a localized benign fibrous and a localized malignant mesothelioma is not always possible (64).

Clinical Manifestations

Approximately 50% of patients with benign fibrous mesotheliomas are asymptomatic, and the tumor is detected on routine chest radiographs (61, 62). In the remaining patients, cough, chest pain, and dyspnea are the most frequent symptoms, each occurring in about 40% of symptomatic patients. About 25% of symptomatic patients are febrile without any evidence of infection (62). The incidence of hypertrophic pulmonary osteoarthropathy in patients with benign fibrous mesotheliomas is high. Approximately 20% of patients with this tumor have hypertrophic pulmonary osteoarthropathy, and the incidence is much higher with larger tumors. In one series, 10 of 11 patients (91%) with lesions greater than 7 cm in diameter had hypertrophic pulmonary osteoarthropathy, whereas none of 41 patients with smaller lesions had the syndrome (61). When the tumors are surgically removed, the symptoms of hypertrophic pulmonary osteoarthropathy are relieved immediately in almost all patients (61).

Another paraneoplastic syndrome that sometimes accompanies benign fibrous mesothelioma is hypoglycemia. Of the approximately 150 extrapancreatic tumors causing hypoglycemia reported by 1975, 10 were benign fibrous mesotheliomas. In a review of 360 cases of benign fibrous mesothelioma, symptomatic hypoglycemia was reported in 4% (62). The mechanism responsible for the hypoglycemia appears to be the production of high levels of insulinlike growth factor II by the tumor (66). The increased production of this insulin-like substance leads to an increased use of glucose by peripheral tissues and perhaps by the tumor. Concomitantly, there is impairment of the counterregulatory response mediated by growth hormone, and hypoglycemia results. The hypoglycemia is relieved with surgical removal of the tumor.

Radiologically, these tumors are manifested as solitary, sharply defined, discrete masses located at the periphery of the lung or related to a fissure (8, 63). The mass is frequently lobulated (8). The mass has an associated pleural effusion about 10% of the time (61, 63) but the presence or absence of an effusion apparently has no effect on the patient's prognosis (8). The mass may occupy the entire hemithorax and may shift the heart and the mediastinum to the contralateral side (63). Calcium is occasionally evident within the mass (63).

The appearance of the benign mesothelioma on CT scan is characteristic (67, 68). The tumors are large, noninvasive and tend to be enhanced by intravenous contrast material, but the enhancement is frequently nonhomogeneous. The intense enhancement of these tumors appears to be due to their high vascularity, while areas of low attenuation are due to foci of myxoid or cystic degeneration and hemorrhage in the lesion (67). There is no associated mediastinal lymphadenopathy.

Diagnosis

A thoracotomy is necessary for diagnosis (8). The existence of benign tumors, such as fibrous mesothelioma, that can produce systemic symptoms underlines the importance of obtaining histologic proof of malignant disease in patients suspected of having malignant tumors before instituting radiotherapy or chemotherapy. Obviously, bronchoscopic and sputum cytologic tests are negative with benign fibrous mesothelioma.

Treatment and Prognosis

The treatment of choice for benign fibrous mesotheliomas is surgical removal. If the tumor originates in the visceral pleura, substantial amounts of lung parenchyma may also have to be removed (61). Surgical resection cures about 90% of these patients (61, 62), but recurrent disease occurs in the remaining 10%. The recurrences may occur more than 10 years after the initial resection. It is recommended that annual chest radiographs be obtained postoperatively in patients with benign fibrous mesotheliomas to detect recurrences early so that they can be surgically removed.

REFERENCES

1. Connelly RR, Spirtas R, Myers MH, et al: Demographic patterns for mesothelioma in the United States. JNCI 1987;78:1053–1060.
2. Borow M, Conston A, Livorness L, Schalet N: Mesothelioma following exposure to asbestos: a review of 72 cases. Chest 1973;64:641–646.
3. Selikoff IJ, Hammond EC, Seidman H: Latency of asbestos disease among insulation workers in the United States and Canada. Cancer 1980;46:2736–2740.
4. Pisani RJ, Colby TV, Williams DE: Malignant mesothelioma of the pleura. Mayo Clin Proc 1988;63:1234–1244.
5. Churg A: Asbestos-related disease in the workplace and the environment: controversial issues. Monog Path 1993;36:52–77.
6. Churg A: Chrysotile, tremolite, and malignant mesothelioma in man. Chest 1988;93:621–628.
7. Oels HC, Harrison EG Jr, Carr DT, Bernatz PE: Diffuse malignant mesothelioma of the pleura: a review of 37 cases. Chest 1971;60:564–570.
8. Antman KH: Clinical presentation and natural history of benign and malignant mesothelioma. Semin Oncol 1981;8:313–320.
9. Wagner JC, Berry G, Timbrell V: Mesothelioma in rats after inoculation with asbestos and other materials. Br J Cancer 1973;28:173–185.
10. Shabad LM, Pylev LN, Krivosheeva LV, et al: Experimental studies on asbestos carcinogenicity. JNCI 1974;52:1175–1187.
11. Aisner J, Wiernik PH: Malignant mesothelioma: current status and future prospects. Chest 1978;74:438–444.
12. Champion P: Two cases of malignant mesotheliomas after exposure to asbestos. Am Rev Respir Dis 1971;103:821–826.
13. Baris YI, Saracci R, Simonato L, et al: Malignant mesothelioma and radiological chest abnormalities in two villages in central Turkey. An epidemiological and environmental investigation. Lancet 1981;1:984–987.
14. Carthew P, Hill RJ, Edwards RE, Lee PN: Intrapleural administration of fibers induces mesothelioma in rats in the same relative order of hazard as occurs in man after exposure. Hum Experiment Tox 1992;11:530–534.
15. Antman KH, Corson JM, Li FP, et al: Malignant mesothelioma following radiation exposure. J Clin Oncol 1983;1:695–700.
16. Roviaro GC, Sartori F, Calabro F, Varoli F: The association of pleural mesothelioma and tuberculosis. Am Rev Respir Dis 1982;126:569–571.
17. Driscoll RJ, Mulligan WJ, Schultz D, Candelaria A: Malignant mesothelioma: a cluster in a Native American pueblo. N Engl J Med 1988;318:1437–1438.
18. Corson JM: Pathology of malignant mesothelioma. In: Antman K, Aisner J, eds. Asbestos Related Malignancy. Orlando, FL: Grune & Stratton, 1987:179–199.
19. Suzuki Y: Pathology of human malignant mesothelioma. Semin Oncol 1981;8:268–282.
20. Hillerdal G: Malignant mesothelioma 1982: review of 4710 published cases. Br J Dis Chest 1983;77:321–343.
21. Lewis RJ, Sisler GE, MacKenzie JW: Diffuse, mixed malignant pleural mesothelioma. Ann Thorac Surg 1980;31:53–60.
22. Branscheid D, Krysa S, Bauer E, Bulzebruck H, Schirren J: Diagnostic and therapeutic strategy in malignant pleural mesothelioma. Brit J Cardiothorac Surg 1991;5:466–472.
23. Kawashima A, Libshitz HI: Malignant pleural mesothelioma: CT manifestations in 50 cases. Am J Roentgenol 1990;155:965–969.
24. Kreel L: Computed tomography in mesothelioma. Semin Oncol 1981;8:302–312.
25. Rusch VW, Godwin JD, Shuman WP: The role of computed tomography scanning in the initial assessment and the follow-up of malignant pleural mesothelioma. J Thorac Cardiovasc Surg 1988;96:171–177.
26. Gottehrer A, Taryle DA, Reed CE, Sahn SA: Pleural fluid analysis in malignant mesothelioma. Chest 1991;100:1003–1006.

27. Klempman S: The exfoliative cytology of diffuse pleural mesothelioma. Cancer 1962;15:691-704.

28. Nurminen M, Dejmek A, Martensson G, Thylen A, Hjerpe A: Clinical utility of liquid-chromatographic analysis of effusions for hyaluronate content. Clin Chem 1994;40:777-780.

29. Hillerdal G, Lindqvist U, Engström-Laurent A: Hyaluronan in pleural effusions and in serum. Cancer 1991;67:2410-2414.

30. Martensson G, Thylen A, Lindquist U, Hjerpe A: The sensitivity of hyaluronan analysis of pleural fluid from patients with malignant mesothelioma and a comparison of different methods. Cancer 1994;73:1406-1410.

31. Law MR, Hodson ME, Turner-Warwick M: Malignant mesothelioma of the pleura: clinical aspects and symptomatic treatment. Eur J Respir Dis 1984;65:162-168.

32. Stevens MW, Leong AS, Fazzalari NL, Dowling KD, Henderson DW: Cytopathology of malignant mesothelioma: a stepwise logistic regression analysis. Diag Cytopath 1992;8:333-342.

33. Menzies R, Charbonneau M: Thoracoscopy for the diagnosis of pleural disease. Ann Intern Med 1991;114:271-276.

34. Hucker J, Bhatnagar NK, Al-Jilaihawi AN, Forrester-Wood CP: Thoracoscopy in the diagnosis and management of recurrent pleural effusions. Ann Thorac Surg 1991;114:271-276.

35. Boutin C, Rey F: Thoracoscopy in pleural malignant mesothelioma: a prospective study of 188 consecutive patients. Part 1: Diagnosis. Cancer 1993;72:389-393.

36. Elmes PC, Simpson MJC: The clinical aspects of mesothelioma. Q J Med 1976;179:427-449.

37. Warnock ML, Stoloff A, Thor A: Differentiation of adenocarcinoma of the lung from mesothelioma: periodic acid-Schiff, monoclonal antibodies B72.3, and Leu M1. Am J Pathol 1988;133:30-38.

38. Wirth PR, Legier J, Wright GL Jr: Immunohistochemical evaluation of seven monoclonal antibodies for differentiation of pleural mesothelioma from lung adenocarcinoma. Cancer 1991;67:655-662.

39. Frisman DM, McCarthy WF, Schleiff P, Buckner SB, Nocito JD Jr, O'Leary TJ: Immunocytochemistry in the differential diagnosis of effusions: use of logistic regression to select a panel of antibodies to distinguish adenocarcinomas from mesothelial proliferations. Modern Path 1993;6:179-184.

40. Brown RW, Clark GM, Tandon AK, Allred DC: Multiple-marker immunohistochemical phenotypes distinguishing malignant pleural mesothelioma from pulmonary adenocarcinoma. Human Path 1993;24:347-354.

41. Coleman M, Henderson DW, Mukherjee TM: The ultrastructural pathology of malignant pleural mesothelioma. Pathol Ann 1989;24:303-353.

42. Jandik WR, Landas SK, Bray CK, Lager DJ: Scanning electron microscopic distinction of pleural mesotheliomas from adenocarcinomas. Modern Path 1993;6:761-764.

43. Burmer GC, Rabinovitch PS, Kulander BG, Rusch V, McNutt MA: Flow cytometric analysis of malignant pleural mesotheliomas. Hum Path 1989;20:777-783.

44. Spirtas R, Connelly RR, Tucker MA: Survival patterns for malignant mesothelioma: the SEER experience. Int J Cancer 1988;15:525-530.

45. Boutin C, Rey F, Gouvernet J, Viallat JR, Astoul P, Ledoray V: Thoracoscopy in pleural malignant mesothelioma: A prospective study of 188 consecutive patients. Cancer 1993;72:394-404.

46. Sugarbaker DJ, Strauss GM, Lynch TJ, Richards W, Mentzer SJ, Lee TH, Corson JM, Antman KH: Node status has prognostic significance in the multimodality therapy of diffuse, malignant mesothelioma. J Clin Oncol 1993;11:1172-1178.

47. Dejmek A, Stromberg C, Wikstrom B, Hjerpe A: Prognostic importance of the DNA ploidy pattern in malignant mesothelioma of the pleura. Analyt Quant Cytol Histol 1992;14:217-222.

48. Ruffie PA: Pleural mesothelioma. Curr Opinion Oncol 1991;3:328-334.

49. Butchart EG, Ashcroft T, Barnsley WC, Holden MP: The role of surgery in diffuse malignant mesothelioma of the pleura. Semin Oncol 1981;8:321-328.

50. Chahinian AP: Therapeutic modalities in malignant pleural mesothelioma. In: Chretien J, Hirsch A, eds. Diseases of the Pleura. New York: Masson, 1983.

51. Rusch VW, Ginsberg RJ: New concepts in the staging of mesotheliomas. In: Deslaurier J, Lacquet LD, eds. Thoracic Surgery: Surgical Management of Pleural Diseases. St Louis: CV Mosby, 1990:340.

52. Law MR, Gregor A, Hodson ME, et al: Malignant mesothelioma of the pleura: a study of 52 treated and 64 untreated patients. Thorax 1984;39:255-259.

53. DaValle MJ, Faber LP, Kittle CF, Jensik RJ: Extrapleural pneumonectomy for diffuse malignant mesothelioma. Ann Thorac Surg 1986;42:612-618.

54. Rusch VW, Piantadosi S, Holmes EC: The role of extrapleural pneumonectomy in malignant pleural mesothelioma. A Lung Cancer Study Group trial. J Thorac Cardiovasc Surg 1991;102:1-9.

55. Wanebo HJ, Martini N, Melamed MR, et al: Pleural mesothelioma. Cancer 1976;38:2481-2488.

56. Aisner J, Wiernik PH: Chemotherapy in the treatment of malignant mesothelioma. Semin Oncol 1981;8:335-343.

57. McCormack PM, Nagasaki F, Hilaris BS, Martini N: Surgical treatment of pleural mesothelioma. J Thorac Cardiovasc Surg 1982;84:834-842.

58. Tansan S, Emri S, Selcuk T, Koc Y, Hesketh P, Heeren T, McCaffrey RP, Barts YI: Treatment of malignant pleural mesothelioma with cisplatin, mitomycin c and alpha interferon. Oncology 1994;51:348-351.

59. Rusch V, Saltz L, Venkatraman E, Ginsberg R, McCormack P, Burt M, Markman M, Kelsen D: A phase II trial of pleurectomy/decortication followed by intrapleural and systemic chemotherapy for malignant pleural mesothelioma. J Clin Oncol 1994;12:1156-1163.

60. Mattson K, Holsti LR, Tammilehto L, Maasilta P, Pyrhonen S, Mantyla M, Kajanti M, Salminen US, Rautonen J, Kivisaari L: Multimodality treatment pro-

grams for malignant pleural mesothelioma using high-dose hemithorax irradiation. Int J Radiation Oncology Biol Phys 1992;24:643–650.

61. Okike N, Bernatz PE, Woolner LB: Localized mesothelioma of the pleura: benign and malignant variants. J Thorac Cardiovasc Surg 1978;75:363–372.

62. Briselli M, Mark EJ, Dickerson GR: Solitary fibrous tumors of the pleura: eight new cases and review of 360 cases in the literature. Cancer 1981;47:2678–2689.

63. Hutchinson WB, Friedenberg MJ: Intrathoracic mesothelioma. Radiology 1963;80:937–945.

64. Ellis K, Wolff M: Mesotheliomas and secondary tumors of the pleura. Semin Roentgenol 1977;12:303–311.

65. Steinetz C, Clarke R, Jacobs GH, Abdul-Karim FW, Petrelli M, Tomashefski JF Jr: Localized fibrous tumors of the pleura: correlation of histopathological, immunohistochemical and ultrastructural features. Path Res Practice 1990;186:344–357.

66. Axelrod L, Ron D: Insulin-like growth factor II and the riddle of tumor-induced hypoglycemia. N Engl J Med 1988;319:1477–1478.

67. Lee KD, Im JG, Choe KO, Kim CJ, Lee BH: CT findings in benign fibrous mesothelioma of the pleura: pathologic correlation in nine patients. AJR 1992;158:983–986.

68. Vandercruysse D, Verschakelen JA, Deneffe G: Localized pleural mesothelioma. J Belge Radiol 1993;76:163–166.

CHAPTER 9

Parapneumonic Effusions and Empyema

Despite the advent of potent antibiotics, bacterial pneumonia still results in morbidity and mortality in the American population. The annual incidence of bacterial pneumonia is estimated to approximate 4 million, with approximately 20% requiring hospitalization (1). Because as many as 40% of hospitalized patients with bacterial pneumonia have an accompanying pleural effusion (2), effusions associated with pneumonia account for a large percentage of pleural effusions. The morbidity and mortality rates in patients with pneumonia and pleural effusions are higher than in patients with pneumonia alone (3). Most pleural effusions associated with pneumonia resolve without any specific therapy directed toward the pleural fluid (2), but about 10% require operative intervention for their resolution. Delay in instituting proper therapy for these effusions is responsible for much of the morbidity, which can be substantial. In one series (4), the median hospital stay was 35 days for patients with community-acquired and 58 days for hospital-acquired pneumonias with culture-positive pleural fluid.

HISTORY

Empyema has been recognized to be a serious problem for centuries. Hippocrates, around 500 BC, recommended treating empyema with open drainage and recognized the bad outlook when the fluid was thin, as demonstrated by the following quotation (5): "Those cases of empyema which are treated by incision or the cautery, if the water flows rapidly all at once certainly prove fatal. When empyema is treated, either by the incision or the cautery, if pure and white pus flows slowly from the wound, the patients recover."

From the time of Hippocrates, the treatment of empyema remained essentially unchanged until the middle of the 19th century. At this time Bowditch (6) in the United States and Trousseau (7) in France popularized the use of thoracentesis and demonstrated that

open drainage was not necessary in many patients. The next advance in the management of empyema came in 1876 when Hewitt (8) described a method of closed drainage of the chest in which a rubber tube was placed into the empyema cavity through a cannula. He was the first to use the water seal for chest tubes.

In the 1890s two articles appeared that described thoracoplasty as a means of obliterating the empyema cavity (9, 10). Thoracoplasty involves resecting the ribs, intercostal muscles, and parietal pleural peel over the cavity and covering the remaining defect by the few remaining muscles, by the scapula, and by subcutaneous tissue and skin. At approximately the same time, the initial reports (11, 12) describing decortication appeared. By 1923 Eggers (13) had reported on a series of 99 patients treated by decortication at the Walter Reed Hospital, of whom two-thirds subsequently healed.

Although Hippocrates had recognized before the birth of Christ that open drainage procedures were dangerous if the empyema fluid was not thick (5) and Paget (14) had emphasized in 1896 that open drainage should not be instituted for empyema before at least the 15th day of the illness, by World War I open drainage was the accepted treatment for all cases of empyema. During World War I there was a high incidence of postpneumonic empyema in American soldiers and the treatment of all such patients with open drainage had disastrous results. In a survey in 1919, the United States Surgeon General found an average mortality of 30.2% in the armed forces for individuals with pleural infections, with a range of up to 70% in some hospitals (15). The primary reason for this very high mortality was that many cases of parapneumonic effusions in military recruits were due to *Streptococcus hemolyticus*, which is associated with a large pleural effusion but without loculation of the pleural space (16). When an open procedure is performed on such patients, there is a high likelihood that the lung will collapse. Graham in 1918 (17) reported that when chest tubes were inserted early in dogs with experimental empyemas, the mortality rate was higher and the dogs died sooner. The Empyema Commission headed by Dr. Evarts Graham soon made the following recommendations, which really form the basis for the treatment of empyema today: (*a*) The pleural fluid should be drained, but one must avoid an open pneumothorax in the acute pneumonic phase; (*b*) care should be taken to avoid a chronic empyema by rapid sterilization and obliteration of the infected cavity; and (*c*) careful attention should be paid to the nutrition of the patient. When these guidelines were observed, the mortality from streptococcal empyema secondary to influenza fell to 4.3% (18, 19).

DEFINITIONS

Any pleural effusion associated with bacterial pneumonia, lung abscess, or bronchiectasis is a **parapneumonic effusion** (20). An **empyema**, by definition, is pus in the pleural space, but how many white blood cells need be present in pleural fluid to make it pus? Weese and associates (21) defined an empyema as pleural fluid with a specific gravity greater than 1.018, a white blood cell count (WBC) greater than 500 cells/mm³, or a protein level greater than 2.5 g/dl. Vianna (22)

Table 9.1. Event or State Precipitating Empyema in 319 Patients

Event or State	Number	Percent
Pulmonary infection	177	55
Following a surgical procedure	66	21
Following trauma	18	6
Esophageal perforation	15	5
Spontaneous pneumothorax	7	2
Following thoracentesis	6	2
Subdiaphragmatic infection	4	1
Septicemia	4	1
Miscellaneous or unknown	22	7
Total	319	100

Data from Yeh TJ, Hall DP, Ellison RG: Empyema thoracis: a review of 110 cases. Am Rev Respir Dis 1963;88:785–790 and Snider GL, Saleh SS: Empyema of the thorax in adults: review of 105 cases. Chest 1968;54:12–17 and Smith JA, Mullerworth MH, Westlake GW, Tatoulis J: Empyema thoracis: 14-year experience in a teaching center. Ann Thorac Surg 1991;51:39–42.

defined an empyema as pleural fluid on which the bacterial cultures are positive or the WBC is greater than 15,000/mm³ and the protein level is above 3.0 g/dl. Because many pleural effusions meeting these criteria resolve without operative intervention (2), I prefer to reserve the term empyema for those pleural effusions with thick, purulent-appearing pleural fluid. Of course, some patients with empyema have no associated pneumonic process, as shown in Table 9.1.

The main decision in managing a patient with a parapneumonic effusion is whether to insert chest tubes. I therefore use the term **complicated parapneumonic effusion** to refer to those effusions that do not resolve without tube thoracostomy. Many complicated parapneumonic effusions are empyemas, but some parapneumonic effusions with nonpurulent-appearing pleural fluid are also complicated parapneumonic effusions.

PATHOPHYSIOLOGIC FEATURES

The evolution of a parapneumonic pleural effusion can be divided into three stages, which are not sharply defined, but gradually merge together (23). First is the **exudative stage**, characterized by the rapid outpouring of sterile pleural fluid into the pleural space. The origin of this fluid is not definitely known, but it is probably the interstitial spaces of the lung. The origin of the pleural fluid in sheep with *Pseudomonas aeruginosa* pneumonia is the interstitial spaces of the lung (24). It is possible that some of the pleural fluid originates in the capillaries in the visceral pleura due to their increased permeability secondary to the contiguous pneumonitis. The pleural fluid in this stage is characterized by a low WBC and lactic acid dehydrogenase (LDH) level and a normal glucose level and pH (25). If appropriate antibiotic therapy is instituted at this stage, the pleural effusion progresses no further, and the insertion of chest tubes is not necessary.

If appropriate antibiotic therapy is not instituted, in some instances bacteria invade the pleural fluid from the contiguous pneumonic process, and the second, **fibropurulent**, stage evolves. This stage is characterized by the accumulation of large amounts of pleural fluid with many polymorphonuclear leukocytes, bacteria, and cellular debris. Fibrin is deposited in a continuous sheet covering both the visceral and parietal pleura in the involved area. As this stage progresses, there is a tendency toward loculation and the formation of limiting membranes. These loculations prevent extension of the empyema, but make drainage of the pleural space with chest tubes increasingly difficult. As this stage progresses, the pleural fluid pH and glucose level become progressively lower and the LDH level progressively higher.

The last stage is the **organization stage**, in which fibroblasts grow into the exudate from both the visceral and parietal pleural surfaces and produce an inelastic membrane called the pleural peel. This inelastic pleural peel encases the lung and renders it virtually functionless. At this stage the exudate is thick, and if the patient has remained untreated, the fluid may drain spontaneously through the chest wall (*empyema necessitatis*) or into the lung, to produce a bronchopleural fistula.

Empyemas may arise without an associated pneumonic process. When 3 series (26–28) totaling 319 cases of empyema are combined (Table 9.1), the majority of patients had pulmonary infections, but postsurgical empyemas were also important. A small percentage of empyemas follow thoracentesis or tube thoracostomy for pneumothorax, hence the necessity for maintaining sterile techniques during these procedures. The pleural effusions associated with esophageal perforation are almost always infected (see Chapter 15). Patients with rheumatoid pleural effusions frequently develop empyema; the genesis of the empyema in this situation is thought to be the formation of a bronchopleural fistula through necrotic subpleural nodules (29).

EXPERIMENTAL EMPYEMA

There has been surprisingly little work done with experimental empyema. It is difficult to produce empyemas in animals. If *Staphylococcus aureus*, *Escherichia coli*, or *Bacteroides fragilis* are injected into the pleural space of guinea pigs, the animals either survive without developing empyema or die of overwhelming sepsis (30). There have been two basic models

for experimental empyema. In the first model umbilical tape is placed into the pleural space in addition to the bacteria and such a combination results in an empyema in some of the animals. The injection of *E. coli* will produce a higher incidence of empyema with a higher mortality than will the injection of *S. aureus* (30). If blood is injected with the bacteria in the presence of the umbilical tape, the incidence of empyema will be higher (31). The injection of *B. fragilis*, even in the presence of umbilical tape and blood, will not lead to an empyema. If 10^4 *B. fragilis* are injected along with 10^4 *S. aureus*, however, the incidence of empyema is 80%, compared with an incidence of 20% with *S. aureus* and 0% with *B. fragilis* alone. The guinea pigs who developed empyema were more likely to have underlying pneumonia (30, 31).

A second model of empyema that has received some study is in the rabbit. In this model sterile pleural effusions are induced by the intrapleural injection of turpentine. Several days later, bacteria are injected into the pleural effusion resulting in an empyema with a low pH and a low glucose level (32). Interestingly, if the rabbits are treated with neither antibiotics nor chest tubes after *Streptococcus pneumoniae* is injected, the animals do not die, and 7 days after the bacterial injection the pleural fluid is no longer purulent (32). If *Klebsiella pneumoniae* is injected (33), the pleural fluid pH will fall below 7.00 and the pleural fluid glucose level will fall below 10 mg/dl, but with the administration of gentamicin there will be complete resolution of the empyema with nonsignificant findings in the pleural cavities and lungs at autopsy. These studies show that at least in the experimental situation, empyemas will resolve without chest tube drainage.

Obviously, neither of the above two experimental models accurately reflect the empyema that occurs naturally. The first model requires that a foreign body be placed in the pleural space. The second model produces gross injury to the pleura before the bacteria are injected and accordingly must markedly alter the defenses of the lung. Recently we have developed a new experimental model of empyema, which we believe is far superior to those previously described. In this rabbit model, *Pasteurella multocida* cultured in agar (rather than broth) are injected into the rabbits. Then 24 hours following the initial injection, procaine penicillin G is administered once per day. In this model, which closely mimics the clinical situation, the rabbits survive for 14 days. At this time, their lung is completely encased with a thick fibrous peel and their pleural spaces are filled with thick pus (34). This model should provide a useful tool for experimental studies of empyema.

BACTERIOLOGIC FEATURES

The bacteriologic features of culture-positive parapneumonic effusions have changed since the introduction of antibiotics. Prior to the antibiotic era, most empyema fluids grew *Streptococcus pneumoniae* or hemolytic streptococci (35). Then between 1955 and 1965, *Staphylococcus aureus* was the bacteria most commonly isolated from pleural fluid (35). In the early 1970s anaerobic organisms were most commonly isolated (36). However, in the 1980s and 1990s it appears that the aerobic organisms again are responsible for the majority of empyema. Brook and Frazier (37) reviewed the microbiology of 197 patients whose pleural fluid was culture positive for bacteria in two military hospitals. In 64% of the cases, only aerobic bacteria were isolated, while in 13% only anaerobic organisms were isolated and in 23% both aerobic and anaerobic organisms were isolated. Alfageme and coworkers (38) recently reviewed the microbiology of 82 patients treated for empyema at a respiratory unit in Spain and reported results similar to those of Brook and Frazier (37). Of their patients 62% had exclusively aerobic bacteria while 12% had exclusively anaerobic bacteria, and 16% had both aerobic and anaerobic organisms.

The organisms isolated from positive pleural fluid cultures in three separate series (36, 37, 39), one each from the last three decades, are tabulated in Table 9.2. These series represent 342 patients from whom 580 organisms were isolated. Aerobic organisms alone were isolated from 181 patients (53%), anaerobic organisms only were isolated from 76 patients (22%), and both aerobic and anaerobic organisms were isolated from 85 patients (25%).

Several conclusions can be made from Table 9.2. First, aerobic organisms are isolated slightly more frequently than anaerobic organisms. Second, *S. aureus* and *S. pneumoniae* account for approximately 70% of all aerobic Gram-positive isolates. Third, when there is a single aerobic Gram-positive organism in the pleural fluid, it almost always is *S. aureus, S. pneumoniae,* or *Streptococcus pyogenes.* Fourth, Gram-positive aerobic organisms are isolated about twice as frequently as are Gram-negative aerobic organisms. Fifth, although *E. coli* is the most commonly isolated Gram-negative aerobic organism, it is rarely by itself responsible for the empyema. Sixth, *Klebsiella* species, *Pseudomonas* species, and *Haemophilus influenzae* are the next three most commonly isolated aerobic Gram-negative organisms and these three organisms account for approximately 75% of all aerobic Gram-negative empyemas with a single organism. Seventh, *Bacteroides* species and *Peptostreptococcus* are the two most commonly isolated anaerobic organisms from infected pleural fluid. Eighth, single anaerobic organisms usually do not cause empyema.

Several other points should be made concerning the bacteriology of infected pleural fluid. One, the incidence of anaerobic isolates is dependent to a large part on the care with which the pleural fluid is cultured from the anaerobes. The relatively high incidence of anaerobes in the series of Bartlett and coworkers (36), is partially explained by the intense interest these investigators had in culturing anaerobes. Two, the organisms cultured depend somewhat on the population studied. If aspiration is responsible for the underlying pneumonia, anaerobic organisms are more likely to be responsible (37). This also explains somewhat the high incidence of anaerobes in Bartlett's series since their patient population was elderly veteran patients. In contrast, young ambulatory patients are more likely to have *S. pneumoniae* responsible, while after thoracotomy, patients are most likely to have *S. aureus.*

The bacteriology of infected pleural fluid in children varies somewhat from that in adults in that *H. influenzae* is more common and anaerobic organisms are less common. In one study of 72 culture-positive pleural fluids (40),

Table 9.2.   Organisms Isolated from Infected Pleural Fluid in Three Separate Series

Organism	Series 1974[a]	1981[b]	1993[c]	Total	Percent
Gram-Positive Organisms					
Staphylococcus aureus	17 (6)[d]	7 (4)	58 (39)	82 (49)	36
Staphylococcus epidermidis	5 (0)	0 (0)	3 (0)	8 (0)	3
Streptococcus pneumoniae	5 (2)	6 (6)	70 (33)	81 (41)	35
Enterococcus faecalis	5 (0)	4 (1)	4 (0)	13 (1)	6
Streptococcus pyogenes	4 (0)	5 (0)	9 (9)	18 (9)	8
Other Streptococci	8 (0)	6 (3)	13 (0)	27 (3)	12
Total	44 (8)	28 (14)	157 (81)	229 (103)	
Gram-Negative Organisms					
Escherichia coli	11 (0)	4 (1)	17 (1)	32 (2)	30
Klebsiella spp.	6 (1)	1 (1)	16 (6)	23 (8)	21
Proteus spp.	2 (0)	1 (0)	5 (1)	8 (1)	7
Pseudomonas spp.	10 (2)	8 (6)	9 (3)	27 (11)	25
Enterobacter spp.	0 (0)	3 (3)	0 (0)	3 (3)	3
Hemophilus influenzae	1 (0)	0 (0)	12 (7)	13 (7)	12
Others	0 (0)	2 (0)	0 (0)	2 (0)	2
Total	30 (3)	19 (11)	59 (18)	108 (32)	
Anaerobic Organisms					
Bacteroides spp.	23 (1)	13 (4)	26 (6)	62 (11)	20
Peptostreptococcus spp.	26 (1)	8 (1)	28 (4)	62 (6)	20
Fusobacterium spp.	16 (3)	7 (2)	20 (4)	43 (9)	14
Prevotella spp.	13 (0)	5 (1)	22 (2)	40 (3)	13
Streptococcus spp.	15 (5)	4 (2)	12 (0)	31 (7)	10
Clostridium spp.	13 (1)	5 (3)	5 (1)	23 (5)	7
Others	34 (1)	4 (2)	14 (0)	52 (4)	16
Total	140 (12)	46 (15)	127 (17)	313 (45)	

[a] Data from Bartlett JG, Gorbach SL, Thadepalli H, Finegold SM: Bacteriology of empyema. Lancet 1974;1:338–340.
[b] Data from Varkey B, Rose HD, Kutty CPK, Politis J: Empyema thoracis during a ten-year period. Arch Intern Med 1981;141:1771–1776.
[c] Data from Brook I, Frazier EH: Aerobic and anaerobic microbiology of empyema. A retrospective review in two military hospitals. Chest 1993;103:1502–1507.
[d] Numbers in parentheses indicate the number of isolates that were recovered in pure culture.

aerobic organisms were found in 48 (67%), anaerobic organisms were found in 17 (24%) and mixed aerobics and anaerobes were found in 7 (10%). The most commonly isolated organisms in this series were *H. influenzae* (15 isolates), *Bacteroides* species (15), *S. pneumoniae* (13), *S. aureus* (10), and anaerobic cocci (9). In another series (41) of 173 culture-positive pleural fluids in children under the age of 15, 38% were due to *S. aureus*, 28% were due to *S. pneumoniae,* 23% were due to *H. influenzae*, and 11% due to other organisms. In this latter series, anaerobic isolates were rare (41).

Incidence of Pleural Effusions with Various Bacterial Pneumonias

Once a patient has a bacterial pneumonia, the incidence of associated pleural effusion and the frequency with which the pleural fluid

becomes infected largely depend on the infecting organism (Table 9.3). Infected pleural fluid is most common in anaerobic pneumonia. In one series of 143 patients with anaerobic infections of the lung (42), 50 (35%) had pleural effusions, and in 47 (94%), the pleural fluid cultures were positive for anaerobic organisms. Aerobic organisms were also cultured from the pleural fluid in 18 (40%) of the patients with positive pleural fluid cultures. Some patients with anaerobic pleural infection have no concomitant parenchymal disease.

Gram-Positive Bacteria

Streptococcus pneumoniae is still responsible for most bacterial pneumonias, and many patients have an associated pleural effusion. Taryle and coworkers (43) studied 53 patients with pneumococcal pneumonia and found that 57% had an associated parapneumonic effu-

Table 9.3. Percentage of Pleural Effusions and of Positive Pleural Fluid Cultures with Various Bacterial Pneumonias

Organism	Reference	Pleural Effusion (%)	Positive Pleural Fluid Culture (%)
Anaerobic	42	35	90
Gram-Positive Aerobic			
Streptococcus pneumoniae	2, 43	40–60	1–5
Staphylococcus aureus			
Adults	46	40	20
Children	45	70	80
Streptococcus pyogenes	47, 48	55–95	30–40
Bacillus anthracis	57	90–100	20
Gram-Negative Aerobic			
Escherichia coli	50	40	80
Pseudomonas	51	50	40
Klebsiella pneumoniae	52	10	20
Haemophilus influenzae			
Adults	55	45	20
Children	53, 54	75	80
Proteus spp.	56	20	50
Legionella spp.	58, 59	30–50	?

sion, whereas my colleagues and I found that 40% of 153 patients with pneumococcal pneumonia had an associated pleural effusion (2). Pleural fluid cultures are usually negative in patients with pneumococcal parapneumonic effusions. Of the 81 patients with pleural effusions in the foregoing 2 series, only 3 (4%) had pleural fluid cultures positive for *S. pneumoniae*. Nevertheless, as shown in Table 9.2, *S. pneumoniae* is responsible for many positive pleural fluid cultures. The explanation for this apparent paradox is the fact that such a large percentage of pneumonias are due to *S. pneumoniae*. The incidence of parapneumonic effusions is greater when patients wait 48 hours or more after the development of symptoms before seeking medical attention (43).

Pneumonia secondary to *S. aureus* is likely to have an accompanying culture-positive pleural effusion. Indeed in one study of the causes of pleural effusion in children, staphylococcal empyema was the most frequent cause (44). Wolfe and associates (44) reviewed 98 children with pleural effusions seen at Duke University between 1952 and 1967 and reported that *S. aureus* was responsible for 35 (36%). In a series of 75 cases of staphylococcal pneumonia in infants and young children (45), over 70% had pleural effusions, and the pleural cultures were positive in nearly 80%. In adults pleural effusions accompany staphylococcal

pneumonia about 40% of the time (46) which is less frequently than in children. Pleural fluid cultures are positive in about 20% of adults with pleural effusions (46).

Pneumonias due to *S. pyogenes* are uncommon, but they are associated with parapneumonic effusion in the majority of cases. Welch and colleagues (47) reported that 95% of 20 patients had an associated pleural effusion, whereas Basiliere and associates (48) reported that 57% of 95 patients with streptococcal pneumonia had a pleural effusion. The pleural fluid cultures are positive in 30 to 40% of those with pleural effusion (47, 48). The pleural effusions secondary to streptococcal pneumonia are more commonly on the left side. Of the 73 pleural effusions in the foregoing series, nearly two thirds were on the left side. Streptococcal pneumonia occurs in epidemics, particularly among military recruits (48). In some patients, the development of the pleuritis is explosive with this organism. Patients can develop large pleural effusions with low glucose levels and pH in less than 12 hours (49).

Gram-Negative Bacteria

Of pneumonias due to Gram-negative aerobic organisms, those caused by *E. coli* are most likely to have complicated parapneumonic effusions. In a series of 20 patients (50), 40% had pleural effusion, and in 6 of these 8 patients, pleural fluid cultures were positive. All 8 patients with pleural effusion in this series had to be treated by tube thoracostomy or open thoracotomy. Rarely, however, is *E. coli* the sole isolate from pleural fluid (Table 9.2). Patients with pseudomonas pneumonia are also likely to have pleural effusions. In one series (51), 50% of patients with pseudomonas pneumonia had pleural effusion, and the cultures were positive in the 2 in which they were obtained. As evident in Table 9.2, *Pseudomonas* species and *E. coli* account for over fifty percent of all aerobic Gram-negative isolations from pleural fluid. Although *K. pneumoniae* is responsible for many Gram-negative pneumonias, pleural effusions are uncommon and are complicated in only a small percentage of patients (52). In recent years, *H. influenzae* has been responsible for an increasing number of pneumonias in both children (41, 53, 54) and adults (55). With *H. influenzae* pneumonia, the pleura is frequently involved, particularly in children (54). In a series of 65 cases in children (54), 49 (75%) had pleural effusions, and the cultures were positive in 36 of 46 (78%). In another series of 24 adult patients (55), 11 (45%) had pleural fluid, and cultures were positive in 2 of 11 (18%). *Proteus* species cause a substantial proportion of Gram-negative pneumonias, but associated pleural effusions are uncommon and, when present, are usually small and uncomplicated (56).

Miscellaneous Pathogenic Organisms

Several unusual organisms should be considered in patients with pneumonia and pleural effusions. *Bacillus anthracis* is a large Gram-positive, spore-forming, rod-shaped organism that may contaminate goat hair, wool, or animal hides (57). This virulent organism causes pulmonary disease when the spores are inhaled into the alveoli, are engulfed by alveolar macrophages, and are carried to the hilar lymph nodes, where they multiply in their vegetative state. After causing flu-like symptoms for several days, the bacteria are disseminated hematogenously. This dissemination is marked by the acute onset of dyspnea, cyanosis, tachycardia, fever, and shock. The characteristic radiologic findings are mediastinal widening, patchy nonsegmental pulmonary infiltrates, and unilateral or bilateral pleural effusions. Because this disease is fatal within 24 hours of hematogenous dissemination unless an appropriate antibiotic (penicillin) is administered, this diagnosis should be considered in all patients with mediastinal widening, parenchymal infiltrates, and pleural effusions (57).

Pleural effusions may also occur in 30 to 50% of patients with pneumonias due to *Legionella* species (58–60). In some cases the organisms can be demonstrated by direct immunofluorescence and/or culture of the pleural fluid (60). Usually, the pleural effusions are small and clinically unimportant, but one reported patient had a multiloculated pleural effusion due to *Legionella* and required a decortication (61). I have seen a patient with Legionnaires' disease with a large pleural effusion in whom tube thoracostomy was necessary.

Clostridial pleuropulmonary infections are uncommon; by 1970 only 17 cases had been reported (62). Almost all patients with clostridial pulmonary infections have a pleural effusion that is culture positive (62). Complicated parapneumonic pleural effusions have also been reported with pneumonias due to *Haemophilus parainfluenzae* (63), *Bacillus cereus* (64), *Citrobacter diversus* (65), *Listeria monocytogenes* (66) and *Francisella tularensis* (67) and can probably occur with any bacterium that is a pathogen in humans.

CLINICAL MANIFESTATIONS

The clinical manifestations of parapneumonic effusions and empyema depend to a large part on whether the patient has an aerobic or an anaerobic infection.

Aerobic Bacterial Pneumonia

The clinical presentation of patients with aerobic bacterial pneumonia and pleural effusion is no different from that of patients with bacterial pneumonia without effusion (2, 43, 68). The patients first manifest an acute febrile illness with chest pain, sputum production, and leukocytosis. In one series (2), the incidence of pleuritic chest pain was 59% in 113 patients without effusion and 64% in 90 patients with pleural effusion. The mean peripheral WBC was 17,100 in patients without effusion and 17,800 in patients with effusion. The longer the patient has symptoms before seeking medical attention, the more likely he is to have a pleural effusion (43). A complicated parapneumonic effusion is suggested by the presence of fever for more than 48 hours after antibiotic therapy is instituted, but of course, the diagnosis of parapneumonic effusion should ideally be established when the patient with pneumonia is first evaluated.

Not all patients with aerobic pneumonias and pleural effusions have acute illnesses. Sahn and associates (69) reported three cases of aerobic empyema in patients who were receiving corticosteroid therapy, and all were afebrile with minimal symptoms referable to the chest. The absence of fever or chest symptoms should not deter one from considering the diagnosis of complicated parapneumonic effusions because, in recent years, a higher percentage of such effusions has occurred in hospitalized patients, many of whom are debilitated or are receiving corticosteroids (35).

Anaerobic Bacterial Infections

In contrast to patients with aerobic bacterial pneumonias, patients with anaerobic bacterial infections involving the pleural space are usually first seen with subacute illnesses. In a series of 47 patients (42), 70% of the patients had symptoms for more than 7 days before presentation, with a median duration of symptoms of 10 days. In this same series of patients (42), 60% had substantial weight loss (mean 29 pounds). Many patients have a history of alcoholism, an episode of unconsciousness, or another factor that predisposes to aspiration. The majority of patients also have poor oral hygiene. Laboratory evaluation reveals leukocytosis (median WBC 23,500/mm^3) and mild anemia (median hematocrit 36%) in the majority of patients (42).

DIAGNOSIS

The possibility of a parapneumonic effusion should be considered during the initial evaluation of every patient with a bacterial pneumonia. It is important to determine at this evaluation whether a complicated parapneumonic

effusion is present because a delay in instituting proper pleural drainage in such patients substantially increases morbidity.

The presence of a significant amount of pleural fluid is usually suggested by the appearance of the lateral chest radiograph. If both diaphragms are visible throughout their length and the posterior costophrenic angle is not blunted, one can assume that a significant amount of pleural fluid is not present. If either of the posterior costophrenic angles is blunted or if a diaphragm is obscured by the infiltrate, however, bilateral decubitus chest radiographs should be obtained. With the suspect side down, free pleural fluid is indicated by the presence of fluid between the chest wall and the inferior part of the lung (see Figure 3.3). The view with the suspect side up is also valuable because, in this position, the free fluid gravitates toward the mediastinum and allows one to assess how much of the increased radiodensity is due to the fluid and how much is due to the parenchymal infiltrate. The amount of free pleural fluid can be semiquantitated by measuring the distance between the inside of the chest wall and the bottom of the lung. If this distance measures less than 10 mm, one can assume that the effusion is not clinically significant, and therefore a thoracentesis is not indicated. My colleagues and I reported that 53 patients with acute bacterial pneumonia had such small effusions, and in each of the patients the pneumonia and the pleural effusion cleared with only antibiotics and left no residual pleural disease (2).

If the thickness of the fluid is greater than 10 mm on the decubitus radiograph, a diagnostic thoracentesis should be performed immediately because it is impossible to separate complicated from uncomplicated effusions without a thoracentesis. During the diagnostic thoracentesis, 30 to 50 ml pleural fluid are withdrawn into a syringe that contains heparin sodium. The pleural fluid is examined grossly for color, turbidity, and odor. Aliquots are sent for determination of the pleural fluid glucose, LDH, amylase and protein levels, pH, and differential and total WBC. Samples of pleural fluid are also sent for bacterial cultures, both aerobic and anaerobic, and for Gram stain as well as for cytologic studies and mycobacterial and fungal smears and cultures, if clinically indicated.

Not all patients with an acute illness, parenchymal infiltrates, and pleural effusion have an acute bacterial pneumonia; pulmonary embolization, acute pancreatitis, tuberculosis, Dressler's syndrome, and other diseases can produce identical pictures. The possibility of pulmonary embolization should always be considered, and lung scans should be obtained if the patient does not have purulent sputum or a peripheral leukocytosis above 15,000/mm³. A normal pleural fluid amylase level rules out pancreatitis, and most patients with acute tuberculous pleuritis have no infiltrate on the decubitus film with the involved side superior.

The pleural fluid with parapneumonic effusions varies from a clear, yellow exudate to thick, foul-smelling pus. If the odor of the pleural fluid is feculent, the patient is likely to have an anaerobic pleural infection (42, 70). Although Sullivan and coworkers (70) reported that 11% of aerobic empyemas were described as foul-smelling, it is probable that these represented mixed aerobic and anaerobic pleural infections in that sophisticated anaerobic culture techniques were not used in this study. Foul-smelling pleural fluid is not always present with anaerobic pleural infection. Only about 60% of anaerobic empyemas have a foul odor (42, 70). If frank pus is obtained with the diagnostic thoracentesis, a pleural fluid pH determination should not be obtained. When thick, purulent material is processed through blood gas machines, it is likely to plug up the machine or damage the membranes. Once laboratory personnel have this experience with one pleural fluid, they are hesitant to process additional pleural fluids. The differential WBC on the pleural fluid usually reveals predominantly polymorphonuclear leukocytes. If many small lymphocytes, mesothelial cells, or macrophages are seen, alternate diagnoses should be considered.

Not all patients with parapneumonic effusions have an acute illness, so the possibility of a parapneumonic effusion should be considered in all patients with pleural effusion. Anaerobic pleural infections are particularly likely to produce subacute or chronic illness (42, 71) and many patients with anaerobic pleural infections do not have associated parenchymal infiltrates (71). Accordingly, aerobic and anaerobic bacterial cultures should be obtained on all exudative pleural effusions.

Loculated Pleural Effusions

Pleural effusions are already loculated in some patients with pneumonia and pleural effusion when they are first evaluated. Although small amounts of freely moving fluid can be demonstrated in most patients with loculated pleural effusion, such is not invariably the case. Loculated pleural effusions manifest as pleural-based masses without air bronchograms on the standard chest radiograph (see Figure 3.5). Frequently, it is difficult to distinguish pleural fluid loculations from peripheral parenchymal infiltrates on standard chest radiographs. Ultrasonic techniques are effective in distinguishing pleural fluid loculations from parenchymal infiltrates (72, 73). As little as 5 ml loculated pleural fluid can be identified by ultrasound. Therefore, if a loculated pleural effusion is suspected, ultrasonic examination of the pleural space should be performed.

Loculated pleural effusion should also be suspected in patients with pneumonia who do not respond clinically within 48 hours to appropriate antibiotic therapy. If one pleural fluid loculation is identified with ultrasound, it is important to examine the entire pleural space ultrasonically because multiple loculations are often present. If pleural fluid is identified by ultrasound, thoracentesis should be performed immediately because if the skin is marked and the patient is sent back to his room, the relationship between the skin and the underlying pleural fluid may be altered with the patient in a different position. If more than one pleural fluid loculation is discovered, all should be diagnostically aspirated because the character of the pleural fluid may vary from one locule to another (42).

The presence of loculated pleural fluid is not by itself an indication for tube thoracostomy. The presence of loculations does indicate that there is or has been an intense inflammatory response in the pleural space. Parapneumonic effusions that are loculated tend to have a lower pH and glucose level and

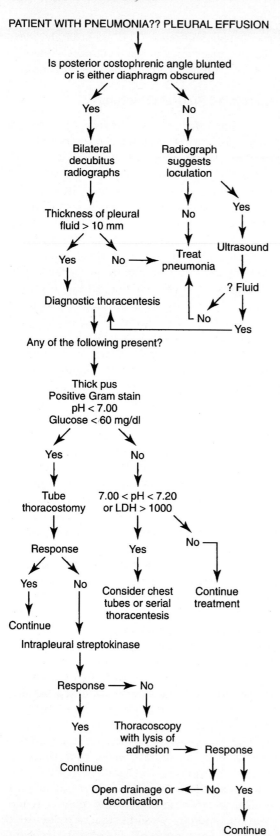

a higher LDH level than do nonloculated parapneumonic pleural effusions (74). Tube thoracostomy with loculated pleural effusions is indicated only if the characteristics of the pleural fluid in one of the locules meet the criteria for tube thoracotomy as outlined subsequently. The pleural fluid from the majority of patients with loculated parapneumonic pleural effusions will indicate that tube thoracostomy should be performed.

Hydropneumothorax versus Lung Abscess

Frequently, on the standard chest radiographs, it is difficult to distinguish a loculated hydropneumothorax with a bronchopleural fistula from a peripheral lung abscess. This differentiation is important because the loculated hydropneumothorax with the bronchopleural fistula needs to be treated with chest tubes immediately in order to prevent discharge of the infected pleural fluid throughout the remainder of the lung. In contrast, only antibiotic therapy is necessary for the peripheral lung abscess. If any doubt exists as to whether the air-fluid level is in the pleural space or the lung parenchyma, ultrasound (72) or computed tomographic (CT) studies (75) should be obtained to make this differentiation (see Chapter 3).

MANAGEMENT

An algorithm for the management of patients with parapneumonic effusions is shown in Figure 9.1. Obviously, the management of each patient must be individualized, but the algorithm should serve as a guide.

Initial Management

The initial management of a patient with pneumonia and pleural effusion involves two major decisions. First, an appropriate antibiotic must be selected. Second, the decision whether to initiate tube drainage of the pleural space must be made. The initial antibiotic selection is usually based on whether the

Figure 9.1. An algorithm for managing patients with parapneumonic effusions.

pneumonia is a community-acquired pneumonia or a hospital-acquired pneumonia and how sick the patient is. For patients hospitalized with community-acquired pneumonias that are not severe, the recommended agents are the second- or third-generation cephalosporins or a β-lactam/β-lactamase inhibitor such as Augmentin with the addition of a macrolide (erythromycin or clarithromycin) if infection with *Legionella* species is likely. For patients hospitalized with severe community-acquired pneumonia, the recommended agents are a macrolide plus a third-generation cephalosporin with anti-*Pseudomonas* activity such as ceftazidime or cefoperazone (1).

Pneumonia acquired in institutions such as nursing homes or hospitals is frequently caused by enteric Gram-negative bacilli, *P. aeruginosa*, or *S. aureus* with or without oral anaerobes. If *S. aureus* is suspected the patient should be treated with nafcillin or vancomycin. If a Gram-negative infection is suspected the patient should be treated with a third generation cephalosporin or a β-lactam/β-lactamase inhibitor plus an aminoglycoside. If the patient is thought to have an anaerobic infection, then the drug of choice is clindamycin. If the Gram stain of the pleural fluid is positive, it should guide the selection of an antibiotic. Because antibiotic levels in the pleural fluid are comparable to those in the serum (76, 77) standard systemic doses of antibiotics for pneumonia provide adequate pleural fluid antibiotic levels. No reason exists to increase the dose of antibiotics merely because a pleural effusion is present.

The decision to institute tube drainage of the pleural space must be based on an examination of the pleural fluid (2). Ideally, one should identify those individuals who require tube drainage of the pleural space as early as possible because if tube thoracostomy is delayed for even a couple of days, the pleural effusion can become loculated (42, 78), and tube drainage becomes difficult. With systemic antibiotics, most parapneumonic effusions resolve without tube drainage of the pleural space (2). In a series reported by my colleagues and myself of 90 patients with parapneumonic effusions, only 9 (10%) required tube thoracostomy (2).

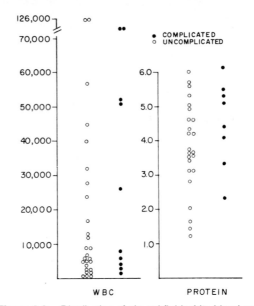

Figure 9.2. Distribution of pleural fluid white blood cell counts (WBC) and protein levels in patients with complicated and uncomplicated parapneumonic effusions. Each circle represents one pleural fluid.

The initial evaluation of a patient with pneumonia and pleural effusion should include a diagnostic thoracentesis if the thickness of the pleural fluid on the decubitus radiograph is more than 10 mm or if the pleural effusion is loculated. If the thickness of the pleural fluid is less than 10 mm on the decubitus radiographs, a diagnostic thoracentesis need not be performed because such small effusions almost always resolve with appropriate systemic antibiotics (2). In deciding whether to institute tube thoracostomy, one should examine the gross appearance of the fluid, the Gram stain of the fluid, and the level of glucose, pH, and LDH in the fluid. The distributions of the pleural fluid WBC and protein levels are comparable in patients with uncomplicated and complicated parapneumonic effusions (Fig. 9.2).

If the diagnostic thoracentesis yields thick pus, the patient has an empyema and tube thoracostomy should be instituted without delay. If the pleural fluid is not thick pus, then one should be guided by the pleural fluid Gram stain and the pleural fluid glucose, pH, and LDH levels. Patients with complicated parapneumonic effusions have a lower pleural fluid glucose and pH and a higher pleural fluid LDH than those with uncomplicated parapneu-

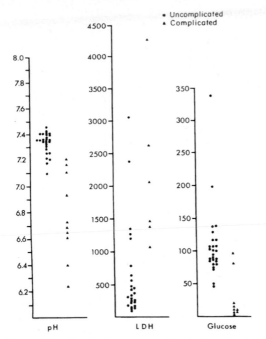

Figure 9.3. Distribution of pleural fluid pH, lactic dehydrogenase (LDH), and glucose levels in uncomplicated and complicated parapneumonic effusions. (From Light RW, Girard WM, Jenkinson SG, George RB: Parapneumonic effusions. Am J Med 1980;69:507–511.)

monic effusions (Fig. 9.3). If the pleural fluid pH is above 7.20, the pleural fluid glucose is above 40 mg/dl, and the pleural fluid LDH is below 1000 IU/L, the parapneumonic effusion is in the exudative stage, and no further diagnostic or therapeutic maneuvers need be directed toward the pleural effusion. In particular, no need exists to perform serial therapeutic thoracenteses because uncomplicated pleural effusions usually resolve spontaneously and leave little or no residual pleural disease if appropriate antibiotics are administered. If the patient remains febrile or if the pleural effusion increases in size once antibiotic therapy is started, a repeat thoracentesis should be performed to verify that the effusion has not become complicated (79). When appropriate antibiotics are started initially, however, it is uncommon for an uncomplicated parapneumonic effusion to become complicated.

If the initial thoracentesis reveals pleural fluid with a pH less than 7.00 or a glucose level less than 40 mg/dl, tube thoracostomy should be performed immediately because parapneumonic effusions with these characteris-

tics are almost always complicated (Fig. 9.3). Similarly, if the Gram stain of the pleural fluid is positive, I recommend the immediate institution of tube thoracostomy. The pleural fluid pH and glucose levels should be used as guides for the placement of chest tubes only in parapneumonic effusions; other pleural effusions, such as those secondary to rheumatoid disease, malignant tumors, and tuberculosis (20) may also have a low pH or a low glucose level and need not always be treated by tube thoracostomy. If one uses the pleural fluid pH as a guide for the placement of chest tubes, it must be measured with the same care as arterial pH (2). The fluid must be collected anaerobically and placed on ice during its transfer to the blood gas laboratory, where the pH should be determined in a blood gas machine. Moreover, because the pleural fluid pH is influenced by the arterial pH (20), the arterial pH should be measured before chest tubes are inserted merely on the basis of the pleural fluid pH. To serve as a definite indication for tube thoracostomy, the pleural fluid pH should be at least 0.30 units less than the arterial pH.

The one situation in which the pleural fluid pH is not reduced in complicated parapneumonic effusion is when the offending organism is of the *Proteus* species. These organisms produce ammonia by their urea-splitting ability, which can lead to an elevated pleural fluid pH. Pine and Hollman reported 3 cases of complicated parapneumonic effusions due to *Proteus* organisms in which the pleural fluid pH exceeded 7.8 (80).

If the initial thoracentesis reveals pleural fluid with a pH between 7.00 and 7.20 or an LDH level above 1000 IU/L, and none of the aforementioned criteria for tube thoracostomy are met, the parapneumonic effusion is either late in Stage I or early in Stage II (2). Accordingly, the patient may or may not need tube thoracostomy, and each patient should be considered individually. If the patient has a large pleural effusion and the pH is close to 7.00, chest tubes should probably be inserted. Alternately, if the effusion is small and the pH is close to 7.20, the patient probably will not require a tube thoracostomy. In borderline cases, serial thoracenteses at 12- to 24-hour intervals are useful (2). If the pleural fluid pH and the glucose level increase and the pleural fluid LDH level falls with serial thoracenteses, the parapneumonic effusion is resolving, and tube thoracostomy is not necessary. In contrast, if the pleural fluid pH and glucose level fall and the LDH level increases, chest tubes should be placed.

In the natural evolution of a parapneumonic effusion, the pleural fluid pH falls before the glucose level falls (20, 32) and therefore the pH is a more sensitive indicator of complicated parapneumonic effusion than the pleural fluid glucose level. The lowered pH with complicated parapneumonic effusions appears to be caused by the metabolism of glucose by the leukocytes in the pleural fluid resulting in increased levels of lactate and carbon dioxide in the pleural fluid (32). When some locules are infected and others are sterile in patients with loculated pleural effusions, the carbon dioxide probably equilibrates across the fibrin membranes separating the different locules more readily than does the glucose. Accordingly, pleural fluid acidosis is present in all locules, even though some locules may contain nearly normal glucose levels (81).

It should be mentioned that there is not universal agreement concerning the usefulness of using the pleural fluid glucose and pH as indicators for tube thoracostomy. Berger and Morganroth (82) reviewed the clinical courses of 26 patients who had a pH less than 7.20 or a positive Gram stain or a positive culture. Sixteen patients were initially treated with intravenous antibiotics alone without tube thoracostomy while the remaining 10 were treated with tube thoracostomy plus intravenous antibiotics. Only two of the 16 patients treated with antibiotics alone subsequently required tube thoracostomy. Three of the four patients with pleural fluid pH less than 7.00 never required tube thoracostomy. The mean duration of hospitalization was longer in the group that received a chest tube immediately. Poe and coworkers (83) reviewed 91 patients with parapneumonic effusions and concluded that measurement of the pleural fluid glucose, pH, and LDH has limited usefulness in predicting the need for eventual chest tube drainage and/or decortication. However, if their data are examined closely (84)

this conclusion is not supported. When patients with frank empyemas are excluded, 10 of 18 patients (56%) who had a pleural fluid pH value below 7.00 and/or a pleural fluid glucose below 40 mg/dl required chest tubes. In contrast, only 8 of 52 patients (15%) who did not meet these criteria required tube thoracostomy ($p < .005$).

In view of the above two series, there is no doubt that some patients with parapneumonic effusions who have a pleural fluid pH below 7.00, a pleural fluid glucose below 40 mg/dl, a positive Gram stain, or a positive pleural fluid culture can be cured with antibiotics alone. Nevertheless, the placement of chest tubes in patients with parapneumonic effusions who have a pleural fluid pH below 7.00, a pleural fluid glucose below 40 mg/dl, or a positive pleural fluid Gram stain is still recommended (84), because these are indicators that it is likely that the parapneumonic process will not resolve with only antibiotics alone. The extra morbidity associated with delayed tube thoracostomy justifies the placement of a few extra chest tubes.

When a patient has a complicated parapneumonic effusion, the pleural fluid often offers clues to the responsible organism. Anaerobic infections often result in putrid pleural fluid. If the initial Gram stain of the pleural fluid is negative, the pleural fluid should be centrifuged, and the sediment should be Gram stained because, by centrifugation, the bacteria as well as the white blood cells and other debris are concentrated in the sediment. Another pleural fluid examination that is sometimes useful is countercurrent immunoelectrophoresis (CIE). With this procedure (see Chapter 4), the presence of bacterial antigens in the pleural fluid can be demonstrated. CIE appears to be particularly useful in identifying the responsible organism in children (85). In a series of 34 children with positive pleural fluid cultures, CIE correctly identified the offending organism in 97% of the patients, even though the Gram stain of the pleural fluid was negative in 25% (85). CIE has not been used as much in adults because many pleural infections are due to anaerobes, and appropriate antigens for all the anaerobic organisms are not available. Another test that may prove to be useful in identifying the bacteria responsible for the effusion is the presence of pneumococcal antigen in the pleural fluid. In one study, pneumococcal antigen was present in the pleural fluid of 8 of 9 patients with pneumococcal pneumonia and pleural effusion, while the Gram stain was positive in only two and the culture was positive in only one (86).

Classification of Complicated Parapneumonic Effusions

It is important to realize that not all complicated parapneumonic effusions are the same. In Table 9.4 I have separated parapneumonic effusions and empyemas into 7 different classes. The higher classes are increasingly difficult to manage. Patients with Class 1 parapneumonic effusions have a **nonsignificant** pleural effusion and do not require a thoracentesis. Patients with Class 2 have a **typical** parapneumonic effusion with negative bacterial studies and normal chemistries. These patients do not require therapeutic thoracentesis or chest tubes. Patients with Class 3 have a **borderline complicated** effusion and the results of serial thoracenteses will dictate whether they will require tube thoracostomy. Patients with Class 4 have a **simple complicated** effusion and are best managed with tube thoracostomy for several days. Patients with Class 5 have a **complex complicated** parapneumonic effusion and should respond to tube thoracostomy plus intrapleural thrombolytics. They usually do not require thoracoscopy or decortication. Patients with Class 6 have a **simple empyema** and require tube thoracostomy. In some of these patients, the underlying lung may fail to expand and a decortication is necessary. Patients with Class 7 have a **complex empyema** and often require thoracoscopy or decortication in addition to chest tubes and thrombolytics.

Chest Tubes

In complicated parapneumonic effusions, adequate drainage of the pleural space is at least as important in the cure as antimicrobial

Table 9.4.   A Classification and Treatment Scheme for Parapneumonic Effusions and Empyema

Class 1: **Nonsignificant pleural effusion**	Small Less than 10 mm thick on decubitus x-ray No thoracentesis indicated
Class 2: **Typical parapneumonic pleural effusion**	More than 10 mm thick Glucose >40 mg/dl, pH > 7.20, Gram stain and culture negative Antibiotics alone
Class 3: **Borderline complicated pleural effusion**	7.00 < pH < 7.20 and/or LDH >1000 and Glucose > 40 mg/dl, Gram stain and culture negative Antibiotics plus serial thoracentesis
Class 4: **Simple complicated pleural effusion**	pH < 7.00 and/or glucose <40 mg/dl and/or Gram stain or culture positive Not loculated, not frank pus Tube thoracostomy plus antibiotics
Class 5: **Complex complicated pleural effusion**	pH < 7.00 and/or glucose < 40 mg/dl and/or Gram stain or culture positive Multiloculated Tube thoracostomy plus thrombolytics (Rarely require thoracoscopy or decortication)
Class 6: **Simple empyema**	Frank pus present Single locule or free-flowing Tube thoracostomy ± decortication
Class 7: **Complex empyema**	Frank pus present Multiple locules Tube thoracostomy + thrombolytics Often require thoracoscopy or decortication

therapy. Chest tubes should be inserted as soon as it is determined that the patient has a complicated parapneumonic effusion, because the longer tube thoracostomy is delayed, the more difficult the pleural drainage becomes. The pleural effusion can progress from free-flowing pleural fluid to loculated pleural fluid within a couple of days (71) as the pleural effusion progresses through the fibropurulent stage. In Bartlett and Finegold's series of 47 anaerobic empyemas, 5 patients died, and all deaths were attributed to a delay in obtaining adequate pleural drainage (42). In Vianna's series of 41 patients (22), none of the patients improved clinically until effective drainage of the pleural space was established.

The chest tube should be positioned in a dependent part of the pleural effusion. Failure of tube thoracostomy is frequently due to having the tube in the wrong place (87). Initially, the chest tube should be connected to an underwater-seal drainage system. If the visceral pleura is covered with a fibrinous peel, the application of negative pressure to the chest tube may help to expand the underlying lung and may hasten the obliteration of the empyema cavity. The management of patients with chest tubes is discussed in Chapter 24.

What size chest tubes should be used to treat complicated parapneumonic effusions? In the past, relatively large (26 to 30 French) have been recommended due to the belief that smaller tubes would become obstructed with the thick fluid. Indeed in a recent edition of the major thoracic surgical text (88), large-bore (28 to 32) French catheters were recommended. There are, however, some data to suggest that such large tubes are unnecessary. There have been two recent series (87, 89) in which a total of 53 patients were treated with smaller catheters (8.3 to 16 French) which were inserted percutaneously after the collection of pleural fluid had been localized by CT scan or by ultrasound. Forty-one of the 53 patients (77%) were successfully managed with these small catheters. Many of the patients had grossly purulent fluid. More than one catheter was inserted in 15 of the 53 (28%) of the patients. These results are certainly as good as those reported in recent surgical series (90, 91) in which much larger tubes were used, but the

cases in the surgical series may have been in a higher category. The advantage of the smaller tube is that it is easier to insert and is less painful to the patient. The percutaneous catheters in the two studies referenced were placed by interventional radiologists and it is quite likely that the excellent results are due to accurate catheter placement.

Successful closed-tube drainage of complicated parapneumonic effusions is evidenced by improvement in the clinical and radiologic status within 24 hours. If the patient has not demonstrated significant improvement within 24 hours of initiating tube thoracostomy, either the pleural drainage is unsatisfactory or the patient is receiving the wrong antibiotic. In such patients, the culture results should be reviewed, and ultrasonic or CT examination of the pleural space should be performed to detect remaining locules of pleural fluid and to determine if the tube is in the proper place. If the chest tube is in the wrong position, it should be replaced. If multiple locules of pleural fluid are demonstrated, a thrombolytic agent should be administered intrapleurally (see next section).

If the patient responds clinically and radiologically to closed-tube drainage of the pleural space, how long should the chest tubes be left in place? In general, chest tubes should be left in place until the volume of the pleural drainage is under 50 ml/24 hours and until the draining fluid becomes clear yellow. If the chest tube ceases to function (no spontaneous fluctuation with respiratory efforts), it should be removed because it serves no useful purpose and can be a conduit for pleural suprainfection.

At times, a patient responds clinically and radiologically to closed-tube drainage, but purulent drainage continues from the chest tube. In this situation, the decision to take a more aggressive approach, e.g., decortication, can be aided by the injection of contrast material through the chest tube into the pleural space (92). When only a tube tract remains, the chest tube is gradually withdrawn over a few days, and the cavity is allowed to fill in with granulation tissue. When a larger cavity (greater than 50 ml) is demonstrated, empyemectomy with decortication or an open drainage procedure should be performed.

In many instances, closed-tube drainage of the pleural space is not sufficient therapy for complicated parapneumonic effusions. In aerobic pleural infection, chest tube drainage yields satisfactory results in approximately 60% of patients (22, 39) whereas in anaerobic pleural infection, results are satisfactory in only about 25% (42, 71). Again, the usual reason for the failure of closed-tube drainage is a delay in its institution or malposition of the tube. In children, tube thoracostomy is curative in a much higher percentage of cases (41). Freij and coworkers had to perform a more extensive procedure in less than 10% of their 148 patients under the age of 15 who underwent tube thoracostomy for complicated parapneumonic effusion (41).

Serial therapeutic thoracenteses probably have no role in the management of patients with complicated parapneumonic effusions. In Bartlett and Finegold's series, the two patients with purulent pleural fluid who were treated only with repeated thoracenteses both died despite intensive antimicrobial therapy (42). Four of seven patients in another series treated with thoracentesis alone died (21). Although serial thoracenteses in patients with complicated parapneumonic effusions occasionally eliminate the necessity for chest tubes, patients with complicated parapneumonic effusions usually do better with chest tubes. Frequently drainage is much more difficult with chest tubes if there is a delay in its initiation due to the interval development of loculations.

Intrapleural Antibiotics

Intrapleural antibiotics were first used to treat an infected pneumonectomy space by Clagett (93) in 1963. Since that time there have been several reports (94–98) regarding the use of intrapleural antibiotics in the treatment of empyema complicating pneumonia. All of these reports have reported positive results, but in none was there a randomized control group.

The most impressive and most recent study was reported by Storm and coworkers in 1992 (98). They had a total of 94 consecutive patients with empyema. The 51 patients who were on one service were treated with daily thoracentesis, saline rinse, systemic antibiotics, and in about 50% of the patients instillation of antibiotics into the pleural space. The 43 patients on the other service were treated with tube thoracostomy and systemic antibiotics. Of the 51 patients on the first service, only 3 (6%) required a rib resection or a decortication. In contrast 33 of the 43 patients (77%) on the other service required either rib resection or decortication. However, it must be pointed out that the patients were not randomized to the two different treatments and the patients in the second group could have been sicker. Nevertheless, these studies raise the possibility that there might be a role for intrapleural antibiotics in the management of complicated parapneumonic effusions. Until such controlled studies documenting their efficacy are completed, however, they are not recommended.

Intrapleural Thrombolytic Agents

Difficulties arise in the drainage of complicated parapneumonic effusions on account of pleural fluid loculations. Many years ago, Tillett and associates (99) proposed the intrapleural injection of streptokinase and streptodornase into patients with empyemas to eliminate the pleural loculations. In the late 1970s, Bergh and colleagues (100) reported the results of the intrapleural injection of streptokinase alone in 12 patients with empyema. They reported radiologic improvement in 10 of their 12 patients.

Since the last edition of this book, there have been at least six articles reporting the results with thrombolytic therapy for loculated complicated parapneumonic effusions (100–106). In the six reports referenced a total of 68 patients were treated and successful results were reported in 60 of the patients (88%). Approximately one-half of the patients were treated with streptokinase and one-half of the patients were treated with urokinase. The thrombolytic agents appear to be more effective if they are administered early in the course of the parapneumonic effusion before fibrosis has developed (106).

From the above studies, it appears that intrapleural thrombolytic agents do have a role in the management of patients with complicated loculated parapneumonic effusions, i.e., Class 5 and Class 7 parapneumonic effusions. It should be emphasized, however, that none of the above studies (100–106) had a control group.

Intrapleural thrombolytic agents are recommended for all patients with Class 5 and Class 7 parapneumonic effusions (Table 9.4). Streptokinase and urokinase appear equally effective. The usual dose of streptokinase is 250,000 U diluted in 100 ml saline while the usual dose of urokinase is 100,000 U diluted in 100 ml saline. After each instillation of the thrombolytic agent, the chest tube is clamped for 1 to 2 hours to allow the thrombolytic agents to attack the fibrin membranes producing the loculations. Successful therapy is heralded by an increase in the amount of drainage from the pleural space. The thrombolytic agents can be administered daily for up to 14 days. One vial of urokinase that contains 250,000 IU costs $258, whereas one vial of streptokinase containing 750,000 U costs $156 (107). One possible advantage for urokinase in comparison to streptokinase is that streptokinase, which is a bacterial protein, forms a complex with plasminogen, which produces an antibody response. Accordingly, if a patient is treated with streptokinase for a loculated effusion, the subsequent administration of the agent might produce an allergic reaction (107). Similar antibodies are not produced with urokinase. The intrapleural injection of thrombolytic agents has no effect on the systemic coagulation parameters (108).

Thoracoscopy with Breakdown of Adhesions

If the patient has a loculated parapneumonic effusion that does not respond to the intrapleural administration of thrombolytic agents, then thoracoscopy should be considered (88). With thoracoscopy, the loculations in the pleural space can be disrupted and the pleural space can be completely drained (109). The chest tube can be positioned optimally with thoracoscopic guidance. In addition, the pleural surfaces can be inspected to determine the necessity for further intervention such as decortication. If at thoracoscopy, the patient is found to have a very thick pleural peel with a large amount of debris and entrapment of the lung, the thoracoscopy incision can be enlarged to allow for decortication (110). It should be emphasized, however, that frequently thoracoscopy does not cure the patient. In one series, 12 of 18 patients (67%) had to have an additional surgical procedure following thoracoscopy (111). In view of this one should be ready to extend the thoracoscopic procedure to a decortication.

Decortication

In this procedure, all the fibrous tissue is removed from the visceral pleura, and all pus is evacuated from the pleural space. Decortication eliminates the pleural sepsis and allows the underlying lung to expand. Decortication is a major thoracic operation requiring a full thoracotomy incision and should therefore not be performed on patients who are markedly debilitated.

Decortication is the procedure of choice in the relatively healthy individual in whom pleural sepsis is not controlled by closed-tube thoracostomy, intrapleural thrombolytic agents, and possibly thoracoscopy. This procedure should be done in appropriate patients as soon as it is recognized that the more conservative therapies are failing (112, 113). This procedure can eliminate the long period, frequently several months, of wound irrigation and dressing changes associated with open drainage. Morin and coworkers (112) performed decortication on 23 adults with empyemas anywhere from 10 to 500 days after the start of the illness. The mean postoperative hospital stay was only 14 days, and the pleural sepsis was controlled in all patients in that no instances of wound infection or recurrent empyemas were seen. In a more recent study (114), the median postoperative stay after decortication in 71 patients was 7 days. The mortality rate in this latter series was 10%, but all the patients who died had other serious medical problems (114).

When managing patients with pleural infections in the acute stages, decortication should only be considered for the control of pleural infection. Decortication should not be performed just to remove thickened pleura because such thickening usually resolves spontaneously over several months (115). If after 6 months the pleura remains thickened and the patient's pulmonary function is sufficiently reduced to limit activities, however, decortication should be considered.

Open Drainage

This method can be employed when closed-tube drainage of the pleural infection is inadequate and the patient does not respond to intrapleural thrombolytic agents (92, 116). This procedure is only recommended when the patient is too ill to tolerate a decortication. Two different types of procedures can be performed. The simplest procedure involves resecting segments of one to three ribs overlying the lower part of the empyema cavity and inserting one or more short, large-bore tubes into the empyema cavity. Following this procedure, the tubes should be irrigated daily with a mild antiseptic solution. The drainage from the tubes can be collected in a colostomy bag placed over the tubes. The advantage of this method over closed-tube drainage is that drainage is more complete, and the patient is freed from his attachment to the chest tube bottles.

A similar but more complicated procedure is open-flap drainage, in which a skin and muscle flap is positioned so it lines the tract between the pleural space and the surface of the chest (112, 116) when two or more overlying ribs are resected. The advantage of this open flap (Eloesser flap) is that it creates a skin-lined fistula that provides drainage without tubes. It can therefore be more easily managed by the patient at home and permits gradual obliteration of the empyema space.

It is important not to convert to an open-drainage procedure too early in the course of a complicated parapneumonic effusion. With an open-drainage procedure, the pleural space is exposed to atmospheric pressure. If the visceral and parietal pleura adjacent to the empyema cavity have not been fused by the inflammatory process, exposure of the pleural space to atmospheric pressure will result in a pneumothorax. Prior to open-drainage procedures, this possibility can be evaluated by leaving the chest tube exposed to atmospheric pressure for a short period and determining radiologi-

cally whether the lung has collapsed. If the lung does collapse in this situation, an open-drainage procedure can still be performed by creating an airtight seal and connecting the large tube to a water-seal drainage apparatus (116). The high mortality with parapneumonic effusions during World War I has been attributed to performing open drainage procedures too early (18).

When a patient is treated by open drainage, he can expect to have an open chest wound for a prolonged period. In one series of 33 patients treated by open-drainage procedures (42), the median time for healing the drainage site was 142 days. With decortication, the period of convalescence is much shorter (112), but decortication is a major surgical procedure that cannot be tolerated by markedly debilitated patients.

SPECIAL SITUATIONS WITH EMPYEMA

Empyema in Children

As mentioned earlier in this chapter, the bacteriology of empyema in children varies somewhat from that in adults. In children the incidence of anaerobic infection is lower while that of *H. influenzae* is higher. Another difference between children and adults is that the complicated parapneumonic effusions can lead to scoliosis in the children. Hoff and coworkers (117) reported that scoliosis of 5° or more was noted in 27 of 61 patients (44%). They also found that 80% of patients presenting with more than 10° of scoliosis required decortication (117).

The criteria for tube thoracostomy, namely a low pleural fluid pH and/or a low pleural fluid glucose, appear to be appropriate for children as well as for adults (117). Additional indicators of a poor outcome in children were significant scoliosis, evidence of parenchymal entrapment, and anaerobic infection. Tube thoracostomy or decortication should be instituted if the patient has two or more of these characteristics of a poor prognosis.

In general the management of children with empyema is very similar to that for adults. The children are usually healthy so there is very little if any role for open drainage procedures. If the pleural fluid is loculated, intrapleural thrombolytic agents should be used (118). If the pleural fluid remains loculated after the intrapleural thrombolytics, then thoracoscopy can be attempted (119). If the sepsis is still not controlled, then the patient should be subjected to decortication (117, 120). Hoff and associates recommend decortication as early as two to three days after the child is hospitalized (117).

Empyema Associated with Bronchopleural Fistula

When an empyema is complicated by the presence of a bronchopleural fistula, adequate pleural drainage is crucial. Pleural fluid that is not drained exteriorly with chest tubes is likely to drain interiorly into the lung. The bacteria then are spread throughout the bronchopulmonary tree and an overwhelming pneumonia can result.

The presence of a bronchopleural fistula should be suspected when a patient with a pleural fluid collection raises more sputum than would be expected from the associated pulmonary disease. If the patient raises large amounts of sputum only when lying in one position, a bronchopleural fistula is strongly suggested. Radiologically, a bronchopleural fistula is manifested by the presence of an air-fluid level in the pleural space when the radiograph is obtained with the patient in the upright position. It is sometimes difficult to determine whether the air-fluid levels are in the lung parenchyma or the pleural space. The utility of ultrasound and CT studies in making this differentiation is discussed in Chapter 3.

It should be emphasized the presence of a bronchopleural fistula in conjunction with infected pleural fluid is a medical emergency. Drainage should be instituted immediately to prevent the possibility of contaminating the entire respiratory system by the infected pleural fluid.

Empyema Distal To an Obstructed Bronchus

One contraindication to the placement of chest tubes in patients with complicated parapneumonic effusions is the presence of a malignant tumor obstructing a lobar or mainstem bronchus. If chest tubes are placed in such patients, the bronchial obstruction will prevent expansion of the lung underlying the pleural effusion and the unfortunate patient will be saddled with a chest tube or an open chest wound for the remainder of his life. When a patient is discovered to have a complicated parapneumonic effusion distal to an obstructed bronchus, appropriate antibiotics should be administered in conjunction with radiotherapy or laser therapy to the affected bronchus. Tube thoracostomy can be instituted if radiotherapy relieves the obstruction. If the obstruction persists, the patient can be sent home with a prescription of appropriate oral antibiotics. In my experience, the continuous administration of oral antibiotics to patients with pleural sepsis and bronchial obstruction allows them to live in symbiosis with their pleural infection without excessive systemic toxicity.

Postpneumonectomy Empyema

Empyemas following thoracic surgical procedures account for approximately 25% of all empyemas (21, 26, 39) and the procedure is usually a pneumonectomy. After a pneumonectomy there is a characteristic evolution of radiological findings and deviations from this suggest the possibility of postpneumonectomy empyema. Immediately after pneumonectomy, the ipsilateral pleural space contains air, the mediastinum is shifted to the ipsilateral side, and the hemidiaphragm is elevated (Fig. 9.4A). The postpneumonectomy space then begins to fill with serosanguineous fluid at a rate of approximately 2 rib spaces a day. In the majority of patients, the pleural space becomes 80 to 90% fluid-filled within 2 weeks and completely filled within 2 to 4 months (121). During this period, the mediastinum progressively shifts ipsilaterally (Fig. 9.4B). Failure of the mediastinum to shift in the postoperative period indicates an abnormality in the postpneumonectomy space (121). Similarly, the most sensitive indicator of late complications in the pneumonectomy space is the return to the midline of a previously shifted mediastinum or a shift of the mediastinum to the contralateral side (Fig. 9.5) (121).

The postoperative occurrence of empyema is a dreaded complication of pneumonectomy. The seriousness of this complication is that it

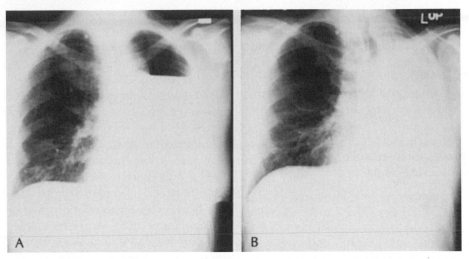

Figure 9.4. Appearance of chest radiograph after pneumonectomy. **A.** Posteroanterior chest radiograph from a patient 1 week after pneumonectomy. Note that the postpneumonectomy space contains an air-fluid level and that the mediastinum is shifted toward the side of the pneumonectomy. **B.** Posteroanterior chest radiograph from the same patient one year after pneumonectomy. The mediastinum has shifted more toward the side with the pneumonectomy, and the hemithorax is completely opacified.

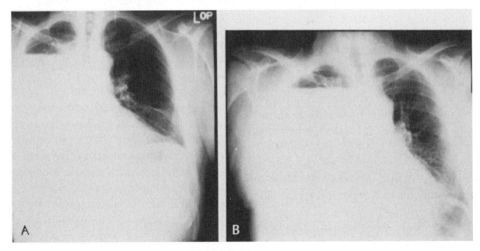

Figure 9.5A. Posteroanterior chest radiograph from a patient who had undergone a right pneumonectomy 2 weeks previously. **B.** Posteroanterior chest radiograph from the same patient a week later. Note the marked interval shift in the mediastinum. This patient had a *Staphylococcus aureus* infection of his pneumonectomy space.

is impossible to eliminate the space containing the infection, and consequently, it is difficult to sterilize the space. Approximately 40% of patients with postpneumonectomy empyema have a bronchopleural or an esophagopleural fistula as a complication (122). Therefore, all patients with this type of empyema should have a barium swallow and a bronchoscopic examination.

The incidence of empyema following pneumonectomy varies from 2 to 10% (123–125).

An infected pneumonectomy space usually becomes manifest in one of four ways: (*a*) a febrile illness with signs of systemic toxicity; (*b*) expectoration of large amounts of pleural fluid; (*c*) an air-fluid level in the pneumonectomy space; or (*d*) the drainage of purulent material from the surgical incision. The time from pneumonectomy to the development of an empyema ranges from 2 days to 7 years, with most evident within 4 weeks (122, 125). The diagnosis should be suspected in any patient who, following this operation, becomes febrile, starts expectorating large amounts of pleural fluid, has purulent drainage from his thoracotomy wound, or who has a mediastinum that is midline or shifted to the contralateral side (Fig. 9.5). The diagnosis is established by a thoracentesis demonstrating bacteria on the Gram stain of the pleural fluid. If more than several weeks have passed since the patient's pneumonectomy, ultrasonic examination of the pleural space should be performed to identify the appropriate location for the thoracentesis. *Staphylococcus aureus* is the bacterium responsible for the majority of postpneumonectomy empyemas (122–124) but Gram-negative organisms such as *Escherichia coli*, *Pseudomonas* species, and *Proteus* species as well as fungi are at times responsible.

All patients with postpneumonectomy empyema should be treated with a chest tube and appropriate antibiotics. Beyond that the treatment is largely dependent upon whether the patient has a bronchopleural fistula. If the patient does not have a bronchopleural fistula, then the treatment of choice is closed-tube drainage of the pleural space in conjunction with antibiotic irrigation (123, 126). A chest tube is inserted into the most dependent portion of the patient's empyema cavity and is connected to an underwater-seal drainage apparatus. The antibiotics to which the offending organisms are susceptible can be instilled by this tube, if a double-lumen tube is used (126), or through a separate, smaller tube inserted into the second or third intercostal space at the midclavicular line. The antibiotics can be infused through the pleural space continuously. Alternatively, with the drainage tube clamped, several hundred milliliters of antibiotic solution can be instilled into the pleural space and allowed to remain for several hours. The pleural fluid is then drained, and the sequence is repeated. When the drained fluid becomes clear, the irrigation fluid is changed to normal saline solution for 24 hours. If the culture of this drainage is sterile, 100 ml concentrated irrigation fluid are left in the pleural space, and the chest tubes are removed.

In two series (123, 126), 12 patients were treated by the foregoing procedure, and the pleural infection was eventually controlled in all these patients. The mean duration of pleural irrigation was less than a month, and although 3 patients had a recurring pleural infection, all were subsequently successfully managed with pleural irrigation. Because closed-tube drainage coupled with antibiotic irrigation of the pleural space appears to be effective in most patients and because it is associated with a shorter hospitalization time than the fenestration procedure described below, it is the treatment of choice for most patients with postpneumonectomy empyema.

An alternate approach to postpneumonectomy empyema involves the creation of a large opening in the chest by resecting several inches of the rib inferior to the thoracotomy incision and one or more ribs superior to it. The procedure is called the Clagett procedure after the surgeon who first described it (93). The superficial fascia is sutured down to the periosteum of the resected ribs to leave a large window in the thoracic wall. Each day, the empyema cavity is irrigated with a mildly antiseptic solution such as half-strength Dakin's solution or chlorhexidine (Hibitane) (124). These irrigations are continued for several weeks until the drainage is no longer purulent and the empyema cavity appears well debrided. At this time, the opening in the chest wall is closed, and a 0.25% solution of neomycin is placed in the cavity.

Goldstraw (124) treated 29 patients with postpneumonectomy empyemas in the foregoing manner and attempted closure in 22 of the patients. In 17 of these 22 patients (77%), closure was successful in that no evidence was seen of a recurrence of the empyema from 5 weeks to 9 years after closure. The 5 patients in whom closure failed initially were subjected to a second fenestration, and a successful closure was eventually obtained in 2 of these patients. Other workers have reported much poorer results with the Clagett procedure. Shamji and colleagues (127) achieved successful closure in only 2 of 31 patients (6%) managed in this manner, whereas Bayes and coworkers (128) reported success in 10 of 28 patients (36%). This treatment is time-consuming, with a mean interval between fenestration and closure of 40 days (124) (range 21 to 74 days), and patients usually have to remain hospitalized for the entire period. The closed irrigation method is the procedure of choice in my opinion.

If a bronchopleural fistula is present, several different procedures can be used to attempt to close the fistula. On occasion the bronchopleural fistula will close with continuous irrigation of the infected pleural space, but usually more extensive procedures must be done. Attempts to close the bronchopleural fistula directly usually fail because of the presence of the pleural infection. Pairolero and associates (129) advocate the intrathoracic transposition of extrathoracic skeletal muscle to facilitate closure of the fistula. They attempted this procedure in 28 patients following open drainage and reported success in 24. The median number of operations was 5.0, with a range of 1 to 19. The median hospitalization time was 34 days with a range of 4 to 137. A related method closes the fistula with an omentopexy (130, 131). Onotera and Unruth (132) reported the successful closure of a 3-mm diameter postpneumonectomy bronchopleural fistula with 1 ml fibrin sealant instilled in the fistula via a thoracoscope. Menard and associates (133) have reported that a tissue adhesive instilled via a bronchoscope is effective in closing postpneumonectomy bronchopleural fistulas in dogs.

REFERENCES

1. Neiderman MS, Bass JB, Campbell GD, Fein AM, Grossman RF, Mandell LA, et al: Guidelines for the initial management of adults with community-acquired pneumonia: diagnosis, assessment of severity, and initial antimicrobial therapy. Am Rev Respir Dis 1993;148:1418–1426.
2. Light RW, Girard WM, Jenkinson SG, George RB: Parapneumonic effusions. Am J Med 1980;69:507–511.
3. Brewin A, Arango L, Hadley WK, Murray JF: High-dose penicillin therapy and pneumococcal pneumonia. JAMA 1974;230:409–413.
4. Finland M, Barnes MW: Duration of hospitalization for acute bacterial empyema at Boston City Hospital during 12 selected years from 1935 to 1972. J Infect Dis 1978;138:520–530.
5. Adams F: The Genuine Works of Hippocrates. New York: William Wood, 1948:266.
6. Bowditch HI: Paracentesis thoracic: An analysis of 25 cases of pleuritic effusion. Am Med Monthly 1853;3–45.
7. Trousseau A: Lectures on Clinical Medicine Delivered at the Hotel-Dieu Paris, JR McCormick (trans). London: The New Sydenham Society, 1987;3:198.
8. Hewitt C: Drainage for empyema. Br Med J 1876;1:317.
9. Estlander JA: Sur le resection des côté dans l'empyème chronique. Rev Mens 1897;8:885.
10. Schede M: Die Behandlung der Empyeme. Verh Innere Med Weisbaden 1890;9:41.
11. Fowler GR: A case of thoracoplasty for the removal of a large cicatricial fibrous growth from the interior of the chest, the result of an old empyema. Med Rec 1893;44:938.
12. Beck C: Thoracoplasty in America and visceral pleurectomy with report of a case. JAMA 1897;28:58.
13. Eggers C: Radical operation for empyema. Ann Surg 1923;77:327.
14. Paget S: The Surgery of the Chest. Bristol, England: John Wright & Co., 1896:204–206.
15. Graham EA: Some Fundamental Considerations in the Treatment of Empyema Thoracis. St. Louis: CV Mosby, 1925:14.
16. Olch PD: Evarts A. Graham in World War I: The empyema commission and service in the American expeditionary forces. J Hist Med Allied Sci 1989;44:430–446.
17. Graham EA, Bell RD: Open pneumothorax: its relations to the treatment of empyema. Am J Med Sci 1918;156:839–871.
18. Empyema Commission: Cases of empyema at Camp Lee, Virginia. JAMA 1918;71:366–373.
19. Stone WJ: The management of postpneumonic empyema based on 310 cases. Am J Med Sci 1919;158.
20. Light RW, MacGregor MI, Ball WC Jr, Luchsinger PC: Diagnostic significance of pleural fluid pH and Pco_2. Chest 1973;64:591–596.
21. Weese WC, Shindler ER, Smith IM, Rabinovich S: Empyema of the thorax then and now. Arch Intern Med 1973;131:516–520.
22. Vianna NJ: Nontuberculous bacterial empyema in patients with and without underlying diseases. JAMA 1971;215:69–75.
23. Andrews NC, Parker EF, Shaw RR, et al: Management of nontuberculous empyema. Am Rev Respir Dis 1962;85:935–936.
24. Wiener-Kronish JP, Sakuma T, Kudoh I, Pittet JF, Frank D, Dobbs L, Vasil ML, Matthay MA: Alveolar epithelial injury and pleural empyema in acute *P. aeruginosa* pneumonia in anesthetized rabbits. J Appl Physiol 1993;75:1661–1669.
25. Light RW: Management of parapneumonic effusions. Arch Intern Med 1981;141:1339–1341.
26. Snider GL, Saleh SS: Empyema of the thorax in adults: review of 105 cases. Chest 1968;54:12–17.
27. Yeh TJ, Hall DP, Ellison RG: Empyema thoracis: a review of 110 cases. Am Rev Respir Dis 1963;88:785–790.
28. Smith JA, Mullerworth MH, Westlake GW, Tatoulis J: Empyema thoracis: 14-year experience in a teaching center. Ann Thorac Surg 1991;51:39–42.
29. Jones FL, Blodgett RC: Empyema in rheumatoid pleuropulmonary disease. Ann Intern Med 1971;74:665–671.

30. Mavroudis C, Ganzel BL, Katzmark S, Polk HC Jr: Effect of hemothorax on experimental empyema thoracis in the guinea pig. J Thorac Cardiovasc Surg 1985;89:42-49.

31. Mavroudis C, Ganzel BL, Cox SK, Polk HC Jr: Experimental aerobic-anaerobic thoracic empyema in the guinea pig. Ann Thorac Surg 1987;43:295-297.

32. Sahn SA, Taryle DA, Good JT Jr: Experimental empyema: time course and pathogenesis of pleural fluid acidosis and low pleural fluid glucose. Am Rev Respir Dis 1979;120:355-361.

33. Shohet I, Yellin A, Meyerovitch J, Rubinstein E: Pharmacokinetics and therapeutic efficacy of gentamicin in an experimental pleural empyema rabbit model. Antimicrob Agents Chemother 1987;31:982-985.

34. Sasse SA, Mulligan MA, Light RW: A new experimental model of empyema in the rabbits. Am J Respir Crit Care Med 1995;151, in press.

35. Finland M, Barnes MW: Changing ecology of acute bacterial empyema: occurrence and mortality at Boston City Hospital during 12 selected years from 1935 to 1972. J Infect Dis 1978;137:274-291.

36. Bartlett JG, Gorbach SL, Thadepalli H, Finegold SM: Bacteriology of empyema. Lancet 1974;1:338-340.

37. Brook I, Frazier EH: Aerobic and anaerobic microbiology of empyema. A retrospective review in two military hospitals. Chest 1993;103:1502-1507.

38. Alfageme I, Munoz F, Pena N, Umbria S: Empyema of the thorax in adults. Etiology, microbiologic findings, and management. Chest 1993;103:839-843.

39. Varkey B, Rose HD, Kutty CPK, Politis J: Empyema thoracis during a ten-year period. Arch Intern Med 1981;141:1771-1776.

40. Brook I: Microbiology of empyema in children and adolescents. Pediatrics 1990;85:722-726.

41. Freij BJ, Kusmiesz H, Nelson JD, McCracken GH: Parapneumonic effusions and empyema in hospitalized children: a retrospective review of 227 cases. Ped Infect Dis 1984;3:578-591.

42. Bartlett JG, Finegold SM: Anaerobic infections of the lung and pleural space. Am Rev Respir Dis 1974;110:56-77.

43. Taryle DA, Potts DE, Sahn SA: The incidence and clinical correlates of parapneumonic effusions in pneumococcal pneumonia. Chest 1978;74:170-173.

44. Wolfe WG, Spock A, Bradford WD: Pleural fluid in infants and children. Am Rev Respir Dis 1968;98:1027-1032.

45. Hendren WH III, Haggerty RJ: Staphylococcic pneumonia in infancy and childhood. JAMA 1958;168:6-16.

46. Kaye MG, Fox MJ, Bartlett JG, Braman SS, Glassroth J: The clinical spectrum of Staphylococcus aureus pulmonary infection. Chest 1990;97:788-792.

47. Welch CC, Tombridge TL, Baker WJ, Kinney RJ: Beta-hemolytic streptococcal pneumonia: report of an outbreak in a military population. Am J Med Sci 1961;242:157-165.

48. Basiliere JL, Bistrong HW, Spence WF: Streptococcal pneumonia: recent outbreaks in military recruit populations. Am J Med 1968;44:580-589.

49. Braman SS, Donat WE: Explosive pleuritis. Manifestation of Group A beta-hemolytic streptococcal infection. Am J Med 1986;81:723-726.

50. Tillotson JR, Lerner AM: Characteristics of pneumonias caused by Escherichia coli. N Engl J Med 1967;277:115-122.

51. Tillotson JR, Lerner AM: Characteristics of nonbacteremic pseudomonas pneumonia. Ann Intern Med 1968;68:295-307.

52. Holmes RB: Friedlander's pneumonia. AJR 1956;75:728-747.

53. Asmar BI, Slovis TL, Reed JO, Dajani AS: Hemophilus influenzae type b pneumonia in 43 children. J Pediatr 1978;93:389-393.

54. Ginsburg CM, Howard JB, Nelson JD: Report of 65 cases of Haemophilus influenzae b pneumonia. Pediatrics 1979;64:283-286.

55. Levin DC, Schwarz MI, Matthay RA, LaForce FM: Bacteremic Haemophilus influenzae pneumonia in adults: a report of 24 cases and a review of the literature. Am J Med 1977;62:219-223.

56. Tillotson JR, Lerner AM: Characteristics of pneumonias caused by Bacillus proteus. Ann Intern Med 1968;68:287-294.

57. Plotkin SA, Brachman PS, Utell M, et al: An epidemic of inhalation anthrax, the first in the twentieth century. Am J Med 1960;29:992-1001.

58. Evans AF, Oakley RH, Whitehouse GH: Analysis of the chest radiograph in Legionnaires' disease. Clin Radiol 1981;32:361-365.

59. Kirby BD, Peck H, Meyer RD: Radiographic features of Legionnaires' disease. Chest 1979;76:562-566.

60. Kroboth FJ, Yu VL, Reddy SC, Yu AC: Clinicoradiographic correlation with extent of Legionnaires' disease. AJR 1983;141:263-268.

61. Randolph KA, Beekman JF: Legionnaires' disease presenting with empyema. Chest 1979;75:404-406.

62. Patel SB, Mahler R: Clostridial pleuropulmonary infections: case report and review of the literature. J Infect 1990;21:81-85.

63. Cooney TG, Harwood BR, Meisner DJ: Haemophilus parainfluenzae thoracic empyema. Arch Intern Med 1981;141:940-941.

64. Bekemeyer WB, Zimmerman GA: Life-threatening complications associated with Bacillus cereus pneumonia. Am Rev Respir Dis 1985;131:466-469.

65. Madrazo A, Henderson MD, Baker L, et al: Massive empyema due to Citrobacter diversus. Chest 1975;68:104-106.

66. Mazzulli T, Salit IE: Pleural fluid infection caused by Listeria monocytogenes: case report and review. Rev Infect Dis 1991;13:564-570.

67. Funk LM, Simpson SQ, Mertz G, Boyd J: Tularemia presenting as an isolated pleural effusion. West J Med 1992;156:415-417.

68. Van De Water JM: The treatment of pleural effusion complicating pneumonia. Chest 1970;57:259-262.

69. Sahn SA, Lakshminarayan S, Char DC: "Silent" empyema in patients receiving corticosteroids. Am Rev Respir Dis 1973;107:873-876.

70. Sullivan KM, O'Toole RD, Fisher RH, Sullivan KN: Anaerobic empyema thoracis. Arch Intern Med 1973;131:521-527.

71. Landay MJ, Christensen EE, Bynum LJ, Goodman C: Anaerobic pleural and pulmonary infections. AJR 1980;134:233-240.

72. McLoud TC, Flower CD: Imaging the pleura: sonography, CT, and MR imaging. AJR 1991;156:1145-1153.

73. Yang PC, Luh KT, Chang DB, Wu HD, Yu CJ, Kuo SH: Value of sonography in determining the nature of pleural effusion: analysis of 320 cases. AJR 1992; 159:29-33.

74. Himelman RB, Callen PW: The prognostic value of loculations in parapneumonic pleural effusions. Chest 1986;90:852-856.

75. Stark DD, Federle MP, Goodman PC, Podrasky AE, Webb WR: Differentiating lung abscess and empyema: radiography and computed tomography. AJR 1983;141:163-167.

76. Taryle DA, Good JT Jr, Morgan EJ III, et al: Antibiotic concentrations in human parapneumonic effusions. J Antimicrob Chemother 1981;7:171-177.

77. Scaglione F, Raichi M, Fraschini F: Serum protein binding and extravascular diffusion of methoxyimino cephalosporins. Time courses of free and total concentrations of cefotaxime and ceftriaxone in serum and pleural exudate. J Antimicrob Agents Chemother 1990;26(Suppl A):1-10.

78. Cham CW, Haq SM, Rahamim J: Empyema thoracis: a problem with late referral? Thorax 1993;48:925-927.

79. Niederman MS, Schachter EN: Serial thoracenteses in parapneumonic effusions. N Engl J Med 1981; 304:847.

80. Pine JR, Hollman JL: Elevated pleural fluid pH in Proteus mirabilis empyema. Chest 1983;84:109-111.

81. Light RW, Moller DJ Jr, George RB: Low pleural fluid pH in parapneumonic effusion. Chest 1975;68: 273-274.

82. Berger HA, Morganroth ML: Immediate drainage is not required for all patients with complicated parapneumonic effusions. Chest 1990;97:731-735.

83. Poe RH, Matthew GM, Israel RH, Kallay MC: Utility of pleural fluid analysis in predicting tube thoracostomy/decortication in parapneumonic effusions. Chest 1991;100:963-967.

84. Light RW: Management of Parapneumonic Effusions. Chest 1991;100:892-893.

85. Lampe RM, Chottipitayasunondh T, Sunakorn P: Detection of bacterial antigen in pleural fluid by counterimmunoelectrophoresis. J Pediatr 1976;88: 557-560.

86. Boersma WG, Lowenberg A, Holloway Y, Kuttschrutter H, Snijder JA, Koeter GH: Rapid detection of pneumococcal antigen in pleural fluid of patients with community acquired pneumonia. Thorax 1993;48:160-162.

87. Kerr A, Vasudevan VP, Powell S, Ligenza C: Percutaneous catheter drainage for acute empyema. Improved cure rate using CAT scan, fluoroscopy, and pigtail drainage catheters. NY State J Med 1991;91: 4-7.

88. Shields TW: Parapneumonic empyema. In: Shields TW, ed. General Thoracic Surgery. 4th ed. Baltimore: Williams & Wilkins, 1994:684-693.

89. Silverman SG, Mueller PR, Saini S, Hahn PF, Simeone JF, Forman BH, Steiner E, Ferrucci JT: Thoracic empyema: management with image-guided catheter drainage. Radiology 1988;169:5-9.

90. Ali I, Unruh H: Management of empyema thoracis. Ann Thorac Surg 1990;50:355-359.

91. Ashbaugh DG: Empyema thoracis. Factors influencing morbidity and mortality. Chest 1991;99:1162-1165.

92. Sherman MM, Subramanian V, Berger RL: Management of thoracic empyema. Am J Surg 1977;133: 474-479.

93. Clagett OT, Geraci JE: A procedure for the management of postpneumonectomy empyema. J Thorac Cardiovasc Surg 1963;45:141-145.

94. Dieter RA Jr, Pifarre R, Neville WE, Magno M, Jasuja M: Empyema treated with neomycin irrigation and closed-chest drainage. J Thorac Cardiovasc Surg 1970;59:496-500.

95. Rosenfeldt FL, McGibney D, Braimbridge MV, Watson DA: Comparison between irrigation and conventional treatment for empyema and pneumonectomy space infection. Thorax 1981;36:272-277.

96. Hutter JA, Harari D, Braimbridge MV: The management of empyema thoracis by thoracoscopy and irrigation. Ann Thorac Surg 1985;39:517-520.

97. Hakim M, Milstein BB: Empyema thoracis and infected pneumonectomy space: case for cyclical irrigation. Ann Thorac Surg 1986;41:85-88.

98. Storm HKR, Krasnik M, Bang K, Frimodt-Moller N: Treatment of pleural empyema secondary to pneumonia: thoracocentesis regimen versus tube drainage. Thorax 1992;47:821-824.

99. Tillett WS, Sherry S, Read CT: The use of streptokinase-streptodornase in the treatment of postpneumonic empyema. J Thorac Surg 1951;21: 275-297.

100. Bergh NP, Ekroth R, Larsson S, Nagy P: Intrapleural streptokinase in the treatment of haemothorax and empyema. Scand J Thorac Cardiovasc Surg 1977;11: 265-268.

101. Henke CA, Leatherman JW: Intrapleurally administered streptokinase in the treatment of acute loculated nonpurulent parapneumonic effusions. Am Rev Respir Dis 1992;145:680-684.

102. Lee KS, Im JG, Kim YH, Hwang SH, Bae WK, Lee BH: Treatment of thoracic multiloculated empyemas with intracavitary urokinase: a prospective study. Radiology 1991;179;771-775.

103. Aye RW, Froese DP, Hill LD: Use of purified streptokinase in empyema and hemothorax. Am J Surg 1991;161:560-562.

104. Moulton JS, Moore PT, Mencini RA: Treatment of loculated pleural effusions with transcatheter intracavitary urokinase. AJR 1989;153:941-945.

105. Robinson LA, Moulton AL, Fleming WH, Alonso A, Galbraith TA: Intrapleural fibrinolytic treatment of multiloculated thoracic empyemas. Ann Thorac Surg 1994;57:803-813.

106. Pollak JS, Passik CS: Intrapleural urokinase in the treatment of loculated pleural effusions. Chest 1994; 105:868-873.

107. Light RW: Pleural disease. Dis Mon 1992;38:265-331.

108. Berglin E, Ekroth R, Teger-Nilsson AL, William-Olsson G: Intrapleural instillation of streptokinase. Effects on systemic fibrinolysis. Thorac Cardiovasc Surg 1981;29:124-126.

109. Ferguson MK: Thoracoscopy for empyema, bronchopleural fistula, and chylothorax. Ann Thorac Surg 1993;56:644-645.

110. Moores DWO: Management of acute empyema. [Editorial]. Chest 1992;102:1316-1317.

111. Ridley PD, Braimbridge MV: Thoracoscopic debridement and pleural irrigation in the management of empyema thoracis. Ann Thorac Surg 1991;51:461-464.

112. Morin JE, Munro DD, MacLean LD: Early thoracotomy for empyema. J Thorac Cardiovasc Surg 1972;64:530-536.

113. Hoover EL, Hsu H-K, Ross JM, Gross AM, Webb H, Ketosugbo A, Finch P: Reappraisal of empyema thoracis: Surgical intervention when the duration of illness is unknown. Chest 1986;90:511-515.

114. Pothula V, Krellenstein DJ: Early aggressive surgical management of parapneumonic empyemas. Chest 1994;105:832-836.

115. Neff CC, vanSonnenberg E, Lawson DW, Patton AS: CT follow-up of empyemas: pleural peels resolve after percutaneous catheter drainage. Radiology 1990;176:195-197.

116. Samson PC: Empyema thoracis: essentials of present-day management. Ann Thorac Surg 1971; 11:210-220.

117. Hoff SJ, Neblett WW, Edwards KM, Heller RM, Pietsch JB, Holcomb GW Jr, Holcomb GW, III: Parapneumonic empyema in children: decortication hastens recovery in patients with severe pleural infections. Ped Infect Dis J 1991;10:194-199.

118. Rosen H, Nadkarni V, Theroux M, Padman R, Klein J: Intrapleural streptokinase as adjunctive treatment for persistent empyema in pediatric patients. Chest 1993;103:1190-1193.

119. Kern JA, Rodgers BM: Thoracoscopy in the management of empyema in children. J Pediatr Surg 1993; 28:1128-1132.

120. Gustafson RA, Murray GF, Warden HE, Hill RC: Role of lung decortication in symptomatic empyemas in children. Ann Thorac Surg 1990;49:940-946.

121. Fraser RG, Pare JAP, Pare PD, Fraser RS, Genereux GP: Diagnosis of Diseases of the Chest. 3rd ed. Philadelphia: WB Saunders, 1991;4:2520-2523.

122. Virkkula L, Eerola S: Treatment of postpneumonectomy empyema. Scand J Thorac Cardiovasc Surg 1974;8:133-137.

123. Karkola P, Kairaluoma MI, Larmi TKI: Postpneumonectomy empyema in pulmonary carcinoma patients. J Thorac Cardiovasc Surg 1976;72:319-322.

124. Goldstraw P: Treatment of postpneumonectomy empyema: the case for fenestration. Thorax 1979; 34:740-745.

125. Ueda H, Shibata K, Kusano T: Postoperative pyothorax. Surgery Today 1992;22:115-119.

126. Rosenfeldt FL, McGibney D, Braimbridge MV, Watson DA: Comparison between irrigation and conventional treatment for empyema and pneumonectomy space infection. Thorax 1981;36:272-277.

127. Shamji FM, Ginsberg RJ, Cooper JD, et al: Open window thoracostomy in the management of postpneumonectomy empyema with or without bronchopleural fistula. J Thorac Cardiovasc Surg 1983; 86:818-822.

128. Bayes AJ, Wilson JA, Chiu RC, et al: Clagett open-window thoracostomy in patients with empyema who had and had not undergone pneumonectomy. Can J Surg 1987;30:329-331.

129. Pairolero PC, Arnold PG, Trastek VF, Meland NB, Kay PP: Postpneumonectomy empyema. The role of intrathoracic muscle transposition. J Thorac Cardiovasc Surg 1990;99:958-968.

130. Saito H, Tatsuzawa T, Kikkawa H, et al: Transpericardial bronchial closure with omentopexy for postpneumonectomy bronchopleural fistula. Ann Thorac Surg 1989;47:312-313.

131. Shirakusa T, Ueda H, Takata S, Yoneda S, Inutsuka K, Hirota N, Okazaki M: Use of pedicled omental flap in treatment of empyema. Ann Thorac Surg 1990;50:420-424.

132. Onotera RT, Unruth HW: Closure of a postpneumonectomy bronchopleural fistula with fibrin sealant (Tisseel). Thorax 1988;43:1015-1016.

133. Menard JW, Prejean CA, Tucker WY: Endoscopic closure of bronchopleural fistulas using a tissue adhesive. Am J Surg 1988;155:415-416.

CHAPTER 10

Tuberculous Pleural Effusions

The diagnosis of tuberculous pleuritis should be considered in any patient with an exudative pleural effusion. A pleural effusion as a manifestation of tuberculosis has been likened to a primary chancre as a manifestation of syphilis. Both are self-limited and of little immediate concern, but both may lead to serious disease many years later.

PATHOGENESIS AND PATHOPHYSIOLOGIC FEATURES

When a tuberculous pleural effusion occurs in the absence of radiologically apparent tuberculosis, it may be the sequel to a primary infection 6 to 12 weeks previously or it may represent reactivation tuberculosis (1). A recent report from England suggested that more pleural effusions were due to reactivation than were postprimary (1). The tuberculous pleural effusion is thought to result from rupture of a subpleural caseous focus in the lung into the pleural space (2). Supporting evidence comes from the operative findings of Stead and co-workers, who reported that they could demonstrate a caseous tuberculous focus in the lung contiguous with the diseased pleura in 12 of 15 patients with tuberculous pleuritis (3). The remaining 3 patients in this series were found to have parenchymal tuberculosis, although these patients did not have caseous foci adjacent to the pleura.

It appears that delayed hypersensitivity plays a large role in the pathogenesis of tuberculous pleural effusion. Several workers (4–7) have reported that when guinea pigs or mice are immunized to tuberculous protein by injecting Freund's adjuvant containing dead tubercle bacilli into their footpads, an intrapleural injection of tuberculin purified protein derivative (PPD) 3 to 5 weeks later causes the rapid appearance (over 12 to 48 hours) of an exudative pleural effusion. The development of the pleural effusion is suppressed when the animals are given antilymphocyte serum (6).

The neutrophil appears to play a key role in the development of experimental tuberculous pleuritis. When bacillus Calmette-Guérin (BCG)-sensitized rabbits are given BCG intrapleurally, the resulting pleural fluid contains predominantly neutrophils for the first 24 hours (8). If the animals are made neutropenic the accumulation of pleural fluid and inflammatory cells, particularly macrophages, is decreased. The intrapleural injection of neutrophils in the neutropenic animals restores the response to control levels. The neutrophils in the pleural space appear to secrete a monocyte chemotaxin that recruits monocytes to the pleural space and thereby contributes to the granuloma formation (8).

In this BCG model of experimental tuberculous pleuritis, macrophages predominate in the pleural fluid from day 2 to day 5 (8). After this period lymphocytes are the predominant cell in the pleural fluid (9). When the lymphocytes first appear in the pleural fluid on approximately day 3, they do not respond to PPD. From day 5 onward, however, reactivity to PPD is found in most cases (10). The reactivity of the lymphocytes in the peripheral blood parallels that of the pleural lymphocytes (10).

It is probable that delayed hypersensitivity also plays a large role in the development of tuberculous pleural effusions in humans. The pleural fluid mycobacterial cultures from the majority of patients with tuberculous pleural effusions are negative (2, 11, 12). T lymphocytes specifically sensitized to tuberculous protein are present in the pleural fluid (13). In one report approximately 1/2000 of the lymphocytes in the pleural fluid was specifically sensitized to tuberculous protein (13). In the same report only 1/15,000 of the lymphocytes in the peripheral blood was specifically sensitized to the tuberculous protein. It is unknown whether the increased percentage of specifically sensitized lymphocytes in the pleural fluid is due to their clonal expansion in the pleural fluid or is due to the migratory loss of PPD-responding T lymphocytes from the blood to the pleural space. When pleural lymphocytes from patients with tuberculous pleural effusions are cocultured with PPD, lymphokines are produced (14). The level of lymphokine production is much greater with pleural lymphocytes than with peripheral blood lymphocytes (14).

Rupture of a subpleural caseous focus into the pleural space allows tuberculous protein to enter the pleural space and to generate the hypersensitivity reaction responsible for most of the clinical manifestations.

Although delayed hypersensitivity to tuberculous protein is probably responsible for most clinical manifestations of tuberculous pleuritis, many patients when first evaluated have a negative reaction to an intermediate PPD skin test. The explanation for this paradox appears to be a combination of two factors. First, in some (15), but not in all (16), patients with tuberculous pleuritis a circulating adherent cell suppresses the specifically sensitized circulating T lymphocytes in the peripheral blood. Second, there may be sequestration of PPD-reactive T lymphocytes in the pleural space involving both Leu-2 (suppressor/cytotoxic) and Leu-3 (helper) positive T cells (16).

Tuberculous pleural effusions are enriched with many potentially immunoreactive cells and substances that comprise the vigorous local cell-mediated immune response (17). Compared with peripheral blood, pleural fluid is enriched with T lymphocytes. The CD4 (helper-inducer):CD8 (suppressor/cytotoxic) ratio is 3:4 in pleural fluid, compared with 1:7 in blood (17). Pleural fluid lymphocytes from patients with tuberculous pleuritis show greater responsiveness to PPD than do peripheral blood lymphocytes (18–20).

The marked, local inflammatory response of tuberculous pleuritis is mediated in part by a number of inflammatory and immunostimulatory factors, including complement degradation products (17), interferon-γ (21), 1,25-dihydroxyvitamin D (22) and interleukin-2 (21). These factors attract and activate macrophages and lymphocytes, and may thereby enhance the elimination of the mycobacteria.

The obvious explanation for the development of the tuberculous pleural effusion is that the delayed hypersensitivity reaction increases the permeability of the pleural capillaries to protein, and the increased protein levels in the pleural fluid result in a much higher level of pleural fluid formation and accordingly result in the accumulation of pleural fluid. Such does not appear to be the mechanism, however, at least in the experimental animal. Apicella and Allen (5) were unable to demonstrate any striking increase in the inflow of protein into the pleural space in their experimental model of delayed-hypersensitivity tuberculous pleuritis. They did, however, demonstrate a dramatic decrease in the clearance of protein from the pleural space (5). Leckie and Tothill reported that the pleural lymphatic flow from patients with tuberculosis was approximately 50% that of patients with congestive heart failure (23). It is probable that the intense inflammatory reaction in the parietal pleura impedes the lymphatic drainage from the pleural space (see Chapter 2) and leads to the accumulation of pleural fluid.

INCIDENCE

In many areas of the world, tuberculosis remains the most common cause of pleural effusions in the absence of demonstrable pulmonary disease (24). For example, in a recent series from Rwanda (24), tuberculosis was diagnosed in 110 of 127 patients (86%) who presented with pleural effusions. In the United States, the annual incidence of tuberculous pleuritis is about 1000 cases (25). Approximately one in thirty patients with tuberculosis will have tuberculous pleuritis (25). One might anticipate that the incidence of tuberculous pleuritis would be relatively low in patients with AIDS and tuberculosis since the patient with AIDS has a compromised immunologic system. However, the opposite appears to be the case. In one series from South Africa, 38% of the HIV positive patients with tuberculosis had a pleural effusion compared with 20% of HIV negative patients (26). In one series of 48 HIV positive patients with tuberculosis from Southern California, 14 (29%) of the patients had a pleural effusion (27).

CLINICAL MANIFESTATIONS

Although tuberculosis is usually considered a chronic illness, tuberculous pleuritis most commonly manifests as an acute illness. In one series of 71 patients, 25 (31%) had initial symptoms of less than a week in duration, whereas 50 (62%) had been symptomatic for less than a month (28). In another series, 31 of 49 patients (62%) had an acute illness that most commonly mimicked acute bacterial pneumonia (2). Most patients (~70%) have a cough, usually nonproductive, and most (~50–75%) have chest pain, usually pleuritic in nature (1, 2, 12). If both cough and pleuritic chest pain are present, the pain usually precedes the cough. Most patients are febrile, but a normal temperature does not rule out the diagnosis. In one series 7 of 49 patients (14%) were afebrile (2). Occasionally, the onset of tuberculosis is less acute, with only mild chest pain, perhaps with a low-grade fever and a nonproductive cough, weight loss, and easy fatigability.

In general, patients with tuberculous pleuritis are younger than patients with parenchymal tuberculosis. In one series, the mean age of patients with tuberculous pleuritis was 28 years, whereas the mean age of patients with parenchymal tuberculosis was 54 years (29). In the United States tuberculous pleuritis is becoming more and more a disease of the older individual. Berger and Mejia (2) in 1973 reported that of their 49 patients with tuberculous pleuritis, 15% of the patients were above the age of 70, and 40% were above the age of 35. Epstein and coworkers (30) in 1987 reported that the median age of their 26 patients with tuberculous pleuritis was 54 years, and one-third of the patients were above the age of 60. Patients with pleural effusions secondary to reactivation tend to be older than those with postprimary pleural effusion (1).

Pleural effusions secondary to tuberculous pleuritis are almost always unilateral and are usually small to moderate in size (2, 12) although they may occupy the entire hemithorax (2, 31). In one series of 46 patients with massive pleural effusions (31) 4% of the effusions were due to tuberculosis. In about a third of patients with pleural effusions second-ary to tuberculosis, coexisting parenchymal disease is radiologically visible. In such patients, the pleural effusion is almost always on the side of the parenchymal infiltrate and invariably indicates active parenchymal disease (2).

NATURAL HISTORY OF UNTREATED TUBERCULOUS PLEURITIS

Tuberculous pleuritis without treatment usually resolves spontaneously, only to return as active tuberculosis at a later date. Patiala, who followed for at least 7 years all 2816 members of the Finnish Armed Forces who developed pleural effusions between 1939 and 1945, found that 43% of this large group of young men developed tuberculosis during the follow-up period (32). Even in the 1-year observation period 5 years following the initial episode, 5% of the total population studied developed active tuberculosis. Confirmatory evidence for this large series comes from the series of Roper and Waring in the United States, who followed 141 military personnel first seen from 1940 to 1944 with a pleural effusion and a positive PPD test (33). Most patients completely resorbed their pleural effusions and became asymptomatic within 2 to 4 months, but 92 of the 141 individuals (65%) subsequently developed some form of active tuberculosis. Manifest tuberculosis did not develop in the lung or elsewhere in any of the patients within 8 months of the onset of the original pleurisy. The incidence of subsequent tuberculosis was 60% in those with initially negative pleural fluid cultures for tuberculosis and 65% in those with initially positive pleural fluid cultures. In addition, the size of the original effusions and the presence or the absence of small radiologic residual pleural disease were not correlated with the subsequent appearance of active tuberculosis (33). The foregoing series emphasize the dangers of a tuberculous pleural effusion.

Because the administration of antituberculous chemotherapy reduces the incidence of subsequent tuberculosis (2, 34), it is important to establish the diagnosis of tuberculous pleuritis and initiate proper treatment. Moreover, patients in whom the diagnosis cannot be established, but in whom the diagnosis is considered likely, should also be treated.

DIAGNOSIS

The diagnosis of tuberculous pleuritis depends upon the demonstration of tubercle bacilli in the sputum, pleural fluid, or pleural biopsy specimen or granulomas in the pleura. The diagnosis can also be established with reasonable certainty by demonstrating that the pleural fluid adenosine deaminase (ADA) level is above 70 U/L or by demonstrating an elevated level of interferon-γ in the pleural fluid. Study of the peripheral blood is not useful; most patients do not have leukocytosis (2). The chest radiograph usually demonstrates only the pleural fluid, but as previously mentioned, about a third of the patients also have a parenchymal infiltrate due to tuberculosis. The observations of Stead and associates that most patients with tuberculous pleuritis have concomitant parenchymal disease that is subclinical radiologically (3), raise the possibility that computed tomographic (CT) studies might be useful in demonstrating such parenchymal disease. Indeed, in one series of 14 patients with no obvious parenchymal abnormality on standard chest radiograph, CT showed parenchymal cavities in 7 and infiltrates in another 4. In 3 cases the site of communication between the parenchymal cavity and the pleural space was demonstrated with CT scan (35), a finding supporting the current theories of the pathogenesis of tuberculous pleuritis. Larger series are necessary to define the rightful place of CT in the diagnosis of tuberculous pleuritis.

Tuberculin Skin Testing

A tuberculin skin test should be performed on all patients with exudative pleural effusions. If the skin test is positive, the only way to exclude the diagnosis of tuberculous pleuritis is to grind up the entire patient and inject him into an army of guinea pigs or to perform an open thoracotomy. Because the patient usually refuses the first alternative and because most patients prefer to take drugs for 9 months rather than to have an open thoracotomy, patients with undiagnosed exudative pleural effusions and a positive PPD test should be treated for pleural tuberculosis.

A negative skin test does not rule out the diagnosis of tuberculous pleuritis (2, 15). In one series of 36 patients with tuberculous pleuritis, 31% had a negative intermediate PPD (2). In another recent series from Hong Kong, more than one-half of the patients tested had a negative PPD (12). Although the pleuritis is thought to be due at least in part to delayed hypersensitivity, circulating adherent cells in the acute phase of the disease may suppress the specifically sensitized T lymphocytes in the peripheral blood and in the skin, but not in the pleural fluid (15). An alternate explanation for the negative skin test is the sequestration of PPD-reactive T lymphocytes in the pleural space (16). If the patient is not anergic, the intermediate PPD will almost always be positive within 8 weeks of the development of symptoms.

Pleural Fluid Analysis

Pleural fluid analysis is useful in the diagnosis of tuberculous pleuritis. The fluid is invariably an exudate. Frequently, the pleural fluid protein level is above 5.0 g/dl, and this finding suggests tuberculous pleuritis. In most patients, the pleural fluid differential white blood cell count (WBC) reveals more than 50% small lymphocytes (2, 27, 36–38). In one series of 49 patients with tuberculous pleuritis (2), only 5 (10%) had fewer than 50% lymphocytes in the pleural fluid. In patients with symptoms of less than 2 weeks' duration, the pleural fluid differential WBC may reveal predominantly polymorphonuclear leukocytes (28), but if serial thoracenteses are performed, the differential WBC will reveal a change to predominantly small lymphocytes (2). The separation of the lymphocytes into T lymphocytes and B lymphocytes is not useful diagnostically (see Chapter 4). If eosinophils are found in the pleural fluid in significant numbers (greater than 10%), one can exclude the diagnosis of tuberculous pleuritis unless the patient has a pneumothorax or has had a previous thoracentesis (see Chapter 4).

A useful study for ruling out tuberculous pleuritis is analysis of the pleural fluid for mesothelial cells (see Figure 4.1A). Four separate series have confirmed that pleural fluid from patients with tuberculosis rarely contains more than 5% mesothelial cells (36, 37, 39, 40). Unfortunately, the absence of mesothelial cells is not diagnostic of tuberculosis because, in any condition in which the pleural surfaces are extensively involved by an inflammatory process, mesothelial cells are not found in the pleural fluid.

Adenosine Deaminase

Measurement of the levels of ADA in the pleural fluid appears to be useful in establishing the diagnosis of tuberculous pleuritis. ADA is the enzyme that catalyzes the conversion of adenosine to inosine. ADA is a predominant T lymphocyte enzyme, and its plasma activity is high in diseases where cellular immunity is stimulated. Ocana and associates (41) measured the pleural fluid ADA levels in 221 pleural or peritoneal effusions (Fig. 10.1). All patients with a pleural fluid ADA level above 70 U/L had tuberculosis, whereas no patient with pleural fluid ADA levels below 40 U/L had tuberculous pleuritis. Fontan Bueso and colleagues (42) reported similar results in a

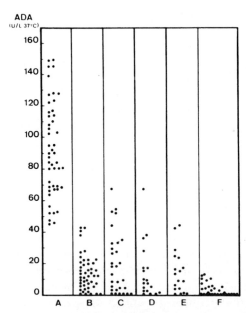

Figure 10.1. Levels of adenosine deaminase (ADA) activity in pleuroperitoneal effusions. *A*, Tuberculosis; *B*, Malignancies; *C*, Pleuropneumonia; *D*, Miscellaneous; *E*, Unknown origin; *F*, Transudates. (From Ocana I, Martinez-Vazquez JM, et al: Adenosine deaminase in pleural fluids: test for diagnosis of tuberculous pleural effusion. Chest 1983;84:51–53.)

group of 138 pleural effusions including 61 due to tuberculosis and 42 due to malignant disease. Recently Valdés and associates (43) have confirmed these findings in a series of 430 pleural effusions (see Figure 4.5).

Some caution should be used when the ADA levels are relied upon to make the diagnosis of pleural tuberculosis. Since Asian patients with tuberculous pleuritis appear to have lower mean levels of ADA (44–46), the test is less useful in the far East. If the patient is immunocompromised and has tuberculous pleuritis, the pleural fluid ADA level may be below 40 U/L (47). Many patients with empyema will have an elevated pleural fluid ADA level (43) as will the majority of patients with rheumatoid pleuritis (48). High pleural fluid ADA levels have also been reported with a very small percentage of neoplasms (49). Analysis of the type of ADA is useful in questionable cases. There are two molecular forms of ADA, a large form and a small form. The tuberculous effusions appear to contain only the large form, whereas other effusions with elevated ADA have both forms, with the small form predominant (49).

In view of the above, it appears that a pleural fluid ADA level above 70 virtually establishes the diagnosis of tuberculosis. If the clinical picture is compatible with tuberculous pleuritis and if the pleural fluid ADA is above 70 U/L, then the diagnosis of tuberculosis is established. Patients with rheumatoid pleuritis or empyema are easily distinguished from those with tuberculous pleurisy. Alternatively, if the pleural fluid ADA level is below 40 U/L and the patient is not immunosuppressed and if the patient is not Asian, the diagnosis of tuberculosis is excluded. Unfortunately, to my knowledge ADA levels are not available commercially in the United States.

Interferon-γ

Another test that is useful in the diagnosis of tuberculous pleuritis is the level of interferon-γ in the pleural fluid (21, 43, 46, 50, 51). Interferon-γ is produced by the CD4[+] lymphocytes from patients with tuberculous pleuritis (51). In one recent report, 33 of 35 patients with tuberculous pleuritis had interferon-γ levels above 140 pg/ml, while only 9 of 110 other pleural fluids had levels that exceed this (Fig. 4.5) (43). Excepting empyemas there was only one nontuberculous pleural fluid that had a interferon-γ level above 200 pg/ml (43). Comparable results have been reported in other series (21, 46, 50, 51), but comparison of the series is difficult because the units have differed from one study to another.

In view of the above, it appears that the pleural fluid interferon-γ level can be used in a manner similar to the pleural fluid ADA level to establish the diagnosis of tuberculous pleuritis with reasonable certainty. The diagnosis of tuberculosis can be established with a pleural fluid interferon-γ level that exceeds 200 pg/ml and a clinical picture compatible with tuberculous pleuritis. Unfortunately, however, interferon-γ levels (like ADA levels) are not available commercially in the United States to my knowledge.

Pleural Fluid Tuberculous Proteins or Antibodies

In recent years the possibility of establishing the diagnosis of tuberculous pleuritis by the demonstration of tuberculous antigens or specific antibodies against tuberculous proteins in the pleural fluid has been investigated. Baig and coworkers (52) demonstrated that the mean levels of tuberculous antigens were higher in the pleural fluid of patients with tuberculous pleuritis than in the pleural fluid of other patients. There was so much overlap, however, that the test was of limited use diagnostically. Yew and coworkers have reported similar results when the level of tuberculostearic acid in pleural fluid was analyzed (53). Six separate reports (54–59) have demonstrated that patients with tuberculous pleural effusions tend to have higher levels of specific antituberculous antibodies in their pleural fluid than do patients with exudative pleural effusions of other etiologies, but again there is too much overlap for the test to be useful diagnostically. Because it appears that passive diffusion from the serum rather than local antibody production in the pleural space is responsible for the antituberculous antibody levels in the pleural fluid (56), it is unlikely that measurement of these antibodies in the pleural fluid will ever be diagnostically useful.

Polymerase Chain Reaction

In the field of infectious diseases, polymerase chain reactions (PCR) have been quite useful in establishing the diagnosis and pathogenesis of viral diseases. It was therefore hypothesized that PCR would be useful in diagnosing tuberculous pleuritis. It appears, however, that PCR is too sensitive in the diagnosis of pleural effusions. de Wit and associates (60) evaluated the diagnostic usefulness of PCR of the pleural fluid in 84 patients with pleural effusions including 53 with tuberculosis. They used a 336 base-pair repetitive sequence from the *Mycobacterium tuberculosis* genome as the DNA target for amplification. Of the 53 patients who were thought to have tuberculous pleuritis, the test was positive in 43, giving a sensitivity of 81%. However, 7 of the 31 other patients also had a positive PCR test on their pleural fluid so the specificity was only 78%. The PCR of the pleural fluid should be considered to be an investigative test until there are more data regarding its specificity.

Other Chemical Tests

Other chemical analyses of the pleural fluid are of limited value in establishing the diagnosis of tuberculous pleuritis. Although in the past it was felt that the pleural fluid glucose level was reduced in most cases of tuberculous pleuritis (61) more recent studies show that the majority of patients with tuberculous pleuritis have a pleural fluid glucose level above 60 mg/dl (2, 30, 62). A low pleural fluid pH was once thought to be suggestive of tuberculous pleuritis (63), and I concluded that tuberculous pleural effusions had a lower pleural fluid pH than malignant pleural effusions in the first paper my colleagues and I wrote on pleural fluid pH (64). Subsequent papers (65, 66), however, and my own observations, indicate that the pleural fluid pH has about the same distribution in malignant as in tuberculous pleural effusions.

The levels of the lysozyme in the pleural fluid have been proposed to be useful diagnostically (42, 67) and there is no doubt that the mean level of lysozyme in the pleural fluid from patients with tuberculous pleuritis is higher than it is in other exudative pleural fluids. A value of 1.2 for the ratio of the pleural fluid to the serum lysozyme has been proposed as a good test for diagnosing tuberculous pleuritis (67). When the utility of this ratio is compared to that of the pleural fluid ADA or interferon-γ level, the lysozyme ratio is distinctly inferior (43). For this reason, the measurement of the lysozyme ratio is not recommended (43).

Pleural Fluid Stains and Cultures

Routine smears for mycobacteria are not indicated because they are almost always negative, unless the patient has a tuberculous empyema (11, 12). Both pleural fluid and sputum should be cultured for mycobacteria when tuberculous pleuritis is suspected. Even if the patient has tuberculous pleuritis, however, both culture results are frequently negative. In one series of 30 patients without concomitant parenchymal infiltrates, only 2 (7%) had positive sputum cultures for tubercle bacilli (2). In most series of patients with tuberculous pleuritis, the pleural fluid cultures are positive for mycobacteria in fewer than 25% (2, 68). For mycobacterial cultures, use of a BACTEC system with bedside inoculation provides higher yields and faster results than do conventional methods. In one study, the median time for the BACTEC cultures to become positive was 18 days (range 3–40) while the median time for conventional cultures was 33.5 days (range 21–48) (69).

Pleural Biopsy

Pleural biopsy has its greatest utility in establishing the diagnosis of tuberculous pleuritis. The demonstration of granuloma in the parietal pleura is suggestive of tuberculous pleuritis; caseous necrosis and acid-fast bacilli (AFB) need not be demonstrated. Although other disorders including fungal diseases, sarcoidosis, tularemia (70) and rheumatoid pleuritis may produce granulomatous pleuritis, more than 95% of patients with granulomatous pleuritis have tuberculosis. Even when granulomas are not demonstrated in the pleural biopsy, the biopsy specimen should be examined for AFB because organisms are occasionally demonstrated when no granulomas are present in the biopsy. The initial pleural biopsy reveals granulomas in approximately 60% of patients with tuberculous pleuritis (68, 71). If three separate pleural biopsies are obtained, the yield increases to approximately 80%. When culture of a biopsy specimen is combined with microscopic examination, the diagnosis can be established in approximately 90% of cases (71).

Diagnostic Problems

In some patients with exudative pleural effusions, no diagnosis is reached despite the examination of several biopsy specimens and cultures. In such patients, an open thoracotomy with pleural biopsy has been recommended by some (3, 72) whereas thoracoscopic examination has been recommended by others (73). Because the treatment for tuberculous pleuritis is benign, however, I feel that one should treat the patient for tuberculous pleuritis without further invasive procedures if there is a reasonable possibility of this diagnosis. Specifically, antituberculous therapy should be instituted in the following situations: (a) if the patient has a pleural fluid ADA level above 70 U/L, (b) if the patient has a pleural fluid interferon-γ level above 200 pg/ml, (c) if the patient has a positive PPD test; or (d) if the patient has a negative PPD test, but fewer than 5% mesothelial cells in the pleural fluid. In the last situation, the PPD test should be repeated in 6 weeks, and antituberculous treatment should be continued only if the skin test has converted to positive at that time. Of course, if the symptoms of the patient worsen while he is receiving antituberculous therapy, more aggressive diagnostic procedures should be initiated. The patient with an exudative pleural effusion, a negative PPD test, and mesothelial cells in his pleural fluid should also have another PPD test in 6 weeks. If it has converted to positive, antituberculous therapy should then be instituted.

TREATMENT

The treatment of tuberculous pleuritis has three goals: (a) to prevent the subsequent development of active tuberculosis; (b) to relieve the patient's symptoms; and (c) to prevent the development of a fibrothorax.

Chemotherapy

The recommendations by the American Thoracic Society for the treatment of all pulmonary and extrapulmonary tuberculosis are as follows (74). The initial phase of a 6-month regimen should consist of a 2-month period of isoniazid (INH), rifampin, and pyrazinamide. Ethambutol should be included in the initial regimen until the results of drug susceptibility studies are available, unless there is little possibility of drug resistance. The second phase of the treatment should be isoniazid and rifampin given for 4 months. Directly observed therapy is recommended. Nine-month regimens using isoniazid and rifampin are also effective when the organisms are fully drug-susceptible.

The above recommendations may be somewhat overkill for tuberculous pleuritis. Less intensive regimens appear to be effective. Dutt and coworkers (75) administered INH 300 mg plus rifampin 600 mg daily for 1 month followed by INH 900 mg plus rifampin 600 mg twice a week for the next 5 months to 198 patients. There was only one failure with this regimen (75). The patient with tuberculous pleuritis appears to have a small bacterial burden because many of the symptoms are due to delayed hypersensitivity. In the series of Patiala and Mattila, the administration of chemotherapy decreased the subsequent incidence of tuberculosis from 28 to 9%, even though the majority of their patients received only one drug for less than 6 months (34). Falk and Stead reported that antituberculous therapy reduced the incidence of subsequent tuberculosis from 19 to 4%, and again, many of their patients did not receive two drugs for even 6 months (76). From the foregoing studies, it appears that 6 months of isoniazid and rifampin administration are sufficient if the patient does not have resistant organisms.

With treatment, the patient's symptoms and radiologic abnormalities gradually abate. The average patient becomes afebrile within 2 weeks, but temperature elevations may persist for as long as 2 months (77). The mean duration for complete resorption of the pleural fluid is about 6 weeks, but it can be as long as 12 weeks (77). The administration of corticosteroids can decrease the duration of fever and the time for pleural fluid resorption (77, 78). Lee and associates in a double-blind, randomized study administered prednisolone, 0.75 mg/kg/day orally, or placebo to 40 patients with tuberculous pleuritis who were all treated with isoniazid, rifampin, and ethambutol. They found that the duration of fever was less in the steroid group (2.4 days mean) than in the control group (9.2 days) and that the pleural fluid was completely absorbed faster in the steroid group (54.5 days) than in the control group (123.2 days). The development of residual pleural thickening was not influenced by the administration of corticosteroids (78). A different report, however, suggested that the administration of corticosteroids resulted in less residual pleural thickening after treatment (1). Therefore, if the patient is more than mildly symptomatic and a definite diagnosis has been established, the administration of 80 mg prednisone every other day until the acute symptoms have subsided is recommended, with a rapid tapering of the dose thereafter.

The incidence of pleural thickening 6 to 12 months after the beginning of treatment is approximately 50% (79). The incidence of residual pleural thickening is not related to the initial pleural fluid findings; patients with a low glucose or a high pleural fluid LDH are not any more likely to have residual pleural thickening (79).

Surgical Procedures

Although the pleura may be thickened when the patient's disorder is first diagnosed, the thickening decreases with treatment, so decortication should not be considered until the patient has been undergoing treatment for at least 6 months. After this period of observation, decortication is rarely necessary. Serial therapeutic thoracenteses also appear to have no beneficial role in the treatment of tuberculous pleuritis. Large and Levick compared the clinical courses of 33 patients who had serial therapeutic thoracenteses with those of 19 patients who had only a single diagnostic thoracentesis (80). These investigators found no difference in the duration of fever or in the radiologic changes at 6 months. Of course, if the patient is symptomatic from a massive pleural effusion, therapeutic thoracentesis is indicated to relieve the symptoms. No reason exists to keep the patient in bed (2), and patients need be isolated only if their sputum tests are positive for mycobacteria.

TUBERCULOUS BRONCHOPLEURAL FISTULA

Tuberculous bronchopleural fistulas are uncommon today because most cases of tuberculosis are easily controlled with modern antituberculous chemotherapy. These fistulas are usually seen in patients with old, healed tuberculosis, especially in patients with a previous therapeutic pneumothorax who were never treated with chemotherapy (81, 82). When such patients develop a bronchopleural fistula, their sputum production usually increases in variable amounts, and superinfection of the pleural space by bacteria sometimes results (81). The diagnosis is suggested by the presence of an air-fluid level in the pleural space, particularly if the level fluctuates with serial chest radiographs (81). The fistula can be confirmed by the injection of methylene blue or a radiopaque dye into the pleural space.

A tuberculous bronchopleural fistula is dangerous to the patient for three reasons. First, the communication between the bronchus and the pleural space allows bacteria to gain access to the pleural space and to cause pleural infection with its attendant toxicity. Second, once the pleural space becomes superinfected, the patient is at risk for a fulminant pneumonia caused by entrance of the infected material from the pleural space into the remainder of the tracheobronchial tree. Third, the tuberculous bacilli in the pleural space are likely to become resistant to antituberculous drugs (81).

The initial treatment of tuberculous bronchopleural fistulas should be the institution of appropriate antituberculous chemotherapy in addition to the insertion of chest tubes into the lower part of the pleural cavity, because a tuberculous bronchopleural fistula does not heal spontaneously (81). Insertion of the chest tubes eliminates the danger of contamination of the contralateral lung by the infected pleural fluid and controls the systemic toxicity from the bacterial infection. Before a definitive surgical procedure is attempted, the patient should be given antituberculous chemotherapy for 90 to 120 days or until sputum tests become negative for AFB.

Definitive surgical treatment consists of decortication, which frequently must be combined with thoracoplasty because the underlying lung has usually been damaged by the tuberculosis to such an extent that it cannot expand to fill the pleural space (81). This is a major operation and is dangerous to the patient with severely damaged lungs. In Jensen's series of 15 patients with tuberculous bronchopleural fistulas, 3 were cured with conservative treatment, 2 were deemed unfit to undergo definitive surgical treatment, and died within a year, and 10 were operated upon with an operative mortality rate of 20% (82).

TUBERCULOUS EMPYEMA

Tuberculous empyema is a rare entity characterized by purulent pleural fluid, which is loaded with tuberculous organisms on AFB stains. It usually develops in fibrous scar tissue resulting from pleurisy, artificial pneumothorax, or thoracoplasty (82). Frequently, the underlying pleura is heavily calcified. The patient usually has a subacute or chronic illness characterized by fatigue, low-grade fever, and weight loss. Radiologically, there may be an obvious pleural effusion, but frequently the chest radiograph only shows pleural thickening. The diagnosis is established with diagnostic thoracentesis, which yields thick pus on which the AFB smear is markedly positive. Treatment is difficult and decortication, extrapleural pneumonectomy, and thoracoplasty have all been recommended. All these procedures have substantial morbidity and some mortality, at least in part because of the compromised pulmonary status of the patient. Because intensive chemotherapy coupled with serial thoracentesis can at times be curative (83), this approach should be attempted initially. It is important to use a multiple (three or more) drug treatment plan and to use agents at their maximal tolerated dosages since these patients have a strong tendency to develop resistant organisms. This is probably because the antituberculous drugs frequently do not reach their normal levels due to the thick fibrous or calcified pleura (84).

ATYPICAL MYCOBACTERIA

Pleural effusions due to atypical mycobacteria are rare. Pleural effusions without parenchymal disease analogous to the postprimary pleural effusion with *Mycobacterium tuberculosis* do not occur, but approximately 5% of patients with parenchymal disease due to either *M. kansasii* or *M. intracellulare* have an associated small pleural effusion, an incidence similar to that seen with parenchymal disease due to *M. tuberculosis* (85). About 15% of patients with parenchymal disease due to *M. intracellulare* have marked pleural thickening (greater than 2 cm), as compared to fewer than 3% of patients with disease due to *M. tuberculosis* or *M. kansasii* (85).

If the cultures of the pleural fluid yield a nontuberculous mycobacterium, one must be cautious in attributing the pleural effusion to that organism. Gribetz and colleagues (86) reviewed the case records of 22 patients whose pleural fluid grew nontuberculous mycobacterium. In 16 of the cases there was another explanation for the pleural effusion, and in only 3 did the nontuberculous mycobacterium appear to be responsible for the pleural effusion. All 3 patients had nontuberculous mycobacterial infection of other tissues. These authors concluded that nontuberculous mycobacteria isolated from pleural fluid should not be considered etiologic, unless there is evidence of the same organism infecting other tissues (86).

Until the AIDS epidemic disseminated nontuberculous mycobacterial infections were very uncommon. However, disseminated disease due to mycobacterium in the *M. intracellulare* or *M. avium* (MAC) is an important cause of infection in patients with AIDS (87). Some autopsy studies have shown that more than 50% of patients dying with AIDS have disseminated disease due to MAC (87). Pleural effusions do occur in some patients with disseminated disease due to MAC (87) and pleural fluid cultures are sometimes positive for MAC. Nevertheless, it is unclear whether the atypical mycobacteria are responsible for the effusion (87). Overall, disease due to MAC accounts for at most only a small percentage of the pleural effusions in patients with AIDS.

REFERENCES

1. Moudgil H, Sridhar G, Leitch AG: Reactivation disease: the commonest form of tuberculous pleural effusion in Edinburgh, 1980–1991. Respir Med 1994; 88:301–304.
2. Berger HW, Mejia E: Tuberculous pleurisy. Chest 1973;63:88–92.
3. Stead WW, Eichenholz A, Stauss H-K: Operative and pathologic findings in twenty-four patients with syndrome of idiopathic pleurisy with effusion, presumably tuberculous. Am Rev Respir Dis 1955;71:473–502.
4. Allen JC, Apicella MA: Experimental pleural effusion as a manifestation of delayed hypersensitivity to tuberculin PPD. J Immunol 1968;101:481–487.
5. Apicella MA, Allen JC: A physiologic differentiation between delayed and immediate hypersensitivity. J Clin Invest 1969;48:250–259.
6. Leibowitz S, Kennedy L, Lessof MH: The tuberculin reaction in the pleural cavity and its suppression by antilymphocyte serum. Br J Exp Pathol 1973;54:152–162.
7. Yamamoto S, Dunn CJ, Willoughby DA: Studies on delayed hypersensitivity pleural exudates in guinea pigs: II. The interrelationship of monocytic and lymphocytic cells with respect to migration activity. Immunology 1976;30:513–519.
8. Antony VB, Sahn SA, Antony AC, Repine JE: Bacillus Calmette-Guérin-stimulated neutrophils release chemotaxins for monocytes in rabbit pleural space in vitro. J Clin Invest 1985;76:1514–1521.
9. Widstrom O, Nilsson BS: Pleurisy induced by intrapleural BCG in immunized guinea pigs. Eur J Respir Dis 1982;63:425–434.
10. Widstrom O, Nilsson BS: Low in vitro response to PPD and PHA in lymphocytes from BCG-induced pleurisy in guinea pigs. Eur J Respir Dis 1982;63:435–441.
11. Bueno CE, Clemente G, Castro BC, Martin LM, Ramos SR, Panizo AG, Glez-Rio JM: Cytologic and bacteriologic analysis of fluid and pleural biopsy specimens with Cope's needle. Arch Intern Med 1990;150:1190–1194.
12. Chan CH, Arnold M, Chan CY, Mak TW, Hoheisel GB: Clinical and pathological features of tuberculous pleural effusion and its long-term consequences. Respiration 1991;58:171–175.
13. Fujiwara H, Tsuyuguchi I: Frequency of tuberculin-reactive T-lymphocytes in pleural fluid and blood from patients with tuberculous pleurisy. Chest 1986; 89:530–532.
14. Shimokata K, Kawachi H, Kishimoto H, et al: Local cellular immunity in tuberculous pleurisy. Am Rev Respir Dis 1982;128:822–824.
15. Ellner JJ: Pleural fluid and peripheral blood lymphocyte function in tuberculosis. Ann Intern Med 1978; 89:932–933.

16. Rossi GA, Balbi B, Manca F: Tuberculous pleural effusions: Evidence for selective presence of PPD-specific T-lymphocytes at site of inflammation in the early phase of the infection. Am Rev Respir Dis 1987;136:575-579.

17. Ellner JJ, Barnes PF, Wallis RS, Modlin RL: The immunology of tuberculous pleurisy. Sem Respir Infect 1988;3:335-342.

18. Ribera E, Espanol T, Martinez-Vazquez, Ocana I, Encabo G: Lymphocyte proliferation and gamma-interferon production after "in Vitro" stimulation with PPD. Differences between tuberculous and nontuberculous pleurisy in patients with positive tuberculin skin test. Chest 1990;97:1381-1385.

19. Lorgat F, Keraan MM, Lukey PT, Ress SR: Evidence for in vivo generation of cytotoxic T cells. PPD-stimulated lymphocytes from tuberculous pleural effusions demonstrate enhanced cytotoxicity with accelerated kinetics of induction. Am Rev Respir Dis 1992;145:418-423.

20. Kurasawa T, Shimokata K: Cooperation between accessory cells and T lymphocytes in patients with tuberculous pleurisy. Chest 1991;100:1046-1052.

21. Shimokata K, Saka H, Murate T, Hasegawa Y, Hasegawa T: Cytokine content in pleural effusion. Chest 1991;99:1103-1107.

22. Barnes PF, Modlin RL, Bikle DD, Adams JS: Transpleural gradient of 1,25-dihydroxyvitamin D in tuberculous pleuritis. J Clin Invest 1989;83:1527-1532.

23. Leckie WJH, Tothill P: Albumin turnover in pleural effusions. Clin Sci 1965;29:339-352.

24. Batungwanayo J, Taelman H, Allen S, Bogaerts J, Kagame A, Van de Perre P: Pleural effusion, tuberculosis and HIV-1 infection in Kigali, Rwanda. AIDS 1993;7:73-79.

25. Mehta JB, Dutt A, Harvill L, Mathews KM: Epidemiology of extrapulmonary tuberculosis. Chest 1991;99:1134-1138.

26. Saks AM, Posner R: Tuberculosis in HIV positive patients in South Africa: A comparative radiological study with HIV negative patients. Clin Radiol 1992;46:387-390.

27. Kramer F, Modilevsky T, Waliany AR, Leedom JM, Barnes PF: Delayed diagnosis of tuberculosis in patients with human immunodeficiency virus infection. Am J Med 1990;89:451-456.

28. Levine H, Szanto PB, Cugell DW: Tuberculous pleurisy: an acute illness. Arch Intern Med 1968;122:329-332.

29. Aho K, Brander E, Patiala J: Studies for primary drug resistance in tuberculous pleurisy. Scand J Respir Dis 1968;63(Suppl):111-114.

30. Epstein DM, Kline LR, Albelda SM, Miller WT: Tuberculous pleural effusions. Chest 1987;91:106-109.

31. Maher GG, Berger HW: Massive pleural effusion: malignant and non-malignant causes in 46 patients. Am Rev Respir Dis 1972;105:458-460.

32. Patiala J: Initial tuberculous pleuritis in the Finnish Armed Forces in 1939-1945 with special reference to eventual post pleuritic tuberculosis. Acta Tuberc Scand 1954;36(Suppl):1-57.

33. Roper WH, Waring JJ: Primary serofibrinous pleural effusion in military personnel. Am Rev Respir Dis 1955;71:616-634.

34. Patiala J, Mattila M: Effect of chemotherapy of exudative tuberculous pleurisy on the incidence of post pleuritic tuberculosis. Acta Tuberc Scand 1964;44:290-296.

35. Hulnick DH, Naidich DP, McCauley DI: Pleural tuberculosis evaluated by computed tomography. Radiology 1983;149:759-765.

36. Yam LT: Diagnostic significance of lymphocytes in pleural effusions. Ann Intern Med 1967;66:972-982.

37. Light RW, Erozan YS, Ball WC: Cells in pleural fluid: their value in differential diagnosis. Arch Intern Med 1973;132:854-860.

38. De Oliveira HG, Rossatto ER, Prolla JC: Pleural fluid adenosine deaminase and lymphocyte proportion: clinical usefulness in the diagnosis of tuberculosis. Cytopathology 1994;5:27-32.

39. Spriggs AI, Boddington MM: The Cytology of Effusions. 2nd ed. New York: Grune & Stratton, 1968.

40. Hurwitz S, Leiman G, Shapiro C: Mesothelial cells in pleural fluid: TB or not TB? S Afr Med J 1980;57:937-939.

41. Ocana I, Martinez-Vazquez JM, Segura R, et al: Adenosine deaminase in pleural fluids: test for diagnosis of tuberculous pleural effusion. Chest 1983;84:51-53.

42. Fontan Bueso J, Verea Hernando H, Garcia-Buela JP, et al: Diagnostic value of simultaneous determination of pleural adenosine deaminase and pleural lysozyme/serum lysozyme ratio in pleural effusion. Chest 1988;93:303-307.

43. Valdes L, San Jose E, Alvarez D, Sarandeses A, Pose A, Chomon B, Alvarez-Dobano JM, Salgueiro M, Rodriguez Suarez JR: Diagnosis of tuberculous pleurisy using the biologic parameters adenosine deaminase, lysozyme, and interferon gamma. Chest 1993;103:458-465.

44. Niwa Y, Kishimoto H, Shimokata K: Carcinomatous and tuberculous pleural effusion. Comparison of tumor markers. Chest 1985;87:351-355.

45. Tamura S, Nishigaki T, Moriwaki Y, et al: Tumor markers in pleural effusion diagnosis. Cancer 1988;61:298-302.

46. Aoki Y, Katoh O, Nakanishi Y, Kuroki S, Yamada H: A comparison study of IFN-gamma, ADA, and CA125 as the diagnostic parameters in tuberculous pleuritis. Resp Med 1994;88:139-143.

47. Hsu WH, Chiang CD, Huang PL: Diagnostic value of pleural adenosine deaminase in tuberculous effusions of immunocompromised hosts. J Formosan Med Assoc 1993;92:668-670.

48. Ocana I, Ribera E, Martinez-Vazquez JM, et al: Adenosine deaminase activity in rheumatoid pleural effusion. Ann Rheum Dis 1988;47:394-397.

49. Ungerer JP, Brobler SM: Molecular forms of adenosine deaminase in pleural effusions. Enzyme 1988;40:7-13.

50. Ribera E, Ocana I, Martinez-Vazquez JM, et al: High level of interferon gamma in tuberculous pleural effusion. Chest 1988;93:308-311.

51. Barnes PF, Mistry SD, Cooper CL, et al: Compartmentalization of a CD4$^+$ T lymphocyte subpopulation in tuberculous pleuritis. J Immunol 1989;142:1114–1119.

52. Baig MME, Pettengell KE, Simgee AE, et al: Diagnosis of tuberculosis by detection of mycobacterial antigens in pleural effusions and ascites. S Afr Med J 1986;69:101–102.

53. Yew WW, Chan CY, Kwan SY, Cheung SW, French GL: Diagnosis of tuberculous pleural effusion by the detection of tuberculostearic acid in pleural aspirates. Chest 1991;100:1261–1263.

54. Banchuin N, Pumprueg U, Pimolpan V, et al: Anti-PPD IgG responses in tuberculous pleurisy. J Med Assoc Thai 1987;70:321–325.

55. Dhand R, Ganguly NK, Vaishnavi C, et al: False-positive reactions with enzyme-linked immunosorbent assay of *Mycobacterium tuberculosis* antigens in pleural fluid. J Med Microbiol 1988;26:241–243.

56. Levy H, Wayne LG, Anderson BE, Barnes PF, Light RW: Anti-mycobacterial antibody levels in pleural fluid reflect passive diffusion from serum. Chest 1989;92:1855.

57. Caminero JA, Rodriguez de Castro F, Carrillo T, Diaz F, Rodriguez Bermejo JC, Cabrera P: Diagnosis of pleural tuberculosis by detection of specific IgG anti-antigen 60 in serum and pleural fluid. Respiration 1993;60:58–62.

58. Van Vooren JP, Farber CM, De Bruyn J, Yernault JC: Antimycobacterial antibodies in pleural effusions. Chest 1990;97:88–90.

59. Murate T, Mizoguchi K, Amano H, Shimokata K, Matsuda T: Antipurified-Protein-Derivative antibody in tuberculous pleural effusions. Chest 1990;97:670–673.

60. de Wit D, Maartens G, Steyn L: A comparative study of the polymerase chain reaction and conventional procedures for the diagnosis of tuberculous pleural effusion. Tubercle Lung Dis 1992;73:262–267.

61. Barber LM, Mazzadi L, Deakins DD, et al: Glucose level in pleural fluid as a diagnostic aid. Dis Chest 1957;31:680–681.

62. Light RW, Ball WC: Glucose and amylase in pleural effusions. JAMA 1973;225:257–260.

63. Holton K: Diagnostic value of some biochemical pleural fluid examinations. Scand J Respir Dis 1968; 63(Suppl):121–125.

64. Light RW, MacGregor MI, Ball WC Jr, Luchsinger PC: Diagnostic significance of pleural fluid pH and Pco$_2$. Chest 1973;64:591–596.

65. Chavalittamrong B, Angsusingha K, Tuchinda M, et al: Diagnostic significance of pH, lactic acid dehydrogenase, lactate and glucose in pleural fluid. Respiration 1979;38:112–120.

66. Good JT Jr, Taryle DA, Maulitz RM, et al: The diagnostic value of pleural fluid pH. Chest 1980;78:55–59.

67. Verea Hernando HR, Masa Jimenez JF, Dominguez Juncal L, et al: Meaning and diagnostic value of determining the lysozyme level of pleural fluid. Chest 1987;91:342–345.

68. Scharer L, McClement JH: Isolation of tubercle bacilli from needle biopsy specimens of parietal pleura. Am Rev Respir Dis 1968;97:466–468.

69. Maartens G, Bateman ED: Tuberculous pleural effusions: increased culture yield with bedside inoculation of pleural fluid and poor diagnostic value of adenosine deaminase. Thorax 1991;46:96–99.

70. Schmid GP, Cantino D, Suffin SC, et al: Granulomatous pleuritis caused by *Francisella tularensis*: possible confusion with tuberculous pleuritis. Am Rev Respir Dis 1983;128:314–316.

71. Levine H, Metzger W, Lacera D, Kay L: Diagnosis of tuberculous pleurisy by culture of pleural biopsy specimen. Arch Intern Med 1970;126:269–271.

72. Arrington CW, Hawkins JA, Richert JH, Hopeman AR: Management of undiagnosed pleural effusions in positive tuberculin reactors. Am Rev Respir Dis 1966;93:587–593.

73. Canto A, Rivas J, Saumench J, et al: Thoracoscopy in the diagnosis of pleural effusion. Thorax 1977;32:550–554.

74. Bass JB Jr, Farer LS, Hopewell PC, O'Brien R, Jacobs RF, Ruben F, Snider DE Jr, Thornton G: Treatment of tuberculosis and tuberculosis infection in adults and children. Am J Respir Crit Care Med 1994;149:1359–1374.

75. Dutt AK, Moers D, Stead WW: Tuberculous pleural effusion: 6-month therapy with isoniazid and rifampin. Am Rev Respir Dis 1992;145:1429–1432.

76. Falk A, Stead WW: US Veterans Administration Armed Forces cooperative studies of tuberculosis: V. Antimicrobial theory in treatment of primary tuberculous pleurisy with effusion: the effect upon the incidence of subsequent tuberculous relapse. Am Rev Tuberc Pulmon Dis 1956;74:897–902.

77. Tani P, Poppius H, Makipaja J: Cortisone therapy for exudative tuberculous pleurisy in the light of the follow-up study. Acta Tuberc Scand 1964;44:303–309.

78. Lee CH, Wang WJ, Lan RS, et al: Corticosteroids in the treatment of tuberculous pleurisy: a double-blind, placebo-controlled, randomized study. Chest 1988;94:1256–1259.

79. Barbas CSV, Cukier A, de Varvalho CRR, Barbas-Fiho JV, Light RW: The relationship between pleural fluid findings and the development of pleural thickening in patients with pleural tuberculosis. Chest 1991;100:1264–1267.

80. Large SE, Levick RK: Aspiration in the treatment of primary tuberculous pleural effusion. Br Med J 1958;1:1512–1514.

81. Johnson TM, McCann W, Davey WN: Tuberculous bronchopleural fistula. Am Rev Respir Dis 1973;107:30–41.

82. Jenssen AD: Chronic calcified pleural empyema. Scand J Respir Dis 1969;50:19–27.

83. Neihart RE, Hof DG: Successful nonsurgical treatment of tuberculous empyema in an irreducible pleural space. Chest 1985;88:792–794.

84. Iseman MD, Madsen LA: Chronic tuberculous empyema with bronchopleural fistula resulting in treat-

ment failure and progressive drug resistance. Chest 1991;100:124–127.

85. Christensen EE, Dietz GW, Ahn CH, et al: Initial roentgenographic manifestations of pulmonary *Mycobacterium tuberculosis, M. kansasii,* and *M. intracellularis* infections. Chest 1981;80:132–136.

86. Gribetz AR, Damsker B, Marchevsky A, Bottone EJ: Nontuberculous mycobacteria in pleural fluid: assessment of clinical significance. Chest 1985;87:495–498.

87. Aronchick JM, Miller WT: Disseminated nontuberculous mycobacterial infections in immunosuppressed patients. Sem Roentgenol 1993;28:150–157.

CHAPTER 11
Pleural Effusions Secondary to Fungi, Actinomycosis, and Nocardiosis

In this chapter, pleural disease resulting from fungal infections is discussed. Although fungal diseases account for only about 1% of all pleural effusions (1, 2), one should correctly establish the diagnosis because effective treatment is available. Actinomycosis and nocardiosis are also included in this chapter because they produce a chronic disease similar to that caused by the fungi, even though they actually are bacteria.

ASPERGILLOSIS

Occasionally, the pleural space becomes infected with the aspergillus species of fungus. The usual infecting organism is *Aspergillus fumigatus* (3), but other species such as *Aspergillus niger* may also be responsible (4). Pleural aspergillosis is uncommon, but 13 cases were observed at one institution during a recent 5-year period (5).

Clinical Manifestations

Pleural aspergillosis usually occurs in one of two settings. Most commonly, it occurs in patients who were treated in the past with artificial pneumothorax therapy for tuberculosis (3, 5, 6). Such patients have signs and symptoms of a chronic infection including weight loss, malaise, a low-grade fever, and a chronic, productive cough (3). The chest radiograph reveals increasing degrees of pleural thickening and usually an air-fluid level in the pleural space indicating the presence of a bronchopleural fistula (3). Fungus balls, although uncommon, may be evident radiographically either in the lungs or the pleural space (3, 7).

The second situation in which pleural aspergillosis occurs is postoperatively after lobectomy or pneumonectomy for tuberculosis or lung cancer (6, 8). A bronchopleural fistula is almost invariably present. The clinical picture is similar to that with a pleural bacterial infection after lung resection (see Chapter 9). On rare occasions, the pleural fluid becomes infected with aspergillus in the immunosuppressed patient with systemic aspergillosis (9). One report cited two patients with pleural effusion that complicated allergic bronchopulmonary aspergillosis (10), but the relationship between the pleural effusion and the allergic aspergillosis was not convincing.

Diagnosis

The diagnosis of pleural aspergillosis should be suspected in any patient with a history of artificial pneumothorax therapy for tuberculosis who has a chronic pleural infection, particularly when a bronchopleural fistula is present. Similarly, the diagnosis should be suspected in any patient with a pleural infection after lung resection. The diagnosis is confirmed by the demonstration of *Aspergillus* on fungal cultures of the pleural fluid. The presence of brown clumps containing fungal hyphae in the pleural fluid suggests the diagnosis (6). Patients with pleural aspergillosis almost always have positive precipitin blood tests for antibodies against *Aspergillus* (3, 6). *Aspergillus* antigens can also be demonstrated in the pleural fluid by radioimmunoassay (11). The presence of calcium oxalate crystals in the pleural fluid suggests an infection due to *A. niger* (4). The presence of the black-pigmented spores of *A. niger* can impart a black color to the pleural fluid (12).

Treatment

The optimal treatment for pleural aspergillosis is early excision of the involved pleura with resection of the upper lobe or the entire ipsilateral lung if necessary (3). When this definitive surgical treatment is undertaken, amphotericin B should be administered systemically before and after the operation because the incidence of postoperative pleural infection with *Aspergillus* is high if systemic antifungal drugs are not administered (3). The reason for performing this extensive operation is that the infection is likely to invade and destroy the underlying lung. The longer the surgical procedure is postponed, the more severe the damage to the underlying lung and the more debilitated the patient becomes (3). The bronchopleural fistulae are often difficult to manage and frequently require muscle transpositions or omentoplasty (5). Even if there is no bronchopleural fistula, muscle transpositions are sometimes necessary because the pleural space cannot be obliterated with just the damaged underlying lung (5).

Some patients with pleural aspergillosis are too debilitated to undergo a surgical procedure, or their pleural aspergillosis is a complication of pulmonary resection. In such patients, a chest tube should be inserted, and the pleural space should be irrigated daily with amphotericin B or nystatin (6, 7, 13). The usual dose of amphotericin B is 25 mg, and the usual dose of nystatin is 75,000 U (7). After instillation of the antifungal agents, the chest tube is clamped for an hour. An open-drainage procedure (see Chapter 9) can be performed for the patient's comfort (7). Although this treatment takes many months, it is successful in most patients (6, 7, 13).

BLASTOMYCOSIS

Infection with *Blastomyces dermatitidis* frequently is associated with pleural disease. In one series of 118 patients with pulmonary blastomycosis, 4 (3%) had pleural effusions (14). In another study of 46 patients with pulmonary blastomycosis, 30% had pleural thickening (15). Four of these patients had a thoracentesis, and the pleural fluid grew *B. dermatitidis* in all four patients. In a more recent study of 63 cases with proven pulmonary blastomycosis, 13 of the patients (21%) had a pleural effusion. The effusions in this series were small and caused only mild-to-moderate blunting of the costophrenic sulci (16).

Patients with pleural blastomycosis have signs and symptoms similar to those with tuberculous pleuritis (see Chapter 10). In addition to the pleural effusion, there may be an associated parenchymal infiltrate (17–20). With pleural blastomycosis, the pleural fluid is an exudate containing predominantly lymphocytes or polymorphonuclear leukocytes (17–20). Microscopic examination of the pleural fluid at times reveals the budding yeasts typical of *B. dermatitidis* (20, 21). Pleural biopsy may reveal noncaseating granulomas (17, 18). Therefore, one should consider the diagnosis of blastomycosis in patients with a clinical picture similar to tuberculous pleuritis, and one should obtain fungal cultures of the pleural fluid in all such patients. All patients reported to have pleural blastomycosis have had positive pleural fluid cultures. The complement-fixation test is the most widely used test for the serologic diagnosis of blastomycosis; however, its clinical value is limited because fewer than 25% of culture-proved cases are detected using this method (22). There is no commercially available skin test for blastomycosis.

Patients with pleural blastomycosis should be treated with itraconazole 400 mg every day for 6 months, ketoconazole 400–800 mg/day for 6 months, or amphotericin B with a total dose of 2 g. It appears that the treatment of choice is itraconazole (23), which will cure virtually all individuals with pulmonary blastomycosis.

COCCIDIOIDOMYCOSIS

Coccidioides immitis is an infectious fungus endemic to the southwestern United States, particularly the San Joaquin Valley in California. The disease is acquired by inhaling the light, fluffy, and infectious arthrospores produced by the mycelial form growing in appropriate soil. Once inhaled, the arthrospores develop into the yeast form that produces disease in humans. Pleural disease of two types occurs in association with coccidioidomycosis (24). The first is associated with the primary benign infection and may or may not have concomitant parenchymal involvement. The second occurs when a coccidioidal cavity adjacent to the pleura ruptures to produce a hydropneumothorax with a bronchopleural fistula.

Primary Infection

The pleura is frequently involved in primary infections with *C. immitis*. As many as 70% of patients have pleuritic chest pain, and about 20% have blunting of the costophrenic angles (25). Approximately 7% of all symptomatic patients with primary coccidioidomycosis have pleural effusions (25). Patients with pleural effusions secondary to coccidioidomycosis are almost always febrile, and over 80% have pleuritic chest pain (25). Nearly 50% of patients have either erythema nodosum or erythema multiforme (25). The chest radiograph reveals parenchymal infiltrates in addition to the pleural effusion in about 50% of patients. The pleural effusion varies in size, but often occupies more than 50% of the hemithorax (25, 26). In one series of 28 patients, all the pleural effusions were unilateral (25).

Pleural fluid analysis reveals an exudate that usually contains predominantly small lymphocytes (25). Although nearly 50% of patients have peripheral eosinophilia, pleural fluid eosinophilia is uncommon and occurred in only 1 of 15 patients in one series (25). The pleural fluid glucose level is almost always above 60 mg/dl (25). The pleural fluid cultures are positive for *C. immitis* in about 20% of patients, but cultures of pleural biopsy specimens are positive in almost all patients (25). In one series, 8 of 8 pleural biopsy cultures were positive, and cocci spherules were identified in 6 of 8 specimens (25). The pleural biopsy may reveal caseating or noncaseating granulomas (25, 26). The cocci skin tests are usually positive, and the mean complement fixation (CF) titer 6 weeks after the onset of symptoms is 1:32 (25).

Most patients with primary coccidioidomycosis and pleural effusion require no systemic antifungal therapy (25). In a series of 28 such patients, 23 (82%) recovered completely without specific therapy. Two patients with disseminated disease died within a short period, whereas the other three patients had minor complications and were treated with amphotericin B. Even though the CF titers are high in patients with pleural coccidioidomycosis (25) and high (greater than 1:16) CF titers are used by some as an indication of dissemination (27), patients with pleural coccidioidomycosis and high CF titers should be treated only if their skin tests are negative or if other evidence of dissemination exists. The treatment of choice is amphotericin B, but in some cases fluconazole 400–800 mg/day for 12 months is effective therapy (23).

Rupture of Coccidioidal Cavity

The second situation in which pleural disease occurs with coccidioidomycosis is when a coccidioidal cavity adjacent to the pleura ruptures into the pleural space to produce a bronchopleural fistula and a hydropneumothorax. Hydropneumothoraces develop in 1 to 5% of patients with chronic cavitary coccidioidomycosis and occasionally occur without a prior cavitation (24). Many patients who experience rupture of a coccidioidal cavity have no history of coccidioidomycosis (28). Accordingly, in endemic areas, all patients with spontaneous hydropneumothoraces should be evaluated for the possibility of coccidioidomycosis.

When a coccidioidal cavity ruptures into the pleural space, the patient usually becomes acutely ill, with systemic signs of toxicity. The pleural fluid cultures are usually positive for *C. immitis* and the CF tests are almost always positive (28). Patients with hydropneumothorax should have a chest tube inserted immediately to drain the air and the fluid from the pleural space. They should also be given amphotericin B systemically. The majority will require additional surgery, such as a partial lobectomy, for control of the cavity. In one series of 23 patients, all but two required surgical treatment in addition to the tube thoracostomy (28). In view of this, it is recommended that patients who have a persistent bronchopleural fistula for more than 7 days be subjected to surgery.

CRYPTOCOCCOSIS

Cryptococcus neoformans, a fungus distributed worldwide, lives in soil, particularly that contaminated by pigeon excreta. On rare occasions, infection with *C. neoformans* produces a pleural effusion. Until 1980, only 30 cryptococcal pleural effusions had been reported (29). With the advent of the AIDS epidemic, pleural effusions secondary to cryptococcosis have become much more frequent. In one series of 12 patients with pulmonary cryptococcal involvement proven by culture, 3 (25%) had a pleural effusion (30). In another series of 75 patients with AIDS and pleural effusion from Paris, 4 (5%) had pleural cryptococcosis (31). Pleural cryptococcosis appears to result from an extension of a primary subpleural cryptococcal nodule into the pleural space (32).

In patients with pleural cryptococcosis, the disease is localized to the hemithorax in about 50% and disseminated in the remaining 50% (29). Over half the patients have serious underlying disease, most commonly leukemia, lymphoma, or AIDS (29, 33). In 27 of the 30 cases reported as of 1980, the pleural effusion was unilateral (29) and most of the effusions associated with AIDS are also unilateral. The size of the pleural effusion ranges from massive to minimal (29). Most patients also have an accompanying parenchymal lesion in the form of a nodule, a mass, or an interstitial infiltrate (29). The pleural fluid is an exudate, usually with a predominance of small lymphocytes. One case report cited an effusion in which the pleural fluid contained 15% eosinophils (34). Cultures of the pleural fluid were positive in 11 of 26 patients in the 1980 series (29). In the remaining patients, the diagnosis was made by histologic study or culture of lung tissue obtained at operation or autopsy (29). Patients with cryptococcal pleural effusion have high titers of cryptococcal antigen in their pleural fluid and serum (29).

It is not clear whether treatment with systemic antifungal agents is necessary for all patients with pleural cryptococcosis. Several patients have recovered without any specific therapy (29, 35, 36). It is therefore recommended that blood and cerebral spinal fluid be studied for cryptococcal antigen. If cryptococcal antigen is detected in either of these fluids, amphotericin B and possibly also 5-fluorocytosine should be administered. Immunosuppressed patients such as those with AIDS, leukemia, lymphoma, diabetes mellitus, sarcoidosis, and patients receiving corticosteroids or immunosuppressant agents should also

be treated. If none of the foregoing conditions are met, it is recommended that the patient be treated only with fluconazole 400 mg/day for 6 months (23). On rare occasions in immunosuppressed individuals, the pleural infection will be so overwhelming that tube thoracostomy is indicated (37).

HISTOPLASMOSIS

Histoplasma capsulatum is a fungus that lives in the mycelial form in soil and is distributed throughout the temperate zones of the world, but is most heavily endemic in the central United States (38). Infection with *H. capsulatum* only rarely produces pleural effusions. Although it has been estimated that 500,000 persons are annually infected in the United States (38), fewer than 20 pleural effusions secondary to histoplasmosis have been reported. In a review of the radiographic manifestations of pulmonary histoplasmosis, only 1 patient of 259 with abnormal chest radiographs had a pleural effusion (39).

Patients with pleural effusions secondary to histoplasmosis usually have a subacute illness characterized by a low-grade fever and pleuritic chest pain. The chest radiograph usually reveals an infiltrate or a subpleural nodule in addition to the pleural effusion (40–43). Pleural fluid analysis reveals an exudate containing predominantly lymphocytes. In two of the reported cases (40, 42) pleural fluid eosinophilia was present. The pleural biopsy may reveal noncaseating granulomas. The diagnosis is made by culturing *H. capsulatum* from the pleural fluid, sputum, or biopsy material by routine fungal cultures or by demonstrating the organism in biopsy material with appropriate stains. A presumptive diagnosis can sometimes be established by demonstrating a high histoplasmosis CF titer or an H band on counterimmunoelectrophoresis. It appears that treatment is not necessary for pleural effusions secondary to histoplasmosis (41, 43, 44). The pleural effusion usually resolves spontaneously over several weeks (40, 41, 45). On rare occasions, however, a patient develops a fibrosing pleuritis for which a decortication should be considered if the patient is symptomatic (41, 46).

An isolated pleural effusion due to infection with *H. capsulatum* has been reported in a patient with AIDS (47). This particular patient presented with fever and bilateral small pleural effusions. Thoracentesis revealed an exudate, and many organisms typical of *H. capsulatum* were seen on the Wright-Giemsa stain of the pleural fluid. This patient appeared to respond to therapy with amphotericin B (47). Pleural effusions can also occur in patients with AIDS and disseminated histoplasmosis (48), but pleural involvement is not a prominent part of the disease picture.

ACTINOMYCOSIS

Actinomyces israelii, an anaerobic or microaerophilic Gram-positive bacterium, is a normal inhabitant of the mouth and oropharynx. Although this organism and *Nocardia asteroides* are actually bacteria, they are usually grouped with fungi because they cause chronic illness.

Clinical Manifestations

Actinomycosis is characterized by the formation of abscesses and multiple sinus tracts (49). The infection arises from endogenous sources such as infected gums, infected tonsils, or carious teeth (49). The pleura is involved in over 50% of patients with thoracic actinomycosis (50). In a series of 15 cases of this disorder, 6 patients had pleural effusions, and an additional 6 patients had marked pleural thickening (51). The pleura is particularly likely to be thickened in areas where parenchymal actinomycosis has extended through the chest wall to produce a chest-wall abscess or a draining sinus. In a more recent series using CT scans, pleural effusions were present in 5 of 8 patients (62.5%) with actinomycosis, although there was enough pleural fluid for thoracentesis in three (52). Pleural thickening was demonstrated with CT scans in all 8 of the patients in this latter series (52).

The pleural fluid with actinomycosis may be either frank pus with predominantly polymorphonuclear leukocytes (53) or serous fluid with predominantly lymphocytes (54). I have seen a patient with thoracic actinomycosis in which the associated pleural effusion was serous and contained more than 50% eosinophils.

Diagnosis

The diagnosis of thoracic actinomycosis should be suspected in any patient with a chronic infiltrative pulmonary disease, particularly when the parenchymal disease crosses lung fissures. The presence of chest wall abscesses or draining sinus tracts suggests the diagnosis, as do bone changes consisting of periosteal proliferation or bone destruction (51). Thoracic actinomycosis sometimes becomes disseminated to produce peripheral abscesses in the skin, subcutaneous tissues, or muscles (55). The diagnosis is suggested by the presence of sulfur granules in the draining exudate or the pleural fluid. These granules are 1 to 2 mm in diameter and consist of clumps of thin bacterial filaments that possess peripheral radiations with or without clubbing at their ends. Sulfur granules may be associated with cutaneous nocardiosis, but their presence in viscera only occurs in actinomycosis.

Gram stains of the exudate should be carefully examined for the presence of the slender, Gram-positive, long-branching filaments characteristic of actinomycosis (55). The definitive diagnosis is established with the demonstration of *A. israelii* by anaerobic cultures. The diagnosis of thoracic actinomycosis cannot be established from cultures of expectorated sputum or bronchoscopic washings because *A. israelii* can frequently be cultured from such specimens in the absence of invasive disease. Bacterial culture of the pleural fluid frequently reveals organisms in addition to *A. israelii* (53, 55). The organism most commonly isolated is *Actinobacillus actinomycetem comitans*, a Gram-negative aerobic coccobacillus (55). It has been suggested that the aerobic Actinobacillus reduces the oxygen level in the lesion to facilitate the growth of *A. israelii* (55).

Treatment

The cornerstone of treatment of actinomycosis is the administration of high doses of antibiotics for prolonged periods. Penicillin is the antibiotic of choice, and a dose of 10 million units/day for 4 to 6 weeks is recommended, followed by 12 to 18 months of therapy with oral penicillin phenoxymethyl potassium (55). Tetracycline, erythromycin, lincomycin, and clindamycin have all been used successfully in the treatment of patients with actinomycosis and a history of penicillin hypersensitivity. The management of the pleural effusion in patients with actinomycosis is similar to that of patients with any other bacterial pneumonia (see Chapter 9). If the pleural fluid is serous and contains predominantly lymphocytes or eosinophils, a tube thoracostomy procedure is not necessary. Alternately, if the pleural fluid is frank pus, tube thoracostomy should be performed (56). Decortication is sometimes necessary for resolution of the process (53).

NOCARDIOSIS

Nocardia asteroides is an aerobic, Gram-positive, filamentous bacteria that has a worldwide distribution and can be cultured from the soil (57).

Clinical Manifestations

The disease produced by this organism is similar to actinomycosis, but there is less abscess and sinus tract formation and more hematogenous dissemination with nocardiosis (49). Nocardiosis also has a greater propensity to occur in AIDS and other immunosuppressed patients than does actinomycosis. Most patients who develop nocardiosis are immunosuppressed (58) and the incidence of nocardiosis is increasing as there are more AIDS and other immunosuppressed individuals. The lung is involved in about 75% of patients with nocardiosis (59), and as many as 50% of patients with pulmonary nocardiosis have pleural effusions (58, 60, 61). Patients with pleural effusions secondary to nocardiosis usually have associated parenchymal infiltrates (58, 60, 62). The pleural fluid is an exudate, which can range from serous fluid to frank pus. Pleural fluid cultures may or may not be positive for *N. asteroides*.

Diagnosis

The diagnosis of nocardiosis should be suspected in patients with subacute or chronic pulmonary infiltrates and pleural effusion, particularly if the patient is immunosuppressed. Support for the diagnosis is obtained from a Gram stain of the sputum, bronchoscopic washings, or pleural fluid revealing the typical Gram-positive, branching, filamentous bacteria or from an acid-fast stain revealing variably acid-fast, filamentous bacteria (57). Definitive diagnosis is made by the demonstration of *N. asteroides* with aerobic bacterial cultures of the sputum, bronchoscopic washings, or pleural fluid. Because *N. asteroides* is a slow-growing organism, the bacterial cultures when nocardiosis is suspected must be flagged so that they can be maintained for at least 2 weeks (62). Not all patients with positive sputum cultures for *N. asteroides* have nocardiosis. In a series of 20 patients with positive sputum cultures for *N. asteroides*, 9 of the patients (45%) did not have radiographic abnormalities (63).

Treatment

The cornerstone of treatment for nocardiosis is administration of sulfonamides. Sulfamethoxazole (1 g three times each day), sulfisoxazole (1–2 g four times each day) or sulfadiazine (6–12 g each day) are all efficacious. The medications are continued for at least 6 weeks after the disease is completely cleared and lifelong therapy has been recommended by some (59). The prognosis with pulmonary nocardiosis is poor. In a review of 89 patients with pulmonary nocardiosis occurring between 1945 and 1968, 88% of those with disseminated disease and 47% of those with localized nocardiosis died (64). The deaths were due to nocardiosis rather than the underlying disease. The recommended management of the pleural effusion with nocardiosis is the same as the management of the pleural effusion with actinomycosis (see the previous section of this chapter).

REFERENCES

1. Storey DD, Dines DE, Coles DT: Pleural effusion: a diagnostic dilemma. JAMA 1976;236:2183–2186.
2. Light RW, Erozan YS, Ball WC: Cells in pleural fluid: their value in differential diagnosis. Arch Intern Med 1973;132:854–860.
3. Hillerdal G: Pulmonary aspergillus infection invading the pleura. Thorax 1981;36:745–751.

4. Reyes CV, Kathuria S, MacGlashan A: Diagnostic value of calcium oxalate crystals in respiratory and pleural fluid cytology: a case report. Acta Cytol 1979;23:65-68.

5. Wex P, Utta E, Drozdz W: Surgical treatment of pulmonary and pleuro-pulmonary Aspergillus disease. Thorac Cardiovasc Surg 1993;41:64-70.

6. Krakowka P, Rowinska E, Halweg H: Infection of the pleura by *Aspergillus fumigatus*. Thorax 1970;25:245-253.

7. Colp CR, Cook WA: Successful treatment of pleural aspergillosis and bronchopleural fistula. Chest 1975;68:96-98.

8. Herring M, Pecora D: Pleural aspergillosis: a case report. Am Surg 1976;42:300-302.

9. Walsh TJ, Bulkley BH: Aspergillus pericarditis: clinical and pathologic features in the immunocompromised patient. Cancer 1982;49:48-54.

10. Murphy D, Lane DJ: Pleural effusion in allergic bronchopulmonary aspergillosis: two case reports. Br J Dis Chest 1981;75:91-95.

11. Weiner MH: Antigenemia detected by radioimmunoassay in systemic aspergillosis. Ann Intern Med 1980;92:793-796.

12. Metzger JB, Garagusi VF, Kerwin DM: Pulmonary oxalosis caused by *Aspergillus niger*. Am Rev Respir Dis 1984;129:501-502.

13. Shirakusa T, Ueda H, Saito T, Matsuba K, Kouno J, Hirota N: Surgical treatment of pulmonary aspergilloma and Aspergillus empyema. Ann Thorac Surg 1989;48:779-782.

14. Blastomycosis Cooperative Study of the Veterans Administration: Blastomycosis. A review of 198 collected cases in Veterans Administration Hospitals. Am Rev Respir Dis 1964;89:659-672.

15. Cush R, Light RW, George RB: Clinical and roentgenographic manifestations of acute and chronic blastomycosis. Chest 1976;69:345-349.

16. Sheflin JR, Campbell JA, Thompson GP: Pulmonary blastomycosis: findings on chest radiographs in 63 patients. Am J Roentgenol 1990;154:1177-1180.

17. Kinasewitz GT, Penn RL, George RB: The spectrum and significance of pleural disease in blastomycosis. Chest 1984;86:580-584.

18. Nelson O, Light RW: Granulomatous pleuritis secondary to blastomycosis. Chest 1977;71:433-434.

19. Jay SJ, O'Neill RP, Goodman N, Penman R: Pleural effusion: a rare manifestation of acute pulmonary blastomycosis. Am J Med Sci 1977;274:325-328.

20. Hargis JL, Bone RC, Miller FC, Wilson FJ: Pulmonary blastomycosis diagnosed by thoracocentesis. Chest 1980;77:455.

21. Arora NS, Oblinger MJ, Feldman PS: Chronic pleural blastomycosis with hyperprolactinemia, galactorrhea, and amenorrhea. Am Rev Respir Dis 1979;120:451-455.

22. Sarosi GA, Armstrong D, Davies SF, et al: Laboratory diagnosis of mycotic and specific fungal infections. Am Rev Respir Dis 1985;132:1373-1380.

23. Davies SF, Sarosi GA: Fungal infections. In: Murray JF, Nadel JA, eds. Textbook of Respiratory Medicine. Philadelphia: WB Saunders, 1994:1161-1200.

24. Drutz DJ, Catanzaro A: Coccidioidomycosis. Am Rev Respir Dis 1978;117:727-771.

25. Lonky SA, Catanzaro A, Moser KM, Einstein H: Acute coccidioidal pleural effusion. Am Rev Respir Dis 1976;114:681-688.

26. Pinckney L, Parker BR: Primary coccidioidomycosis in children presenting with massive pleural effusion. AJR 1978;130:247-249.

27. Sarosi GA, Armstrong D, Barbee RA, et al: Treatment of fungal diseases. Am Rev Respir Dis 1979;120:1393-1397.

28. Cunningham RT, Einstein H: Coccidioidal pulmonary cavities with rupture. J Thorac Cardiovasc Surg 1982;84:172-177.

29. Young EJ, Hirsh DD, Fainstein V, Williams TW: Pleural effusions due to *Cryptococcus neoformans*: a review of the literature and report of two cases with cryptococcal antigen determinations. Am Rev Respir Dis 1980;121:743-747.

30. Chechani V, Kamhloz SL: Pulmonary manifestations of disseminated cryptococcosis is patients with AIDS. Chest 1990;98:1060-1065.

31. Cadranel JL, Chouaid C, Denis M, Lebeau B, Akoun GM, Mayaud CM: Causes of pleural effusion in 75 HIV-infected patients. Chest 1993;104:655.

32. Salyer WR, Salyer DC: Pleural involvement in cryptococcosis. Chest 1974;66:139-140.

33. Wasser L, Talavera W: Pulmonary cryptococcosis in AIDS: Chest 1987;92:692-695.

34. Epstein R, Cole R, Hunt KK Jr: Pleural effusion secondary to pulmonary cryptococcosis. Chest 1972;61:296-298.

35. Duperval R, Hermans PE, Brewer NS, Roberts GD: Cryptococcosis, with emphasis on the significance of isolation of *Cryptococcus neoformans* from the respiratory tract. Chest 1977;72:13-19.

36. Warr W, Bates JH, Stone A: The spectrum of pulmonary cryptococcosis. Ann Intern Med 1968;69:1109-1116.

37. Tenholder MF, Ewald FW Jr, Khankhanian NK, Crosby JH: Complex cryptococcal empyema. Chest 1992;101:586-588.

38. Goodwin RA Jr, Des Prez RM: Histoplasmosis. Am Rev Respir Dis 1978;117:929-956.

39. Connell JV Jr, Muhm JR: Radiographic manifestations of pulmonary histoplasmosis: a 10-year review. Radiology 1976;121:281-285.

40. Brewer PL, Himmelwright JP: Pleural effusion due to infection with *Histoplasma capsulatum*. Chest 1970;58:76-79.

41. Schub HM, Spivey CG Jr, Baird GD: Pleural involvement in histoplasmosis. Am Rev Respir Dis 1966;94:225-232.

42. Campbell GD, Webb WR: Eosinophilic pleural effusion. Am Rev Respir Dis 1964;90:194-201.

43. Weissbluth M: Pleural effusion in histoplasmosis. J Pediatr 1976;88:894-895.

44. Quasney MW, Leggiadro RJ: Pleural effusion associated with histoplasmosis. Ped Infect Dis J 1993;12:415-418.

45. Ericsson CD, Pickering LK, Salmon GW: Pleural effusion in histoplasmosis. J Pediatr 1977;90:326-327.

46. Kilburn CD, McKinsey DS, Recurrent massive pleural effusion due to pleural, pericardial, and epicardial fibrosis in histoplasmosis. Chest 1991;100:1715–1717.

47. Marshall BC, Cox JK Jr, Carroll KC, Morrison RE: Histoplasmosis as a cause of pleural effusion in the acquired immunodeficiency syndrome. Am J Med Sci 1990;300:98–101.

48. Ankobiah WA, Vaidya K, Powell S, Carrasco M, Allam A, Chechani V, Kamholz SL: Disseminated histoplasmosis in AIDS. Clinicopathologic features in seven patients from a non-endemic area. NY State J Med 1990;90(5):234–238.

49. Peabody JW Jr, Seabury JH: Actinomycosis and nocardiosis: a review of basic differences in therapy. Am J Med 1960;28:99–115.

50. Bates M, Cruickshank G: Thoracic actinomycosis. Thorax 1957;12:99–124.

51. Flynn MW, Felson B: The roentgen manifestations of thoracic actinomycosis. AJR 1970;110:707–716.

52. Kwong JS, Muller NL, Godwin JD, Aberle D, Grymaloski MR: Thoracic actinomycosis: CT findings in eight patients. Radiology 1992;183:189–192.

53. Karetzky MS, Garvey JW: Empyema due to *Actinomycosis naeslundi*. Chest 1974;65:229–230.

54. Barker CS: Thoracic actinomycosis. Canad Med Assoc J 1954;71:332–334.

55. Varkey B, Landis FB, Tang TT, Rose HD: Thoracic actinomycosis: dissemination to skin, subcutaneous tissue and muscle. Arch Intern Med 1974;134:689–693.

56. McQuarrie DG, Hall WH: Actinomycosis of the lung and chest wall. Surgery 1968;64:905–911.

57. Neu HC, Silva M, Hazen E, Rosenheim SH: Necrotizing nocardial pneumonitis. Ann Intern Med 1967;66:274–284.

58. Feigin DS: Nocardiosis of the lung: chest radiographic findings in 21 cases. Radiology 1986;159:9–14.

59. Uttamchandani RB, Daikos GL, Reyes RR, Fischl MA, Dickinson GM, Yamaguchi E, Kramer MR: Nocardiosis in 30 patients with advanced human immunodeficiency virus infection: clinical features and outcome. Clin Infect Dis 1994;18:348–353.

60. Rubin E, Shin MS: Pleural and extrapleural disease in nocardia infections. Can Assoc Radiol J 1984;35:189–191.

61. Kramer MR, Uttamchandani RB: The radiographic appearance of pulmonary nocardiosis associated with AIDS. Chest 1990;98:382–385.

62. Palmer DL, Harvey RL, Wheeler JK: Diagnostic and therapeutic considerations in Nocardia asteroides infection. Medicine 1974;53:391–401.

63. Frazier AR, Rosenow EC III, Roberts GD: Nocardiosis: a review of 25 cases occurring during 24 months. Mayo Clin Proc 1975;50:657–663.

64. Presant CA, Wiernik PH, Serpick AA: Factors affecting survival in nocardiosis. Am Rev Respir Dis 1974;108:1444–1448.

CHAPTER 12

Pleural Effusion Due to Parasitic Infection

Pleural effusions secondary to parasitic infections are uncommon in the United States, but in some countries, they account for a sizeable percentage of all pleural effusions. With worldwide travel more prevalent, one can anticipate that the incidence of pleural effusions secondary to parasitic disease will gradually increase in the United States.

AMEBIASIS

Amebiasis, the disease caused by *Entamoeba histolytica*, occurs throughout the world. Humans acquire the disease by ingesting the cyst, which is the infectious form of the organism. After ingestion by the host, eight daughter trophozoites develop and colonize the proximal large intestine. The trophozoites, which can proliferate, are the potentially invasive form. These trophozoites may migrate through the portal system to the liver, where the liberation of cytolytic enzymes gives rise to liver abscesses. The trophozoite can also revert to a cyst. When the cyst is passed in the stool, it can be ingested by another individual, to complete the parasite's life cycle. Trophozoites can also be passed in the stool, but are not infectious (1).

The prevalence of amebiasis is most dependent upon the level of sanitation in the community, as would be expected from the life cycle of this parasite. About 5% of the population in the United States are carriers. Amebiasis is most prevalent in the southeastern United States, but is reported with low frequency from every state. Amebic abscess is not unusual in the United States. For example, there were 30 patients seen with hepatic amebiasis at the Santa Clara Valley Medical Center in San Jose, CA, during the period of 1981–1988. None of the patients, however, was born in the United States (2).

Pathogenesis

Pleural effusions arise by two mechanisms in association with amebic liver abscess. The first occurs when an amebic abscess produces diaphragmatic irritation and a sympathetic pleural effusion in a manner analogous to that seen with pyogenic liver abscesses (3, 4) (see Chapter 15). Amebic liver abscesses also produce pleural effusions when the abscess ruptures through the diaphragm into the pleural space (3–5). In this situation, the pleural fluid is described as "chocolate sauce" or "anchovy paste" (6). Such pleural fluid does not contain purulent material, but is rather a mixture of blood, cytolyzed liver tissue, and small, solid particles of liver parenchyma that have resisted dissolution (6).

Clinical Manifestations and Diagnosis

The sympathetic effusion seen with amebic liver abscess is more common than rupture of an abscess through the diaphragm into the pleural space (2, 3). Approximately 20–35% of patients with an amebic liver abscess will have a sympathetic pleural effusion (1, 2). Patients with the sympathetic effusion frequently experience pleuritic chest pain referred to the tip of the scapula or the shoulder. Most patients have a tender, enlarged liver (7). Eosinophilia is not associated with extraintestinal amebiasis. The level of alkaline phosphatase is elevated in more than 75% of patients, while the levels of transaminases are elevated in 50% (1). The chest radiograph reveals a pleural effusion of small to moderate size, often with a concomitant elevation of the hemidiaphragm and platelike atelectasis at the base (2–4). The pleural fluid in this situation has not been well characterized, but is an exudate (2).

The diagnosis of amebiasis should be considered in all patients with right-sided pleural effusions for which no other explanation is obvious. Ultrasonic studies and computed tomography (CT) scanning can demonstrate the hepatic abscess, but cannot differentiate pyogenic from amebic abscesses (8). The diagnosis is aided with the use of serological tests. The gel-diffusion test is positive in 85–95% of patients with acute invasive disease and reverts to negative after 6–12 months. With the indirect hemagglutination tests, an antibody titer of 1:128 or more is seen in 95% of cases, but the titer remains elevated for up to 10 years (9).

Treatment

The treatment of choice is metronidazole, 2.4 g/day orally, for 10 days. If the patient is dyspneic from the pleural effusion, a single therapeutic thoracentesis is usually sufficient to control the symptoms. Over 90% of patients can be cured with the foregoing regimen. If the patient is severely ill, dehydroemetine, a cardiotoxic amebicide available from the Centers for Disease Control and Prevention, Atlanta, GA, may be given concomitantly (9).

Transdiaphragmatic Rupture of Liver Abscess

The transdiaphragmatic rupture of an amebic liver abscess is usually signaled by an abrupt exacerbation of pain in the right upper quadrant and may be accompanied by a tearing sensation (3). These symptoms are followed by the development of rapidly progressive respiratory distress and sepsis, occasionally with shock (3). The pleural effusion is frequently massive, with opacification of the entire hemithorax and shift of the mediastinum to the contralateral side (3). The rupture is into the right pleural space in over 90% of patients. The symptoms are sometimes subacute or chronic in nature (5). The diagnosis of amebic abscess with transdiaphragmatic rupture is suggested by the discovery of anchovy paste or chocolate sauce pleural fluid on diagnostic thoracentesis. Amebas can be demonstrated in the pleural fluid in fewer than 10% of patients. Concomitant rupture into the airways occurs in about 30% of patients (3), and this complication is usually manifested by the expectoration of chocolate sauce sputum, which may be confused with hemoptysis by the patient and the physician.

The diagnosis is established by the characteristic appearance of the pleural fluid and can be confirmed by serologic tests for amebiasis. Ultrasound or CT scanning of the abdomen can delineate the extent of the intrahepatic disease and the presence or absence of a subphrenic abscess. Patients with transdiaphragmatic rupture should be treated with the same drugs as patients with sympathetic pleural effusions due to amebic hepatic abscess. Patients with transdiaphragmatic rupture should also undergo a tube thoracostomy procedure (3–5). Large-bore tubes are recommended because the pleural fluid can be thick (3). The combination of the drugs and the chest tubes results in clinical cure in the majority of patients (3, 4).

About a third of patients with transhepatic rupture also have a bacterial infection of their pleural space (4, 5). Such patients should be treated with the appropriate antibiotics. In addition, an open drainage procedure or decortication is frequently necessary, indications for which are outlined in Chapter 9. In patients who undergo decortication, the visceral pleura is found to be covered with a thick membrane (5), but this membrane can easily be stripped off the visceral pleura (5). Even when no bacterial superinfection is present, decortication should be performed if the lung has not fully expanded in 10 days (5). The prognosis with transdiaphragmatic rupture is excellent if the patient is not too debilitated initially or if the diagnosis is not delayed (3–5).

ECHINOCOCCOSIS (HYDATID DISEASE)

Echinococcosis is caused by the tapeworm *Echinococcus granulosus*. The definitive host for this small tapeworm is the dog or wolf. When dog feces containing the parasite's eggs are ingested by humans, larvae emerge in the duodenum, enter the blood, and usually lodge in either the liver or the lung. In these tissues, the parasite gradually grows, and years may pass before symptoms appear. It takes about 6 months for the cyst to reach a diameter of 1 cm, and thereafter it in increases in size by 2–3 cm/year (10). The dog becomes infected by eating meat containing the larvae. Echinococcosis is seen in most sheep- and cattle-raising areas of the world including Australia, New Zealand, Argentina, Uruguay, Chile, parts of Africa, Eastern Europe, and the Middle East. The disease is particularly common in Lebanon and Greece.

Pathogenesis

Pleural involvement with hydatid disease can occur in one of four situations (11, 12): (a) a hepatic hydatid cyst or, on rare occasions, a splenic cyst may rupture through the diaphragm into the pleural space; (b) a pulmonary hydatid cyst may rupture into the pleural space; (c) on rare occasions, the pleura may be primarily involved by the slowly enlarging cyst (11); or (d) a pulmonary or hepatic hydatid cyst may be accompanied by a pleural effusion (13, 14). The incidence of pulmonary and hepatic cyst rupture into the pleural space is equivalent (11). Fewer than 5% of hepatic or pulmonary hydatid cysts are complicated by intrapleural rupture (11, 12, 15). Approximately 5% of patients with a hepatic or a pulmonary hydatid cyst have a pleural effusion (13). The characteristics of the pleural fluid in this situation have not been characterized.

Clinical Manifestations and Diagnosis

When a hepatic cyst ruptures into the pleural space, the patient usually becomes acutely ill, with sudden tearing chest pain, dyspnea, and shock from the antigenic challenge to the body (16). In about 50% of patients with rupture into the pleural space, simultaneous rupture into the tracheobronchial tree occurs (16). Such patients may cough up large quantities of pus and membranes of the cyst. When a pulmonary cyst ruptures into the pleural space, similar symptoms are frequently present. In addition, a bronchopleural fistula often produces a hydropneumothorax that may become secondarily infected.

The diagnosis of pleural echinococcosis is established by the demonstration of echinococcal scolices with hooklets in the pleural fluid (17). A CT scan demonstrating multiple round cysts is very suggestive of the diagnosis (18). Eosinophils are frequently present in the pleural fluid unless it becomes secondarily infected (12, 17, 19). The Casoni skin test is positive in

about 75% of patients (16), and the Weinberg complement-fixation (CF) test is positive in a higher percentage.

Treatment

An immediate thoracotomy is recommended for patients who have rupture of a hepatic or pulmonary cyst into the pleural space (16). When a hepatic cyst has ruptured, the objectives of surgical treatment are to remove the parasite, to drain the hepatic cavity, and to re-expand the lung immediately (16). If the surgical procedure is delayed, a decortication may also be required (16). An exploratory thoracotomy should also be performed when a pulmonary hydatid cyst ruptures into the pleural space, to remove the parasite, to excise the original cyst, and to close the bronchopleural fistula. Experimental evidence from both animal and clinical studies suggests that benzimidazole compounds, such as mebendazole or albendazole, may be effective in treating hydatid cysts. The treatment of choice appears to be albendazole 400 mg twice a day for 28 days (20). These compounds are recommended when all the cysts cannot be removed, or when rupture of a cyst has occurred.

PARAGONIMIASIS

Paragonimiasis is caused by the lung flukes *Paragonimus westermani* and *Paragonimus miyazakii* (21), which have a fascinating life cycle. Humans acquire the disease by eating raw or undercooked crabs or crayfish containing the larvae of these parasites (22, 23). Once ingested, the larvae bore through the intestinal wall and enter the peritoneal cavity. They then migrate upward in the peritoneal cavity to the diaphragm, bore through the diaphragm, and then, after traversing the pleural space, bore through the visceral pleura and enter the lung (22, 23). In the lung, the larvae lodge near small bronchi and mature into the adult lung fluke, persisting in the lungs for years while producing about 10,000 eggs daily. The eggs produced by the mature flukes are expectorated or swallowed, and excreted in the feces. Once in water, the eggs develop into ciliated miracidia that infect freshwater snails. Another larval form develops in the snails and is eventually liberated as cercariae that penetrate crayfish and crabs, to complete the cycle (22, 23).

Pathogenesis and Incidence

The pleural disease associated with paragonimiasis is thought to arise when the parasites traverse the pleural space and penetrate the visceral pleura. Pleural disease is common with paragonimiasis (24, 25). In a series of 71 cases of pleuropulmonary paragonimiasis from Korea (25), 43 patients (61%) had pleural disease. Of the 43 patients with pleural disease, 20 had unilateral pleural effusions, 6 had bilateral pleural effusion, 6 had unilateral hydropneumothorax, 6 had bilateral hydropneumothorax, and 5 had pleural thickening (25). In another series from Japan, 9 of 13 patients (69%) had a pleural effusion (24).

Although paragonimiasis is confined mainly to residents of the Far East, there was an increased incidence of this disease in the United States in the 1980s with the influx of refugees from Southeast Asia (22, 26). Johnson and Johnson reported a series of 25 cases of paragonimiasis that occurred in Indochinese refugees between March 1980 and December 1982. Seventeen cases occurred in Minneapolis, while eight cases occurred in Seattle (26). Twelve of the patients (48%) had pleural effusions. The effusions were bilateral in three individuals and were massive in six. Non-Oriental individuals in the United States have developed paragonimiasis from ingesting infected crayfish (27) or crabs (28).

Diagnosis

The diagnosis of pleural paragonimiasis should be suspected in Oriental patients or in patients with pleural effusion who have recently traveled to the Orient. The diagnosis of paragonimiasis is made either by detecting eggs in sputum, stool, fluid from bronchoscopic lavage, or biopsy specimens, or by a positive anti-*Paragonimus* antibody test (25). Enzyme-linked immunosorbent assay (ELISA) is highly sensitive and specific in detecting antibodies, while eggs are demonstrable in less than 50% of cases (25).

The characteristics of the pleural fluid are virtually pathognomonic for paragonimiasis. The pleural fluid with paragonimiasis is an exudate with a low glucose level (less than 10 mg/dl), a low pH (less than 7.10), and a high lactic acid dehydrogenase (LDH) level (more than 1000 IU/L) (22, 26). Cholesterol crystals are usually present in the pleural fluid. Most patients with pleural paragonimiasis have significant eosinophilia in their pleural fluid (21, 22, 26). The only other disease that produces an eosinophilic exudate with a low glucose level and a low pH is the Churg-Strauss syndrome (29).

Yokogawa and coworkers have reported that pleural fluid IgE levels are elevated and are higher than the simultaneous serum IgE levels in patients with pleural paragonimiasis (21). Subsequently, Ikeda and associates (30) used ELISA to measure *P. westermani*-specific IgE and IgG in seven patients. They reported that the levels of parasite-specific IgE and IgG were significantly higher in the pleural effusion than in the serum in all patients (30). This latter study suggests that the measurement of parasite-specific IgE and IgG is useful diagnostically, and indicates that these antibodies are produced in the pleural space.

Treatment

The treatment of choice is praziquantel, 25 mg/kg body weight 3 times a day for 3 days. Bithionol, 35 to 50 mg/kg on alternate days for 10 to 15 doses is also effective, but its toxic gastrointestinal effects can be troublesome (28). If pleural disease has been present for such a prolonged period that the pleural surfaces are abnormally thickened, penetration of the drugs into the pleural space is insufficient to eradicate the infection, and thoracotomy with decortication may be necessary (22, 31).

OTHER PARASITIC INFECTIONS

Pleural disease due to other parasites is uncommon. A rare patient with *Pneumocystis carinii* pneumonia has a pleural effusion, but the effusion hardly ever dominates the clinical picture. Since *P. carinii* infection usually occurs in patients with AIDS, this entity is discussed in Chapter 13. Patients who die from malaria frequently have pleural effusions (7). The pleural effusions in this circumstance are probably secondary to the pulmonary edema and have little, if any, clinical significance (7). There have been case reports of pleural effusions due to *Trichomonas* (32), loiasis (33), and sporotrichosis (34).

REFERENCES

1. Reed SL: Amebiasis: an update. Clin Infect Dis 1992; 14:385–393.
2. Lyche KD, Jensen WA, Kirsch CM, Yenokida GG, Maltz GS, Knauer CM: Pleuropulmonary manifestations of hepatic amebiasis. West J Med 1990;153: 275–278.
3. Ibarra-Perez C: Thoracic complications of amebic abscess of the liver. Chest 1981;79:672–676.
4. Cameron EWJ: The treatment of pleuropulmonary amebiasis with metronidazole. Chest 1978;73:647–650.
5. Rasaretnam R, Paul ATS, Yoganathan M: Pleural empyema due to ruptured amoebic liver abscess. Br J Surg 1974;61:713–715.
6. Daniels AC, Childress ME: Pleuropulmonary ambiasis. Calif Med 1956;85:369–375.
7. Sharma OP, Maheshwari A: Lung diseases in the tropics. Part 2: Common tropical lung diseases: diagnosis and management. Tubercle Lung Dis 1993; 74:359–370.
8. Boultbee JE, Simjee AE, Rooknoodeen F, Englebrecht HE: Experiences with grey scale ultrasonography in hepatic amoebiasis. Clin Radiol 1979;30:683–689.
9. Petersen C, Mills J: Parasitic infections. In: Murray JF, Nadel JA, eds. Textbook of Respiratory Medicine. 2nd ed. Philadelphia: WB Saunders, 1994:1201–1243.
10. von Sinner WN: Ultrasound, CT and MRI of ruptured and disseminated hydatid cysts. Euro J Radiol 1990; 11:31–37.
11. Rakower J, Milwidsky H: Hydatid pleural disease. Am Rev Respir Dis 1964;90:623–631.
12. Barzilai A, Pollack S, Kaftori JK, et al: Splenic echinococcal cyst burrowing into left pleural space. Chest 1977;72:543–545.
13. Jerray M, Benzarti M, Garrouche A, Klabi N, Hayouni A: Hydatid disease of the lung. Am Rev Respir Dis 1992;146:185–189.
14. von Sinner W: Pleural complications of hydatid disease (*Echinococcus granulosus*). Rofo: Fortschritte Auf Dem Gebiete Der Rontgenstrahlen Und Der Nuklearmedizin. 1990;152:718–722.
15. Balikian JP, Mudarris FF: Hydatid disease of the lungs: a roentgenologic study of 50 cases. AJR 1974; 122:692–707.
16. Xanthakis DS, Katsaras E, Efthimiadis M, Papadakis G, et al: Hydatid cyst of the liver with intrathoracic rupture. Thorax 1981;36:497–501.
17. Jacobson ES: A case of secondary echinococcosis diagnosed by cytologic examination of pleural fluid and needle biopsy of pleura. Acta Cytol 1973;17:76–79.
18. Gouliamos AD, Kalovidouris A, Papailiou J, Vlahos L, Papavasiliou C: CT appearance of pulmonary hydatid disease. Chest 1991;100:1578–1581.
19. Yacoubian HD: Thoracic problems associated with hydatid cyst of the dome of the liver. Surgery 1976; 79:544–548.
20. Wen H, New RRC, Craig PS: Diagnosis and treatment of human hydatidosis. Br J Clin Pharmac 1993;35: 565–574.
21. Yokogawa M, Kojima S, Araki K, et al: Immunoglobulin E: raised levels in sera and pleural exudates of patients with paragonimiasis. Am J Trop Med Hyg 1976;25:581–586.
22. Minh V-D, Engle P, Greenwood JR, et al: Pleural paragonimiasis in a southeast Asian refugee. Am Rev Respir Dis 1981;124:186–188.
23. Eikas J, Kim PK: Clinical investigation of paragonimiasis. Acta Tuberc Scand 1960;39:140–147.
24. Nawa Y: Recent trends of *Paragonimiasis westermani* in Miyazaki Prefecture, Japan. Southeast Asian J Trop Med Public Health 1991;22(Suppl):342–344.
25. Im JG, Whang HY, Kim WS, Han MC, Shim YS, Cho SY: Pleuropulmonary paragonimiasis: radiologic findings in 71 patients. AJR 1992;159:39–43.
26. Johnson RJ, Johnson JR: Paragonimiasis in Indochinese refugees: roentgenographic findings with clinical correlations. Am Rev Respir Dis 1983;128:534–538.
27. Pachucki CT, Levandowski RA, Brown VA, et al: American paragonimiasis treated with praziquantel. N Engl J Med 1984;311:582–584.
28. Sharma OP: The man who loved drunken crabs: a case of pulmonary paragonimiasis. Chest 1989;95: 670–672.
29. Erzurum SE, Underwood GA, Hamilos DL, Waldron JA: Pleural effusion in Churg-Strauss syndrome. Chest 1989;95:1357–1359.
30. Ikeda T, Oikawa Y, Owhashi M, Nawa Y: Parasite-specific IgE and IgG levels in the serum and pleural effusion of *Paragonimiasis westermanii* patients. Am J Trop Med Hyg 1992;47:104–107.
31. Dietrick RB, Sade RM, Pak JS: Results of decortication in chronic empyema with special reference to paragonimiasis. J Thorac Cardiovasc Surg 1981;82: 58–62.
32. Walzer PD, Rutherford I, East R: Empyema with trichomonas species. Am Rev Respir Dis 1978;118: 415–418.
33. Klion AD, Eisenstein EM, Smirniotopoulos TT, Neumann MP, Nutman TB: Pulmonary involvement in loiasis. Am Rev Respir Dis 1992;145:961–963.
34. Morrissey R, Caso R: Pleural sporotrichosis. Chest 1983;84:507.

CHAPTER 13

Pleural Effusion Due to AIDS, Other Viruses, *Mycoplasma pneumoniae*, and Rickettsiae

Over the past decade the AIDS epidemic has had a profound impact on the practice of medicine. Accordingly, the first part of this chapter deals with pleural effusions in patients with AIDS. Since the organism responsible for AIDS is a virus, we have also included pleural diseases due to viruses in this chapter.

In addition, the pleural effusions resulting from infection with *Mycoplasma pneumoniae* and the rickettsial agent *Coxiella burnetii* are also discussed. Disease secondary to the latter two agents is discussed in this chapter because they produce clinical pictures simulating viral pneumonias.

PLEURAL EFFUSIONS IN PATIENTS WITH AIDS

Pleural effusions are uncommon in patients with AIDS. The incidence was 1.7% in one large series of 4511 patients who were HIV positive and admitted to the Metropolitan Hospital Center in New York (1). The distribution of the diseases responsible for pleural effusions in patients with AIDS varies widely from series to series. In a series of 30 patients from New York, 12 (40%) had parapneumonic effusion or empyema, 6 (20%) had tuberculosis, 2 (7%) had Kaposi's sarcoma, 3 (10%) had end-stage renal disease with volume overload, 3 (10%) had miscellaneous diseases, while 4 (13%) had an undetermined etiology for their pleural effusion (1). In another series of 61 patients from Paris, more than 50% of the effusions were due to Kaposi's sarcoma (2). In this series 32 of the patients (52%) had Kaposi's sarcoma, 11 (18%) had aerobic bacteria, 9 (15%) had *Mycobacterium tuberculosis*, 6 (10%) had opportunistic infections, and 3 (5%) had effusions due to other malignancies (2). In contrast, in a series from Rwanda (3), tubercu-

losis was responsible for the pleural effusion in 82 of 91 (90%) of patients who were HIV positive and had a pleural effusion. Lastly, in a series from South Carolina, *Pneumocystis carinii* pneumonia and hypoalbuminemia were responsible for a significant percentage of the pleural effusions (4). In this series of 59 patients the causes of the pleural effusion were bacterial pneumonia 18 (31%), hypoalbuminemia 11 (19%), *Pneumocystis carinii* pneumonia 9 (15%), *M. tuberculosis* 5 (8%), cardiac failure 3 (5%), other opportunistic infections 4 (6%) and miscellaneous 9 (16%) (4).

Kaposi's Sarcoma

Kaposi's sarcoma (KS) is one of the more common causes of pleural effusion in patients with AIDS. KS occurs in 20 to 25% of individuals with AIDS (5, 6). KS occurs almost exclusively in homosexual patients with AIDS (6). Cutaneous violaceous plaques are the most common presentation of KS. Pleuropulmonary KS occurs in approximately 20% of patients with cutaneous KS (6). Most patients with pleuropulmonary KS present with progressive shortness of breath, nonproductive cough, and fever. Patients with pulmonary KS generally have abnormal chest roentgenograms characterized by bilateral infiltrates (6). The incidence of pleural effusion with pulmonary KS is approximately 50% (6). Most patients with a pleural effusion due to KS also have bilateral parenchymal infiltrates (6). The pleural effusions may be unilateral or bilateral. Autopsy studies demonstrate multiple cherry red to purple lesions on the visceral but not on the parietal pleural surface (6).

The diagnosis of pleural KS is difficult. The pleural fluid is an exudate that is usually serosanguineous or hemorrhagic. The differential cell count shows a mononuclear cell-predominant pattern (6). The pleural fluid glucose and pH levels are usually normal, but were reduced in one patient (6). Cytologic examination of the pleural fluid is not helpful because the diagnosis requires a characteristic architectural appearance and not a particular neoplastic cell type (5). The pleural effusion in about 20% of patients is a chylothorax (6). Pleural biopsies usually do not establish the diagnosis of KS probably because there is not parietal pleural involvement (6). It is probable that the diagnosis could be established with thoracoscopy given the characteristic appearance of the KS lesions on the visceral pleura (6). One report (7) suggested that the diagnosis of pleural KS could be made by immunohistochemical staining of the cells in the pleural fluid with CD34 antibody, a newly recognized marker for vascular neoplasia.

The prognosis of a patient with pleuropulmonary KS is poor. In one study, the average interval from diagnosis of pulmonary KS to death was 4 ± 3 months (6). The presence of the pleural effusion is a significant problem for many patients with pleuropulmonary KS. In one series, recurrent massive, progressive effusion dominated the final days of a substantial percentage of patients and contributed significantly to their death in about 50% (6).

The treatment of pulmonary KS is difficult. Tube thoracostomy with the instillation of tetracycline is usually not successful (6). If the diagnosis is made with thoracoscopy, insufflated talc is probably the treatment of choice. Otherwise, pleurodesis via talc in a slurry or a pleuroperitoneal shunt are probably the best alternatives.

Parapneumonic Effusion and Empyema and AIDS

Community acquired bacterial pneumonia occurs frequently in patients with AIDS. It appears that patients with AIDS are probably more likely to develop pleural complications with their pneumonias than are other patients. They are more likely to have bacteremia with their pneumonia (8). In one series of 45 cases, pleural effusion occurred in 10 and empyema occurred in three (8). The distribution of organisms responsible for community acquired

bacterial pneumonia in AIDS is very similar to that of patients without AIDS (9). The management of the patient with AIDS and a parapneumonic effusion or an empyema is the same as that for any patient.

Pneumocystis carinii Pneumonia and AIDS

Although pleural effusions due to *P. carinii* account for only a small percent of pleural effusions in patients with AIDS, they do occur. By 1993 a total of seven cases of pleural effusion due to *P. carinii* infection had been reported (10, 11). In most cases the diagnosis was established by visualization of *Pneumocystis* in pleural fluid stained with Gomori's methenamine-silver. All seven of the reported patients were receiving aerosolized pentamidine, and five of the seven had documented underlying *Pneumocystis* pneumonia. Two patients presented with primary pleural infection with *Pneumocystis*. It appears that *Pneumocystis* pleural disease is an anatomic extension of smoldering subpleural *Pneumocystis* pneumonia and the prognosis is not worse than with pneumonia alone. Four of the seven patients with pleural *Pneumocystis* have also had a bronchopleural fistula (10).

The pleural fluid is an exudate with pleural *Pneumocystis*. The pleural fluid lactic acid dehydrogenase (LDH) has been above 400 IU and the ratio of the pleural fluid to serum LDH has exceeded 1.0. Interestingly, the pleural fluid protein level has been below 3.0 gm/dl in all patients. The pleural fluid glucose and pH are not reduced and the differential cell count can reveal either neutrophils or mononuclear cells (10). The treatment of pleural *Pneumocystis* is the same as the treatment of pulmonary *Pneumocystis*.

Tuberculous Pleural Effusions and AIDS

In some series, tuberculosis is the most common etiology for pleural effusions associated with AIDS (3). The fact that the patient has AIDS appears to have very little influence on the clinical picture of the patient with tuberculous pleuritis, but there are some differences. The percentage of tuberculosis cases that have pleural effusions in patients with AIDS is higher in patients with CD4 counts above 200 than in those with CD4 counts below 200/µl (12). The purified protein derivative (PPD) skin test is less frequently positive in patients with AIDS who have tuberculous pleuritis. In one series the PPD was positive in 76% of patients without AIDS but in only 41% of patients with AIDS (13). In patients without AIDS, the pleural fluid acid-fast bacillus (AFB) stain is only rarely positive (~1%), but in one series the AFB pleural fluid smear was positive in 15% of patients with AIDS (13). The incidence of granuloma on pleural biopsy is comparable in patients with and without AIDS (13). Cultures of the pleural biopsy specimen are positive more frequently (more than 50%) than cultures of the pleural fluid (~10%). The pleural fluid ADA levels are less useful diagnostically in the immunocompromised individual. Patients with AIDS and tuberculous pleuritis may have adenosine deaminase (ADA) levels below 40 IU/L (14). However, levels of interferon-γ in the pleural fluid are increased in patients with AIDS and pleural tuberculosis as they are in other patients with pleural tuberculosis (15). Tuberculous pleuritis is discussed in more detail in Chapter 10.

Miscellaneous Pleural Effusion in Patients with AIDS

Other opportunistic diseases such as cryptococcosis (16), histoplasmosis (17), nocardiosis (18), or atypical mycobacteria (19) at times are responsible for a pleural effusion in the patient with AIDS. In their terminal stages, some patients with AIDS develop hypoproteinemia and this may lead to a transudative pleural effusion (4). Patients with AIDS may also develop hypervolemia due to heart failure or renal failure, which can lead to a pleural effusion (1). The diagnosis and management of pleural effusions due to these different entities are described in the appropriate chapters in this book.

Approach to the Patient with AIDS and Pleural Effusion

AIDS patients with a pleural effusion should have a diagnostic thoracentesis. If the diagnosis is not apparent after the thoracentesis, the patient should have a pleural biopsy if the pleural fluid is an exudate. A pleural biopsy specimen should be sent for mycobacterial culture. If no diagnosis is established with this procedure, careful consideration of the diagnosis of tuberculosis should be made. If the patient has a positive PPD (greater than 5mm) or if there are no mesothelial cells in the pleural fluid, chemotherapy with isoniazid and rifampin for 9 months is recommended. If the patient is receiving aerosolized pentamidine, silver stains of the pleural fluid should be obtained to rule out *Pneumocystis*. If the patient has cutaneous Kaposi's sarcoma, consideration should be given to a diagnostic thoracoscopy with talc insufflation. If the patient does not have KS, but is symptomatic from the pleural effusion, strong consideration should be given to creating a chemical pleurodesis with talc slurry or a tetracycline derivative or to implanting a pleuroperitoneal shunt, as described in Chapter 7.

VIRUSES

Viral infections probably account for a larger percentage of pleural effusions than generally realized. The diagnosis usually depends upon isolation of the virus or the demonstration of a significant increase in the antibodies to the virus. Because most pleural effusions secondary to viruses are self-limiting, paired sera from patients in the acute and convalescent phases of disease are not usually obtained for diagnosis. Moreover, most hospitals are not equipped to culture viruses.

The most interesting epidemic of pleural effusions attributed to viral infection occurred in Turkey in 1955, when 559 individuals at a military base developed a pleural effusion in conjunction with an acute illness characterized by fever, cough, malaise, anorexia, and shortness of breath (20). None of the patients had parenchymal infiltrates, but about 30% had an enlarged hilar shadow. The peripheral white blood cell count (WBC) was normal or reduced with an increased percentage of lymphocytes. The differential WBC on the pleural fluid revealed mostly mononuclear cells. The disease was self-limited, and almost all patients recovered completely within 90 days. Because all bacterial cultures were negative, as were serologic tests for Q fever, and because the patients recovered without any specific therapy, it was concluded that the disease was due to a viral infection (20). This report is important because it documents that viral infections can cause pleural effusions, and in large numbers. One wonders what fraction of undiagnosed pleural effusions is due to viral infections.

Small pleural effusions frequently accompany primary atypical pneumonia. Fine and coworkers prospectively studied 59 patients with nonbacterial pneumonia that satisfied serologic criteria for association with either a mycoplasma, viral, or cold-agglutinin-positive pneumonia (21). Twelve of these patients (20%) had small pleural effusions, which in four patients could only be demonstrated on lateral decubitus radiographs. This finding compares with a 45% incidence of pleural effusions in patients with acute bacterial pneumonia (22). In the series of Fine and associates, 6 of 29 (21%) patients with mycoplasma pneumonia, 1 of 7 (14%) with adenoviral pneumonia, 1 of 4 (25%) with influenza pneumonia, and 4 of 19 (21%) with only increased titers of cold agglutinins had pleural effusions (21).

In patients with viral infections, the pleural effusions are usually small (20, 21), but occasionally may be large (23). The pleural fluid is an exudate (21), and usually mononuclear cells are predominant on the pleural fluid differential WBC (20, 24). I have seen a patient with a viral pneumonia, however, in whom the initial thoracentesis revealed predominantly polymorphonuclear leukocytes, but a subsequent thoracentesis 48 hours later revealed predominantly mononuclear cells. The diagnosis of pleural effusions secondary to viral infections is established by documenting increasing titers with the specific serologic tests or by culturing viruses from the pleural fluid (23, 25). At times, with pleural effusions secondary to herpes infections or cytomegalovirus, the cytologic findings in the pleural fluid consisting of intranuclear inclusions and multinuclear giant cells with gelatinous nuclear changes suggest the diagnosis (26, 27).

Adenovirus Pneumonia

After *Mycoplasma pneumoniae*, adenoviruses are the second leading cause of primary atypical pneumonia. Pleural effusions occur in 3 to 15% of patients with adenoviral pneumonia (28, 29). The pleural effusions are usually small, but may be large (28). When adenovirus infection results in a pleural effusion, a concomitant parenchymal infiltrate is usually present (29).

Infectious Hepatitis

Pleural effusions occasionally occur in conjunction with infectious hepatitis and at times precede the development of icterus (24, 30–34). In a review of 2500 patients with viral hepatitis (30), 4 patients (0.16%) had pleural effusions. In another prospective study of 156 patients with hepatitis (34), however, 70% of the patients had at least a small pleural effusion. Patients with pleural effusions secondary to viral hepatitis do not have parenchymal infiltrates. The pleural fluid is an exudate with predominantly mononuclear cells (24, 35). The pleural effusion frequently resolves before the hepatitis (31). One must be careful in handling pleural fluid when infectious hepatitis is suspected because the infectious hepatitis B e antigen has been demonstrated in pleural fluid secondary to hepatitis (33, 35).

Infectious Mononucleosis

Pleural effusions occasionally occur in the course of infectious mononucleosis (36–38). Lander and Palayew reviewed the chest radiographs of 59 patients with infectious mononucleosis and reported that 3 (5%) had pleural effusions (36). Two of the patients had bilateral interstitial infiltrates and small bilateral pleural effusions, whereas the third patient had a moderate-sized, left-sided pleural effusion without any parenchymal infiltrates (36). The pleural effusions are exudates and usually take several months to resolve (37, 38).

Hantavirus Infections

The hantavirus pulmonary syndrome is a recently described entity which is due to infection with a previously unknown hantavirus species (39, 40). As of December 1, 1993, laboratory evidence of acute hantavirus infection had been confirmed in 48 patients in 14 states who had a similar clinical syndrome.

The majority of cases have occurred in the Four Corners Region where New Mexico, Arizona, Colorado, and Utah meet. The deer mouse *Peromyscus maniculatus* has been identified as the likely principal reservoir of this virus.

The hantavirus pulmonary syndrome is characterized by a brief prodromal illness followed by rapidly progressive, noncardiogenic pulmonary edema (39, 40). The median age of infected individuals is about 30, and 50% of the patients have been Native American Indians (39). Most patients present with fever or chills, gastrointestinal complaints such as nausea or vomiting, abdominal pain, or diarrhea. Myalgias are also reported by most patients as is cough, but dyspnea tends to be a late-developing symptom, occurring just prior to respiratory decompensation.

Patients who present with the hantavirus pulmonary syndrome have many abnormal laboratory tests. They characteristically have the triad of thrombocytopenia, a left shift in the myeloid series, and large immunoblastoid lymphocytes. The PaO_2/FIO_2 is usually severely reduced and 50% of the patients require mechanical ventilation. The chest radiograph of patients who progress to respiratory failure initially shows bibasilar infiltrates, which rapidly spread to include all four quadrants of the lung. The heart size is normal. Patients with the hantavirus pulmonary syndrome tend to decompensate rapidly with refractory hypoxemia and hypotension. The mean duration of hospitalization before death is only about 3 days.

Pleural effusions are present in about 40% of patients with the hantavirus pulmonary syndrome. The pleural fluid has not been well characterized, but it is probably an exudate. When the pulmonary edema fluid is analyzed, its protein content is more than 80% that of the serum which indicates that the patients have a noncardiogenic pulmonary edema (39). At autopsy, patients dying of the hantavirus pulmonary syndrome have large serous effusions with severe edema of the lungs. It is probable that the pleural effusion results from interstitial fluid traversing the visceral pleura to the pleural space.

It is important to make the diagnosis of the hantavirus pulmonary syndrome early, since antiviral therapy requires time to be beneficial.

Rapid diagnosis is now available at the University of New Mexico, which has developed a test for antibodies in a three-antigen recombinant immunoblot assay for IgM and IgG. The treatment of choice appears to be intravenous ribavirin. Intravenous ribavirin, however, is not licensed for use in the United States and must be administered under a Centers for Disease Control and Prevention (CDC) protocol (39).

Other Viral Infections

Pleural effusions have also been reported to result from infection with respiratory syncytial virus (41), influenza viruses (21), measles after the administration of inactivated virus vaccine (42), cytomegalovirus (24), herpes simplex virus (26), and Lassa fever virus (23). Pleural effusions probably result from infection by many other viruses as well.

MYCOPLASMA PNEUMONIAE

This organism is actually a small bacterium rather than a virus. It is included in this chapter because the disease it produces more closely resembles a viral than a bacterial disease. Pleural effusions occur in 5 to 20% of patients with pneumonias due to *M. pneumoniae* (21, 43). The effusions are usually small (21), but can be large (43–45). The diagnosis, suggested by increased titers of cold agglutinins, is established by increasing specific antibody titers. It may take several weeks for a fourfold rise in specific antibody titer to become evident, however. In one report, *M. pneumoniae* was isolated from the pleural fluid of 2 patients with pleural effusion and pneumonia (46). The treatment of choice is tetracycline or erythromycin administration. No specific treatment need be directed toward the pleural effusion, but a diagnostic thoracentesis should be performed to ensure that a complicated parapneumonic effusion is not present.

RICKETTSIAE (Q FEVER)

The primary rickettsial agent associated with pleural effusions is *Coxiella burnetii*, which is the agent responsible for Q fever. This disease is sometimes manifested as a primary atypical pneumonia. Q fever is acquired by the inhalation of contaminated dust particles or by drinking infected, unpasteurized milk. Because the infection is prevalent among livestock in the United States, farmers and stockyard workers are particularly likely to contract the disease. Patients with Q fever pneumonia present with the clinical picture of primary atypical pneumonia with high fever, cough, headache, and myalgias. Nearly half of the patients have no respiratory symptoms, although one-third have pleuritic chest pain (47). Pleural involvement is relatively common with Q fever pneumonia. In one series of 164 cases from the Basque country of Spain, 12% had a pleural effusion (47). In another review 5 of 25 patients (20%) with chest radiographic abnormalities due to Q fever had a pleural effusion, and in 1 of these the effusion was large (48). The pleural fluid is an exudate and the differential reveals predominantly mononuclear cells (49) or eosinophils (50). In one report the pleural fluid ADA level was increased to 64 IU/L with Q fever (49). The diagnosis is usually established by demonstrating fourfold rises in antibody titers of sera that become apparent in most patients within 2 weeks of the onset of the illness. The treatment of choice is tetracycline or doxycycline, which appear to be superior to erythromycin (47).

REFERENCES

1. Lababidi HMS, Gupta K, Newman T, Fuleihan FJD: A retrospective analysis of pleural effusion in human immunodeficiency virus infected patients. Chest 1994;106:86S.
2. Cadranel JL, Chouaid C, Denis M, Lebeau B, Akoun GM, Mayaud CM: Causes of pleural effusion in 75 HIV-infected patients [letter]. Chest 1993;104:655.
3. Batungwanayo J, Taelman H, Allen S, Bogaerts J, Kagame A, Van de Perre P: Pleural effusion, tuberculosis and HIV-1 infection in Kigali, Rwanda. AIDS 1993;7:73-79.
4. Joseph J, Strange C, Sahn SA: Pleural effusions in hospitalized patients with AIDS. Ann Intern Med 1993;118:856-869.
5. Ognibene FP, Shelhamer JH: Kaposi's sarcoma. In Pulmonary Effects of AIDS. Clin Chest Med 1988;9:459-463.
6. O'Brien RF, Cohn DL: Serosanguineous pleural effusions in AIDS-associated Kaposi's sarcoma. Chest 1989;96:460-466.
7. Yang GC, Brooks JJ, Roberts S, Gupta PK: The detection of acquired immunodeficiency syndrome-associated Kaposi sarcoma cells in pleural effusion by CD34 immunostain. Cancer 1993;72:2260-2265.
8. Rodriguez Barradas MC, Musher DM, Hamill RJ, Dowell M, Bagwell JT, Sanders CV: Unusual manifestations of pneumococcal infection in human immunodeficiency virus-infected individuals: the past revisited. Clin Infect Dis 1992;14:192-199.
9. Miller RF, Foley NM, Kessel D, Jeffrey AA: Community acquired lobar pneumonia in patients with HIV infection and AIDS. Thorax 1994;49:367-368.
10. Horowitz ML, Schiff M, Samuels J, Russo R, Schnader J: Pneumocystis carinii pleural effusion. Pathogenesis and pleural fluid analysis. Am Rev Respir Dis 1993;148:232-234.
11. Jayes RL, Kamerow HN, Hasselquist SM, Delaney MD, Parenti DM: Disseminated pneumocystosis presenting as a pleural effusion. Chest 1993;103:306-308.
12. Jones BE, Young SMM, Antoniskis D, Davidson PT, Kramer F, Barnes PF: Relationship of the manifestations of tuberculosis to CD4 cell counts in patients with human immunodeficiency virus infection. Am Rev Respir Dis 1993;148:1292-1297.
13. Relkin F, Aranda CP, Garay SM, Smith R, Berkowitz KA, Rom WN: Pleural tuberculosis and HIV infection. Chest 1994;105:1338-1341.
14. Hsu WH, Chiang CD, Huang PL: Diagnostic value of pleural adenosine deaminase in tuberculous effusions of immunocompromised hosts. J Formosan Med Assoc 1993;92:668-670.
15. Villena V, Lopez-Encuetra A, Echave-Sustaeta J, Martin-Escribano P, Ortuno-de-Solo B, Estenoz-Alfaro J: Diagnosis of pleural tuberculosis using pleural interferon gamma. Am J Resp Crit Care Med 1994;149:A1103.
16. Newman TG, Soni A, Acaron S, Huang CT: Pleural cryptococcosis in the acquired immune deficiency syndrome. Chest 1987;91:459-460.
17. Ankobiah WA, Vaidya K, Powell S, Carrasco M, Allam A, Chechani V, Kamholz SL: Disseminated histoplasmosis in AIDS. Clinicopathologic features in seven patients from a non-endemic area. NY State J Med 1990;90:234-238.
18. Uttamchandani RB, Daikos GL, Reyes RR, Fischl MA, Dickinson GM, Yamaguchi E, Kramer MR: Nocardiosis in 30 patients with advanced human immunodeficiency virus infection: clinical features and outcome. Clin Infect Dis 1994;18:348-353.
19. Aronchick JM, Miller WT: Disseminated nontuberculous mycobacterial infections in immunosuppressed patients. Sem Roentgenol 1993;28:150-157.
20. Alptekin F: An epidemic of pleurisy with effusion in Bitlis, Turkey: study of 559 cases. US Armed Forces Med J 1958;9:1-11.
21. Fine NL, Smith LR, Sheedy PF: Frequency of pleural effusions in mycoplasma and viral pneumonias. N Engl J Med 1970;283:790-793.
22. Light RW, Girard WM, Jenkinson SG, George RB: Parapneumonic effusions. Am J Med 1980;69:507-511.
23. Monath TP, Maher M, Casals J, et al: Lassa fever in the Eastern Province of Sierra Leone, 1970-1972. II. Clinical observations and virological studies on selected hospital cases. Am J Trop Med Hyg 1974;23:1140-1149.

24. Gross PA, Gerding DN: Pleural effusion associated with viral hepatitis. Gastroenterology 1971;60:898–902.

25. Cho CT, Hiatt WO, Behbehami AM: Pneumonia and massive pleural effusion associated with adenovirus type 7. Am J Dis Child 1973;126:92–94.

26. Goodman ZD, Gupta PK, Frost JK, Erozan YS: Cytodiagnosis of viral infections in body cavity fluids. Acta Cytol 1979;23:204–208.

27. Charles RE, Katz RL, Ordonez NG, MacKay B: Varicella-zoster infection with pleural involvement. Am J Clin Pathol 1986;85:522–526.

28. Speer ME, Schaffer RL, Barrett FF: Adenovirus type 7 pneumonia associated with a large pleural effusion. South Med J 1977;70:119–120.

29. Simila S, Ylikorkala O, Wasz-Hockert O: Type 7 adenovirus pneumonia. J Pediatr 1971;79:605–611.

30. Katsilabros L, Triandafillou G, Kontoyiannis P, Katsilabros N: Pleural effusion and hepatitis. Gastroenterology 1972;63:718.

31. Cocchi P, Silenzi M: Pleural effusion in HB$_s$AG-positive hepatitis. J Pediatr 1976;89:329–330.

32. Owen RL, Shapiro H: Pleural effusion, rash, and anergy in icteric hepatitis. N Engl J Med 1974;291:963–964.

33. Tabor E, Russell RP, Gerety RJ, et al: Hepatitis B surface antigen and e antigen in pleural effusion: a case report. Gastroenterology 1977;73:1157–1159.

34. Sposito M, Petroni VA, Valeri L: Importanza diagnostica dei piccoli versamenti pleurici nella virus epatite. Epatologia 1966;12:228–231.

35. Lee HS, Yang PM, Liu BF, Lee CL, Hsu HC, Su IJ, Chen DS: Pleural effusion coinciding with acute exacerbations in a patient with chronic hepatitis B. Gastroenterology 1989;96:1604–1606.

36. Lander P, Palayew MJ: Infectious mononucleosis: a review of chest roentgenographic manifestations. J Can Assoc Radiol 1974;25:303–306.

37. Fermaglich DR: Pulmonary involvement in infectious mononucleosis. J Pediatr 1975;86:93–95.

38. Sarkar TK: Infectious mononucleosis with pleural effusion. Chest 1969;56:359–360.

39. Levy H, Simpson SQ: Hantavirus pulmonary syndrome. Am J Respir Crit Care Med 1994;149:1710–1713.

40. Duchin JS, Koster FT, Peters CJ, Simpson GL, Tempest B, Zaki SR, Ksiazek TG, Rollin PE, Nichol S, Umland ET, et al: Hantavirus pulmonary syndrome: a clinical description of 17 patients with a newly recognized disease. The Hantavirus Study Group. N Engl J Med 1994;330:949–955.

41. Milder JE, McDearmon SC, Walzer PD: Presumed respiratory syncytial virus pneumonia in an adolescent compromised host. South Med J 1979;72:1195–1198.

42. Fulginiti VA, Eller JJ, Downie AW, Kempe CH: Altered reactivity to measles virus. JAMA 1967;202:1075–1080.

43. Mansel JK, Rosenow EC III, Smith TF, Martin JW Jr: *Mycoplasma pneumoniae* pneumonia. Chest 1989;95:639–646.

44. Decancq HG Jr, Lee FA: *Mycoplasma pneumoniae* pneumonia. JAMA 1965;194;1010–1011.

45. Grix A, Giammona ST: Pneumonitis with pleural effusion in children due to *Mycoplasma pneumoniae*. Am Rev Respir Dis 1974;109:665–671.

46. Nagayama Y, Sakurai N, Tamai K, et al: Isolation of *Mycoplasma pneumoniae* from pleural fluid and/or cerebrospinal fluid: report of four cases. Scand J Infect Dis 1987;19:521–524.

47. Sobradillo V, Ansola P, Baranda F, Corral C: Q fever pneumonia: a review of 164 community-acquired cases in the Basque country. Eur Respir J 1989;2:263–266.

48. Gordon JK, MacKeen AD, Marrie TJ, Fraser DB: The radiographic features of epidemic and sporadic Q fever pneumonia. J Can Assoc Radiol 1984;35:293–296.

49. Esteban C, Oribe M, Fernandez A, Ramos J, Capelastegui A: Increased adenosine deaminase activity in Q fever pneumonia with pleural effusion. Chest 1994;105:648.

50. Murphy PP, Richardson SG: Q fever pneumonia presenting as an eosinophilic pleural effusion. Thorax 1989;44:228–229.

CHAPTER 14

Pleural Effusion Due to Pulmonary Embolization

The disorder most commonly overlooked in the workup of a patient with pleural effusion is pulmonary embolization. The possibility of pulmonary embolization should be excluded in every patient with a pleural effusion of uncertain origin.

INCIDENCE

Moser has estimated that at least 500,000 persons have a pulmonary embolic event each year in this country (1). Because pleural effusions occur in 30 to 50% of patients with pulmonary emboli (2–4) over 100,000 pleural effusions secondary to pulmonary emboli should occur annually. Therefore, one should expect to see more cases of pleural effusions secondary to pulmonary embolization than to bronchogenic carcinoma. Nevertheless, in most large series, pulmonary embolization accounts for fewer than 5% of the pleural effusions (5, 6). This discrepancy probably occurs because the diagnosis is frequently not considered in patients with undiagnosed pleural effusions. Indeed in a recent epidemiological study from the Czech Republic, pulmonary embolism was the fourth leading cause of pleural effusion (7).

It is likely that pulmonary embolism is responsible for a substantial fraction of undiagnosed pleural effusions. Gunnels followed 27 patients with exudative pleural effusions in whom no diagnosis was established after an initial workup including pleural biopsy (8). Of the 19 patients that did not have malignant disease, 2 subsequently died, and both had pulmonary emboli at autopsy. One wonders how many of the remaining 17 patients might have had pulmonary emboli if this diagnosis had been considered. Along the same lines, Storey and coworkers reported a series of 133 patients with pleural effusions in which only 3 were due to pulmonary emboli, but causes were not determined in 25 patients (6). In this article, the authors do not suggest obtaining lung scans in patients with undiagnosed pleural effusions. Again, one wonders how many of the 25 patients would have been switched from the undetermined category to the pulmonary embolus category if lung scans or pulmonary arteriograms had been routinely obtained.

PATHOPHYSIOLOGIC MECHANISMS

Pulmonary embolization appears to produce a pleural effusion by two distinct mechanisms. First, the obstruction of the pulmonary vasculature can lead to the development of right-sided heart failure and increased pressures in the capillaries in the parietal pleura. This increased pressure increases pleural fluid formation (see Chapter 2) and can lead to pleural fluid accumulation (9). The pleural fluid is a transudate with this mechanism. In the series of Bynum and Wilson of 29 patients with pleural effusions secondary to pulmonary embolization, 7 (24%) had transudative pleural effusions (10).

The second mechanism by which pulmonary emboli can produce pleural effusion is by increasing the permeability of the capillaries in the lung. The interstitial fluid that results from this increased permeability traverses the visceral pleura and leads to the accumulation of pleural fluid. In the experimental situation it has been shown (11) that more than 20% of the fluid formed in the lung with increased-permeability pulmonary edema is cleared through the pleural space. It is probable that ischemia of the capillaries in the visceral pleura plays at most a minor role because these capillaries are supplied by the bronchial circulation (12). Leckie and Tothill (13) have demonstrated that patients with exudative pleural effusion secondary to pulmonary emboli have a large amount of protein entering and leaving the pleural space. The main factor responsible for the increased permeability of the pulmonary capillaries is probably the release of inflammatory mediators from the platelet-rich thrombi. The release of the mediators can increase the permeability of the capillaries in either the visceral pleura or the lung. Ischemia of the capillaries distal to the embolus may also contribute to the increased permeability.

CLINICAL MANIFESTATIONS

Symptoms and Signs

The symptoms of patients with pulmonary emboli and pleural effusion are no different from the symptoms of patients with pulmonary emboli and no pleural effusion. Over 75% of patients have pleuritic chest pain (14) which is almost invariably on the side of the effusion (2). Indeed, the presence of pleuritic chest pain in a patient with pleural effusion is suggestive of pulmonary embolus. In one series pulmonary emboli were present in 12 of 22 patients (55%) below the age of 40 who presented as outpatients with pleural effusion and pleuritic chest pain (15). Dyspnea, also present in more than 70% of patients (14, 16), is usually out of proportion to the size of the pleural effusion. Cough and apprehension are present in approximately 50% of patients (14, 16). Nearly 50% of these patients are febrile (16) but less than 10% have temperatures above 38.5°C (14, 16). Approximately 15% have hemoptysis (14). Most patients have a respiratory rate above 20/min, and tachycardia above 100/min occurs in about 30% (14). In the Perspective Investigation of Pulmonary Embolism Diagnosis (PIOPED) study, 113 of 117 patients (97%) with no pre-existing cardiac or pulmonary disease had dyspnea or tachypnea or pleuritic chest pain (14).

Chest Radiograph

When a pleural effusion is secondary to pulmonary emboli, an associated parenchymal infiltrate may or may not be present. In one series of 62 patients with pleural effusions secondary to pulmonary embolism, 28 (45%) had no associated infiltrate (2), but in another series of 20 patients (17) only 1 (5%) did not

have an associated infiltrate. In a third series of 10 patients with pulmonary emboli and bilateral pleural effusions, only 3 (30%) had parenchymal infiltrates (18). Infiltrates are usually in the lower lobes, are pleural-based, and are convex toward the hilum. Patients with an embolic occlusion of segmental pulmonary arteries are more likely to have infiltrates than those with an embolic occlusion of the central arteries (17).

The pleural effusions secondary to pulmonary emboli are small, with the mean size equal to about 15% of the hemithorax (2). In the PIOPED study 48 of the 56 effusions (86%) were manifest only as blunting of the costophrenic angle and in no patient did the pleural effusion occupy more than one-third of a hemithorax (14). If parenchymal infiltrates are present, the pleural effusions are larger. In one series, the pleural effusion occupied greater than 15% of the hemithorax in 74% of the patients with parenchymal infiltrates, but in only 21% of those without parenchymal infiltrates (2). The pleural effusions are usually unilateral even if bilateral pulmonary emboli are present (2). but occasionally may be bilateral (2, 18).

Pleural Fluid Findings

In patients with pulmonary emboli, analysis of the pleural fluid is not helpful in establishing the diagnosis because the pleural fluid associated with pulmonary emboli can vary widely. Nevertheless, a thoracentesis should be performed in patients suspected of having pulmonary emboli to exclude other causes of pleural effusion such as tuberculosis, malignant disease, or pneumonia with a parapneumonic effusion.

As mentioned previously, the pleural fluid may be either a transudate or an exudate, depending upon the mechanism of its production. The pleural fluid is not always blood-tinged or bloody. The pleural fluid red blood cell count (RBC) is below 10,000/mm^3 in about 30% of effusions secondary to pulmonary emboli, whether transudates or exudates. The pleural fluid RBC exceeds 100,000/mm^3 in fewer than 20% of such effusions (10). The pleural fluid white blood cell count (WBC) ranges from under 100 to over 50,000 cells/

mm³ (10). The differential WBC may reveal predominantly polymorphonuclear leukocytes or lymphocytes (10). Spriggs and Boddington have reported that pleural effusions secondary to pulmonary emboli frequently have large numbers of mesothelial cells or eosinophils (19).

DIAGNOSIS

The diagnosis of pulmonary embolization should be considered in every patient with a pleural effusion. Because the patient may or may not have fever, chest pain, or a parenchymal infiltrate, and because the pleural fluid may be either a transudate or an exudate, a perfusion lung scan should be obtained in all patients with pleural effusions when the origin of the effusion is not apparent. Even patients with pleural effusions and obvious congestive heart failure may have pulmonary emboli. In an autopsy series of 290 patients with congestive heart failure and pleural effusions, 60 (21%) had pulmonary emboli (20).

Lung Scans

The perfusion lung scan must be interpreted with caution in the patient with pleural effusion (Fig. 14.1). A large effusion severely restricts the ability of the lung to expand and causes a shift of perfusion to the contralateral lung (21). Small, mobile effusions of any origin may gravitate to different regions of the pleural space, depending upon the position of the patient at the time of the examination. For

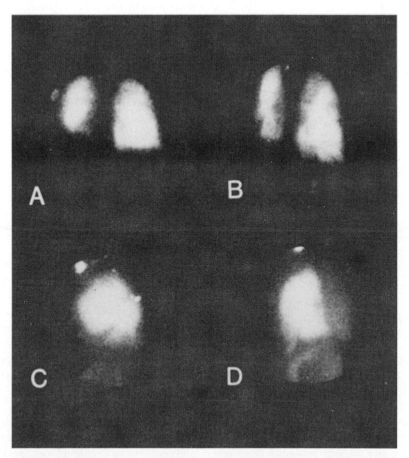

Figure 14.1. Influence of pleural fluid on lung scans. Posterior perfusion lung scans with the patient upright (**A**) and in the left lateral decubitus (**B**) position from a patient with a left pleural effusion. Note the marked difference in the configuration of the left lung as the patient's position is changed, owing to shifts in the pleural fluid. Left lateral scans with the same patient upright (**C**) and supine (**D**). The perfusion defect seen posteriorly with the patient upright disappears when the patient is supine. (Courtesy of Norah Milne, M.D.)

example, fluid may enter the major fissures when the patient lies down, to produce a perfusion defect on the lung scan, when no comparable defect is seen on the erect chest radiograph. Similarly, mismatching of the ventilation and perfusion lung scans can be produced by the pleural fluid itself when the scans are obtained in different positions (Fig. 14.1) (21). For these reasons, a therapeutic thoracentesis (see Chapter 23) should be performed prior to obtaining the lung scan whenever feasible.

If the perfusion scan is abnormal, a ventilation lung scan should be obtained. Typically, the lung scans are interpreted as being normal or suggesting pulmonary emboli with a high probability, an intermediate probability, or a low probability. In the PIOPED study 87% of the patients (102/116) had an arteriographically proven embolus if the lung scan showed a high probability, 33% had emboli (105/322) if the lung scan had intermediate probability, 16% if the lung scan showed low probability (39/238) and 9% if the lung scan was normal or near normal (5/55) (22). Therefore, if the lung scan shows a high probability, the patient probably has a pulmonary embolus; while if the lung scan shows a low probability or is normal, the patient probably does not have an embolus. However, the most common lung scan result in patients suspected of having pulmonary embolus is intermediate, and additional studies should be done to diagnose pulmonary embolus if this is the result. In many patients a pulmonary arteriogram is required to determine definitively whether a pulmonary embolus is present.

Impedance Plethysmogram and Venogram

Another approach for establishing the diagnosis of pulmonary emboli is to study the veins in the legs. The basis for this approach is that over 90% of pulmonary emboli originate from the deep venous system in the legs. Therefore, if the deep venous system of the legs is normal, the patient probably does not have a pulmonary embolus. Electrical impedance plethysmography (IPG) has been extensively evaluated during the last decade for its utility as a screening test for pulmonary embolism. It does not appear sufficiently sensitive to serve as a good screening test for pulmonary emboli. In one series of 83 patients with pulmonary emboli demonstrated angiographically, only 36 (43%) had a positive IPG (23). Similarly, in another series of 41 patients with pulmonary emboli, only 71% had positive venograms of the lower extremities (24). Accordingly, it appears that neither IPG nor lower-extremity venograms are good screening tests for patients suspected of having pulmonary emboli.

TREATMENT

The treatment of the patient with pleural effusion secondary to pulmonary embolization is the same as for any patient with pulmonary emboli. Initially, the patient should be given intravenous heparin or thrombolytic therapy with subsequent oral anticoagulants or subcutaneous heparin, 5000 U every 8 to 12 hours. With treatment, pleural effusions gradually resolve, particularly if no infiltrates are present. In one series, the effusions had cleared completely after 7 days of therapy in 18 of 28 patients (64%) without parenchymal infiltrates, but in none of 30 patients with parenchymal infiltrates (2).

The presence of bloody pleural fluid is not a contraindication to the administration of heparin or thrombolytic agents. Bynum and Wilson treated three patients who had pleural fluid RBC greater than 100,000/mm^3 with intravenous heparin, and in none did the effusion increase in size (10).

If the pleural effusion increases in size with therapy, or if a contralateral pleural effusion develops, the patient probably has recurrent emboli or another complication. In one series, two patients developed an enlarged ipsilateral effusion and one had recurrent pulmonary emboli, whereas the other had developed infected pleural fluid (2). Two other patients developed contralateral pleural effusions, and both had recurrent emboli.

On rare occasions, the administration of anticoagulants to patients with pulmonary emboli can lead to the development of a hemothorax. Rostand and coworkers (24) reviewed 11 such cases and reported that the clotting studies were within an acceptable range when the hemothorax occurred in 7 of the patients. Hemothorax developed within the 1st week of anticoagulation in 9 of the 11 reported cases and developed on the side of the embolus in each of these patients. In 2 patients the hemothorax developed while they were receiving long-term anticoagulation. When a pleural effusion increases in size in a patient with pulmonary emboli, a diagnostic thoracentesis should be performed to rule out a complicated parapneumonic effusion or a hemothorax. If bloody pleural fluid is obtained, the hematocrit of the pleural fluid should be determined. If the hematocrit on the pleural fluid is greater than 50% that of the peripheral blood, anticoagulation should be discontinued, and chest tubes should be inserted (see Chapter 20).

REFERENCES

1. Moser KM: Pulmonary embolism. In: Textbook of Respiratory Medicine. Murray JF, Nadel JA, eds. Philadelphia: WB Saunders, 1994;2:1652-1678.

2. Bynum LJ, Wilson JE III: Radiographic features of pleural effusions in pulmonary embolism. Am Rev Respir Dis 1978;117:829-834.

3. Worsley DF, Alavi A, Aronchick JM, Chen JTT, Greenspan RH, Ravin CE: Chest radiographic findings in patients with acute pulmonary embolism: observations from the PIOPED study. Radiology 1993;189:133-136.

4. Stein PD, Athanasoulis C, Greenspan RH, Henry JW: Relation of plain chest radiographic findings to pulmonary arterial pressure and arterial blood oxygen levels in patients with acute pulmonary embolism. Am J Cardiol 1992;69:394-396.

5. Lowell JR: Pleural Effusions. A Comprehensive Review. Baltimore: University Park Press, 1977.

6. Storey DD, Dines DE, Coles DT: Pleural effusion: a diagnostic dilemma. JAMA 1976;236:2183-2186.

7. Marel M, Arustova M, Stasny B, Light RW: Incidence of pleural effusion in a well-defined region: Epidemiologic study in Central Bohemia. Chest 1993;104: 1486-1489.

8. Gunnels JJ: Perplexing pleural effusion. Chest 1978; 74:390-393.

9. Mellins RB, Levine OR, Fishman AP: Effect of systemic and pulmonary venous hypertension on pleural and pericardial fluid accumulation. J Appl Physiol 1970;29:564-569.

10. Bynum LJ, Wilson JE III: Characteristics of pleural effusions associated with pulmonary embolism. Arch Intern Med 1976;136:159-162.

11. Wiener-Kronish JP, Broaddus VC, Albertine KH, et al: Relationship of pleural effusions to increased permeability pulmonary edema in anesthetized sheep. J Clin Invest 1988;82:1422-1429.

12. Albertine KH, Wiener-Kronish JP, Roos PJ, Staub NC: Structure, blood supply, and lymphatic vessels of the sheep's visceral pleura. Am J Anat 1982;165;277-294.

13. Leckie WJH, Tothill P: Albumin turnover in pleural effusions. Clin Sci 1965;29:339-352.

14. Stein PD, Terrin ML, Hales CA, Palevsky HI, Saltzman HA, Thompson T, Weg JG: Clinical, laboratory, roentgenographic, and electrocardiographic findings in patients with acute pulmonary embolism and no pre-existing cardiac or pulmonary disease. Chest 1991;100:598-603.

15. Branch WR, McNeil BJ: Analysis of the differential diagnosis and assessment of pleuritic chest pain in young adults. Am J Med 1983;75:671-679.

16. Bell WR, Simon TL, DeMets DL: The clinical features of submassive and massive pulmonary emboli. Am J Med 1977;62:355-360.

17. Dalen JE, et al.: Pulmonary embolism, pulmonary hemorrhage and pulmonary infarction. N Engl J Med 1977;296:1431-1435.

18. Rabin CB, Blackman NS: Bilateral pleural effusion: its significance in association with a heart of normal size. J Mt Sinai Hosp 1957;24:45-63.

19. Spriggs AI, Boddington MM: The Cytology of Effusions. 2nd ed. New York: Grune & Stratton, 1968.

20. Race GA, Scheifley CH, Edward JE: Hydrothorax in congestive heart failure. Am J Med 1957;22:83-89.

21. Baum S, Vincent NR, Lyons KP, et al: Atlas of Nuclear Medicine Imaging. New York: Appleton-Century-Crofts, 1981.

22. The PIOPED Investigators: Value of the ventilation/perfusion scan in acute pulmonary embolism. JAMA 1990;263:2753-2759.

23. Hull RD, Hirsh J, Carter CJ, et al: Pulmonary angiography, ventilation lung scanning, and venography for clinically suspected pulmonary embolism with abnormal perfusion lung scan. Ann Intern Med 1983;98: 891-899.

24. Rostand RA, Feldman RL, Block ER: Massive hemothorax complicating heparin anticoagulation for pulmonary embolus. South Med J 1977;70:1128-1130.

CHAPTER 15

Pleural Effusion Secondary to Diseases of the Gastrointestinal Tract

Disease of the gastrointestinal tract is sometimes associated with pleural effusion. In this chapter, the exudative pleural effusions resulting from pancreatic disease, intra-abdominal abscesses, esophageal perforation, abdominal operations, diaphragmatic hernia, variceal sclerotherapy, hepatic transplantation, and disease of the biliary tract are discussed. The transudative pleural effusion occurring with cirrhosis and ascites is discussed in Chapter 6.

PANCREATIC DISEASE

Three different types of nonmalignant pancreatic disease can have an accompanying pleural effusion: acute pancreatitis, chronic pancreatitis with pseudocyst, and pancreatic ascites.

Acute Pancreatitis

The reported incidence of pleural effusion with acute pancreatitis ranges from 3 to 17% (1, 2). Most of the reported series have been retrospective, and probably at least 20% of patients with acute pancreatitis have pleural effusions. Pleural effusions appear to be more common in patients with pancreatitis due to alcohol abuse than in those with pancreatitis due to biliary tract disease (2). The incidence of pleural effusion is higher in patients with more severe pancreatitis and in those with a pancreatic pseudocyst (2). The majority of pleural effusions secondary to acute pancreatic disease are unilateral and left-sided, but they may be right-sided or bilateral. In a review of 80 pleural effusions secondary to pancreatic disease, Kaye found that 48 were left-sided, 24 were right-sided, and 8 were bilateral (1).

The exudative pleural effusion accompanying acute pancreatitis results primarily from the transdiaphragmatic transfer of the exudative fluid arising from acute pancreatic inflammation (2). Numerous lymphatic networks join the peritoneal and pleural aspects of the diaphragm (1). Anatomically, the tail of the pancreas is in direct contact with the diaphragm. Hence the exudate resulting from acute pancreatic inflammation, rich in pancreatic enzymes, enters the lymphatic vessels on the peritoneal side of the diaphragm and is conveyed to the pleural side of the diaphragm. Because this fluid contains high levels of pancreatic enzymes, the permeability of the lymphatic vessels is increased, and fluid leaks from the pleural lymphatic vessels into the pleural space. The high enzymatic content of the pancreatic exudate may also cause partial or complete obstruction of the pleural lymphatic vessels, which leads to more pleural fluid formation (1). Of course, the diaphragm itself may be inflamed from the adjacent inflammatory process, and this inflammation may increase the permeability of the capillaries in the diaphragmatic pleura. This mechanism cannot be entirely responsible for the pleural fluid accumulation, however, because the pleural fluid amylase concentration is almost always higher than the simultaneous serum amylase.

In the patient with acute pancreatitis, the clinical picture is usually dominated by abdominal symptoms including pain, nausea, and vomiting. At times, however, respiratory symptoms consisting of pleuritic chest pain and dyspnea may dominate the clinical picture. The chest radiograph may reveal, in addition to the small-to-moderate-sized pleural effusion, an elevated, sluggish, or immobile diaphragm and basilar infiltrates (3). The clinical picture may look much like that of pneumonia or pulmonary embolism complicated by pleural effusion. A pleural fluid amylase determination should be obtained for all patients with acute chest symptoms and an exudative pleural effusion, as well as in those with abdominal symptoms and a pleural effusion.

The diagnosis is established in most cases by demonstrating an elevated pleural fluid amylase level. Kaye reviewed 40 patients with pleural effusions secondary to pancreatic disease and found that the pleural fluid amylase level was elevated in 90% (1). Ball and I reported five patients with pleural effusions secondary to pancreatic disease (4), and in one of the patients, the pleural fluid amylase was originally within normal limits for serum. Subsequent pleural fluid amylase levels were elevated, however. The pleural fluid amylase level is usually higher than the serum amylase (1, 4) and remains elevated longer than the serum amylase. The pleural fluid amylase level in patients with acute pancreatitis and pleural effusion tends to be lower than that in patients with chronic pancreatic disease (2).

Other tests on the pleural fluid are not diagnostic for pleural effusions secondary to pancreatic disease. The pleural fluid is an exudate with high protein and lactic acid dehydrogenase (LDH) levels. Frequently, the pleural fluid is serosanguineous, and it can be bloody. The pleural fluid glucose level is comparable to that of the serum (4). The pleural fluid differential white blood cell count (WBC) usually reveals predominantly polymorphonuclear leukocytes, and the pleural fluid WBC can vary from 1,000 to 50,000 cells/mm^3 (4).

In the patient with acute pancreatitis, the pleural effusion usually resolves as the pancreatic inflammation subsides. If the pleural effusion does not resolve within 2 weeks of treatment of the pancreatic disease, the possibility of a pancreatic abscess or a pancreatic pseudocyst must be considered.

Pancreatic Abscess

Pancreatic abscess usually follows an episode of acute pancreatitis. Typically, the acute pancreatitis initially responds to therapy, but 10 to 21 days later the patient becomes febrile with abdominal pain and leukocytosis (5). The diagnosis is also suggested if a patient with acute pancreatitis does not respond to the usual therapy within several days (5). It is important to establish the diagnosis because the mortality rate approaches 100% if the abscess is not drained surgically (5). Both

ultrasound (5) and abdominal computed tomography (CT) scanning (6) are useful in establishing the diagnosis of pancreatic abscess preoperatively. Pleural effusion occurs commonly in patients with pancreatic abscess. In one series of 63 patients, 38% had pleural effusions (5). Although pleural fluid findings were not described in this series, another patient with a pleural effusion associated with pancreatic abscess had a high pleural fluid amylase level (7).

The other complication that can cause a pleural effusion to persist in patients with acute pancreatitis is a pancreatic pseudocyst.

Pancreatic Pseudocyst and Chronic Pancreatic Pleural Effusion

A pancreatic pseudocyst is not a true cyst, but rather a collection of fluid and debris rich in pancreatic enzymes near or within the pancreas. The walls consist of granulation tissue without an epithelial lining (8). About 10% of patients with acute pancreatitis have a clinically significant pseudocyst (9). Approximately 5% of patients with a pancreatic pseudocyst will have a pleural effusion (9). Pleural effusions due to pancreatic pseudocysts are relatively uncommon. By 1990 only 96 cases had been reported in the English literature (9). Between 1983 and 1989 there were only seven cases at the Moffitt-Long and San Francisco General Hospitals (9).

The mechanism responsible for the pleural effusion in patients with a chronic pseudocyst is the development of a direct sinus tract between the pancreas and the pleural space (7, 10). When the pancreatic ductal system is disrupted, the extruded pancreatic fluid sometimes passes through the aortic or esophageal hiatus into the mediastinum. Once in the mediastinum, the process either can be contained, to form a mediastinal pseudocyst, or it may decompress into one or both pleural spaces. Once fluid enters the pleural space, the pancreaticopleural fistula is likely to result in a massive chronic pleural effusion.

Most patients with chronic pancreatic pleural effusion are males and over 90% have their pancreatic disease due to alcoholism (9, 11). Chest symptoms usually dominate the clinical picture of the patient with chronic pancreatic disease and a pleural effusion (11). These patients complain of chest pain and shortness of breath. In one series of 101 patients from Japan, 42 complained of dyspnea and 29 complained of chest and back pain, while only 23 complained of upper abdominal pain (11). The explanation for the lack of abdominal symptoms is that the pancreaticopleural fistula decompresses the pseudocyst. Weight loss is common in patients with chronic pancreatic pleural effusions (9). The pleural effusion is usually large, sometimes occupying the entire hemithorax. In the majority of cases the effusion is unilateral left-sided, but about 20% are unilateral right-sided, and 15% are bilateral (9, 11). If a therapeutic thoracentesis is performed, the pleural effusion will reaccumulate rapidly. In one patient, more than 13 L pleural fluid were removed during three separate thoracenteses over a short period (12). Because chest symptoms dominate the clinical picture and some patients have no history of prior pancreatic disease, the diagnosis is easily missed unless the pleural fluid amylase is measured.

The diagnosis of a chronic pancreatic pleural effusion should be suspected in any individual with a large pleural effusion who appears to be chronically ill or has a history of pancreatic disease or abdominal trauma (13). Many patients have no history of pancreatic disease (9). The best screening test for chronic pancreatic pleural effusion is to measure the pleural fluid amylase. The pleural fluid amylase is usually markedly elevated (more than 1000 U/L) (13), whereas the serum amylase may be normal or mildly elevated (13). An elevated pleural fluid amylase level is not diagnostic of pancreatic disease as it also occurs with a ruptured esophagus and with malignant pleural effusions. The origin of the amylase with esophageal rupture is salivary rather than pancreatic (14). The clinical picture with esophageal rupture, discussed later in this chapter, is usually sufficiently characteristic to make the diagnosis apparent if it is considered, but at times it can be confused with acute pancreatitis.

The other main diagnosis to consider in a patient with a chronic pleural effusion with a high amylase level is malignant disease. Approximately 10% of patients with a malignant pleural effusion have an elevated pleural fluid amylase level (4). The differentiation can be made by obtaining amylase isoenzymes on the pleural fluid. With malignant effusions, the amylase is of the salivary rather than the pancreatic type (15).

The diagnosis can usually be established by CT of the chest and abdomen, which frequently shows both the pseudocyst and the sinus tract (9). Endoscopic retrograde cholangiopancreatography (ERCP) also plays an important role in the evaluation and management of patients with pancreaticopleural fistula. ERCP is useful in delineating the ductal structure, the pseudocyst, and the fistulous connection to the pleura via the sinus tract (9). The greatest utility for ERCP is in defining the precise anatomical relationship preoperatively so that a direct and expeditious surgical procedure can be planned.

The initial therapy of a patient with a pancreatic pseudocyst and a pleural effusion should probably be nonoperative. The theory behind conservative therapy is that if pancreatic secretions are minimized, the pseudocyst will regress and the sinus tract will close. Accordingly a nasogastric tube is inserted and the patient is given intravenous hyperalimentation. It is probable that the patients are also benefited if they are given somatostatin or octreotide, a synthetic analog of somatostatin (16). Somatostatin has numerous inhibitory actions on gastrointestinal functions, one of which is its inhibitory effect on pancreatic exocrine secretion (9). It has been shown that somatostatin decreases the output from external pancreatic fistulas by over 80% (17). Some authors recommend serial thoracentesis and subsequent tube thoracostomy if the effusions recur, but there in no evidence that such procedures are beneficial.

If after 2 weeks the patient remains symptomatic and the pleural fluid continues to accumulate, surgical intervention should be considered. Approximately 50% of patients will require surgery. Surgery is more likely to be required in patients with more severe pancreatic disease (16). Prior to surgery an endoscopic retrograde pancreatogram and an abdominal CT scan should be performed to aid in planning the surgical procedure (18). For example, if a leak from the duct or pseudocyst is demonstrated in the distal portion of the gland, distal pancreatectomy will be curative. If a direct pancreatic duct leak is found in the more proximal portion of the gland, without a pseudocyst, a direct anastomosis between the leak and a Roux-en-Y jejunal loop or a Whipple resection should be considered. Conversely, if a large cyst is present within the body of the gland, internal drainage should be performed either into the stomach or with a Roux-en-Y jejunal loop. Procedures that do not focus on removal of the disrupted portion of the gland or on drainage of the pseudocyst usually fail. If the preoperative ERCP is unsuccessful, pancreatography may be performed at the time of surgery (9).

An alternative approach to the patient with a pancreatic pseudocyst is to drain the pseudocyst percutaneously. Under CT control a catheter is introduced through the anterior abdominal wall through the anterior and then the posterior stomach wall and then into the pseudocyst cavity. Side holes are cut into the part of the catheter that lies in the pseudocyst and in the stomach. Maintenance of this drainage for 15 to 20 days is thought to create a fistulous tract, between the pseudocyst and stomach, akin to surgical marsupialization. In one series 20 of 26 patients (77%) were cured by this procedure (19). To my knowledge there are no randomized studies comparing the results with surgery and with percutaneous drainage of the pseudocyst.

The prognosis of patients with pancreaticopleural fistula appears to be favorable (9). In the series of 96 patients reviewed by Rockey and Cello the overall mortality rate was 5%, and 3 patients died of unrelated illnesses during their follow-up period. Both patients who died as a direct result of the pancreatic process were managed conservatively and died of sepsis (9).

In patients with chronic pleural effusions secondary to pancreatic disease, the pleural surfaces may become thickened, and in several patients, decortications have been performed (20). Because the pleural thickening gradually improves spontaneously, however, decortication should be delayed for at least 6 months following definitive treatment of the pancreatic disease in order to ascertain

whether the pleural disease will resolve spontaneously.

One rare complication of pancreatic pleural effusion is the development of a bronchopleural fistula. Kaye reported one such patient in whom the development of the bronchopleural fistula was heralded by the expectoration of copious quantities of clear yellow fluid (1). In this situation, chest tubes should be inserted immediately to drain the pleural space and to protect the lung from the fluid with its high enzymatic content.

Pancreatic Ascites

Some patients with pancreatic disease develop ascites characterized by high amylase and protein levels (16, 21). The genesis of the ascites is leakage of fluid from a pseudocyst directly into the peritoneal cavity or a sinus tract from the pseudocyst into the peritoneal cavity. If such a patient should happen to have a defect in his diaphragm, he will develop a large pleural effusion as a result of the flow of fluid from the peritoneal to the pleural cavity in the same way that pleural effusions develop secondary to ascites from cirrhosis (see Chapter 6). Approximately 20% of patients with pancreatic ascites have a pleural effusion (21).

Most patients with pancreatic ascites and pleural effusion are initially thought to have cirrhosis and ascites. The diagnosis is easily established if amylase determinations are made on the peritoneal and pleural fluid in such patients (21). The treatment for pancreatic ascites is the same as for pancreatic pleural effusion, except serial paracenteses rather than serial thoracenteses are performed (21).

SUBPHRENIC ABSCESS

Subphrenic abscess continues to be a significant clinical problem despite the development of potent antibiotics.

Incidence

In most large medical centers, between 6 and 15 subphrenic abscesses are seen each year (22–24). Subphrenic abscesses are discussed in this chapter because a pleural effusion is present in approximately 80% of cases.

Pathogenesis

Approximately 80% of subphrenic abscesses follow intra-abdominal surgical procedures (25, 26). Splenectomy is likely to be complicated by a left subphrenic abscess (26), as is gastrectomy. Deck and Berne noted a high incidence of subphrenic abscess after exploratory laparotomy for trauma; in their study, 59% of subphrenic abscesses occurred after such an operation (27). Overall, about 1% of abdominal operations are complicated by subphrenic abscess (24). Sanders reviewed the incidence of subphrenic abscesses following 1566 abdominal surgical procedures at the Radcliffe Infirmary in 1965 and found 15 patients with subphrenic abscess (24). Sanders also reviewed the cases of 23 patients with pleural effusion following intra-abdominal surgical procedures during the same period. He found that 12 of the 23 had definite subphrenic abscesses, and felt that another 5 possibly had subphrenic abscesses.

Subphrenic abscess may also occur without antecedent abdominal surgical procedures. It may result from processes such as gastric, duodenal, or appendiceal perforation, diverticulitis, cholecystitis, pancreatitis, or trauma (25). In such patients, the diagnosis of subphrenic abscess is frequently not considered. In one series of 22 patients in whom abscesses occurred without antecedent abdominal operations, the diagnosis was established prior to death in only 41% (25).

The pathogenesis of the pleural effusion associated with subphrenic abscess is probably related to inflammation of the diaphragm. Although Carter and Brewer proposed that the pleural effusion arose from the transdiaphragmatic transfer of abscess material by the lymphatic vessels (22), this hypothesis is unlikely because fluid from these pleural effusions is only rarely culture-positive. If the pleural effusion arose from the transdiaphragmatic transport of abscess material, bacteria as well as leukocytes should be transported. The diaphragmatic inflammation resulting from the adjacent abscess probably increases the permeability of the capillaries in the diaphragmatic pleura and causes pleural fluid to accumulate.

Clinical Manifestations

The clinical picture with subphrenic abscess can be dominated by either chest or abdominal symptoms. In the series of 125 cases of Carter and Brewer, chest findings dominated the clinical picture in 44% of patients (22). The main chest symptom is pleuritic chest pain. Radiographic abnormalities include pleural effusion, basal pneumonitis, compression atelectasis, and an elevated diaphragm on the affected side. Pleural effusions occur in 60 to 80% of patients (22, 23, 26–28), and are usually small to moderate in size, but may be large, occupying more than 50% of the hemithorax.

Most patients with postoperative subphrenic abscesses have fever, leukocytosis, and abdominal pain (22, 23, 27), but frequently no localizing signs or symptoms are present. The symptoms and signs of subphrenic abscess are variable. In a series of 60 patients, 37% had no abdominal pain, 21% had no abdominal tenderness, 15% had no temperature elevation greater than 39°C, and 8% had no leukocytosis above 10,000/mm^3 (23). The interval between the surgical procedure and the development of the subphrenic abscess is usually 1 to 3 weeks, but can be as long as 5 months (25, 26).

Examination of the pleural fluid from patients with subphrenic abscesses usually reveals an exudate with predominantly polymorphonuclear leukocytes. Although the pleural fluid WBC may approach or may even exceed 50,000/mm^3, the pleural fluid pH and glucose level remain above 7.20 and 60 mg/dl, respectively. It is distinctly uncommon for the pleural fluid to become infected (22). However, empyemas have resulted from contamination of the pleural space when the abscesses were drained percutaneously (29).

Diagnosis

The diagnosis of subphrenic abscess should be suspected in any patient who develops a pleural effusion several days or more after an abdominal surgical procedure or in any other undiagnosed patient who has an exudative pleural effusion containing predominantly polymorphonuclear leukocytes. The chest radiographs from such a patient are shown in Figure 15.1. This patient had left-sided chest pain and a low-grade fever without any abdominal symptoms. Thoracentesis revealed an exudate with a WBC of 29,000, an LDH level of 340 IU/L, a glucose level of 117 mg/dl, and a pH of 7.36. He was treated with parenteral antibiotics for a presumed parapneumonic effusion with little clinical response. Two subsequent thoracenteses revealed similar pleural fluid findings. Two weeks after admission, a gallium scan revealed increased uptake of the gallium in the left upper quadrant (Fig. 15.2). At laparotomy, this patient was found to have a left subphrenic abscess resulting from a colonic perforation secondary to a colonic carcinoma. At no time did this patient have more than mild left upper quadrant tenderness.

Routine chest or abdominal radiographs frequently establish the diagnosis of subphrenic abscess. A pathognomonic radiologic finding is an air-fluid level below the diaphragm outside the gastrointestinal tract. These air-fluid levels are best demonstrated with heavily exposed abdominal films that include the diaphragm, with the patient upright and in the lateral decubitus position (26). In one series of 82 patients, these routine radiographs demonstrated air within the abscess in 70% (26). In over 25% of the patients with air in the abscess, this finding had been overlooked on the initial radiologic interpretation (26). A second radiographic sign sometimes seen on routinely obtained radiographs is displacement of intra-abdominal viscera. Contrast studies including upper gastrointestinal series and barium enemas are helpful in demonstrating extraluminal location of gas, leakage, and deformity or displacement of normal structures. Some investigators have recommended water-soluble contrast material for these studies because of the possibility of perforation or leakage and because retained barium can make subsequent CT scans and ultrasound studies more difficult.

In recent years, CT scans, ultrasound studies, and gallium scans have all proved useful in diagnosing subphrenic abscesses. As demonstrated in Figure 15.2, gallium scans can be helpful in establishing the diagnosis. Gallium scans are not always positive when subphrenic abscesses are present, however. In one series, 4 of 11 patients (36%) with subphrenic abscesses had negative gallium scans (27). Abdominal CT scans are probably the best means by which to establish the diagnosis of subphrenic abscess (30). One advantage of CT scans over gallium scans is that, with CT scans, the precise anatomic location and extent of the abscess can be defined (26). Ultrasonic examination effectively demonstrates fluid-filled abscess cavities, but it is technically difficult in the left subphrenic region because of overlying lung, ribs, and gas in the gastrointestinal tract (26). In one series, ultrasonic examinations were negative in 41% of 22 patients with subphrenic abscesses (27). When a right-sided subphrenic abscess is suspected, combined liver and lung scans are useful in documenting fluid collections between the liver and the lung (31). Because the pleural effusion itself also produces defects between the lung and the liver, however, this procedure is of limited use in the patient with a subphrenic abscess and a pleural effusion.

Treatment and Prognosis

The two main aspects of treatment are the administration of appropriate antibiotics and drainage. Sepsis is an ever present threat to the patient with subphrenic abscess. In a series of 125 cases, 29 patients (23%) developed positive blood cultures, and the mortality rate of these 29 patients was 93% (22). Most subphrenic abscesses contain more than a single organism; *Escherichia coli*, *Staphylococcus aureus*, and anaerobic organisms are most commonly isolated (28). Haaga and Weinstein recommend CT-guided percutaneous aspiration of subphrenic abscesses to identify the responsible organisms before undertaking definitive surgical procedures (32).

Drainage of the subphrenic abscess can be accomplished either percutaneously or with surgery. Since the results seem comparable with the two procedures (33, 34), it is recommended that percutaneous drainage be used in

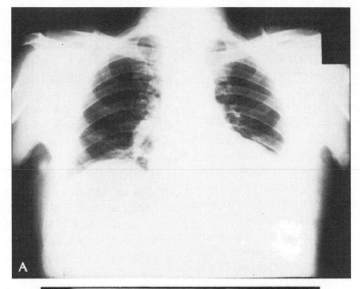

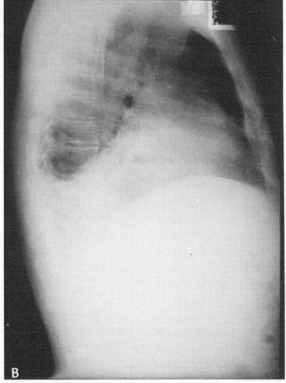

Figure 15.1.   A, Posteroanterior chest radiograph, and **B**, left lateral radiograph, demonstrating elevated left diaphragm and blunting of the left diaphragm posteriorly.

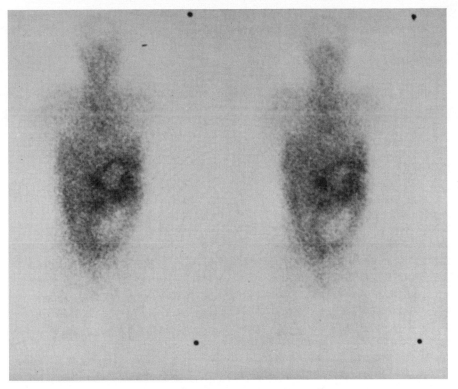

Figure 15.2. Gallium scan from the patient whose radiographs are shown in Figure 15.1. Note the increased activity in the left upper abdominal quadrant with the "cold" spot in the center of the area with the increased uptake.

most cases. Surgical drainage of subphrenic abscesses can be either extraserosal, in which case the peritoneal cavity is not entered, or transperitoneal (28). Extraserosal drainage is indicated if preoperative evaluation reveals a single, well-localized abscess. The transperitoneal approach is recommended if multicentricity is suspected, if the localization of the abscess is not definite, or if a reasonable likelihood of other intra-abdominal pathologic conditions exists. Antibiotics should be given before the drainage procedure is attempted to prevent bacteremia during this procedure.

Mortality rates among patients with subphrenic abscesses remain high, ranging from 20 to 45% (22, 23, 25, 28). Because much of the mortality is due to delayed diagnosis or lack of a diagnosis before autopsy, the possibility of a subphrenic abscess must be considered in every patient with an exudative pleural effusion containing predominantly polymorphonuclear leukocytes. In such patients, heavily penetrated abdominal radiographs should be examined for extravisceral gas, and one should consider obtaining an abdominal CT scan.

INTRAHEPATIC ABSCESS

Pleural effusions accompany intrahepatic abscesses in about 20% of patients (35). The pathogenesis of the pleural fluid and the pleural fluid findings with intrahepatic abscess are similar to those for subphrenic abscess, as previously discussed. Because the mortality rate of patients with untreated liver abscesses approaches 100% (36), the diagnosis of intrahepatic abscess should be considered in every patient with a right-sided exudative pleural effusion with predominantly polymorphonuclear leukocytes on the pleural fluid differential. Amebic liver abscesses are discussed in Chapter 12.

Clinical Manifestations

Most patients with pyogenic intrahepatic abscesses have fever and anorexia (36), and approximately 50% give a history of shaking chills. Abdominal pain is common, but it frequently is not localized to the right upper quadrant. Most patients have an enlarged, tender liver. Laboratory tests usually reveal leukocytosis, anemia, elevated alkaline phosphatase levels, and hyperbilirubinemia. Because none of these findings are invariably present in patients with pyogenic liver abscesses, however, the diagnosis of liver abscess should be pursued in all patients with right-sided exudative pleural effusions containing polymorphonuclear leukocytes.

Diagnosis

The best way to establish the diagnosis of pyogenic liver abscess is by abdominal CT scan (37). With CT scanning, abscesses with diameters as small as 0.5 cm can be readily appreciated. In contrast, the lower limit of resolution by liver scan is about 2 cm (37). Another advantage of CT scanning is that it better defines the exact anatomic location of the abscess and identifies multiple small abscesses, and thereby allows better preoperative planning (37). Abdominal ultrasound studies can also identify fluid-filled intrahepatic lesions (38), but because CT scanning provides more precise anatomic information, it is the procedure of choice. Not all fluid-filled intrahepatic lesions are pyogenic abscesses; cysts, hematomas, and amebic abscesses can produce identical findings on ultrasound studies and CT scans. The definitive diagnosis can be established by percutaneous aspiration guided by CT scanning or ultrasound.

Treatment

The treatment of pyogenic abscess consists of the administration of appropriate parenteral antibiotics and drainage of the abscess. One method of drainage is surgical exploration with the insertion of intrahepatic drains followed by serial CT scans to evaluate the efficacy of the drainage (37). An alternate approach is closed aspiration guided by ultrasound studies (36) or CT scans (39). In one series of 25 patients, 24 were managed solely with antibiotics and aspiration (39). Eighteen abscesses were aspirated only once while four were aspirated twice, two were aspirated three

times and one was aspirated four times (39). If closed aspiration is used, however, it is imperative to perform serial ultrasonic examinations or CT scans to verify the effectiveness of the treatment. If the patient remains ill or if the abscess cavity is not decreasing in size, surgical exploration should be performed without delay.

INTRASPLENIC ABSCESS

Splenic abscess is an unusual entity. In the 30 years between 1950 and 1980 there were only 11 cases diagnosed at Johns Hopkins Hospital (40). In a more recent series from the University of California at Davis Medical Center (41), nine patients were seen between 1980 and 1990. In this latter series, all patients had an associated pleural effusion, but in prior series only 20 to 50% of patients with splenic abscess had a left-sided pleural effusion (40, 42). In most patients, the splenic suppuration arises from primary hematogenous seeding such as with endocarditis. Splenic abscess appears to be more common in individuals with diseases producing splenic abnormalities, such as chronic hemolytic anemia or hemoglobin S (40).

Most but not all patients have localized pain in the left upper quadrant. One combination that is particularly suggestive of the diagnosis is a left pleural effusion plus thrombocytosis. In the series of Ho and Wisner, 7 of 9 patients (78%) had this combination (41). The diagnosis can be made preoperatively by spleen scan, gallium scan, ultrasonography, or CT. The treatment is splenectomy plus antibiotics (41).

ESOPHAGEAL PERFORATION

Esophageal rupture should always be considered in the differential diagnosis of pleural effusions, because if this entity is not rapidly treated, the mortality rate approaches 100%.

Incidence

Esophageal perforation is uncommon. Michel and associates reported only 85 cases at the Massachusetts General Hospital over a 21-year period (43), whereas Abbott and co-workers found 47 cases at the 4 teaching hospitals associated with Emory University School of Medicine over a 20-year period (44). Recently, the incidence of esophageal perforation has increased dramatically, primarily because of the higher incidence of iatrogenic perforation associated with gastrointestinal endoscopy (45, 46). The diagnosis of esophageal rupture should be considered initially in every patient with a pleural effusion who looks acutely ill because the mortality rate increases markedly if treatment is delayed for more than 24 hours (46, 47).

Pathogenesis and Pathophysiologic Mechanisms

Esophageal perforation most commonly arises as a complication of esophagoscopic examination. In one series of 108 cases, 67% occurred as a complication of esophagoscopy (48). Esophageal perforation is particularly common with esophagoscopy when one has attempted to remove a foreign body or to dilate an esophageal stricture (48). Overall, between 0.15 and 0.70% of all esophagoscopic examinations are complicated by esophageal perforation (43, 49). The insertion of a Blakemore tube for esophageal varices can also be complicated by esophageal rupture; this mechanism accounted for 11% of all esophageal perforations in one series (43). Frequently, the diagnosis of esophageal perforation is missed in patients with Blakemore tubes because they are so ill with multiple problems (43).

Esophageal perforations may also arise from foreign bodies themselves, carcinomas, gastric intubation, chest trauma, and chest operations. Finally, esophageal rupture may occur as a complication of vomiting (Boerhaave's syndrome). Spontaneous rupture almost always involves the lower esophagus just above the diaphragm.

The clinical symptoms of esophageal perforation are due to contamination of the mediastinum by oropharyngeal contents to produce an acute mediastinitis. When the mediastinal pleura ruptures, a pleural effusion develops, frequently complicated by a pneumothorax. Most of the morbidity from esophageal perforation is due to the infection of the mediastinum and the pleural space by the oropharyngeal bacterial flora (50).

Clinical Manifestations

With esophageal perforation secondary to esophagoscopic examination, the endoscopist usually does not realize that the esophagus has been perforated (49). Since, however, such patients usually complain of persistent chest or epigastric pain within several hours of the procedure (51), such complaints should serve as indications for an emergency contrast study of the esophagus.

Patients with spontaneous rupture of the esophagus usually have a history of vomiting followed by chest pain (44) and they frequently describe a sensation of tearing or bursting in the lower part of the chest or the epigastrium. The chest pain is characteristically excruciating and is often unrelieved by opiates. Small amounts of hematemesis are present in more than 50% of these patients (44). Dyspnea is frequently a prominent symptom. The presence of subcutaneous emphysema that first appears in the suprasternal notch suggests esophageal perforation, but this emphysema appears late in the course of perforation. In Abbott's series of 47 patients, only 4 (9%) had subcutaneous emphysema within the first 4 hours (44). The clinical picture may be much less dramatic than that described. Chandrasekhara and Levitan described a patient with a ruptured esophagus and symptoms present for 5 days who had only mild distress (52).

In patients with esophageal perforation, the chest radiograph reveals a pleural effusion in about 60% and a pneumothorax in about 25% (43). Most patients with spontaneous rupture have a pleural effusion (53). The pleural effusion is usually left-sided, but it may be right-sided or bilateral. Other radiographic findings may include widening of the mediastinum and visible air within the mediastinal compartments.

Diagnosis

On account of the high mortality rate (as high as 60% (53)) when treatment is delayed for more than 24 hours, the diagnosis of esophageal rupture should be entertained any time one sees a patient with an exudative pleural effusion, particularly when the patient appears acutely ill. Examination of the pleural fluid is helpful in suggesting the diagnosis of esophageal perforation because it is characterized by (*a*) a high amylase level, (*b*) a low pH, (*c*) the presence of squamous epithelial cells, and sometimes (*d*) ingested food particles.

An elevated pleural fluid amylase level appears to be the best indication of esophageal rupture. In the experimental model, the pleural fluid amylase level is elevated within 2 hours of esophageal rupture (41). In one clinical series, all 7 patients with esophageal rupture had elevated pleural fluid amylase levels (44). The origin of the amylase is salivary rather than pancreatic because the saliva, with its high amylase content, enters the pleural space through the defect in the esophagus (14). To my knowledge, in only two reported cases have pleural fluid amylase levels been within normal limits with esophageal perforation and pleural effusion (54, 55). One of these patients (55) had Sjogren's syndrome and essentially no production of saliva. The other (54) had a chronic perforation due to esophageal carcinoma.

The pleural fluid pH is usually decreased with esophageal rupture (56, 57). In fact, Dye and Laforet concluded that a pleural fluid pH below 6.0 was highly suggestive of esophageal rupture and attributed the low pleural fluid pH to the leakage of acidic gastric juice through the esophageal tear (57). Both of these conclusions appear to be wrong. Patients with severe infections of the pleural space and an intact esophagus frequently have a pleural fluid pH below 6.0.

Good and associates demonstrated, in an experimental model, that the pleural fluid pH falls just as rapidly after esophageal perforation when the esophagogastric junction is ligated (58). These authors concluded that leukocyte metabolism was the major contributor to the low pleural fluid pH with esophageal rupture. Nevertheless, the presence of a pleural fluid pH below 7.0 increases the likelihood that the patient has a ruptured esophagus.

Another useful test in diagnosing esophageal perforation is examination of the Wright stain of the pleural fluid for squamous epithelial cells (59). Eriksen demonstrated the presence of squamous epithelial cells in the pleural fluid from all 14 patients with esophageal perforation. Again, as with amylase, the squamous epithelial cells enter the pleural space through the esophageal perforation. Obviously, the demonstration of food particles in pleural fluid is diagnostic of esophageal perforation.

The diagnosis of esophageal perforation is established when esophageal disruption is confirmed by contrast studies of the esophagus. The contrast agent of choice is probably Hexabrix (meglumine and sodium ioxaglate 320 mg I/ml) (60). Barium has a greater radiographic density, better mucosal adherence, and minimal irritation to the tracheobronchial tree, but it is not absorbed once it leaks into the mediastinum or pleura and produces a marked inflammatory reaction in the pleura. When water soluble agents, such as Hexabrix or Gastrografin, are injected in the pleural space, they are almost completely absorbed after 24 hours (60) and neither create much of an inflammatory response. Hexabrix is considered the agent of choice because Gastrografin creates marked bronchospasm when it is aspirated and Hexabrix does not create such a reaction (60). The contrast studies are positive in about 85% of patients (43, 46). If the perforation is small or has already closed spontaneously, the esophagogram may not be diagnostic. It has been suggested that contrast studies of the esophagus when perforation is suspected be done in the decubitus position (45). In this position the contrast material fills the whole length of the esophagus and thereby allows the actual site of the perforation and its interconnecting cavities to be demonstrated in almost all patients (45).

If the esophageal perforation is not demonstrated by the contrast study of the esophagus, a chest CT scan may facilitate the diagnosis (61). White and coworkers performed chest CT scans on 12 patients with esophageal perforation. They found esophageal thickening in nine patients, periesophageal fluid in 11 patients, extraluminal air in 11 patients, and pleural effusion in nine. The site of the perforation was visible on CT scan in two patients.

The finding that most commonly pointed to esophageal rupture was extraluminal air (61).

Treatment

The treatment of choice for esophageal rupture is exploration of the mediastinum with primary repair of the esophageal tear and drainage of the pleural space and mediastinum (44–49). Large doses of parenteral antibiotics should be given to treat the mediastinitis and pleural infection. Although conservative treatment consisting of antibiotics and nasogastric suction is adequate in some patients with esophageal perforation (43, 48, 62), in patients with pleural effusion or pneumothorax complicating esophageal perforation, mediastinal exploration should be performed. It is crucial to perform the mediastinal exploration as an emergency as soon as the diagnosis is established because a delay of even 12 hours increases the mortality rate (53). If exploration of the mediastinum is delayed for more than 48 hours after rupture, primary repair is usually not possible because the damaged tissue cannot hold the sutures. Such patients are probably best managed with T tube intubation of the esophageal defect (63).

ABDOMINAL SURGICAL PROCEDURES

The incidence of small pleural effusions after abdominal operations is high. George and I reported a series of 200 patients who had bilateral decubitus chest radiographs 48 to 72 hours following abdominal surgical procedures (64). Pleural effusions were identified in 97 patients (49%). In a more recent series Nielsen and coworkers (65) reported that 89 of 128 patients (69%) undergoing upper abdominal surgery had pleural effusions in the first 4 days postoperatively. Most of the pleural effusions are small; only 21 patients (22%) in our series had pleural fluid that measured more than 10 mm in thickness on the decubitus films (64). Larger left-sided pleural effusions are particularly common after splenectomy. Postoperative pleural effusions are more common in patients undergoing upper abdominal surgical procedures (64), in patients with postoperative atelectasis (64, 65), and in those with free abdominal fluid at the time of operation (64). In our series (64), a thoracentesis was performed on 20 patients, and in 16 of these, the pleural fluid was an exudate (64). The pleural effusions in all but a single patient resolved spontaneously without any specific therapy. One patient had a staphylococcal pleural infection. This study showed that pleural effusions frequently occur after abdominal surgical procedures and are usually related to diaphragmatic irritation or atelectasis. If the pleural effusion measures more than 10 mm in thickness on the decubitus film, a diagnostic thoracentesis should be done to rule out pleural infection. Although pulmonary embolization and subphrenic abscess can cause pleural effusion postoperatively, most effusions occurring within the first 72 hours after abdominal surgery are not due to these factors and resolve spontaneously.

DIAPHRAGMATIC HERNIA

Hernias through the diaphragm are important in the differential diagnosis of pleural effusions from two viewpoints. First, they may mimic a pleural effusion. Second, pleural effusions are usually present with a strangulated diaphragmatic hernia.

Diaphragmatic hernia should be considered whenever an apparent pleural effusion has an atypical shape or location. Air in the herniated intestine usually is the clue to this diagnosis. Occasionally, an upper gastrointestinal series and a small bowel follow-through study in conjunction with a barium enema are necessary for accurate diagnosis.

The possibility of a strangulated diaphragmatic hernia should always be considered in patients with a left pleural effusion and signs of an acute abdominal catastrophe (66, 67). At least 90% of strangulated diaphragmatic hernias are traumatic in origin, and at least 95% are on the left side because the liver protects the right diaphragm. Strangulation can occur months to years after the original injury, which is usually an automobile accident. Strangulation typically occurs suddenly and progresses rapidly. Left shoulder pain is generally present from diaphragmatic irritation. Serosanguineous exudative pleural fluid with predominantly polymorphonuclear leukocytes is almost always present. The diagnosis is usually suggested by air-fluid levels in the viscera strangulated in the left pleural space. Contrast studies of the gastrointestinal tract are sometimes necessary to make the diagnosis. Immediate surgical treatment is imperative to prevent gangrene of the strangulated viscera (66, 67).

ENDOSCOPIC VARICEAL SCLEROTHERAPY

Over the past decade endoscopic variceal sclerotherapy (EVS) has become one of the principal forms of therapy for patients who have bled from ruptured esophageal varices. Frequently, EVS is followed by the development of a pleural effusion. Saks and coworkers (68) reviewed the chest radiographs following 38 different EVS procedures and reported that 50% of the procedures were followed by the development of a pleural effusion, whereas Bacon and associates (69) reported pleural effusions following 48% of 65 procedures. The sclerosant used in both the above series was 5% sodium morrhuate. Parikh and coworkers (70) reported that the incidence of pleural effusion was only 19% in 31 patients in whom absolute alcohol was used as the sclerosant. Left, right, and bilateral effusions occur with approximately equal frequency (71). Most of the effusions are small.

In the Bacon study, 11 pleural fluids were analyzed and all were exudates, primarily by the LDH criteria (69). There is no relationship between the incidence of fever, the patient's fluid status, or the presence of ascites and the occurrence of postsclerotherapy effusions (69). Patients who develop pleural effusion are more likely to experience chest pain requiring medication after the procedure (69). It is hypothesized that the development of the pleural effusion is related to extravasation of the sclerosant into the esophageal mucosa, which results in an intense inflammatory reaction in the mediastinum and pleura (69). No treatment is necessary for the pleural effusion secondary to EVS. However, if the effusion persists for more than 24 to 48 hours and is accompanied by fever or if the effusion occupies more than 25% of the hemithorax, a thoracentesis should be done to rule out an infection or an esophagopleural fistula (71).

The latter diagnosis is suggested by a high pleural fluid amylase level.

BILIOUS PLEURAL EFFUSIONS

Bilious pleural effusions are a rare complication of biliary tract disorder. With all cases of bilious pleural effusions, there is a fistula from the biliary tree to the pleural space. Historically, the most common cause has been thoracoabdominal trauma (72); other causes have included parasitic liver disease, suppurative complications of biliary tract obstruction, and postoperative strictures of bile ducts (73). Bilious pleural effusions have also been reported to occur after percutaneous biliary drainage (74) or after an internal stent was placed for an obstructed biliary system (75). In two cases with spontaneous biliary pleural fistula, the tract was large enough to allow the passage of gallstones into the pleural space (73, 76).

When bile is instilled into the pleural space of rabbits, an inflammatory reaction is produced. The influx of fluid plus the rapid resorption of the bile results in the pleural fluid having a much lower bilirubin than one would anticipate (74). In one patient who developed a pleural effusion as a complication of percutaneous biliary drainage, the pleural fluid bilirubin was only 2.1 mg/dl (74). However, the pleural fluid bilirubin has exceeded 25 mg/dl in some patients (74).

The diagnosis of a bilious pleural effusion should be suspected in any patient with an obstructed biliary system. It is important to remember that the pleural fluid may not appear to be bile, although the ratio of the pleural fluid to serum bilirubin is greater than 1.0 (74). The appropriate treatment for this condition is the re-establishment of the biliary drainage. Most patients who have a bilious pleural effusion after trauma will require decortication and diaphragmatic repair (72). The incidence of empyema with bilious pleural effusions approaches 50%, and one should constantly be aware of this complication.

PLEURAL EFFUSIONS AFTER LIVER TRANSPLANT

Almost all patients who undergo an orthotopic liver transplantation develop a pleural effusion postoperatively. Spizarny and associates (77) reviewed the chest radiographs of 42 patients undergoing liver transplantation and found that 40 of 42 patients (95%) developed a right-sided pleural effusion within 72 hours of transplantation. One of the remaining two patients had a left-sided effusion. Afessa and coworkers (78) reported that pleural effusions were present postoperatively in 77% of their 44 patients undergoing liver transplantation. The pleural effusions are bilateral in about one-third of patients but the amount of fluid on the right side is greater than that on the left side (78).

The pleural effusion after liver transplantation may be large. In one series of liver transplants in 48 children, effusions large enough to cause clinically detectable respiratory compromise occurred in 23 (19 right-sided and 4 left-sided) (79). Fifteen of the patients in this latter series were treated with chest tubes (79).

The pathogenesis of the pleural effusions after liver transplant is not definitely known. It has been suggested that the effusion is due to injury or irritation of the right hemidiaphragm caused by the extensive right upper quadrant dissection and retraction. The natural history of a pleural effusion after transplant is that it increases in size over the first three postoperative days and then gradually resolves over a period ranging from several weeks to several months (77). In one series, the effusion increased in size in the period beyond the first 3 days in 10 patients. Seven of the 10 patients had subdiaphragmatic pathology, including 4 with hematomas, 1 with a biloma, and 2 with abscesses. Accordingly, patients with enlarging pleural effusions after liver transplantation should be evaluated for subdiaphragmatic pathology.

To my knowledge there has been no systematic analysis of the pleural fluid in these patients. Indeed in the series referenced above, there was no mention of the findings with thoracentesis.

REFERENCES

1. Kaye MD: Pleuropulmonary complications of pancreatitis. Thorax 1968;23:297-306.
2. Gumaste V, Singh V, Dave P: Significance of pleural effusion in patients with acute pancreatitis. Am J Gastro 1992;87:871-874.
3. Roseman DM, Kowlessar OD, Sleisenger MH: Pulmonary manifestations of pancreatitis. N Engl J Med 1960;263:294-296.
4. Light RW, Ball WC: Glucose and amylase in pleural effusions. JAMA 1973;225:257-260.
5. Miller TA, Lindenauer SM, Frey CF, Stanley JC: Pancreatic abscess. Arch Surg 1974;108:545-551.
6. Kolmannskog F, Kolbenstvedt A, Aakhus T: Computed tomography in inflammatory mass lesions following acute pancreatitis. J Comput Assist Tomogr 1981;5:169-172.
7. Tombroff M, Loicq A, De Koster j-P, et al: Pleural effusion with pancreaticopleural fistula. Br Med J 1973;1:330-331.
8. Shetty AN: Pseudocysts of the pancreas: an overview. South Med J 1980;73:1239-1242.
9. Rockey DC, Cello JP: Pancreaticopleural fistula. Report of 7 patients and review of the literature. Medicine 1990;69:332-344.
10. Anderson WJ, Skinner DB, Zuidema GD, Cameron, JL: Chronic pancreatic pleural effusions. Surg Gynecol Obstet 1973;137:827-830.
11. Uchiyama T, Suzuki T, Adachi A, Hiraki S, Iizuka N: Pancreatic pleural effusion: case report and review of 113 cases in Japan. Am J Gastro 1992;87:387-391.
12. Miridjianian A, Ambruoso VN, Derby BM, Tice DA: Massive bilateral hemorrhagic pleural effusions in chronic relapsing pancreatitis. Arch Surg 1969;98:62-66.
13. Pottmeyer EW III, Frey CF, Matsuno S: Pancreaticopleural fistulas. Arch Surg 1987;122:648-654.
14. Sherr HP, Light RW, Merson MH, et al: Origin of pleural fluid amylase in esophageal rupture. Ann Intern Med 1972;76:985-986.
15. Kramer MR, Saidana MJ, Cepero RJ, Pitchenik AE: High amylase levels in neoplasm-related pleural effusion. Ann Intern Med 1989;110:567-569.
16. Parekh D, Segal I: Pancreatic ascites and effusion. Risk factors for failure of conservative therapy and the role of octreotide. Arch Surg 1992;127:707-712.
17. Pederzoli P, Bassi C, Falconi M, Albrigo R, Vantini I, Micciolo R: Conservative treatment of external pancreatic fistulae with parenteral nutrition along or in combination with continuous intravenous infusion of somatostatin, glucagon or calcitonin. Surg Gynecol Obstet 1986;163:428-432.
18. Krasnow AZ, Collier BD, Isitman AT, et al: The value of preoperative imaging techniques in patients with chronic pancreatic pleural effusions. Int J Pancreatol 1987;2:269-276.
19. Lang EK, Paolini RM, Pottmeyer A: The efficacy of palliative and definitive percutaneous versus surgical drainage of pancreatic abscesses and pseudocysts: A prospective study of 85 patients. South Med J 1991;84:55-64.
20. Shapiro DH, Anagnostopoulos CE, Dineen JP: Decortication and pleurectomy for the pleuropulmonary complications of pancreatitis. Ann Thorac Surg 1970;9:76-80.
21. Lipsett PA, Cameron JL: Internal pancreatic fistula. Am J Surg 1992;163:216-220.

22. Carter R, Brewer LA: Subphrenic abscess: a thoraco-abdominal clinical complex. Am J Surg 1964;108:165-174.

23. DeCosse JJ, Poulin TL, Fox PS, Condon RE: Subphrenic abscess. Surg Gynecol Obstet 1974;138:841-846.

24. Sanders RC: Post-operative pleural effusion and subphrenic abscess. Clin Radiol 1970;21:308-312.

25. Sherman NJ, Davis JR, Jesseph JE: Subphrenic abscess: a continuing hazard. Am J Surg 1969;117:117-123.

26. Connell TR, Stephens DH, Carlson HC, Brown ML: Upper abdominal abscess: a continuing and deadly problem. AJR 1980;134:759-765.

27. Deck KB, Berne TV: Selective management of subphrenic abscesses. Arch Surg 1979;114:1165-1168.

28. van der Sluis RF: Subphrenic abscess. Surg Gynecol Obstet 1984;158:427-435.

29. Samelson SL, Ferguson MK: Empyema following percutaneous catheter drainage of upper abdominal abscess. Chest 1992;1612-1614.

30. Alexander ES, Proto AV, Clark RA: CT differentiation of subphrenic abscess and pleural effusion. AJR 1983;145:47-51.

31. Gold RP, Johnson PM: Efficacy of combined liver-lung scintillation imaging. Radiology 1975;117:105-111.

32. Haaga JR, Weinstein AJ: CT-guided percutaneous aspiration and drainage of abscesses. AJR 1980;135:1187-1194.

33. Stylianos S, Martin EC, Starker PM, Laffey KJ, Bixon R, Forde KA: Percutaneous drainage of intra-abdominal abscesses following abdominal trauma. J Trauma 1989;29:584-588.

34. Hemming A, Davis NL, Robins RE: Surgical versus percutaneous drainage of intra-abdominal abscesses. Am J Surg 1991;161:593-595.

35. Rubin RH, Swartz MN, Malt R: Hepatic abscess: changes in clinical, bacteriologic and therapeutic aspects. Am J Med 1974;57:601-610.

36. Perera MR, Kirk A, Noone P: Presentation, diagnosis and management of liver abscess. Lancet 1980;3:629-632.

37. Buchman TG, Zuidema GD: The role of computerized tomographic scanning in the surgical management of pyogenic hepatic abscess. Surg Gynecol Obstet 1981;153:1-9.

38. Newlin N, Silver TM, Stuck KJ, Sandler MA: Ultrasonic features of pyogenic liver abscesses. Radiology 1981;139:155-159.

39. Baek SY, Lee MG, Cho KS, Lee SC, Sung KB, Auh YH: Therapeutic percutaneous aspiration of hepatic abscesses: effectiveness in 25 patients. Am J Roentgenol 1993;160:799-802.

40. Sarr MG, Zuidema GD: Splenic abscess:presentation, diagnosis and treatment. Surgery 1982;92:480-485.

41. Ho HS, Wisner DH: Splenic abscess in the intensive care unit. Arch Surg 1993;842-848.

42. Johnson JF, Raff MJ, Barnwell PA, Chun CH: Splenic abscess complicating infectious endocarditis. Arch Intern Med 1983;143:905-912.

43. Michel L, Grillo HC, Malt RA: Operative and nonoperative management of esophageal perforations. Ann Surg 1981;194:57-63.

44. Abbott OA, Mansour KA, Logan WD, et al: Atraumatic so-called "spontaneous" rupture of the esophagus. J Thorac Cardiovasc Surg 1970;59:67-83.

45. Demeester TR: Perforation of the esophagus. Ann Thorac Surg 1986;42:231-232.

46. Bladergroen MR, Lowe JE, Postlethwait RW: Diagnosis and recommended management of esophageal perforation and rupture. Ann Thorac Surg 1986;42:235-239.

47. Graeber GM, Niezgoda JA, Albus RA, et al: A comparison of patients with endoscopic esophageal perforations and patients with Boerhaave's syndrome. Chest 1987;92:995-998.

48. Keszler P, Buzna E: Surgical and conservative management of esophageal perforation. Chest 1981;80:158-162.

49. Quintana R, Bartley TD, Wheat MW Jr: Esophageal perforation: analysis of 10 cases. Ann Thorac Surg 1970;10:45-53.

50. Maulitz RM, Good JT Jr, Kaplan RL, et al: The pleuropulmonary consequences of esophageal rupture: an experimental model. Am Rev Respir Dis 1979;120:363-367.

51. Skinner DB, Little AG, DeMeester TR: Management of esophageal perforation. Am J Surg 1980;139:760-764.

52. Chandrasekhara R, Levitan R: Spontaneous rupture of the esophagus. Arch Intern Med 1970;126:1008-1009.

53. Finley RJ, Pearson FG, Weisel RD, et al: The management of non-malignant intrathoracic esophageal perforations. Ann Thorac Surg 1980;30:575-581.

54. Faling LJ, Pugatch RD, Robbins AH: Case report: the diagnosis of unsuspected esophageal perforation by computed tomography. Am J Med Sci 1981;281:31-34.

55. Rudin JS, Ellrodt AG, Phillips EH: Low pleural fluid amylase associated with spontaneous rupture of the esophagus. Arch Intern Med 1983;143:1034-1035.

56. Good JT Jr, Taryle DA, Maulitz RM, et al: The diagnostic value of pleural fluid pH. Chest 1980;78:55-59.

57. Dye RA, Laforet EG: Esophageal rupture: diagnosis by pleural fluid pH. Chest 1974;66:454-456.

58. Good JT Jr, Antony VB, Reller LB, et al: The pathogenesis of the low pleural fluid pH in esophageal rupture. Am Rev Respir Dis 1983;127:702-704.

59. Eriksen KR: Oesophagopleural fistula diagnosed by microscopic examination of pleural fluid. Acta Chir Scand 1964;128:771-777.

60. Ginai AZ: Experimental evaluation of various available contrast agents for use in the gastrointestinal tract in case of suspected leakage: effects on pleura. Br J Radiol 1986;59:887-894.

61. White CS, Templeton PA, Attar S: Esophageal perforation: CT findings. AJR 1993;160:767-770.

62. Shaffer JA Jr, Valenzuela G, Mittai RK: Esophageal perforation. A reassessment of the criteria for choos-

ing medical or surgical therapy. Arch Intern Med 1992;152:757-761.

63. Naylor AR, Walker WS, Dark J, Cameron EW: T tube intubation in the management of seriously ill patients with oesophagopleural fistulae. Brit J Surg 1990;77:40-42.

64. Light RW, George RB: Incidence and significance of pleural effusion after abdominal surgery. Chest 1976; 69:621-626.

65. Nielsen PH, Jepsen SB, Olsen AD: Postoperative pleural effusion following upper abdominal surgery. Chest 1989;96:1133-1135.

66. Keshishian JM, Cox SA: Diagnosis and management of strangulated diaphragmatic hernias. Surg Gynecol Obstet 1962;115:626-632.

67. Aronchick JM, Epstein DM, Gefter WB, Miller WT: Chronic traumatic diaphragmatic hernia: the significance of pleural effusion. Radiology 1988;168:675-678.

68. Saks BJ, Kilby AE, Dietrich PA, et al: Pleural and mediastinal changes following endoscopic injection sclerotherapy of esophageal varices. Radiology 1983; 149:639-642.

69. Bacon BR, Bailey-Newton RS, Connors AF Jr: Pleural effusions after endoscopic variceal sclerotherapy. Gastroenterology 1985;88:1910-1914.

70. Parikh SS, Amarapurkar DN, Dhawan PS, Kalro RH, Desai HG: Development of pleural effusion after sclerotherapy with absolute alcohol. Gastrointest Endosc 1993;39:404-405.

71. Edling JE, Bacon BR: Pleuropulmonary complications of endoscopic variceal sclerotherapy. Chest 1991;99: 1252-1257.

72. Ivatury RR, O'Shea J, Rohman M: Post-traumatic thoracobiliary fistula. J Trauma 1984;24:438-441.

73. Delco F, Domenigheti G, Kauzlaric D, Donati D, Mombelli G: Spontaneous biliothorax (thoracobilia) following cholecystopleural fistula presenting as an acute respiratory insufficiency. Chest 1994;106:961-963.

74. Strange C, Allen ML, Freedland PN, et al: Biliopleural fistula as a complication of percutaneous biliary drainage: experimental evidence for pleural inflammation. Am Rev Respir Dis 1988;137:959-961.

75. Dasmahapatra HK, Pepper JR: Bronchopleurobiliary fistula: a complication of intrahepatic biliary stent migration. Chest 1988;94:874-875.

76. Cunningham LW, Grobman M, Paz HL, Hanlon CA, Promisloff RA: Chylecystopleural fistula with cholelithiasis presenting as a right pleural effusion. Chest 1990;97:751-752.

77. Spizarny DL, Gross BH, McLoud T: Enlarging pleural effusion after liver transplantation. J Thorac Imaging 1993;8:85-87.

78. Afessa B, Gay PC, Plevak DJ, Swensen SJ, Patel HG, Krowka MJ: Pulmonary complications of orthotopic liver transplantation. Mayo Clin Proceed 1993;68: 427-434.

79. Bilik R, Yellen M, Superina RA: Surgical complications in children after liver transplantation. J Pediat Surg 1992;27:1371-1375.

CHAPTER 16
Pleural Disease Due to Collagen Vascular Diseases

RHEUMATOID PLEURITIS

Rheumatoid disease is occasionally complicated by an exudative pleural effusion that characteristically has a low pleural fluid glucose level.

Incidence

Patients with rheumatoid arthritis have an increased incidence of pleural effusion. In a review of 516 patients with rheumatoid arthritis, Walker and Wright found 17 cases of pleural effusions (3.3%) without other obvious causes (1). Pleural effusions were more common in men (7.9%) than in women (1.6%). These authors also found a high incidence of chest pain in their patients with rheumatoid arthritis; 28% of the men and 18% of the women gave a history of pleuritic chest pain (1). In a separate study, Horler and Thompson studied 180 patients with rheumatoid disease and found that 9 (5%) had an otherwise unexplained pleural effusion (2). In this latter study, 8 of 52 males (15%) but only 1 of 128 females (1%) had rheumatoid pleural effusions.

Pathologic Features

Examination of the pleural surfaces in patients with rheumatoid pleuritis at the time of thoracoscopy reveals a visceral pleura with varying degrees of nonspecific inflammation. In contrast, the parietal pleural surface has in most cases a "gritty" or frozen appearance. The parietal surface looks slightly inflamed and thickened with numerous small vesicles or granules about 0.5 mm in diameter (3).

Histopathologically, the most constant finding is a lack of a normal mesothelial cell covering (3). Instead there is a pseudostratified layer of epithelioid cells that focally forms multinucleated giant cells of a type different from those of Langerhans or foreign body giant cells (3). The histologic features in nodular areas are those of a rheumatoid nodule with palisading cells, fibrinoid necrosis, and both lymphocytes and plasma cells (4, 5). This picture is virtually diagnostic of rheumatoid pleuritis, but it is only occasionally seen in closed pleural biopsy specimens because the rheumatoid nodules usually involve the visceral pleura. This specific histologic picture may not even be seen with tissue obtained from open thoracotomy (6). At times, the thickened pleura contains cholesterol clefts (5).

Clinical Manifestations

Rheumatoid pleural effusions classically occur in the older male patient with rheumatoid arthritis and subcutaneous nodules. Almost all patients with rheumatoid pleural effusions are over 35 years of age, approximately 80% are male, and approximately 80% have subcutaneous nodules (1, 2, 6, 7). Typically, the pleural effusion appears when the arthritis has been present for several years. When two series totaling 29 patients are combined (1, 7), the pleural effusion preceded the development of arthritis in 2 patients by 6 weeks and 6 months, occurred simultaneously (within 4 weeks) with arthritis in 6 patients, and occurred after the development of arthritis in the remaining 21 patients. In this last group of patients, the mean interval between the development of arthritis and the pleural effusion was about 10 years.

The reported frequency of chest symptoms in patients with rheumatoid pleural effusions has varied markedly from one series to another. In one series of 24 patients, 50% of the patients had no symptoms referable to the chest (8). In a second series of 17 patients, 15 complained of pleuritic chest pain (1), while in a third series, 4 of 12 complained of pleu-

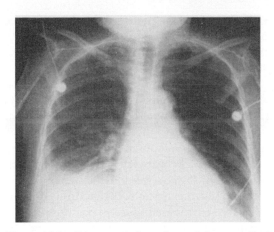

Figure 16.1. Posteroanterior radiograph from a patient with long-standing rheumatoid arthritis. Note the right pleural effusion and the destructive changes in the shoulders. (Courtesy of Dr. Harry Sassoon.)

ritic chest pain, and of these, 3 were febrile (7). Other patients complain of dyspnea secondary to the presence of fluid. In one reported patient, the pleural effusion was large enough to cause respiratory failure (9).

The chest radiograph in most patients reveals a small-to-moderate-sized pleural effusion occupying less than 50% of the hemithorax (Fig. 16.1). The pleural effusion is most commonly unilateral, and no predilection exists for either side (6). In approximately 25% of patients, the effusion is bilateral (1). The effusion may eventually alternate from one side to the other or may come and go on the same side. As many as one-third of these patients may have associated intrapulmonary manifestations of rheumatoid arthritis (1).

Diagnosis

The diagnosis of a rheumatoid pleural effusion is not difficult if the patient is a middle-aged man with rheumatoid arthritis and subcutaneous nodules.

Pleural Fluid Examination

Examination of the pleural fluid is useful in establishing the diagnosis because the fluid is an exudate characterized by a low glucose level (<40 mg/dl), a low pH (<7.20), a high lactic acid dehydrogenase (LDH) level (>700 IU/L), low complement levels, and high rheumatoid factor titers (≥1:320), which are at least as high as those in serum (7) (see Chapter

4). Occasionally, the pleural fluid glucose is not reduced when the patient is first seen, but serial pleural fluid glucose determinations reveal progressively lower pleural fluid glucose levels. In the patient with arthritis and pleural effusions, the main differential diagnosis is between rheumatoid pleuritis and lupus pleuritis. Patients with lupus pleuritis have higher pleural fluid glucose levels (>60 mg/dl), higher pleural fluid pH (>7.35), and lower pleural fluid LDH levels (<500 IU/L) than patients with rheumatoid pleuritis (7). Other immunologic tests are discussed in Chapter 4, but they are not generally recommended.

The pleural fluid differential can reveal predominantly polymorphonuclear or mononuclear leukocytes, depending on the acuteness of the process. The cytologic picture from most patients with rheumatoid pleural effusion is very suggestive of the diagnosis (8). The cytological picture with rheumatoid pleuritis is characterized by three distinct features: (*a*) slender, elongated multinucleated macrophages, (*b*) round giant multinucleated macrophages, and (*c*) necrotic background material (8). When Naylor reviewed the cytological picture of 24 patients with rheumatoid pleuritis seen at the University of Michigan over a 32-year period, the pleural fluid from each patient had a least one of the above three characteristics (8). Twenty-three fluids demonstrated granular necrotic material, 17 multinucleated giant macrophages, and 15 elongated macrophages (8). These features were not seen in any of 10,000 other pleural fluids due to diverse causes (8).

The pleural fluid from patients with rheumatoid pleuritis may contain "ragocytes" or rheumatoid arthritis (RA) cells. The term *ragocyte* was coined by Delbarre and colleagues (10) who described small, spherical, cytoplasmic inclusions in neutrophilic leukocytes, and occasionally in monocytes, in unstained wet films of the sediment obtained from the synovial fluid of patients with various types of arthritis. These inclusions were reminiscent of raisin seeds, hence the adoption of the prefix "rago," which is derived from the Greek word for grape. The inclusion bodies have been shown to represent phagocytic vacuoles or phagosomes, which are of greater size than normal lysosomes of granular leukocytes (11).

The presence of these cells is not useful diagnostically because pleural effusions of other etiologies, particularly those with a low glucose level, contain these cells (8, 12).

Concomitant Infection

When a patient is seen with rheumatoid arthritis and a pleural effusion characterized by a low glucose level (<20 mg/dl), a low pH (<7.20), and a high LDH level, one must rule out pleural infection, which can produce pleural fluid with the same characteristics (see Chapter 9). Hindle and Yates first reported a pyopneumothorax in a patient with a rheumatoid pleural effusion (13). At thoracotomy, it was found that a necrobiotic nodule in the visceral pleura had broken down, producing a bronchopleural fistula. Jones and Blodgett subsequently reported that 5 of 10 patients with rheumatoid pleural effusion followed for a 5-year period developed empyemas (14). These investigators found that empyemas were more common in patients who had been treated with corticosteroids, and they attributed the pleural infection to the creation of bronchopleural fistulas through necrobiotic subpleural rheumatoid nodules.

When patients with apparent rheumatoid pleural effusions are seen, it is important to obtain both aerobic and anaerobic cultures of the pleural fluid. In addition, the pleural fluid should be centrifuged, and the sediment should be Gram stained because stains made in this manner are more sensitive than those made on uncentrifuged pleural fluid.

Glucose Levels

The most striking characteristic of the rheumatoid pleural effusion is its low glucose content. In a review of 76 patients with rheumatoid pleuritis, 48 patients (63%) had pleural fluid glucose levels below 20 mg/dl, whereas 63 patients (83%) had pleural fluid glucose levels below 50 mg/dl (6). The explanation for the low pleural fluid glucose in this condition is not known precisely. If the serum level of glucose is increased in patients with rheumatoid pleural effusions, little change is seen in the pleural fluid glucose levels (15–17), but similar results are obtained in patients with other diseases and low pleural fluid glucose levels (18). In contrast, when patients with rheumatoid pleural effusions are given oral urea (17) or intravenous D-xylose (16) loads, the pleural fluid and serum levels of these substances equilibrate over several hours.

Carr and McGuckin have suggested that the rheumatoid inflammatory process alters the normal state of one or more enzymes that constitute the carbohydrate transport mechanism of cellular membranes (17). This interpretation should be viewed with some caution. The relationship between the serum and pleural fluid glucose levels is dictated not only by the ease with which glucose passes from the serum into the pleural fluid, but also by the rate at which the pleural surfaces and fluid use the glucose. Because the pleural fluid glucose level falls within 30 minutes from 2000 to 236 mg/dl after the intrapleural injection of glucose in patients with rheumatoid pleuritis (15), there must be either rapid glucose uptake by the pleura or no great barrier to its diffusion.

The pleural surfaces with rheumatoid pleuritis appear to be active metabolically, as manifested by the high pleural fluid LDH and the low pleural fluid glucose levels, although the metabolic activity of rheumatoid pleural fluid is virtually nil even when glucose is added (16). The thickened pleura in rheumatoid pleuritis probably limits the movement of glucose into the pleural space, and because glucose consumption by the pleural surfaces is high, an equilibrium is formed in which the pleural fluid glucose level is much lower than the serum glucose level.

Cholesterol Levels

Another interesting characteristic of rheumatoid pleural effusions is their tendency to contain cholesterol crystals or high levels of cholesterol. Ferguson first reported two patients with rheumatoid pleural effusions in whom the pleural fluid contained numerous cholesterol crystals (5). Subsequently, Naylor reported that 5 of 24 rheumatoid pleural fluids (21%) contained cholesterol crystals (8). Some rheumatoid pleural effusions contain high levels of cholesterol without cholesterol crystals (6).

Lillington and coworkers measured the lipid levels in 7 rheumatoid pleural effusions and found levels above 1000 mg/dl in 4 of the 7 fluids (6). One of the two patients that I have seen with cholesterol crystals in the pleural fluid had rheumatoid pleuritis. The cholesterol crystals impart a sheen to the fluid when viewed with the naked eye under proper lighting. High cholesterol levels make the pleural fluid turbid. The significance of the presence of high levels of cholesterol or cholesterol crystals in the pleural fluid is unknown. Cholesterol pleural effusions are discussed more extensively in Chapter 21.

Biopsy

Closed pleural biopsies have a limited role in the diagnosis of rheumatoid pleuritis. Although a pleural biopsy specimen may reveal a rheumatoid nodule diagnostic of rheumatoid pleuritis in an occasional patient, the pleural biopsy usually only reveals chronic inflammation or fibrosis. Pleural biopsy is not recommended in the typical case of rheumatoid pleuritis. In atypical cases, however, such as in patients without arthritis or in those with a normal pleural fluid glucose level, pleural biopsy should be performed to rule out malignant disease and tuberculosis.

Prognosis and Treatment

The natural history of rheumatoid pleuritis is variable. In the series of Walker and Wright, 13 of 17 patients (76%) had spontaneous resolution of their pleural effusions within 3 months, although 1 of the 13 patients had a subsequent recurrence (1). One patient had a spontaneous resolution after 18 months of observation, whereas another had a persistent effusion for more than 2 years. One patient developed progressive severe pleural thickening and eventually had to undergo a decortication. The last patient developed an empyema.

Little information is available in the literature on the efficacy of therapy in rheumatoid pleural disease. Some patients have appeared to respond to systemic corticosteroids (1) whereas in others no beneficial effects were observed (19–21). The degree of activity in the pleural space and in the joints is not necessarily parallel. In one report, the administration of methotrexate was associated with improvement in the arthritis but the development of a pleural effusion (22). The main goal of therapy

should be to prevent the progressive pleural fibrosis that may necessitate a decortication in a small percentage of patients (1, 4, 20, 23, 24). There are no controlled studies evaluating the efficacy of corticosteroids or nonsteroidal anti-inflammatory drugs in the treatment of rheumatoid pleural effusion. It is recommended that patients be treated with nonsteroidal anti-inflammatory drugs such as aspirin or ibuprofen for 8 to 12 weeks initially. If the pleural effusion persists and if the joint symptoms are not well controlled, then appropriate therapy should be directed toward the rheumatologic problem. If the only symptomatic problem is the pleural disease, then the patient should have a therapeutic thoracentesis and possibly an intrapleural injection of corticosteroids. There have been two reports concerning the intrapleural injection of corticosteroids; the first (21) had two patients and the intrapleural corticosteroids were ineffective; the second (25) had one patient who seemed to respond to one injection of 120 mg depomethylprednisolone.

Decortication should be considered in patients with thickened pleura who are symptomatic with dyspnea. Computed tomographic examination is useful in delineating the extent of the pleural thickening. In patients with pleural effusions, the significance of the pleural thickening can be gauged by measuring the pleural pressure serially during a therapeutic thoracentesis (see Chapter 23). If the pleural pressure drops rapidly as pleural fluid is removed, the lung is trapped by the pleural disease (26), and decortication should be considered. The decortication procedure is difficult in patients with rheumatoid pleuritis because it is not easy to develop a plane between the lung and the fibrous peel. Therefore, air leaks persist longer than usual after decortication (24). Nevertheless, decortication can substantially improve the quality of life of some patients with dense pleural fibrosis secondary to rheumatoid disease.

As mentioned earlier, patients with rheumatoid pleural effusions have a high incidence of complicated parapneumonic effusions. The management of such patients is the same as for any patient with complicated parapneumonic effusion (see Chapter 9). The incidence of persistent bronchopleural fistula is higher in the patient with rheumatoid disease, and more exploratory thoracotomies are required (24).

SYSTEMIC LUPUS ERYTHEMATOSUS (SLE)

Both systemic and drug-induced lupus erythematosus may affect the pleura.

Incidence

The pleura is involved more frequently in SLE than in any other collagen disease. In a review of 138 patients with SLE, Harvey and associates found that 16% had pleural effusions and that 56% complained of pleuritic chest pain some time during the course of their illness (27). Winslow and colleagues reviewed the chest radiographs of 57 cases of SLE and found pleural effusions without other apparent cause in 21 (37%) (28). Alarcon-Segovia and Alarcon reviewed 48 patients with SLE and found that 21 (44%) had pleural effusions some time during their course (29). These figures may overestimate the incidence of pleural effusions with SLE because almost all these patients had severe disease. A comparable incidence of pleural effusions has been reported with drug-induced SLE (30).

Pathologic Features

Surprisingly little has been written concerning the pathologic features of the pleura with SLE. In an autopsy series of 54 patients with SLE, acute fibrinous pleuritis was seen in about 40% and evidence of previous pleural inflammation in the form of pleural fibrosis and thickening was seen in about 33% (31). Pleural biopsy usually reveals chronic inflammation, although on rare occasions, hematoxylin bodies can be demonstrated in pleural biopsy specimens (32).

Clinical Manifestations

Most patients with pleural effusions secondary to SLE are female (7, 28), and any age group can be affected. Pleuritic chest pain is the most common symptom of the pleural disease. All 9 patients in the series by Halla and associates had pleuritic chest pain (7), as did 12 of the 14 patients in a more recent series (33). Thirteen of the 23 patients (57%) in these

two series were febrile. The majority of patients with lupus pleuritis have arthritis or arthralgias before the pleuritis. The pleuritis frequently dominates the clinical picture (33) and may precede any other symptoms (28).

The pleural effusions secondary to SLE are usually small, but at times they may occupy nearly the entire hemithorax. The pleural effusions are bilateral in about 50% of patients, left-sided only in 17%, right-sided only in 17%, and alternate from one side to another in 17% (28). The effusion may be the only abnormality on the chest radiograph, but frequently the cardiac silhouette is enlarged (34). Nonspecific alveolar infiltrates, usually basilar, or atelectasis may also be seen (33, 34).

It is important to recognize that a lupuslike syndrome may develop after taking many different drugs (Table 16.1). The first five drugs in this table have been definitely incriminated in producing the lupuslike syndrome (35). They cause SLE in many individuals and elicit antinuclear antibodies (ANA) in a still higher percentage of patients. The remainder of the

Table 16.1.   Drugs Associated with Lupuslike Syndromes

Definitely Associated
  Hydralazine
  Procainamide
  Isoniazid
  Phenytoin
  Chlorpromazine
Possibly Associated
  Carbamazepine
  D-Penicillamine
  Ethosuximide
  Ethylphenacemide
  Guanoxan
  Griseofulvin
  Mephenytoin
  Methyldopa
  Methylthiouracil
  Methysergide
  Oral contraceptives
  Para-aminosalicylic acid (PAS)
  Penicillin
  Phenylbutazone
  Propylthiouracil
  Primidone
  Reserpine
  Streptomycin
  Sulfonamides
  Tetracycline
  Troxidone

drugs occasionally induce a lupuslike syndrome and are not associated with an increase in the ANA (35). The incidence of pleuritic chest pain and pleural effusion is comparable in patients with drug-induced SLE and naturally occurring SLE. The main clinical difference between drug-induced SLE and idiopathic SLE is the lower incidence of renal involvement with the former. The symptoms associated with drug-induced SLE characteristically abate within days of discontinuing the offending drug (30).

Of course, patients with SLE may have pleural effusions for other reasons than SLE. Patients with the nephrotic syndrome may have hypoproteinemia and pleural effusions on this basis. In addition, patients with SLE may have uremia, pneumonia, pulmonary emboli, congestive heart failure, or other disorders that can produce pleural effusions.

Diagnosis

The possibility of lupus pleuritis should be considered in any patient with an exudative pleural effusion of unknown etiology.

Pleural Fluid Examination

The pleural fluid is usually a yellow or serosanguineous exudate. The differential white blood cell count (WBC) on the pleural fluid may reveal a preponderance of polymorphonuclear leukocytes or mononuclear cells (33).

Halla and coworkers (7) reported that measurement of the pleural fluid glucose, LDH, and pH levels were useful in distinguishing rheumatoid pleural effusions from lupus effusions. They reported that patients with lupus pleuritis had a pleural fluid glucose level above 80 mg/dl, an LDH level below 500 IU/L, and a pH above 7.20, whereas patients with rheumatoid pleuritis had a glucose level below 25 mg/dl, an LDH above 700 IU/L, and a pH below 7.20. These biochemical tests do not always separate lupus and rheumatoid pleuritis because an occasional patient with lupus pleuritis will have a low pleural fluid glucose, a high pleural fluid LDH, or a low pleural fluid pH (33). In one report of a pleural effusion due to procainamide, the pleural fluid was an exudate with a WBC of 53,200/mm^3, an LDH

of 4296 IU/L, a pH of 7.195, and a glucose of 79 mg/dl (36).

The most useful test for establishing the diagnosis of lupus pleuritis is the measurement of the antinuclear antibody (ANA) level in the pleural fluid. Two older reports suggested that elevated pleural fluid ANA levels were both sensitive and specific in the diagnosis of lupus pleuritis (33, 37). However, the methodology for the performance of the ANA tests has been changed since these articles were written. Specifically, the substrate antigens in the past were derived from animal cell lines, while those used presently are derived from human cell lines (38).

In a recent study of 82 patients including 8 with known SLE, the pleural fluid ANA levels were less useful than had been reported previously. The pleural fluid ANA titers were increased to 1:320 or above in six patients with lupus pleuritis (38) and were below 1:160 in 2 patients with SLE and effusions due to other factors. In the six patients with lupus pleuritis, the ANA titers in the pleural fluid and in the serum tended to be within one dilution of each other. However, the pleural fluid ANA titers were above 1:40 in 8 of the 74 patients (10.8%) who did not appear to have lupus and in 3 of the patients the titers were ≥ 1:160. The staining pattern in the patients with lupus pleuritis tended to be homogeneous while it tended to be speckled in the patients without lupus, but again there was some overlap. The patients with lupus also tended to have higher titers for specific antinuclear antibodies to ssDNA, dsDNA, smooth muscle, and ribonucleoprotein (38).

On the basis of the above studies, it appears that a pleural fluid ANA titer greater than 1:320 is very suggestive of lupus pleuritis. If the staining pattern is homogenous, the patient in all probability has lupus. If the patient has lupus and the pleural fluid ANA titer is below 1:320, an alternate explanation for the pleural effusion should be sought.

The demonstration of LE cells in pleural fluid is thought to be diagnostic of lupus pleuritis (39). At times, LE cells are present in the pleural fluid before they are present in the peripheral blood (40). In one study 8 of 29 pleural fluids from patients with lupus pleuritis *spontaneously* had LE cells (39). The LE cells are not always obvious and their presence was detected only upon re-review in four of the patients. The labor intensive LE preparation on peripheral blood is now obsolete and should not be ordered on pleural fluid (39).

Biopsy

Pleural biopsy is useful in establishing the diagnosis of lupus pleuritis if immunofluorescence is combined with light-microscopic examination. Chandrasekhar and coworkers performed immunofluorescent studies on pleural biopsy specimens from 36 patients with exudative pleural effusions (41). These researchers found that their three patients with drug-induced SLE had a specific immunofluorescent pattern characterized by diffuse and speckled staining of the nuclei of the cells in the pleural biopsy with either anti-IgG, anti-IgM, or anti-C3.

Other workers have reported that pleural specimens obtained at autopsy from patients with SLE have the same specific nuclear immunofluorescence (42). Many pleural biopsy specimens have positive immunofluorescence outside the nuclei (43); only positive nuclear immunofluorescence is thought to be diagnostic of SLE. It is my impression, however, that these stains are rarely used in establishing the diagnosis of lupus pleuritis.

Treatment

In contrast to rheumatoid pleuritis, the pleuritis with SLE definitely responds to corticosteroid administration. Hunder and colleagues treated 6 patients with lupus pleuritis with corticosteroids and reported that the pleural effusions in 5 of the 6 patients rapidly cleared once therapy was begun, and the sixth effusion gradually subsided over 6 months (44). In the series of Winslow and coworkers, 11 patients were treated with corticosteroids and the effusions cleared rapidly in 10 of these patients (28). In contrast, only 10 of 16 effusions cleared spontaneously without corticosteroids. In view of the responsiveness of the pleuritis to corticosteroids and the much lower incidence of side effects with alternate-day corticosteroid therapy, corticosteroid therapy should be initiated with 80 mg prednisone every other day, with rapid dose tapering once the symptoms are controlled. Of course, if the patient has drug-induced SLE, adequate therapy consists of withdrawing the drug.

At times the pleural effusion is large and does not respond to corticosteroid therapy. In such a situation, the alternatives are similar to those for malignant pleural effusion and include chemical pleurodesis with a tetracycline derivative (45) or talc (46) or the implantation of a pleuroperitoneal shunt.

OTHER COLLAGEN VASCULAR DISEASES

Pleural effusions occasionally occur in the course of several other collagen vascular diseases.

Immunoblastic Lymphadenopathy

This disease, which is also called angioimmunoblastic lymphadenopathy, is characterized by the acute onset of constitutional symptoms, generalized lymphadenopathy, hepatosplenomegaly, anemia, and polyclonal hypergammaglobulinemia (19). Between its original description in 1973 (47) and 1979, more than 200 cases were reported (48). It affects primarily the elderly of either sex, with the median age of the reported cases exceeding 60 years. Pathologically, this disorder is characterized by extensive infiltration of lymph nodes with atypical lymphocytes, proliferation of arborizing small vessels, and the deposition of amorphous acidophilic material (19). It is thought to be a nonneoplastic hyperimmune proliferation of the B lymphocytes, possibly related to a lack of suppressor T lymphocytes (48, 49).

Approximately 12% of patients with immunoblastic lymphadenopathy have pleural effusions (49). The pleural fluid is said to be an exudate with a preponderance of mononuclear cells but no other particularly characteristic finding. In one series of 10 patients, 50% had pleural effusions, but the same patients also had ascites and pedal edema (48). In this series, the characteristics of the pleural fluid were not described, and the pleural effusions might have been transudates. Other findings on the chest radiograph include interstitial infiltrates and mediastinal or hilar adenopathy each in 15 to 20% of patients (48). The diagnosis is made by biopsy examination of an enlarged lymph node. In general, the prognosis is poor, with more than a 65% mortality rate in 2 years (49). Both corticosteroids and cytotoxic therapy have been tried, with equivocal results (19, 49).

Sjögren's Syndrome

This syndrome is a chronic inflammatory disease characterized by dryness of the mouth, eyes, and other mucous membranes (19). It is frequently associated with other collagen vascular diseases, most notably rheumatoid arthritis, but sometimes systemic lupus erythematosus, dermatomyositis, or scleroderma. Pathologically, lymphocytic infiltration of the lacrimal and salivary glands occurs. It appears that Sjögren's syndrome can have an associated pleural effusion.

In a review of the pulmonary manifestations of Sjögren's syndrome, 31 of 349 patients (9%) had pulmonary involvement, and of these, 5 (1%) had pleural effusions (50). Of these 5 patients, 3 had rheumatoid arthritis or systemic lupus erythematosus, but 2 had no other connective tissue disease (50). In another series, however, none of 62 patients with Sjögren's syndrome had a pleural effusion (51). The pleural fluid has been described in one patient with Sjögren's syndrome (52). The fluid was a lymphocyte predominant exudate with normal pH and glucose level (52).

Familial Mediterranean Fever

This disease, also known as familial paroxysmal polyserositis, is a rare cause of paroxysmal attacks of fever and pleuritic chest pain, sometimes with pleural effusion (53, 54). The hallmark of the disease is the recurrent, acute, self-limited febrile episodes of peritonitis, pleuritis, synovitis, or an erysipelaslike syndrome. Familial Mediterranean fever is an autosomal recessive disease that occurs almost exclusively in Armenians and Sephardic Jews who have their origin in the Mediterranean countries.

The initial attack usually occurs before age 20 and is typically dominated by peritoneal symptoms and signs. The initial attack is characterized by pleuritic chest pain and fever in fewer than 10% of patients, but approximately 40% have an attack of febrile pleurisy during the course of their disease (53). Chest radiographs during the acute pleuritic attacks reveal elevation of the ipsilateral diaphragm, and frequently, small pleural effusions (54). The pleural fluid contains predominantly polymorphonuclear leukocytes (55). The radiographic abnormalities and the symptoms are usually completely gone within 48 hours. Approximately 25% of the patients also have amyloidosis (52). The attacks are recurrent, with irregular intervals of days to months between. Because the administration of colchicine, 0.5 mg orally twice daily, decreases the frequency of the attacks (56, 57), it is worthwhile to establish this diagnosis in patients with recurrent episodes of polyserositis.

Churg-Strauss Syndrome

This syndrome is a disorder characterized by hypereosinophilia and systemic vasculitis occurring in individuals with asthma and allergic rhinitis (58). Typically, this disease begins with allergic rhinitis with the subsequent development of asthma and peripheral blood eosinophilia. The systemic vasculitis with the Churg-Strauss syndrome resembles that of periarteritis nodosa, but severe renal disease is uncommon. The classic histologic picture consists of a necrotizing vasculitis, eosinophilic tissue infiltration, and extravascular granulomas, but all three components are found in a minority of cases.

Pleural involvement is common with the Churg-Strauss syndrome. In Lanham's review of the literature in 1984 (58), 18 of 61 patients (30%) in whom chest radiograph results were reported had a pleural effusion. The pleural fluid findings with the Churg-Strauss syndrome may be unique. Erzurum and associates (59) reported 1 patient with bilateral effusions and pleural fluid with an LDH of 2856 IU/L, a pH of 7.08, a glucose less than 10 mg/dl, and 10,400 WBC with 95% eosinophils. The only other disease with comparable pleural findings is paragonimiasis.

The Churg-Strauss syndrome responds well to treatment with steroids, although some patients benefit from the addition of immunosuppressive agents. The vasculitic illness is usually of limited duration, but relapses can occur, and they should be detected and treated early (58).

Wegener's Granulomatosis

This disease, characterized by necrotizing granulomatous vasculitis of the small vessels, typically involves the upper and lower respiratory tracts and produces glomerulonephritis (19). Radiologically, the most common patterns in the lung are solitary or multiple nodular densities, either poorly defined or sharply circumscribed (60). An associated small pleural effusion is frequently seen (60, 61).

In one series of 11 patients, 6 (55%) had small pleural effusions (61), whereas in another series of 18 patients, 4 (22%) had pleural effusions (60). The pleural fluid in patients with Wegener's granulomatosis has not been well characterized, but it is probably an exudate. Because effective treatment for this disease is now available (19), it is important to consider this diagnosis in patients with parenchymal infiltrates and a pleural effusion.

Eosinophilia-Myalgia Syndrome

In the late 1980s an epidemic of the eosinophilia-myalgia syndrome was linked to the dietary ingestion of contaminated L-tryptophan. The clinical manifestations of the eosinophilia-myalgia syndrome include myalgias, arthralgias, skin rashes, muscle pain, edema, fatigue, neuropathy, and marked peripheral eosinophilia (62). Over half of the patients with the eosinophilia-myalgia syndrome have respiratory complaints, with dyspnea occurring most frequently.

Pleural effusions can occur with the eosinophilia-myalgia syndrome. Strumpf and coworkers reported a series of four patients with pulmonary infiltrates, pleural effusions, hypoxemia, peripheral eosinophilia, and symptoms of dyspnea, fatigue, and weakness (63). The pleural effusions are usually bilateral and are sterile exudates (63). Although some patients have improved with the discontinuation of L-tryptophan or corticosteroid therapy, the response is often incomplete and the disease may be chronic and progressive.

Miscellaneous Diseases

Occasionally, patients with other collagen vascular diseases such as polyarteritis nodosa, scleroderma, ankylosing spondylitis, Behçet's syndrome, or dermatomyositis have a pleural effusion, but it appears that the pleural effusions in such patients result from complications of the disease, such as heart failure, pneumonia, or pulmonary embolism, rather than from the primary disease.

REFERENCES

1. Walker WC, Wright V: Rheumatoid pleuritis. Ann Rheum Dis 1967;26:467–474.
2. Horler AR, Thompson M: The pleural and pulmonary complications of rheumatoid arthritis. Ann Intern Med 1959;51:1179–1203.
3. Faurschou P, Francis D, Faarup P: Thoracoscopic, histological, and clinical findings in nine case of rheumatoid pleural effusion. Thorax 1985;40:371–375.
4. Feagler JR, Sorensen GD, Rosenfeld MG, Osterland CK: Rheumatoid pleural effusion. Arch Pathol 1971;92:257–266.
5. Ferguson GC: Cholesterol pleural effusion in rheumatoid lung disease. Thorax 1966;21:577–582.
6. Lillington GA, Carr DT, Mayne JG: Rheumatoid pleurisy with effusion. Arch Intern Med 1971;128:764–768.
7. Halla JT, Schronhenloher RE, Volanakis JE: Immune complexes and other laboratory features of pleural effusions. Ann Intern Med 1980;92:748–752.
8. Naylor B: The pathognomonic cytologic picture of rheumatoid pleuritis. Acta Cytol 1990;34:465–473.
9. Pritikin JD, Jensen WA, Yenokida GG, Kirsch CM, Fainstat M: Respiratory failure due to a massive rheumatoid pleural effusion. J Rheumat 1990;17:673–675.
10. Delbarre F, Kahan A, Amor B, Krassinine G: La ragocyte synovial: Son intérèt pour le diagnosic des maladies rheumatismales. Presse Méd 1964;72:2129–2132.
11. Sahn SA: Immunologic diseases of the pleura. Clin Chest Med 1985;6:103–112.
12. Faurschou P: Decreased glucose in RA-cell-positive pleural effusion: correlation of pleural glucose, lactic dehydrogenase and protein concentration to the presence of RA-cells. Eur J Respir Dis 1984;65:272–277.
13. Hindle W, Yates DAH: Pyopneumothorax complicating rheumatoid lung disease. Ann Rheum Dis 1965;24:57–60.
14. Jones FL, Blodgett RC: Empyema in rheumatoid pleuropulmonary disease. Ann Intern Med 1971;74:665–671.
15. Ball GV, Whitfield CL: Studies on rheumatoid disease pleural fluid. Arthritis Rheumat 1966;9:846.
16. Dodson WH, Hollingsworth JW: Pleural effusion in rheumatoid arthritis. N Engl J Med 1966;275:1337–1342.
17. Carr DT, McGuckin WF: Pleural fluid glucose. Am Rev Respir Dis 1968;97:302–305.
18. Russakoff AH, LeMaistre CA, Dewlett HJ: An evaluation of the pleural fluid glucose determination. Am Rev Respir Dis 1962;85:220–223.

19. Hunninghake GW, Fauci AS: Pulmonary involvement in the collagen vascular diseases. Am Rev Respir Dis 1979;119:471–503.

20. Mays EE: Rheumatoid pleuritis: observations in eight cases and suggestions for making the diagnosis in patients without the "typical findings." Dis Chest 1968;53:202–214.

21. Russell ML, Gladman DD, Mintz S: Rheumatoid pleural effusion: lack of response to intrapleural corticosteroid. J Rheumatol 1986;13:412–415.

22. Abu-Shakra M, Nicol P, Urowitz MB: Accelerated nodulosis, pleural effusion, and pericardial tamponade during methotrexate therapy. J Rheumat 1994; 21:934–937.

23. Brunk JR, Drash EC, Swineford O: Rheumatoid pleuritis successfully treated with decortication. Report of a case and review of the literature. Am J Med Sci 1966;251:545–551.

24. Yarbrough JW, Sealy WC, Miller JA: Thoracic surgical problems associated with rheumatoid arthritis. J Thorac Cardiovasc Surg 1975;68:347–354.

25. Chapman PT, O'Donnell JL, Moller PW: Rheumatoid pleural effusion: response to intrapleural corticosteroid. Rheumatology 1992;19:478–480.

26. Light RW, Jenkinson SG, Minh V, George RB: Observations on pleural pressures as fluid is withdrawn during thoracentesis. Am Rev Respir Dis 1980;121:799–804.

27. Harvey AM, Shulman LE, Tumulty PA, et al: Systemic lupus erythematosus: review of the literature and clinical analysis of 138 cases. Medicine 1954;33:291–437.

28. Winslow WA, Ploss LN, Loitman B: Pleuritis in systemic lupus erythematosus: its importance as an early manifestation in diagnosis. Ann Intern Med 1958;49:70–88.

29. Alarcon-Segovia D, Alarcon DG: Pleuro-pulmonary manifestations of systemic lupus erythematosus. Dis Chest 1961;39:7–17.

30. Blomgren SE, Condemi JJ, Vaughan JH: Procainamide-induced lupus erythematosus. Am J Med 1972;52:338–348.

31. Purnell DC, Baggenstoss AH, Olsen AM: Pulmonary lesions in disseminated lupus erythematosus. Ann Intern Med 1955;42:619–628.

32. Gueft B, Laufer A: Further cytochemical studies in systemic lupus erythematosus. Arch Pathol 1954;57:201–226.

33. Good JT Jr, King TE, Antony VB, Sahn SA: Lupus pleuritis: clinical features and pleural fluid characteristics with special reference to pleural fluid antinuclear antibodies. Chest 1983;84:714–718.

34. Gould DM, Dayes ML: Roentgenologic findings in systemic lupus erythematosus. J Chronic Dis 1955;2:136–145.

35. Harpey J-P: Lupus-like syndromes induced by drugs. Ann Allergy 1974;33:256–261.

36. Smith PR, Nacht RI: Drug-induced lupus pleuritis mimicking pleural space infection. Chest 1992;101:268–269.

37. Leechawengwong M, Berger HW, Sukumaran M: Diagnostic significance of antinuclear antibodies in pleural effusion. Mt Sinai J Med 1979;46:137–139.

38. Khare V, Baethge B, Lang S, Wolf RE, Campbell GD Jr: Antinuclear antibodies in pleural fluid. Chest 1994;106:866–871.

39. Naylor B: Cytological aspects of pleural, peritoneal and pericardial fluids from patients with systemic lupus erythematosus. Cytopathology 1992;3:1–8.

40. Carel RS, Shapiro MS, Shoham D, Gutman A: Lupus erythematosus cells in pleural effusion. Chest 1977;72:670–672.

41. Chandrasekhar AJ, Robinson J, Barr L: Antibody deposition in the pleura: a finding in drug-induced lupus. J Allergy Clin Immunol 1978;61:399–402.

42. Pertschuk LP, Moccia LF, Rosen Y, et al: Acute pulmonary complications in systemic lupus erythematosus. Immunofluorescence and light microscopic study. Am J Clin Pathol 1977;68:553–557.

43. Andrews BS, Arora NS, Shadforth MF, et al: The role of immune complexes in the pathogenesis of pleural effusions. Am Rev Respir Dis 1981;124:115–120.

44. Hunder GG, McDuffie FC, Hepper NGG: Pleural fluid complement in systemic lupus erythematosus and rheumatoid arthritis. Ann Intern Med 1972;76:357–362.

45. McKnight KM, Adair NE, Agudelo CA: Successful use of tetracycline pleurodesis to treat massive pleural effusion secondary to systemic lupus erythematosus. Arth Rheum 1991;34:1483–1484.

46. Vargas FS, Milanez JR, Filomeno LT, Fernandez A, Jatene A, Light RW: Intrapleural talc for the prevention of recurrence in benign or undiagnosed pleural effusion. Chest 1994;106:1771–1775.

47. Lukes RJ, Tindle BH: Immunoblastic lymphadenopathy: a hyperimmune entity resembling Hodgkin's disease. N Engl J Med 1975;292:1–8.

48. Cullen MH, Stansfield AG, Oliver RTD, et al: Angioimmunoblastic lymphadenopathy: report of ten cases and review of the literature. Quart J Med 1979;181:151–177.

49. Shaw RA, Schonfeld SA, Whitcomb ME: A perplexing case of hilar adenopathy. Chest 1981;80:736–740.

50. Strimlan CV, Rosenow EC, Divertie MG, Harrison EG: Pulmonary manifestations of Sjögren's syndrome. Chest 1976;70:354–361.

51. Bloch KJ, Buchanan WW, Wohl MJ, Bunim JJ: Sjögren's syndrome. Medicine 1965;44:187–231.

52. Alvarez-Sala R, Sanchez-Toril F, Garcia-Martinez J, Zaera A, Masa JF: Primary Sjögren's syndrome and pleural effusion. Chest 1989;96:1440–1441.

53. Sohar E, Gafni J, Pras M, Heller H: Familial Mediterranean fever. Am J Med 1967;43:227–253.

54. Ehrenfeld EN, Eliakim M, Rachmilewitz M: Recurrent polyserositis (familial Mediterranean fever; periodic disease). Am J Med 1961;31:107–123.

55. Merker H-J, Hersko C, Shibolet S: Serosal exudates in familial Mediterranean fever. Am J Clin Pathol 1967;48:23–29.

56. Zemer D, Revach M, Pras M, et al: A controlled trial of colchicine in preventing attacks of familial Mediterranean fever. N Engl J Med 1974;291:932–934.

57. Dinarello CA, Colchicine therapy for familial Mediterranean fever. A double-blind trial. N Engl J Med 1974;291:934–937.

58. Lanham JG, Elkon KB, Pusey CD, Hughes GR: Systemic vasculitis with asthma and eosinophilia: a clinical approach to the Churg-Strauss syndrome. Medicine 1984;63:65–81.

59. Erzurum SE, Underwood GA, Hamilos DL, Waldron JA: Pleural effusion in Churg-Strauss syndrome. Chest 1989;95:1357–1359.

60. Fauci AS, Wolff SM: Wegener's granulomatosis: studies in eighteen patients and a review of the literature. Medicine 1973;52:535–561.

61. Gonzales L, Van Ordstrand HS: Wegener's granulomatosis: review of 11 cases. Radiology 1973;295–300.

62. Martin RW, Duffy J, Engel AG, et al: The clinical spectrum of the eosinophilia-myalgia syndrome associated with L-tryptophan ingestion. Ann Intern Med 1990;113:124–134.

63. Strumpf IJ, Drucker RD, Ander KH, Cohen S, Fajolu O: Acute eosinophilic pulmonary disease associated with the ingestion of L-tryptophan-containing products. Chest 1991;99:8–13.

CHAPTER 17
Pleural Effusion Due to Drug Reactions

Adverse reactions to drugs produce only a small percentage of all pleural effusions. Because the pleural disease in most cases rapidly resolves when the drug is discontinued, however, it is important to consider the possibility of drug-induced pleural disease in all patients with pleural effusions. The lupuslike syndromes associated with various drugs are described in Chapter 16. In this chapter, the pleural diseases resulting from the administration of nitrofurantoin, dantrolene, methysergide, bromocriptine, amiodarone, interleukin-2, procarbazine, and methotrexate are discussed. These are the only drugs convincingly incriminated in the production of pleural disease other than drugs that produce the lupuslike syndrome. Additional drugs will probably be implicated in the future.

NITROFURANTOIN

Nitrofurantoin (Furadantin) is widely used in the treatment of urinary tract infections. Israel and Diamond first reported that the administration of nitrofurantoin could be associated with the development of an acute febrile illness with pulmonary infiltrates and pleural effusion (1). A subsequent review of the literature and the records of the company that produces nitrofurantoin in 1969 revealed that approximately 200 cases of this syndrome had been reported (2). There have now been over 2000 cases reported (3). It is thought that nitrofurantoin injures the lung through the production of oxygen radicals (4).

Pulmonary reactions to nitrofurantoin may develop in two distinct patterns characterized by the length of treatment prior to the development of the syndrome (4). The acute presentation occurs within 1 month of initiating therapy with the drug. The symptoms with the acute presentation include dyspnea, nonproductive cough, and fever. The chest radiograph is usually abnormal. In one series of 335 patients (5), 186 (56%) had infiltrates, 65 (19%) had infiltrates and effusion, 14 (3%) had only an effusion, and 70 (21%) had a normal chest radiograph.

Most patients with acute pleuropulmonary reactions to nitrofurantoin have both peripheral eosinophilia (greater than $350/mm^3$) and lymphopenia (less than $1000/mm^3$) (6). The only reported pleural fluid analysis showed 17% eosinophils in the patient's pleural fluid (6).

The chronic syndrome occurs when the patient has been taking nitrofurantoin for 2 months to 5 years and is much less frequent than the acute syndrome. The presentation is insidious, with the gradual onset of dyspnea on exertion and a nonproductive cough (4). Patients with the chronic syndrome always have abnormal chest radiographs; diffuse bibasilar infiltrates are the most common abnormality (5). Pleural effusions, less common with the chronic form, occur in fewer than 10% of patients. No patients with the chronic syndrome have had a pleural effusion without an infiltrate (4).

The diagnosis of nitrofurantoin pleuropulmonary reaction should be suspected in all patients with a pleural effusion who are taking nitrofurantoin. If the drug is discontinued, the patient with the acute syndrome usually improves clinically within 1 to 4 days, and the chest radiograph becomes normal within a week (5). Symptoms and signs with the chronic syndrome improve much more slowly (5).

DANTROLENE

Dantrolene sodium (Dantrium) is a long-acting skeletal muscle relaxant used in treating patients with spastic neurologic disorders. The chemical structure of dantrolene is similar to that of nitrofurantoin (7, 8). The chronic administration of dantrolene can lead to an eosinophilic pleural effusion (7, 8). At our institution, which has a large population of patients with spinal cord injury for whom dantrolene is frequently prescribed, we have seen more than 10 instances of pleural effusions due to dantrolene during the past 10 years. In one report four patients developed an eosinophilic pleural effusion 2 months to 3 years after the initial administration of dantrolene (7). The pleural effusions in all patients were unilateral, and no associated pulmonary infiltrates were seen. In the reported series of four patients, one had a pericardial friction rub and another had a pericardial rub with a pericardial effusion (7). Two of the patients were febrile, and two had pleuritic chest pain.

All reported patients have had at least 5% eosinophils in their peripheral blood (7). The pleural fluid is an exudate with normal glucose and amylase levels. The differential white blood cell count on the pleural fluid has revealed at least 35% eosinophils in all cases. When dantrolene is discontinued, the patients improve symptomatically within days, but it takes several months for the pleural effusions to resolve completely. The mechanism by which dantrolene produces the eosinophilic pleural effusion is unknown.

METHYSERGIDE

Methysergide (Sansert) is a serotonin antagonist used to treat migraine headaches. The association of methysergide administration with the development of retroperitoneal fibrosis and fibrosing mediastinitis is well established (9). One report described 13 cases of "pleurisy" secondary to methysergide treatment (10). It is not clear what these authors meant by "pleurisy," but apparently all the patients had pleural effusions or pleural thickening (10). The pleurisy developed 1 month to 3 years after methysergide therapy was initiated, and in 5 patients it was bilateral. Only 1 of the 13 patients had concomitant retroperitoneal fibrosis. No description of the pleural fluid was reported. When methysergide was discontinued, the patients' symptoms and signs improved. At follow-up 6 months or more after discontinuance of the drug, pleural fibrosis was not detectable or was slight in 7 patients, moderate in 3, and severe in 2. The 2 patients with severe fibrosis were those who had continued to take methysergide for the longest period (18 and 36 months) after the onset of this pleurisy (10). Therefore, the oc-

currence of a pleural effusion or pleural thickening in a patient taking methysergide is a strong indication for the prompt discontinuance of the drug.

BROMOCRIPTINE AND OTHER DOPAMINE AGONISTS

Dopamine agonists including bromocriptine mesylate, mesulergine, lisuride, and cabergoline are sometimes used in the long-term treatment of Parkinson's disease. These drugs may also be serotonin antagonists, as is methysergide, which is discussed in the previous section. The long-term administration of any of these drugs can lead to pleuropulmonary changes (11-14). Rinne reviewed the chest radiographs of 123 patients taking bromocriptine for Parkinson's disease and found that 7 patients (6%) had pleural effusions, pleural thickening, and pulmonary infiltrates (11).

As of 1988 there had been a total of 23 patients reported who developed pleuropulmonary disease while taking bromocriptine (12). All the patients have been men, and the majority have had a history of long-term cigarette smoking. The prevalence of symptomatic pleuropulmonary disease among individuals taking bromocriptine is 2 to 5% (12). Patients had taken the drug for 6 months to 4 years before symptoms developed. The chest radiograph reveals unilateral or bilateral pleural thickening or effusion with or without pulmonary infiltrates. An occasional patient has only pulmonary infiltrates. Analysis of the pleural fluid reveals an exudate with predominantly lymphocytes and frequently eosinophils (12, 15).

The natural history of pleuropulmonary disease during bromocriptine treatment is unclear. The disease progresses only in some of the patients who continue taking the drug (12). Upon discontinuance, the majority of patients improve, but complete resolution of the process is rare. It is recommended that annual chest radiographs be obtained in patients who are taking any of these dopamine agonists on a long-term basis. If the radiograph reveals pleural or parenchymal infiltrates, strong consideration should be given to stopping bromocriptine.

AMIODARONE

Amiodarone is a relatively new antiarrhythmic drug that may produce severe and potentially lethal pulmonary toxicity. The current incidence of pulmonary toxicity in patients receiving amiodarone is 5 to 10% (16), and 5 to 10% of those with pulmonary toxicity die of pulmonary fibrosis. The pulmonary toxicity is characterized by the insidious onset of nonproductive cough, dyspnea, weight loss, and occasionally fever. The chest radiograph reveals parenchymal infiltrates, which are predominantly interstitial (16). The toxicity rarely begins before 2 months of therapy, and rarely in patients receiving less than 400 mg/day.

Pleural effusions occur as a manifestation of amiodarone toxicity, but they are uncommon (17–19). Gonzalez-Rothi and coworkers (17) reviewed 11 cases of pleural disease attributed to amiodarone and found that all 11 had concomitant parenchymal involvement. Subsequently, a case has been reported in which there was no parenchymal involvement (18). The pleural fluid is an exudate (17–19) and may have predominantly lymphocytes (19), macrophages (18), or polymorphonuclear leukocytes (17). Pleural fluid eosinophilia has not been reported with amiodarone toxicity. The pleural abnormalities resolve when the amiodarone is discontinued.

INTERLEUKIN-2 (IL-2)

Recombinant interleukin-2 (IL-2) is sometimes used in the treatment of malignancy, most commonly melanoma or renal cell carcinoma. The administration of IL-2 is accompanied by multiple acute but generally reversible toxic effects including fever, chills, lethargy, diarrhea, anemia, thrombocytopenia, eosinophilia, confusion, and diffuse erythroderma, among others (20).

One of the primary side effects of IL-2 administration is the development of pulmonary infiltrates and pleural effusion (20, 21). Vogelzang and associates (20) reviewed the chest radiographs of 54 patients who were receiving high-dose IL-2 with or without lymphokine-activated killer cell therapy for advanced cancer, and reported that 28 (52%) had a pleural effusion (20). Other abnormalities on the chest radiograph included pulmo-

nary edema in 41% and focal infiltrates in 22%. The abnormalities were more frequent in patients receiving bolus doses rather than constant intravenous therapy (20). These pulmonary reactions were clinically significant in that 19 patients (35%) either developed dyspnea at rest or required intubation. The pleural effusions tend to improve, but they persisted in 17% of patients 4 weeks following therapy. In a second study, 26 of 54 patients (48%) developed a pleural effusion after IL-2 therapy (21). In this latter series 80% of the patients had either alveolar edema or interstitial edema. Two of the patients without parenchymal infiltrates had a pleural effusion (21).

The pathogenesis of the pleural effusion with IL-2 therapy is probably related to the generalized capillary leak syndrome that sometimes occurs after IL-2 therapy. It is likely that the pleural fluid originates from the leaky capillaries in the lung. Therefore, the pleural fluid would be expected to be an exudate, but to my knowledge there is no published description of the pleural fluid characteristics. It is unclear as to why the pleural effusion persists so much longer than does the pulmonary edema.

PROCARBAZINE

Procarbazine hydrochloride (Matulane), a methylhydralazine derivative, is effective in the treatment of Hodgkin's disease and other lymphomas. Two detailed case reports have described pleuropulmonary reactions consisting of chills, cough, dyspnea, and bilateral pulmonary infiltrates with pleural effusions occurring after treatment with procarbazine (22, 23). In both instances, rechallenge with procarbazine again produced the infiltrates and pleural effusions. Both patients had peripheral eosinophilia. When the drug was discontinued, the patients' symptoms and radiologic changes resolved within several days (22, 23). This syndrome appears to be identical to that associated with nitrofurantoin.

METHOTREXATE

One report exists of pleural effusion occurring after methotrexate therapy for trophoblastic tumors (24). Walden and coworkers treated 317 patients with methotrexate, 50 mg intramuscularly followed by folinic acid for tropho-blastic disease, and reported that 14 of the patients developed pleuritic chest pain after the second to the fifth injection (24). Four of the patients also developed pleural effusions, but no peripheral eosinophilia was noted. The mechanism of the pleuritis in those patients is unknown.

OTHER DRUGS

Several other drugs have been incriminated as causing pleural effusions.

Ergotamine

In one report (25), a woman who had been taking ergotamine for 12 years developed an exudative right-sided pleural effusion and bilat-eral pleural thickening. Open thoracotomy revealed dense pleural fibrosis. Discontinua-tion of ergotamine was associated with resolu-tion of the pleural disease.

Metronidazole

Kristenson and Fryden (26) reported an interesting patient who developed fever and pleural effusions on two different occasions within a day of starting a course of oral metronidazole. On the initial occasion pulmo-nary infiltrates were also present.

Mitomycin

Small pleural effusions are frequently present in patients who have interstitial infil-trates secondary to mitomycin therapy (27).

Isotretinoin

There is one report (28) of a 49-year-old female who developed an eosinophilic pleural effusion 7 months after starting isotretinoin for systemic sclerosis. When the isotretinoin was stopped, the chest radiograph became normal within 3 months. The manufacturer of isotret-inoin has on file three other cases of pleural effusion occurring in patients who took isotre-tinoin for acne.

Propylthiouracil (PTU)

Middleton and associates (29) have re-ported one patient who developed left pleu-ritic chest pain and an eosinophilic pleural effusion 3 weeks after starting PTU. A thora-centesis 5 weeks after starting therapy re-vealed 16% eosinophils. She continued taking the PTU for 2 more weeks and the effusion enlarged and the eosinophils increased to 45%. The effusion then resolved after PTU was discontinued (29).

REFERENCES

1. Israel HL, Diamond P: Recurrent pulmonary infiltra-tion and pleural effusion due to nitrofurantoin sensi-tivity. N Engl J Med 1962;266:1024-1026.
2. Hailey FJ, Glascock HW Jr, Hewitt WF: Pleuropneu-monic reactions to nitrofurantoin. N Engl J Med 1969;281:1087-1090.
3. Rosenow EC III: Drug-induced bronchopulmonary pleural disease. J Allergy Clin Immunol 1987;80:780-787.
4. Cooper JA, White DA, Matthay RA: Drug-induced pulmonary disease. Am Rev Respir Dis 1986;133:488-505.
5. Holmberg L, Boman G: Pulmonary reactions to nitrofurantoin: 447 cases reported to the Swedish adverse drug reaction committee, 1966-1976. Eur J Respir Dis 1981;62:180-189.
6. Geller M, Flaherty DK, Dickie HA, Reed CE: Lym-phopenia in acute nitrofurantoin pleuropulmonary reactions. J Allergy Clin Immunol 1977;59:445-448.
7. Petusevsky ML, Faling J, Rocklin RE, et al: Pleuroperi-cardial reaction to treatment with dantrolene. JAMA 1979;242:2772-2774.
8. Mahoney JM, Bachtel MD: Pleural effusion associated with chronic dantrolene administration. Ann Pharma-cother 1994;28:587-589.
9. Graham JR: Cardiac and pulmonary fibrosis during methysergide therapy for headache. Am J Med Sci 1967;254:1-12.
10. Kok-Jensen A, Lindeneg O: Pleurisy and fibrosis of the pleura during methysergide treatment of hemi-crania. Scand J Respir Dis 1970;51:218-222.
11. Rinne UK: Pleuropulmonary changes during long-term bromocriptine treatment for Parkinson's dis-ease. Lancet 1981;1:44.
12. McElvaney NG, Wilcox PG, Churg A, Fleetham JA: Pleuropulmonary disease during bromocriptine treat-ment of Parkinson's disease. Arch Intern Med 1988;148:2231-2236.
13. Bhatt MH, Keenan SP, Fleetham JA, Calne DB: Pleu-ropulmonary disease associated with dopamine ago-nist therapy. Ann Neurol 1991;30:613-616.
14. Frans E, Dom R, Demedts M: Pleuropulmonary changes during treatment of Parkinson's disease with a long-acting ergot derivative, cabergoline. Eu-rop Respir J 1992;5:263-265.
15. Kinnunen E, Viljanen A: Pleuropulmonary involve-ment during bromocriptine treatment. Chest 1988;94:1034-1036.
16. Martin WJ II, Rosenow EC III: Amiodarone pulmo-nary toxicity. Chest 1988;93:1067-1074.

17. Gonzalez-Rothi RJ, Hannan SE, Hood I, Franzini DA: Amiodarone pulmonary toxicity presenting as bilateral exudative pleural effusions. Chest 1987;92:179–182.

18. Stein B, Zaatari GS, Pine JR: Amiodarone pulmonary toxicity. Clinical, cytologic and ultrastructural findings. Acta Cytol 1987;31:357–361.

19. Akoun GM, Milleron BJ, Badaro DM, et al: Pleural T-lymphocyte subsets in amiodarone-associated pleuropneumonitis. Chest 1989;95:596–597.

20. Vogelzang PJ, Bloom SM, Mier JW, Atkins MB: Chest roentgenographic abnormalities in IL-2 recipients. Incidence and correlation with clinical parameters. Chest 1992;101:746–752.

21. Saxon RR, Klein JR, Bar MH, Blanc P, Gamsu G, Webb WR, et al: Pathogenesis of pulmonary edema during interleukin-2 therapy: correlation of chest radiographic and clinical findings in 54 patients. AJR 1991;156:281–285.

22. Jones SE, Moore M, Blank N, Castellino RA: Hypersensitivity to procarbazine (Matulane) manifested by fever and pleuropulmonary reaction. Cancer 1972; 29:498–500.

23. Ecker MD, Jay B, Keohane MF: Procarbazine lung. AJR 1978;131:527–528.

24. Walden PAM, Mitchell-Heggs PF, Coppin C, et al: Pleurisy and methotrexate treatment. Br Med J 1977; 2:867.

25. Taal BG, Spierings ELH, Hilvering C: Pleuropulmonary fibrosis associated with chronic and excessive intake of ergotamine. Thorax 1983;38:396–398.

26. Kristenson M, Fryden A: Pneumonitis caused by metronidazole. JAMA 1988;260:184.

27. Gunstream SR, Seidenfield JJ, Sobonya RE, McMahon LJ: Mitomycin-associated lung disease. Cancer Treat Rep 1983;67:301–304.

28. Bunker CB, Sheron N, Maurice PD, Kocjan G, Johnson NM, Dowd PM: Isotretinoin and eosinophilic pleural effusion [letter]. Lancet 1989;1:435–436.

29. Middleton KL, Santella R, Couser JI Jr: Eosinophilic pleuritis due to propylthiouracil. Chest 1993;103: 955–956.

CHAPTER 18
Pleural Effusion Due to Miscellaneous Diseases

ASBESTOS EXPOSURE

The exposure to asbestos definitely appears to be associated with the occurrence of benign inflammatory exudative pleural effusions.

Incidence

Epler and coworkers reviewed the medical histories of 1135 asbestos workers whom they had followed for several years and found that 35 of the workers (3%) had pleural effusions for which there was no other ready explanation (1). In contrast, no unexplained effusions were seen in the control group of 717 subjects. These authors found a direct relationship between the level of asbestos exposure and the development of a pleural effusion. In patients with heavy, moderate, and mild asbestos exposure, the incidence of pleural effusion was 9.2, 3.9, and 0.7 effusions per 1000 person-years, respectively (1). Pleural effusions occur sooner after asbestos exposure than do pleural plaques or pleural calcification. In the foregoing series, many patients developed pleural effusions within 5 years of the initial exposure, and almost all did so within 20 years of the initial exposure. This finding is in direct contrast to the occurrence of pleural plaques and pleural calcifications, which usually do not occur until at least 20 years after the initial exposure. Other investigators, however, have reported a much longer period between the initial exposure and the development of the effusion. Hillerdal and Ozesmi (2) reviewed 60 patients with asbestos-related pleural effusions and found that the mean latency after the initial exposure was 30 years, and that only 4 of their patients had developed a pleural effusion within 10 years of the initial exposure.

Pathogenesis and Pathologic Features

The pathogenesis of the pleural effusion that occurs after asbestos exposure is not known, but is probably similar to that of pleural plaques, described in Chapter 22. In the series of Epler and associates, 20% of the affected individuals had pleural plaques (1), whereas in the Hillerdal series (2) 39 of 60 patients (65%) had bilateral pleural plaques. It is likely that the presence of submicroscopic asbestos particles in the pleural space provides a constant stimulation to the pleural mesothelial cells (3). When mesothelial cells are cultured in the presence of asbestos particles they synthesize and release a protein fraction with chemotactic activity for neutrophils, which appears to be interleukin-8 (IL-8) (4). When crocidolite is instilled into the pleural spaces of rabbits, chemotactic activity rapidly appears in the pleural fluid, and this chemotactic activity is significantly inhibited by a neutralizing antibody to human IL-8 (4). In addition, when rat mesothelial cells are incubated in the presence of crocidolite or chrysotile asbestos fibers, they secrete the fibroblast chemoattractant fibronectin (5).

The gross pathologic findings in patients with pleural effusions secondary to asbestos exposure are not well defined. Mattson performed thoracoscopy on 9 patients with asbestos-related pleural effusion and found that the lung surface was completely normal in all patients, but the parietal pleura was inflamed (6). In contrast, Gaensler and Kaplan reported that both the visceral pleura and the parietal pleura of their patients were thickened, and an irregular pleural symphysis was seen in all patients (7). Perhaps the difference between these series is that pleural disease had been present longer in the second group. Microscopic examination of the pleura reveals chronic fibrosing pleuritis with varying degrees of inflammation and vascularity, depending on the acuteness of the process (7, 8).

Clinical Manifestations

Patients with pleural effusions secondary to asbestos exposure have surprisingly few symptoms (1, 2). In Hillerdal's series of 60 patients, 47% had no symptoms, 34% had chest pain, 6% had dyspnea, and the remainder had various other symptoms (2). Mattson reported that his patients often complained of feeling heavy in their chest (6). Most of Gaensler's patients complained of pleuritic chest pain or progressive dyspnea, but these patients were referred for symptoms rather than having their disorder diagnosed on the basis of serial chest radiographs (7).

The chest radiograph usually reveals a small-to-moderate-sized pleural effusion, which is bilateral in about 10% of patients (1). Many patients have pleural plaques, whereas fewer than 5% have pleural calcifications, and approximately 50% have some evidence of parenchymal asbestosis (1, 7).

The pleural fluid with asbestos-related pleural effusion is an exudate that is serous or serosanguineous (6). The pleural fluid white blood cell count (WBC) can be as high as $28,000/mm^3$, and the pleural fluid differential WBC can reveal either predominantly polymorphonuclear leukocytes or mononuclear cells (2). Pleural fluid eosinophilia appears to be a characteristic of asbestos-related pleural effusions. In one series, more than 50% eosinophils were found in 5 of 11 pleural effusions, and an additional two effusions had more than 15% eosinophils (6). In a second series (2), 26% of 66 asbestos-related effusions had pleural fluid eosinophilia. Most asbestos-related pleural effusions contain mesothelial cells (2).

Diagnosis

The diagnosis of asbestos-related pleural effusion is one of exclusion. Patients with a strong history of exposure to asbestos and a pleural effusion should be closely evaluated for mesothelioma or metastatic bronchogenic carcinoma because these diseases occur much more commonly in individuals exposed to asbestos. If these diseases as well as tuberculosis and pulmonary embolism are ruled out, the patient probably has an asbestos-related pleural effusion and should be watched. The work history of any patient with an undiagnosed exudative pleural effusion should be evaluated for exposure to asbestos. If such exposure is found and the patient is asymptomatic with a small pleural effusion, the effusion is probably due to asbestos exposure.

Prognosis

The natural history of the patient with an asbestos-related pleural effusion is one of chronicity with frequent recurrences and sometimes the development of fibrosis of the parietal pleura (1, 6–8). The pleural effusion on the average lasts several months, but eventually it clears and leaves no residual pleural disease in the majority of patients (2). In the series of 35 patients followed by Epler and colleagues for a mean period of 9.7 years, 29% of the patients developed recurrent benign effusions, more commonly on the contralateral side (1). In about 20% of patients, massive pleural fibrosis follows the asbestos-related pleural effusion, whereas in an additional 20%, the ipsilateral costophrenic angle remains blunted after the effusion has resolved. Malignant mesotheliomas at times follow asbestos-related pleural effusions. Three of the 61 patients (5%) in the series of Epler and associates developed a mesothelioma during the follow-up period. These mesotheliomas occurred 6, 9, and 16 years after the initial pleural effusion (1).

POSTCARDIAC INJURY (DRESSLER'S) SYNDROME

The postcardiac injury syndrome is characterized by the onset of fever, pleuropericarditis, and parenchymal infiltrates in the weeks following injury to the pericardium or myocardium (9, 10). This syndrome has been described following myocardial infarction, cardiac surgery, blunt chest trauma, percutaneous left ventricular puncture, pacemaker implantation, and angioplasty.

Incidence

The incidence of the postcardiac injury syndrome was thought by Dressler to be 3 to 4% after an acute myocardial infarction (9). Subsequent studies have demonstrated that the incidence is probably less than 1% (11), but the incidence is much higher in patients with large transmural infarctions in which the pericardium is involved (12). In one series, 15% of patients with an acute myocardial infarction and pericarditis developed the post-myocardial infarction syndrome during the follow-up period (12). The incidence of the syndrome is much higher following surgical procedures involving the pericardium (10, 13) than after an acute myocardial infarction. Engle and associates reported that 30% of 257 children undergoing cardiac operations developed the syndrome (10). Miller and coworkers reported an incidence of 17.8% in 944 patients undergoing cardiac surgery at Johns Hopkins Hospital during a 1-year period (14).

Etiologic Factors

The cause of the syndrome is unknown, but it appears to have an immunologic basis. Damage to the pericardium may initiate the immunologic events in susceptible individuals. In patients undergoing surgical procedures involving the pericardium, a close relationship exists between the development of the syndrome and the presence of antiheart antibodies. Engle and colleagues prospectively followed 257 patients undergoing cardiac operations and found that 67 (26%) had high titers of antiheart antibodies, and all these patients developed the syndrome (10). None of 102 patients without a rise in antibody titers developed the syndrome, and only 4 of 93 patients with intermediate titers developed the syndrome. In a second study conducted by De Scheerder and coworkers, antibodies were measured to actin and myosin preoperatively and postoperatively in 62 patients undergoing coronary artery bypass surgery (15). Eight patients (13%) developed the postcardiac injury syndrome and all eight had more than a 60% increase in their antibodies to both actin and myosin postoperatively. Thirty-eight patients did not develop the syndrome and none

of these patients had more than a 50% rise in either of the antibodies. The remaining patients developed an incomplete syndrome and had intermediate increases in their antibody titers. No such clear-cut relationship has been demonstrated between antiheart antibodies and the syndrome in patients with myocardial infarction. Liem and coworkers were unable to find any association between the development of the syndrome and the presence of antiheart muscle antibodies in 136 patients with an acute myocardial infarction (11). In postoperative patients, it is unclear whether the antiheart antibodies precipitate or result from the syndrome.

Other factors also appear to be associated with the development of the postcardiac injury syndrome. Epidemiologic studies indicate that there is a seasonal variation in the postcardiac injury syndrome with the highest incidence corresponding to the time of the highest prevalence of viral infection in the community (16). It has been hypothesized than a concurrent viral infection may trigger the immune response (15). In patients undergoing cardiac surgery, the incidence is approximately the same after all types of surgery (14). Younger patients and patients who are asymptomatic preoperatively are more likely to develop the syndrome (14). There is also a higher incidence of the syndrome if the patient has a history of pericarditis or if the patient had taken corticosteroids previously (14).

Clinical Manifestations

This syndrome is characterized by fever, chest pain, pericarditis, pleuritis, and pneumonitis occurring after cardiac trauma or an acute myocardial infarction. The symptoms following myocardial infarction usually develop in the 2nd or 3rd week; an occasional patient develops symptoms within the 1st week (17), and a larger percentage develops symptoms only after the 3rd week. The syndrome is seen at an average of 3 weeks following cardiac operations, but can occur anywhere between 3 days and 1 year (18). The two cardinal symptoms of the syndrome are fever and chest pain (9, 18). The chest pain often precedes the onset of fever and varies from crushing and agonizing, mimicking myocardial ischemia, to a dull ache, to pleuritic chest pain (9). Almost all patients have a pericardial friction rub, and many also have a pericardial effusion. As many as 75% of patients with these syndromes have pulmonary infiltrates, either linear or in patches, mostly located in the base of the lungs (19). Laboratory evaluation reveals leukocytosis (10,000–20,000/mm^3) and an elevated erythrocyte sedimentation rate in most patients (9, 18).

Pleural involvement is common in the postcardiac injury syndrome. Dressler reported that 68% of 35 patients with the postmyocardial infarction syndrome had pleural effusions (9). Stelzner and coworkers (19) reported that 29 of 35 patients (83%) had a pleural effusion. The effusion was unilateral in 18 and bilateral in 11 in the latter series (19). In general, the pleural effusion is small, and pericarditis is the dominant feature. The pleural fluid is an exudate with a normal pH and a normal glucose level (19). The pleural fluid is frankly bloody in about 30% of patients, and the differential WBC may reveal predominantly polymorphonuclear leukocytes or mononuclear cells, depending on the acuteness of the process (19). In certain instances the pleural fluid will contain mostly small lymphocytes (20).

Diagnosis

The diagnosis of the syndrome should be considered in any patient who develops a pleural effusion following myocardial infarction or a cardiac operation, particularly when signs of pericarditis are present. The diagnosis of the syndrome is established by the clinical picture and by ruling out congestive heart failure, pulmonary embolism, and pneumonia. Congestive heart failure as a cause of the pleural effusion is excluded by the demonstration of an exudative pleural fluid. A perfusion lung scan should be obtained to exclude the diagnosis of pulmonary embolization. If the perfusion lung scan is positive or equivocal, one should consider obtaining a pulmonary arteriogram because anticoagulation is contraindicated in the postmyocardial infarction

syndrome (9). Patients with the syndrome are at risk for developing hemopericardium.

Treatment

This syndrome usually responds to treatment with anti-inflammatory agents such as aspirin or indomethacin. In the more severe forms of the syndrome, corticosteroids may be necessary (21). It is important to establish the diagnosis of the postcardiac injury syndrome in patients who have undergone coronary artery bypass procedures because the pericarditis may cause graft occlusion. Urschel and associates reported that graft occlusion occurred in 12 of 14 patients (86%) who developed the syndrome after coronary artery bypass operations and who were treated symptomatically (18). When 31 subsequent patients were treated with prednisone, 30 mg/day for a week and tapering doses for 5 weeks thereafter, in addition to aspirin 600 mg four times daily, only 5 (16%) of the grafts became occluded (18).

PERICARDIAL DISEASE

A substantial percentage of patients with pericardial disease will develop a pleural effusion, which is usually left-sided. Weiss and Spodick (22) reviewed the charts of 133 consecutively discharged patients with pericardial disease. Thirty-five of the patients (26%) had a roentgenographically demonstrable pleural effusion and no other lung disease. Twenty-one of the patients had inflammatory pericardial disease without congestive heart failure, and 15 of these patients had only a left-sided pleural effusion, 3 had more fluid on the left than on the right, and in 3 the effusions were the same size on both sides. Of the 5 patients with inflammatory pericarditis and congestive heart failure, the effusions were equal bilaterally in 2, greater on the right side in 2, and left-sided in 1. Two of the 3 patients with constrictive pericarditis had a unilateral left-sided effusion. Tomaselli and associates (23) reviewed 30 cases of constrictive pericarditis and found that a pleural effusion was present in 18 (60%). In 12 of the 18 patients the effusion was bilateral and approximately symmetric. Three effusions were left-sided, and 3 were right-sided.

The mechanism responsible for the pleural effusion associated with pericardial disease is not clear. The obvious explanation is that the pulmonary and systemic capillary pressures are elevated secondary to the pericardial disease, resulting in a transudative pleural effusion. It is still not clear why the effusions are more commonly left-sided in patients with inflammatory pericardial disease or why at least some patients with constrictive pericarditis have exudative pleural effusions (23). The pericardial inflammation itself is probably related to the development of the pleural effusion (22).

The characteristics of the pleural fluid seen in conjunction with pericardial disease are not well described. Tomaselli and coworkers (23) reported that the fluid was exudative in 3 patients and transudative in 1 patient with constrictive pericarditis. I would guess that the pleural fluid with inflammatory pericardial disease is also exudative.

Obviously, the treatment of choice for the pleural effusion secondary to pericardial disease is to treat the pericardial disease.

AFTER CORONARY ARTERY BYPASS SURGERY

There is a very high incidence of pleural effusions after coronary artery bypass graft (CABG) surgery. In one study of 152 patients who had undergone CABG surgery, the incidence of pleural effusion on routine chest radiographs 7 days postoperatively was 42% (24). In a subsequent study 47 patients underwent chest ultrasound on the 7th, 14th and 30th postoperative day. In this latter study the prevalence of pleural effusion was 89.4% on the 7th postoperative day, 76.6% on the 14th postoperative day, and 57.4% on the 30th postoperative day (25).

The pleural effusions that occur after CABG surgery tend to be unilateral on the left side. In the study using ultrasound (25) in which 42 of 47 patients had pleural effusion on the 7th postoperative day, 17 (40%) of the effusions were unilateral on the left, 24 (57%) were bilateral, and 1 (2%) was unilateral on the right. By the 30th postoperative day, there were 27 patients with effusions and 18 (67%) of these were unilateral left-sided, 8 (30%) were bilateral, and 1 (4%) was unilateral right-sided (25). The effusions are usually small. In the study of Peng and coworkers, only 6 of the 51 patients with pleural effusion (12%) had a pleural effusion that occupied more than two intercostal spaces (24).

The etiology of the pleural effusion after CABG surgery is probably related to trauma to the pleura during the time of surgery (25). Patients undergoing internal mammary grafting are more likely to have a pleural effusion than those undergoing only saphenous vein grafting (25). Patients with a pericardial effusion postoperatively are more likely to have a pleural effusion, but it is likely that both are a result of trauma rather than being responsible for the other (25). It is unlikely that the effusions are due to the postcardiac injury syndrome since the highest incidence of pleural effusion is within the first week of surgery (25). The pleural effusion is probably not due to congestive heart failure because the group with pleural effusions do not have a higher incidence of an enlarged heart (24) or a lower ejection fraction (25) than do the group without pleural effusion.

The proper management of the patient with a pleural effusion after CABG surgery is usually observation. Since most patients have pleural effusion, a diagnostic thoracentesis is not usually warranted. However, if the patient is febrile or has a large effusion, a diagnostic thoracentesis should be performed. If the effusion develops more than a few days after surgery, important diagnostic considerations are pulmonary embolism, the postcardiac injury syndrome, and heart failure. If the pleural effusion develops after the first week, a diagnostic thoracentesis should be performed with the major diagnostic considerations being pleural infection, heart failure, pulmonary embolism, and the postcardiac injury syndrome.

Occasionally patients will develop symptomatic left-sided pleural effusions several months after CABG surgery (26–28). The effusions are sometimes quite large and can occur 3 weeks to 12 months postoperatively. Some such effusions are due to persistent bleeding into the pleural space at the site of harvest of the internal mammary graft (26) while others are due to a trapped lung (27). Such patients should undergo a therapeutic thoracentesis, which is curative in some cases. If the effusion rapidly recurs, consideration should be given to performing a decortication if there is evidence that the lung is trapped.

AFTER LUNG TRANSPLANTATION

Pleural effusions are common after lung transplantation. Normally 80% of the fluid which enters the interstitial spaces of the lungs is cleared from the lung via the lymphatics, while 20% is cleared through the pleural space (see Chapter 2). In the patient with a lung transplant, however, the lymphatics are transected and accordingly almost all the fluid that enters the lung exits through the pleural space.

Pleural effusions usually are not evident in the immediate posttransplant period because the patients have chest tubes. The amount of fluid that drains through the chest tube may be very large, particularly if the patient has the reperfusion syndrome. In one patient with a severe reperfusion syndrome the chest tube drained more than 600 ml/hour (29). Interestingly, although the fluid draining from the chest tube in the immediate postoperative period presumably represents interstitial fluid, there have been no systematic studies on the diagnostic usefulness of cellular or chemical measurements on this fluid.

It appears that patients who develop complications after their lung transplants are likely to have a pleural effusion. In one series in children radiologic findings were correlated with histopathologic diagnoses in 62 instances (30). Pleural effusions occurred with 14 of 19 (74%) episodes of acute rejection, 7 of 8 (88%) instances of chronic rejection, 6 of 11 (55%) episodes of infection, 3 of 4 (75%) instances with lymphoproliferative diseases, and 15 of 20 (75%) episodes in which the histopathology was nonspecific. The high prevalence of effusion with the different entities posttransplantation is probably due to the fact that a larger percentage of interstitial fluid exits through the pleural space in the patient with lung transplantation.

The omental flap used to prevent dehiscence of the bronchial anastomosis may result in a "pseudo-effusion" on the chest radiograph. The omentum with its blood supply is introduced into the chest cavity through a small incision in the diaphragm. It is particularly likely to mimic an effusion on a supine radiograph (31).

MEIGS' SYNDROME

Meigs originally described a syndrome characterized by the presence of ascites and pleural effusions in patients with benign solid ovarian tumors (32). When the ovarian tumor was removed, the ascites and the pleural effusion both resolved. Subsequent to this original report, it has become apparent that a similar syndrome can occur with benign cystic ovarian tumors, with benign tumors of the uterus (fibromyomata), with low-grade ovarian malignant tumors without evidence of metastases (33), and with endometrioma (34). Meigs still prefers to reserve his name for only those cases in which the primary neoplasm is a benign solid ovarian tumor (33). Nevertheless, I classify any patient with a pelvic neoplasm associated with ascites and pleural effusion, in whom surgical extirpation of the tumor results in permanent disappearance of the ascites and pleural effusion, as having Meigs' syndrome.

Etiologic Factors

The pathogenesis of the ascitic fluid in patients with Meigs' syndrome appears to be a generalized secretion of fluid from the primary tumor. Such tumors secrete a large amount of fluid even when they have been resected and placed in dry containers (33). Only large tumors appear to be associated with free peritoneal fluid at the time of surgical procedures. Samanth and Black found that only tumors with diameters greater than 11 cm were associated with free peritoneal fluid (35). Approximately 15% of ovarian fibromas are associated with free ascitic fluid (36), but not all patients with ascites have pleural effusions. I believe that the genesis of the pleural fluid in Meigs' syndrome is similar to that with ascites and cirrhosis (see Chapter 6); that is, fluid passes through pores in the diaphragm. Evidence for this pathogenesis includes the similar characteristics of the ascitic and pleural fluid, the rapid reaccumulation of the fluid following thoracentesis, and the absence of pleural effusions in some patients with ovarian tumors and ascites (36). Other investigators have concluded that the pleural fluid arises from the transdiaphragmatic transfer of ascitic fluid by the lymphatic vessels (36–38).

The tumor most commonly responsible for Meigs' syndrome is the ovarian fibroma, followed by ovarian cysts, thecomas, granulosal cell tumors, and leiomyomas of the uterus (33).

Clinical Manifestations

Patients with Meigs' syndrome usually have a chronic illness characterized by weight loss, pleural effusion, ascites, and a pelvic mass (36). It is important to remember that not all such patients have disseminated pelvic malignant disease. Patients with Meigs' syndrome may even have markedly elevated serum CA 125 levels (39). The pleural effusion is right-sided in about 70% of patients, is left-sided in 10%, and is bilateral in 20% (38). The only symptom referable to the pleural effusion is shortness of breath. The ascites may not be evident on physical examination.

The pleural fluid is usually an exudate. Although several authors have stated that the pleural fluid with Meigs' syndrome is a transudate (36, 40), this opinion appears to be based on the gross appearance of the fluid rather than on its protein levels. Most pleural fluids secondary to Meigs' syndrome have a protein level above 3.0 g/dl (36, 40–44). The pleural fluid usually has a low WBC (fewer than 1000/mm^3) and occasionally is bloody (36, 43).

Diagnosis and Management

The diagnosis of Meigs' syndrome should be considered in all women who have pelvic masses, ascites, and pleural effusions. If in such patients the cytologic examination of the ascitic and pleural fluid is negative, an exploratory laparotomy or at least a diagnostic laparoscopy should be performed with surgical removal of the primary neoplasm. The diagnosis is confirmed when the ascites and the pleural fluid resolve postoperatively and do not recur. Postoperatively, the pleural fluid

disappears from the chest rapidly and is usually completely gone within 2 weeks (36).

YELLOW NAIL SYNDROME

The yellow nail syndrome consists of the triad of deformed yellow nails, lymphedema, and pleural effusions. Until 1986, only 97 patients had been reported with this syndrome (45). About twice as many females as males are affected (46). Eighty-nine percent of the reported cases have had yellow nails, and the yellow nails were the presenting manifestation in 37%. Lymphedema of various degrees was encountered in 80% of the reported cases and was the initial manifestation in 34%. Pleural effusions were found in 36% of all cases (45). The 3 separate entities may become manifest at widely varying times. For example, 1 patient developed lymphedema in childhood, chronic nail changes at age 78, and a pleural effusion in her ninth decade (47).

The basic abnormality in this syndrome appears to be hypoplasia of the lymphatic vessels. Lymphangiograms of the lower extremity demonstrate hypoplasia of at least some lymphatic vessels in most patients with the syndrome (47). Emerson has postulated that pleural effusions may develop when a lower respiratory tract infection or pleural inflammation damages previously adequate but impaired lymphatic vessels (48). Subsequently, the lymphatic drainage of the pleural space is insufficient to maintain a fluid-free pleural space. In one report biopsy of the parietal pleura revealed abnormally dilated lymphatics, neogenesis of lymphatic channels, and edematous tissues in some areas, suggesting some deficit in lymphatic drainage (49). The albumin turnover in the pleural fluid is not greatly decreased in patients with this syndrome, however (50).

With this syndrome, the nails are yellow, thickened, and smooth and may show transverse ridging (51). They are excessively curved from side to side, and the actual color is pale yellow to greenish. Onycholysis (separation of nail from bed) is frequently present, and nail growth is slow (51).

The pleural effusions are bilateral in about 50% of patients and vary in size from small to massive (51). Once pleural effusions have occurred with this syndrome, they persist and recur rapidly after a thoracentesis (47). The pleural fluid is usually a clear yellow exudate with a normal glucose level and predominantly lymphocytes in the pleural fluid differential WBC (47, 48, 51). The pleural biopsy reveals fibrosis, nonspecific inflammation, or lymphocytic cellular infiltrates, none of which are diagnostic of the disease (46).

The diagnosis is made when a patient has a chronic pleural effusion in conjunction with yellow nails or lymphedema. No specific treatment exists for the syndrome, but if the effusion is large and produces dyspnea, pleurodesis with a tetracycline derivative or talc (see Chapter 7) or thoracoscopy with talc insufflation or pleural abrasion should be considered (49, 51). One patient with pleural effusion secondary to the yellow nail syndrome has been treated successfully with a pleuroperitoneal shunt (52). There is one case report where the nail deformities improved after they were treated with topical vitamin E (53).

SARCOIDOSIS

Sarcoidosis is occasionally complicated by pleural effusion (54–58). The incidence of pleural effusion with sarcoidosis is probably about 1 to 2% (54, 57), although it has been reported to be as high as 7% (55). Patients with sarcoid pleural effusion usually have extensive parenchymal sarcoidosis and frequently also have extrathoracic sarcoidosis (54, 55). The symptoms of pleural involvement with sarcoidosis are variable; many patients have no symptoms (54), although an equal number have pleuritic chest pain or dyspnea.

The pleural effusions with sarcoidosis are bilateral in approximately one-third of cases and are unilateral in the remainder. The pleural effusions are usually small, but may be large. The pleural fluid is generally an exudate with predominantly small lymphocytes on the differential WBC (54, 56–58). In one case (59), 90% of the cells in the pleural fluid were eosinophils at the time of the initial thoracentesis. In one report, all seven patients were described as having transudative pleural effusions with no pleural fluid protein concentration above 2.5 g/dl (55). This report is so much at variance with other reports (54, 56–

58) concerning the protein levels in the pleural fluid, however, that it can probably be ignored. Needle biopsy of the pleura or open pleural biopsy reveals noncaseating granulomas in the pleura.

The diagnosis of a sarcoid pleural effusion should be suspected in any patient with bilateral parenchymal infiltrates and a pleural effusion. A pleural biopsy demonstrating noncaseating granulomas is further support for the diagnosis, but most patients with pleural effusions and noncaseating granulomas on their pleural biopsy have tuberculosis rather than sarcoidosis. Fungal disease involving the pleura (see Chapter 11) must also be considered when noncaseating granulomas are seen on pleural biopsy examination. If a patient has typical, symmetric bilateral hilar adenopathy, parenchymal infiltrates, a negative purified protein derivative (PPD) test, and noncaseating granulomas in tissue besides the pleura, however, he probably has sarcoidosis. An elevated serum angiotensin-converting enzyme level gives strong support to the diagnosis. The administration of corticosteroids to patients with pleural sarcoidosis leads to a rapid amelioration of symptoms (if any) and a resolution of the pleural effusion (56, 58).

Necrotizing sarcoid granulomatosis is a disease in which the primary pathologic abnormality is a sarcoidlike granuloma but which is also characterized by vasculitis and necrosis (60). By 1989 about 80 cases had been described. Clinically, patients may be asymptomatic or may present with cough, fever, sweats, malaise, dyspnea, hemoptysis, or pleuritic pain. Extrapulmonary findings are usually absent. Roentgenographically, the majority of patients manifest multiple well-defined nodules or ill-defined opacities. There seems to a greater pleural component with necrotizing sarcoid granulomatosis than with typical sarcoid. In one recent report, seven patients presented with pleuritic chest pain (60). Pleural involvement was seen on CT scanning in six patients and two patients had pleural effusion. The pleural fluid findings with necrotizing sarcoid granulomatosis have not been described. The prognosis of patients with necrotizing sarcoid granulomatosis is favorable and most patients improve rapidly after corticosteroid therapy is initiated (60).

FETAL PLEURAL EFFUSION

The ability to diagnose fetal abnormalities prenatally has been extended by diagnostic ultrasound. One abnormality now diagnosed on occasion is fetal pleural effusion. The prevalence of fetal pleural effusion is approximately 1 in 10,000 deliveries (61). The prevalence is approximately twice as high in males as in females (62).

Fetal pleural effusion is associated with a high perinatal mortality. In a review of 78 cases, the mortality was 36%. The mortality rate was 37% for those treated conservatively while it was 33% for those treated with pleuroamniotic shunts (61). The high perinatal mortality rate in cases of fetal pleural effusion is related to three factors: development of nonimmune hydrops, prematurity, and pulmonary hypoplasia (61). The intrathoracic compression of the developing lung produces pulmonary hypoplasia. This pulmonary hypoplasia can sometimes result in perinatal death.

The pathogenesis of the fetal pleural effusion is not known and is possibly multifactorial. There is some evidence that the fetal pleural effusions are actually chylothoraces. Benacerraf and Frigoletto (63, 64) analyzed the pleural fluid from two fetuses and reported abundant lymphocytes in both, but one had almost all T lymphocytes, whereas the other had a mixture of T and B lymphocytes. The presence of the lymphocytes was suggestive of a chylous effusion. In addition, most neonatal pleural effusions are chylothoraces (65). Analysis of the pleural fluid for chylomicrons is not useful in diagnosing fetal chylothorax because the fetuses are not eating any lipids.

In a recent review of isolated fetal pleural effusion, 82 cases were found in the medical literature (61). The fetal pleural effusions were bilateral in 48 of 82 cases (59%), right-sided in 14 (17%), and left-sided in 20 (24%) (61). Polyhydramnios was noted in 35 of 82 (42%). The reason for the polyhydramnios is not clear, but it has been suggested that the increased intrathoracic pressure may interfere with normal fetal swallowing.

The optimal management for fetuses with pleural effusions is controversial (61). If the pleural effusions are not treated, some will resolve spontaneously while others will deteriorate to generalized hydrops. Some infants will die from pulmonary hypoplasia after delivery, whereas others survive. As mentioned above, in a recent review, the mortality rates of those treated surgically and those treated conservatively was comparable (61). In a second review, however, the percentage of fetuses with a good outcome was significantly higher if they were subjected to invasive treatment (66).

The following management scheme as recommended by Hagay and coworkers is suggested for the management of fetal pleural effusion (61). When a pleural effusion is discovered in a fetus, a repeat ultrasound is obtained in 2–3 weeks. If the effusion has decreased in size, then the fetus is followed with scans every 2–3 weeks. If the effusion is stable or if the effusion has increased in size, then a diagnostic amniocentesis should be performed for chromosomal analysis and culture of amniotic fluid to screen for bacterial or viral infection. At the same time, a diagnostic thoracentesis should be performed and the pleural fluid sent for culture, cell analysis, and biochemical study. The lung size and the fetal lung distensibility are assessed via ultrasound before and after the thoracentesis. Fetuses who have less than normal lung expansion are then subjected to surgical intervention.

The possible surgical interventions for fetal pleural effusion are pleuroamniotic shunt or repeated therapeutic thoracentesis. Rodeck et al. (67) reported their results with the implantation of pleuroamniotic shunts in eight human fetuses with pleural effusion. These shunts were established with double-pigtail nylon catheters with external and internal diameters of 0.21 and 0.15 mm, respectively. The shunts were introduced transamniotically under ultrasound visualization through the fetal midthoracic wall into the effusion. All eight fetuses in this series had large pleural effusions with hydramnios. Twelve pleuroamniotic shunts were placed in these fetuses. One shunt was noted to be free in the amniotic cavity 1 week after insertion, and a second shunt was inserted. The remaining 11 shunts functioned until delivery (median 2.5 weeks; range 1 to 14 weeks). In six fetuses, the pleural effusions almost completely resolved and the hydramnios disappeared. Three of the six had hydrops that resolved after the insertion of the shunt. All six infants survived and five had no respiratory difficulty at birth. Fetal hydrothoraces did not resolve in two patients, both of whom had hydrops and died shortly after delivery. In a second study Blott and coworkers (68) inserted shunts into 11 fetuses between 24 and 35 weeks' gestation and reported that the effusions were successfully drained in all cases and that 8 of the 11 fetuses survived.

An alternative approach to the management of the fetal pleural effusion is to perform serial thoracenteses. Benacerraf and coworkers (63, 64) performed 3 to 5 thoracenteses between 20 and 24 weeks' gestation on two fetuses with massive pleural effusions. The effusion did not recur after the last thoracentesis and normal babies resulted from both pregnancies.

The prognosis of fetuses who have pleural effusion and who receive pleuroamniotic shunting appears to be good. Thompson and coworkers studied 17 infants who had undergone pleuroamniotic shunting for a fetal pleural effusion at a median age of 12 months. They reported that respiratory symptoms and respiratory function were no different in these 17 infants than in a control group (69).

UREMIA

At autopsy, fibrinous pleuritis is found in approximately 20% of patients dying of uremia (70). During life, this fibrinous pleuritis can be manifested as pleuritic chest pain with pleural rubs (71), pleural effusions (71-73), or progressive pleural fibrosis producing severe restrictive ventilatory dysfunction (73-75). The pathogenesis of the pleural disease associated with uremia is not known, but it is probably similar to that for the pericarditis that is seen with uremia. The pleural effusion and the restrictive pleuritis have been likened to the hemorrhagic pericarditis and constrictive pericarditis seen with uremia.

The incidence of pleural effusions with uremia is approximately 3% (72). No close relationship exists between the degree of uremia and the occurrence of a pleural effusion (72). More than 50% of these patients are symptomatic, with fever (50%), chest pain (30%), cough (35%), and dyspnea (20%) the most common symptoms (72). The pleural effusions are bilateral in about 20% of patients and may be large. In a series of 14 patients with uremic pleural effusions, more than 50% of the hemithorax was occupied by pleural fluid in 6 patients (43%) (72). Another patient had opacification of the entire hemithorax with mediastinal shift contralaterally.

The pleural fluid in uremic pleuritis is an exudate that is frequently serosanguineous or frankly hemorrhagic (71-73). The glucose level is normal, and the differential WBC reveals predominantly lymphocytes in the majority of patients (72). Pleural biopsy specimens invariably reveal chronic fibrinous pleuritis.

The diagnosis of uremic pleuritis is one of exclusion in the patient with chronic renal failure. Specifically, fluid overload (in such a case the fluid is a transudate), chronic pleural infection, malignant disease, and pulmonary embolism need to be excluded. There is one report (76) that suggests that measurement of the pleural fluid levels of neopterin might be useful in diagnosing uremic pleural effusions. In this report 8 of 9 patients (89%) with a uremic pleural effusion had a pleural fluid neopterin level above 200 nmol/L while none of 85 other patients with pleural effusions of varying etiologies had levels this high (76).

Dialysis is the treatment of choice for patients with uremic pleuritis. With dialysis, the effusion gradually disappears within 4 to 6 weeks in about 75% of patients. In the remaining 25%, the effusion persists, progresses, or recurs.

In an occasional patient, the pleural thickening is progressive and leads to severe restrictive ventilatory dysfunction and marked shortness of breath (73-75). At least three such patients have undergone a decortication procedure, and the operation was not complicated by severe bleeding in any of these patients (73-75). All three patients reported marked symptomatic improvement, and one patient's vital capacity increased from 850 ml preoperatively to 1600 ml 9 months postoperatively. Based on these reports and the progressive nature of uremic pleuritis, decortication should be considered in uremic patients with pleural thickening and severe respiratory symptoms.

TRAPPED LUNG

A fibrous peel may form over the visceral pleura in response to pleural inflammation. This peel can prevent the underlying lung from expanding (77, 78). The lung is therefore said to be trapped. When the lung is trapped, the pleural pressure becomes more negative as the chest wall is pulled in. The negative pleural pressure increases pleural fluid formation and decreases pleural fluid absorption (see Figure 2.1) resulting in a chronic pleural effusion.

The incidence of pleural effusion secondary to trapped lung is not known, but it is probably much higher than generally recognized. The event producing the initial pleural inflammation is usually a pneumonia or a hemothorax, but spontaneous pneumothorax, thoracic operations including coronary artery bypass surgery (27), uremia, and collagen vascular disease can all cause the initial pleural inflammation. The presence of a transudative pleural effusion for many months on occasion can lead to the formation of a visceral pleural peel and a trapped lung.

Patients with pleural effusions secondary to trapped lung have either shortness of breath due to restrictive ventilatory dysfunction or an asymptomatic pleural effusion. Symptoms of acute pleural inflammation such as pleuritic chest pain or fever are distinctly uncommon, but the patient often gives a history of such events in the past. One characteristic of the pleural effusion secondary to trapped lung is that the amount of fluid is remarkably constant from one study to another (77). Following thoracentesis, the fluid reaccumulates rapidly to its previous level.

Although one would expect that the pleural fluid with trapped lung would be exudative because the pleural surfaces are involved, the pleural fluid is usually a borderline exudate. The ratio of pleural fluid to serum protein is about 0.5, and the ratio of the pleural fluid lactic acid dehydrogenase (LDH) level to the serum LDH level is about 0.6. The pleural fluid glucose level is normal, and the pleural fluid WBC is usually less than $1000/mm^3$, with the differential WBC revealing predominantly mononuclear cells.

The diagnosis of pleural effusion secondary to trapped lung should be suspected in any patient with a stable chronic pleural effusion, particularly with a history of pneumonia, pneumothorax, hemothorax, or thoracic operation. The injection of 200 to 400 ml air at the time of a diagnostic thoracentesis frequently permits demonstration of the thickened visceral pleura. Measurements of the pleural pressure as fluid is withdrawn during therapeutic thoracentesis (see Chapter 23) are useful in supporting this diagnosis. The initial pleural pressure is low, and the rate of decline of pleural pressure as fluid is removed is high in patients with trapped lung. If the initial pleural pressure is below -10 cm H_2O, or if the pleural pressure falls more than 20 cm $H_2O/1000$ ml fluid removed, the diagnosis is suggested if the patient does not have bronchial obstruction or malignant disease coating the pleura (78).

The definitive diagnosis of trapped lung requires a thoracotomy and decortication with the demonstration that the underlying lung will expand to fill the pleural space. This operation also cures the patient, but such a surgical procedure is probably not indicated in the asymptomatic or minimally symptomatic patient with trapped lung. Such patients can be observed if the clinical picture, pleural fluid findings, and pleural pressure measurements are all compatible with the diagnosis (78).

THERAPEUTIC RADIATION EXPOSURE

Pleural effusions can occur as a complication of radiotherapy to the chest. Bachman and Macken followed 200 patients treated with between 4000 and 6000 rads to the hemithorax for breast carcinoma (79). These researchers reported that 11 patients (5.5%) developed pleural effusions with no other obvious explanation. The pleural effusions, therefore, were attributed to the radiation (79). All patients developed their pleural effusions within 6 months of completing radiation therapy, and every patient had concomitant radiation pneumonitis (79). The pleural fluid with radiation pleuritis has not been well characterized, but one report characterized the fluid as an exudate with many vacuolated mesothelial cells (80). Most pleural effusions were small, but at least one occupied nearly 50% of the hemithorax. In 4 of the 11 patients, the fluid gradually disappeared spontaneously in 4 to 23 months. In the remaining patients, the pleural effusions persisted, gradually decreasing in size over the follow-up period of 10 to 40 months.

Pleural effusions can also occur as a late complication of radiotherapy to the chest. Morrone and associates (81) reported one case of bilateral pleural effusion that developed in a patient 19 years after receiving mediastinal radiotherapy for Hodgkin's disease. The effusions were exudates with predominantly lymphocytes. Thoracoscopy revealed that there were enlarged lymphatic vessels in the visceral pleura. In a second report, a patient developed bilateral pleural effusions 8 years after receiving radiotherapy for Hodgkin's disease. In this instance thoracoscopy demonstrated diffuse thickening of the pleura (82).

OVARIAN HYPERSTIMULATION SYNDROME

This uncommon syndrome is characterized by ovarian enlargement, ascites, pleural effusion, hypovolemia, hemoconcentration, and oliguria (83). A rare complication is the occurrence of thromboembolism related to hemoconcentration (83).The ovarian hyperstimulation syndrome is a serious complication of ovulation induction with human chorionic gonadotropin (HCG) and occasionally clomiphene. The severe form with ascites and/or pleural effusion occurs in approximately 2% of patients undergoing ovulation induction for in vitro fertilization (83).

The pathogenesis of this syndrome is not clear. The syndrome does not appear to develop if ovulation does not occur (84). At one time it was thought that the ovarian hyperstimulation syndrome resulted from high local concentrations of estrogen in the ovaries causing altered capillary permeability and ascites, which in turn led to the pleural effusion. This does not appear to be the sole explanation, however, because the syndrome can still be produced in rabbits when the ovaries are exteriorized (85). This indicates that there must be systemic effects involved in the fluid shifts into the peritoneal and pleural cavities. Essentially, the patient develops a massive capillary leak syndrome.

The pleural fluid has not been well characterized, but is probably an exudate because the ascitic fluid has a protein level comparable to serum (86, 87). The pleural effusion can be a significant problem, as evidenced by one patient (88) who had 8500 ml pleural fluid aspirated from her pleural space over 14 days. The treatment of the ovarian hyperstimulation syndrome is primarily observation, with careful attention paid to the intravascular fluid status of the patient. Hypovolemia can lead to renal failure and even death.

The incidence of the syndrome can be reduced if the serum estrogen levels and the number of ovarian follicles are monitored. If the serum estrogen levels are very high or if there are more than 15 ovarian follicles with a high proportion of small and intermediate size follicles, HCG should be withheld (83).

POSTPARTUM PLEURAL EFFUSION

Pleural effusions may develop in the immediate postpartum period or a week or more after delivery. The pathogenesis of the pleural effusions at these two different times periods is different.

Immediate Postpartum

The prevalence of small pleural effusions in the immediate postpartum period is uncertain (89, 90). Hughson and associates (89) retrospectively studied 112 patients who had delivered vaginally and had posteroanterior and lateral chest radiographs within 24 hours of delivery. They reported that 46% of the patients had small pleural effusions, which were bilateral in 75%. The same workers then conducted a prospective study of 30 similar patients who were requested to have a lateral decubitus radiograph if fluid was suggested on the standard radiographs. In this group of 30 women, 20 (67%) had a pleural effusion, and in 11 the effusion was bilateral. Ten of the women had a decubitus radiograph, and free fluid was demonstrated in 7. The results by Hughson and associates (89), however, could not be duplicated by Udeshi and coworkers

(90) who prospectively studied 50 women within 1–45 hours of delivery by ultrasound. These workers reported that only one patient (2%) had a pleural effusion and that this patient had severe preeclampsia with clinically apparent pulmonary edema (90). In a subsequent study, Wallis et al. prospectively studied 34 patients with preeclampsia with ultrasound and reported that 6 (26.5%) of the patients had a pleural effusion (91). There was no difference in the severity of the preeclampsia between those women with and without pleural effusion (91). Since ultrasound is more sensitive than the chest radiograph, it is likely that the true incidence is closer to that reported by the latter two groups. The mechanism responsible for the pleural effusion is unknown. No therapeutic intervention is necessary in the absence of symptoms or signs of illness (89).

Delayed Postpartum

There have been two reports (92, 93) with a total of four patients that have documented the occurrence of a systemic illness with pleural effusions and pulmonary infiltrates occurring in the first few weeks after delivery. All four of the patients had biologically false positive tests for syphilis early in the course of their pregnancy. Three of the four patients had severe preeclampsia and had a cesarean section. All four patients had either lupus anticoagulant or anticardiolipin antibodies or both in conjunction with a negative antinuclear antibody test (92, 93). Two of the four patients had serious cardiac manifestations and two of the four patients had intravascular thrombosis within 4 weeks of delivery. Patients who experience pleuropulmonary complications in the first few weeks after delivery should be evaluated for antiphospholipin antibodies. Patients with positive assays may benefit from immunosuppressive therapy and prophylactic anticoagulation to prevent thromboembolic disease (92, 93).

AMYLOIDOSIS

On rare occasions amyloidosis can produce an exudative pleural effusion (94–96). Most pleural effusions seen in patients with amyloidosis are transudates and are secondary to the cardiomyopathy associated with that disease.

The pleural biopsy may be positive for amyloid even though the pleural fluid is transudative (96). Knapp and colleagues (94) reported two patients with amyloidosis secondary to multiple myeloma who had pleural biopsies that demonstrated amyloid. The pleural effusion was exudative in one of the two patients. Graham and Ahmad (95) reported one patient with an exudative pleural effusion and a positive pleural biopsy for amyloid who had primary amyloidosis. The mechanism for the exudative pleural effusion with pleural amyloidosis is unknown, but it is possibly related to obstruction of the lymphatics in the parietal pleura by the amyloid infiltration.

MILK OF CALCIUM PLEURAL EFFUSION

"Milk of calcium" is a colloidal suspension of precipitated calcium salts. It has been seen in various cystic spaces, such as the gallbladder, renal caliceal diverticula, adrenal cysts, and breast cysts (97). Milk of calcium can also collect in the pleural space. The radiographic picture is characteristic, showing a half-moon or hemispherical calcium-fluid level (97).

Im and associates reported five patients with pleural milk of calcium who showed a loculated pleural collection with double contour on radiography and homogeneous calcification on computed tomography (CT) scan (97). Four of the five patients gave a history of pleurisy more than 10 years previously. Aspirated materials from the pleural space consisted of thick yellow fluid containing gritty particles. The concentration of calcium in the aspirated material was greater than 500 mg% (97). The five patients were essentially asymptomatic from the milk of calcium fluid collections and received no therapy for the pleural effusion (97).

ELECTRICAL BURNS

Individuals who have suffered major electrical burns may develop a pleural effusion secondary to the burn. If the contact point for the electrical burn is over the chest, the underlying pleura is damaged. Accordingly, a pleural effusion develops within the first week of the accident, and an accompanying pneumonitis may be seen (98). The pleural fluid is an exudate that gradually resolves over a period of several months.

ACUTE RESPIRATORY DISTRESS SYNDROME

There appears to be a high prevalence of small pleural effusions in patients with the acute respiratory distress syndrome (ARDS). Tagliabue and associates reviewed the CT findings in 74 patients with ARDS (99). They reported that pleural effusions were present in 37 (50%). On the chest radiograph, the effusion was apparent in 25 of the 37 (41%). The effusions were bilateral in 21, unilateral right-sided in 6, and unilateral left-sided in 10. The effusions were small in 22 and moderate in 15. The pleural fluid in patients with the ARDS probably originates from the interstitial spaces of the lung. If a significant amount of fluid is detected in a patient with ARDS, a diagnostic thoracentesis should be performed to verify that the fluid is not infected.

IATROGENIC PLEURAL EFFUSIONS

At times, physicians are responsible for the development of pleural effusions in their patients. The iatrogenic effusions secondary to various pharmaceutic agents, radiation therapy, endoscopic esophageal sclerotherapy, the ovarian hyperstimulation syndrome, and fluid overload are discussed elsewhere in this book as are those that occur following coronary artery bypass surgery and abdominal surgery. In this section, I discuss the iatrogenic pleural effusions that result from misplacement of percutaneously inserted catheters or enteral feeding tubes, those associated with translumbar aortography, and those resulting from rupture of silicone bag mammary prosthesis.

A common iatrogenic cause of pleural effusion is the misplacement of a percutaneously inserted catheter into the mediastinum or the pleural space. Both internal jugular (100) and subclavian vein catheterization (101, 102) can be complicated by the development of a pleural effusion. Reinsertion of a central venous catheter over a guidewire has been associated with a fatal hydrothorax (103). The pleural fluid may be pure blood resulting from laceration or puncture of one of the vessels (102).

Alternatively, the pleural fluid may be clear or just slightly blood-tinged and may have the same composition as the fluid administered intravenously. Of course, if blood is administered through the central venous line, the pleural fluid can be bloody when no substantial leak of intravascular blood into the pleural space exists (104). The diagnosis of a misplaced central venous line should be considered in all patients with such lines who rapidly develop pleural effusions. A diagnostic thoracentesis reveals fluid that is either similar to the intravenous fluid or is frank blood. In either case, the central catheter should be withdrawn. If fresh blood is present, a chest tube should be inserted immediately, and if bleeding persists, an exploratory thoracotomy may be necessary (102).

In the last several years, the development of soft, flexible, small-bore polyurethane feeding tubes has made nasogastric and nasoenteric feeding more practical and comfortable for patients. The increasing awareness by physicians of the importance of malnutrition and metabolic support has led to an increase in the use of such tubes. Their use has been associated with significant pleural complications, however.

Pneumothorax is the most common complication (105), but the infusion of the enteral formula into the pleural space and/or the development of an empyema also occur relatively frequently (105). The stylets used for ease of insertion provide stiffness and strength to the tubing and allow easier advancement of the device. With the stylet in place, the tubing becomes stiff and is able to perforate structures relatively easily. There are frequently no clinical clues that the tube has entered the bronchial tree instead of the esophagus. The risk of this complication is much greater if the patient has an endotracheal tube in place or if he is obtunded (105). To prevent this complication, these tubes should only be inserted by experienced individuals, and the tube should be immediately removed if the patient starts coughing. If any resistance is felt, no further attempts should be made to advance the tube. Before feeding is initiated, the position of the tip of the tube should be confirmed radiographically (106). The standard tests for the placement of nasogastric tubes such as the insufflation of air with auscultation over the left upper quadrant or the aspiration of fluid are often misleading with the small nasogastric tubes (106).

If the tube enters the pleural space and the enteral solutions enter the pleural space, tube thoracostomy should be performed after the nasogastric tube has been removed. In such a situation, the possibility of an empyema should be evaluated because the incidence of empyema is high when these small tubes enter the pleural space (105).

Pleural effusion may also complicate translumbar aortographic examination (107). Small pleural effusions requiring decubitus radiographs for their demonstration frequently occur after translumbar aortographic studies (107) and are thought to be secondary to the passage of the needle through the most inferior part of the pleural space. An exudative pleural effusion may result from irritation of the pleural space by the extravasated contrast medium. The pleural effusion following translumbar aortographic examination is sometimes frankly bloody and probably results from blood leaking from the aorta into the pleural space. In such situations, a therapeutic thoracentesis is usually sufficient treatment because the leak stops spontaneously (107).

There have been at least three case reports of a pleural effusion developing after rupture of a silicone bag mammary prosthesis (108–110). One patient developed left-sided pleuritic chest pain 24 hours after she had sustained a blow of moderate severity on the left anterior chest wall. Five years previously, she had had bilateral augmentation mammoplasties with insertion of silicone bag prostheses. On physical examination, the breasts appeared equal in size. The chest radiograph revealed a large left pleural effusion. Thoracentesis revealed slightly turbid fluid with a protein of 4.6 g/dl and a LDH of 372 IU/L. A subsequent pleural biopsy revealed a dense mixed cellular infiltrate with several granulomas with large multinucleated giant cells suggestive of a foreign body reaction. Two liters of pleural fluid were aspirated, and an oily layer was observed on the top of the fluid consistent with the presence of silicone gel in the aspirate. After the aspiration, the pleural effusion did not recur. Two other patients

(109, 110) developed pleural effusions approximately 1 year after their implants had ruptured. In one patient there was viscid, yellowish pasty material that could only be obtained with a 14-gauge needle (109). The other fluid was yellow and scanning electron microscopy was necessary to demonstrate material with the electron energy pattern of silicone (110). These three reports demonstrate that silicone can reach the pleural space, but once there it does not elicit much of an inflammatory reaction.

OTHER CAUSES OF PLEURAL EFFUSIONS

On rare occasions pleural effusions result from rupture of a benign germ cell tumor into the pleural space. Hiraiwa and associates reported one patient who developed a right pleural effusion after rupture of a benign mediastinal teratoma (111). Interestingly, the pleural fluid level of carcinoembryonic antigen (CEA) was elevated to 160 µg/L. I have seen another case in which the pleural fluid amylase level was elevated due to high amylase levels in the germ cell tumor.

Syphilis, on rare occasions, can cause a pleural effusion. There was one case report (112) of a patient with an exudative pleural effusion with predominantly lymphocytes in the fluid and granuloma on the pleural biopsy who turned out to have syphilis (112).

REFERENCES

1. Epler GR, McLoud TC, Gaensler EA: Prevalence and incidence of benign asbestos pleural effusion in a working population. JAMA 1982;247:617–622.
2. Hillerdal G, Ozesmi M: Benign asbestos pleural effusion: 73 exudates in 60 patients. Eur J Respir Dis 1987;71:113–121.
3. Sargent EN, Jacobson G, Gordonson JS: Pleural plaques: a signpost of asbestos dust inhalation. Semin Roentgenol 1977;12:287–297.
4. Boylan AM, Ruegg C, Kim KJ, Hebert CA, Hoeffel JM, Pytela R, Sheppard D, Goldstein IM, Broaddus VC: Evidence of a role for mesothelial cell-derived interleukin 8 in the pathogenesis of asbestos-induced pleurisy in rabbits. J Clin Invest 1992;89: 1257–1267.
5. Kuwahara M, Kuwahara M, Verma K, Ando T, Hemenway ER, Kagan K: Asbestos exposure stimulates pleural mesothelial cells to secrete the fibroblast chemattractant, fibronectin. Am J Respir Cell Mol Biol 1994;10:167–176.

6. Mattson S-B: Monosymptomatic exudative pleurisy in persons exposed to asbestos dust. Scand J Respir Dis 1975;56:263–272.

7. Gaensler EA, Kaplan AI: Asbestos pleural effusion. Ann Intern Med 1971;74:178–191.

8. Hillerdal G: Non-malignant asbestos pleural disease. Thorax 1981;36:669–675.

9. Dressler W: The post-myocardial infarction syndrome. Arch Intern Med 1959;103:28–42.

10. Engle MA, Zabriskie JB, Senterfit LB, Ebert PA: Post-pericardiotomy syndrome: a new look at an old condition. Mod Concepts Cardiovasc Dis 1975; 44:59–64.

11. Liem KL, ten Veen JH, Lie KI, et al: Incidence and significance of heart-muscle antibodies in patients with acute myocardial infarction and unstable angina. Acta Med Scand 1979;206:473–475.

12. Toole JC, Silverman ME: Pericarditis of acute myocardial infarction. Chest 1975;67:647–653.

13. McCabe JC, Ebert PA, Engle MA, Zabriskie JB: Circulating heart-reactive antibodies in the postpericardiotomy syndrome. J Surg Res 1973;14:158–164.

14. Miller RH, Horneffer PJ, Gardner TJ, Rykiel MF, Pearson TA: The epidemiology of the postpericardiotomy syndrome: A common complication of cardiac surgery. Am Heart J 1988;116:1323–1329.

15. De Scheerder I, De Buyzere M, Robbrecht J, De Langhe M, Delanghe J, Bogaert AM, Clement D: Postoperative immunologic response against contractile proteins after coronary bypass surgery. Br Heart J 1986;56:440–444.

16. Khan AH: The postcardiac injury syndromes. Clin Cardiol 1992;15:67–72.

17. Kossowsky WA, Epstein PJ, Levine RS: Post-myocardial infarction syndrome: an early complication of acute myocardial infarction. Chest 1973;63: 35–40.

18. Urschel HC Jr, Razzuk MA, Gardner M: Coronary artery bypass occlusion secondary to postcardiotomy syndrome. Ann Thorac Surg 1976;22: 528–531.

19. Stelzner TJ, King TE Jr, Antony VB, Sahn SA: The pleuropulmonary manifestations of the postcardiac injury syndrome. Chest 1983;84:383–387.

20. Kim YK, Mohsenifar Z, Koerner SK: Lymphocytic pleural effusion in postpericardiotomy syndrome. Am Heart J 1988;115:1077–1079.

21. Gregoratos G: Pericardial involvement in acute myocardial infarction. Cardiol Clin 1990;8:601–618.

22. Weiss JM, Spodick DH: Association of left pleural effusion with pericardial disease. N Engl J Med 1983;308:696–697.

23. Tomaselli G, Gamsu G, Stulbarg MS: Constrictive pericarditis presenting as pleural effusion of unknown origin. Arch Intern Med 1989;149:201–203.

24. Peng M-J, Vargas FS, Cukier A, Terra-Filho M, Teixeira LR, Light RW: Postoperative pleural changes after coronary revascularization. Chest 1992;101: 327–330.

25. Vargas FS, Cukier A, Hueb W, Teixeira LR, Light RW: Relationship between pleural effusion and pericardial involvement after myocardial revascularization. Chest 1994;105:1748–1752.

26. Kollef MH, Peller T, Knodel A, Cragun WH: Delayed pleuropulmonary complications following coronary artery revascularization with the internal mammary artery. Chest 1988;94:68–71.

27. Kollef MH: Trapped-lung syndrome after cardiac surgery: a potentially preventable complication of pleural injury. Heart & Lung 1990;19:671–675.

28. Kollef MH: Symptomatic pleural effusion after coronary artery revascularization: unsuspected pleural injury from internal mammary artery resection. South Med J 1993;86:585–588.

29. Raju S, Heath BJ, Warren ET, Hardy JD: Single- and double-lung transplantation. Problems and possible solutions. Ann Surg 1990;211:681–691.

30. Medina LS, Siegel MJ, Bejarano PA, Glazer HS, Anderson DJ, Mallory GB Jr: Pediatric lung transplantation: radiographic-histopathologic correlation. Radiology 1993;187:807–810.

31. O'Donovan PB: Imaging of complications of lung transplantation. Radiographics 1993;13:787–796.

32. Meigs JV, Cass JW: Fibroma of the ovary with ascites and hydrothorax. Am J Obstet Gynecol 1937;33:249–267.

33. Meigs JV: Pelvic tumors other than fibromas of the ovary with ascites and hydrothorax. Obstet Gynecol 1954;3:471–486.

34. Yu J, Grimes DA: Ascites and pleural effusions associated with endometriosis. Obstet Gynecol 1991;78:533–534.

35. Samanth KK, Black WC III: Benign ovarian stromal tumors associated with free peritoneal fluid. Am J Obstet Gynecol 1970;107:538–545.

36. Meigs JV: Fibroma of the ovary with ascites and hydrothorax. Meigs' syndrome. Am J Obstet Gynecol 1954;67:962–987.

37. Lemming R: Meigs' syndrome and pathogenesis of pleurisy and polyserositis. Acta Med Scand 1960; 168:197–204.

38. Majzlin G, Stevens FL: Meigs' syndrome: case report and review of literature. J Int Coll Surg 1964;42: 625–630.

39. Lin JY, Angel C, Sickel JZ: Meigs syndrome with elevated serum CA 125. Obstet Gynecol 1992;80: 563–566.

40. O'Flanagan SJ, Tighe BF, Egan TJ, Delaney PV: Meigs' syndrome and pseudo-Meigs' syndrome. J R Soc Med 1987;80:252–253.

41. Hurlow RA, Greening WP, Krantz E: Ascites and hydrothorax in association with stroma ovarii. Br J Surg 1976;63:110–112.

42. Jimerson SD: Pseudo-Meigs' syndrome: an unusual case with analysis of the effusions. Obstet Gynecol 1973;42:535–537.

43. Neustadt JE, Levy RC: Hemorrhagic pleural effusion in Meigs' syndrome. JAMA 1968;204:179–180.

44. Solomon S, Farber SJ, Caruso LJ: Fibromyomata of the uterus with hemothorax. Meigs' syndrome? Arch Intern Med 1971;127:307–309.

45. Nordkild P, Kromann-Andersen H, Struve-Christensen E: Yellow nail syndrome—the triad of yellow nails, lymphedema and pleural effusions. Acta Med Scand 1986;219:221-227.

46. Cordasco EM Jr, Beder S, Coltro A, Bavbek S, Gurses H, Mehta AC: Clinical features of the yellow nail syndrome. Cleve Clin J Med 1990:57:472-476.

47. Beer DJ, Pereira W Jr, Snider GL: Pleural effusion associated with primary lymphedema: a perspective on the yellow nail syndrome. Am Rev Respir Dis 1978;117:595-599.

48. Emerson PA: Yellow nails, lymphoedema, and pleural effusions. Thorax 1966;21:247-253.

49. Lewis M, Kallenbach J, Zaltzman M, et al: Pleurectomy in the management of massive pleural effusion associated with primary lymphoedema: demonstration of abnormal pleural lymphatics. Thorax 1983;38:637-639.

50. Mambretti-Zumwalt J, Seidman JM, Higano N: Yellow nail syndrome: complete triad with pleural protein turnover studies. South Med J 1980;73:995-997.

51. Hiller E, Rosenow EC III, Olsen AM: Pulmonary manifestations of the yellow nail syndrome. Chest 1972;61:452-458.

52. Brofman JD, Hall JB, Scott W, Little AG: Yellow nails, lymphedema and pleural effusion. Treatment of chronic pleural effusion with pleuroperitoneal shunting. Chest 1990;97:743-745.

53. Williams HC, Buffham R, du Vivier A: Successful use of topical vitamin E solution in the treatment of nail changes in yellow nail syndrome. Arch Dermatol 1991;127:1023-1028.

54. Chusid EL, Siltzbach LE: Sarcoidosis of the pleura. Ann Intern Med 1974;81:190-194.

55. Wilen SB, Rabinowitz JG, Ulreich S, Lyons HA: Pleural involvement in sarcoidosis. Am J Med 1974;57:200-209.

56. Sharma OP, Gordonson J: Pleural effusion in sarcoidosis: a report of six cases. Thorax 1975;30:95-101.

57. Beekman JF, Zimmet SM, Chun BK, et al: Spectrum of pleural involvement in sarcoidosis. Arch Intern Med 1976;136:323-330.

58. Nicholls AJ, Friend JAR, Legge JS: Sarcoid pleural effusion: three cases and review of the literature. Thorax 1980;35:277-281.

59. Durand DV, Dellinger A, Guerin C, et al: Pleural sarcoidosis: one case presenting with an eosinophilic effusion. Thorax 1984;39:468-469.

60. Chittock DR, Joseph MG, Paterson NA, McFadden RG: Necrotizing sarcoid granulomatosis with pleural involvement. Clinical and radiographic features. Chest 1994;106:672-676.

61. Hagay Z, Reece A, Roberts A, Hobbins JC: Isolated fetal pleural effusion: a prenatal management dilemma. Obst Gynec 1993;81:147-152.

62. Eddleman KA, Levine AB, Chitkara U, Berkowitz RL: Reliability of pleural fluid lymphocyte counts in the antenatal diagnosis of congenital chylothorax. Obstet Gynecol 1991;78:530-532.

63. Benacerraf BR, Frigoletto FD Jr: Mid-trimester fetal thoracentesis. J Clin Ultrasound 1985;13:202-204.

64. Benacerraf BR, Frigoletto FD Jr, Wilson M: Successful midtrimester thoracentesis with analysis of the lymphocyte population in the pleural effusion. Am J Obstet Gynecol 1986;155:398-399.

65. Chernick V, Reed MH: Pneumothorax and chylothorax in the neonatal period. J Pediatr 1970;76:624-632.

66. Weber AM, Philipson EH: Fetal pleural effusion: a review and meta-analysis for prognostic indicators. Obstet Gynecol 1992;79:281-286.

67. Rodeck CH, Fisk NM, Fraser DI, Nicolini U: Long-term in utero drainage of fetal hydrothorax. N Engl J Med 1988;319:1135-1138.

68. Blott M, Nicolaides KH, Greenough A: Pleuroamniotic shunting for decompression of fetal pleural effusions. Obstet Gynecol 1988;102:288-290.

69. Thompson PJ, Greenough A, Nicolaides KH: Respiratory function in infancy following pleuro-amniotic shunting. Fetal Diagn Ther 1993;8:79-83.

70. Hopps HC, Wissler RW: Uremic pneumonitis. Am J Pathol 1955;31:261-273.

71. Nidus BD, Matalon R, Cantacuzino D, Eisinger RP: Uremic pleuritis: a clinicopathological entity. N Engl J Med 1969;281:255-256.

72. Berger HW, Rammohan G, Neff MS, Buhain WJ: Uremic pleural effusion: a study in 14 patients on chronic dialysis. Ann Intern Med 1975;82:362-364.

73. Galen MA, Steinberg SM, Lowrie EG, et al: Hemorrhagic pleural effusion in patients undergoing chronic hemodialysis. Ann Intern Med 1975;82:359-361.

74. Gilbert L, Ribot S, Frankel H, et al: Fibrinous uremic pleuritis: a surgical entity. Chest 1975;67:53-56.

75. Rodelas R, Rakowski TA, Argy WP, Schreiner GE: Fibrosing uremic pleuritis during hemodialysis. JAMA 1980;243:2424-2425.

76. Chiang CS, Chiang CD, Lin JW, Huang PL, Chu JJ: Neopterin, soluble interleukin-2 receptor and adenosine deaminase levels in pleural effusions. Respiration 1994;61:150-154.

77. Moore PJ, Thomas PA: The trapped lung with chronic pleural space, a cause of recurring pleural effusion. Milit Med 1967;132:998-1002.

78. Light RW, Jenkinson SG, Minh V, George RB: Observations on pleural pressures as fluid is withdrawn during thoracentesis. Am Rev Respir Dis 1980;121:799-804.

79. Bachman AL, Macken K: Pleural effusions following supervoltage radiation for breast carcinoma. Radiology 1959;72:699-709.

80. Fentanes de Torres E, Guevara E: Pleuritis by radiation: report of two cases. Acta Cytol 1981;25:427-429.

81. Morrone N, Silva Volpa VLG, Dourado AM, Mitre F, Coletta EN: Bilateral pleural effusion due to mediastinal fibrosis induced by radiotherapy. Chest 1993;104:1276-1278.

82. Rodriguez-Garcia JL, Fraile G, Moreno MA, Sanchez-Corral JA, Penalver R: Recurrent massive pleural

effusion as a late complication of radiotherapy in Hodgkin's disease. Chest 1991;100:1165–1166.

83. Rizk B, Aboulghar M: Modern management of ovarian hyperstimulation syndrome. Hum Reprod 1991; 6:1082–1087.

84. Engel T, Jewelewicz R, Dyrenfurth I, et al: Ovarian hyperstimulation syndrome. Am J Obstet Gynecol 1972;112:1052–1060.

85. Polishuk WZ, Schenker JG: Ovarian overstimulation syndrome. Fertil Steril 1969;20:241–249.

86. Morgan H, Paredes RA, Lachelin GCL: Severe ovarian hyperstimulation after clomiphene citrate in a hypothyroid patient. Case report. Br J Obstet Gynaecol 1983;90:977–982.

87. Neuwirth RS, Turksoy RN, Vandewiele RL: Acute Meigs' syndrome secondary to ovarian stimulation with human menopausal gonadotropins. Am J Obstet Gynecol 1965;91:977–981.

88. Yuen BH, McComb P, Sy L, et al: Plasma prolactin, human chorionic gonadotropin, estradiol, testosterone, and progesterone in the ovarian hyperstimulation syndrome. Am J Obstet Gynecol 1979;133:316–320.

89. Hughson WG, Friedman PJ, Feigin DS, Resnick R, Moser KM: Postpartum pleural effusion: a common radiologic finding. Ann Intern Med 1982;97:856–858.

90. Udeshi UL, McHugo JM, Selwyn CJ: Postpartum pleural effusion. Br J Obstet Gynaecol 1988;95:894–897.

91. Wallis MG, McHugo JM, Carruthers DA, Selwyn Crawford J: The prevalence of pleural effusions in pre-eclampsia: an ultrasound study. Brit J Obstet Gynaec 1989;96:431–433.

92. Kochenour NK, Branch DW, Rote NS, et al: A new postpartum syndrome associated with antiphospholipid antibodies. Obstet Gynecol 1987;69:460–468.

93. Ayres MA, Sulak PJ: Pregnancy complicated by antiphospholipid antibodies. South Med J 1991;84:266–269.

94. Knapp MJ, Roggli VL, Kim J, et al: Pleural amyloidosis. Arch Pathol Lab Med 1988;112:57–60.

95. Graham DR, Ahmad D: Amyloidosis with pleural involvement. Eur Respir J 1988;1:571–572.

96. Kavuru MS, Adamo JP, Ahmad M, Mehta AC, Gephardt GN: Amyloidosis and pleural disease. Chest 1990;98:20–23.

97. Im JG, Chung JW, Han MC: Milk of calcium pleural collections: CT findings. J Comp Assist Tomography 1993;17:613–616.

98. Baxter CR: Present concepts in the management of major electrical injury. Surg Clin North Am 1970; 50:1401–1418.

99. Tagliabue M, Casella TC, Zincone GE, Fumagalli R, Salvini E: CT and chest radiography in the evaluation of adult respiratory distress syndrome. Acta Radiologica 1994;35:230–234.

100. Hopkinson RB, Parkin CE: Hydrohemothorax following percutaneous internal jugular vein cannulation recognized by intravenous pyelography. Anesth Analg (Cleve) 1978;57:507–511.

101. Usselman JA, Seat SG: Superior caval catheter displacement causing bilateral pleural effusions. AJR 1979;133:738–739.

102. Holt S, Kirkman N, Myerscough E: Haemothorax after subclavian vein cannulation. Thorax 1977;32:101–103.

103. Armstrong CW, Mayhall CG: Contralateral hydrothorax following subclavian catheter replacement using a guidewire. Chest 1983;84:231–233.

104. Mattox KL, Fisher RG: Persistent hemothorax secondary to malposition of a subclavian venous catheter. J Trauma 1977;17:387–388.

105. Roubenoff R, Ravich WJ: Pneumothorax due to nasogastric feeding tubes. Report of four cases, review of the literature, and recommendations for prevention. Arch Intern Med 1989;149:184–188.

106. Miller KS, Tomlinson JR, Sahn SA: Pleuropulmonary complications of enteral tube feedings. Chest 1985; 88:231–233.

107. Bilbrey GL, Hedberg CL: Hemorrhagic pleural effusion secondary to aortography: a case report. J Thorac Cardiovasc Surg 1967;54:85–89.

108. Stevens UM, Burdon JG, Niall JF: Pleural effusion after rupture of silicone bag mammary prosthesis. Thorax 1987;42:825–826.

109. Taupmann RE, Adler S: Silicone pleural effusion due to iatrogenic breast implant rupture. South Med J 1993;86:570–571.

110. Hirmand H, Hoffman LA, Smith JP: Silicone migration to the pleural space associated with silicone-gel augmentation mammaplasty. Ann Plast Surg 1994;32:645–647.

111. Hiraiwa T, Hayashi T, Kaneda M, Sakai T, Namikawa S, Kusagawa M, Kusano I: Rupture of a benign mediastinal teratoma into the right pleural cavity. Ann Thorac Surg 1991;51:110–112.

112. Impens N, Warson F, Roels P, Schandevyl W: A rare cause of pleurisy. Eur J Respir Dis 1986;68:388–389.

CHAPTER 19
Pneumothorax

A pneumothorax is air in the pleural space, that is, air between the lung and the chest wall. Pneumothoraces can be divided into **spontaneous pneumothoraces**, which occur without antecedent trauma or other obvious cause, and **traumatic pneumothoraces**, which occur as a result of direct or indirect trauma to the chest. A subcategory of traumatic pneumothorax is **iatrogenic pneumothorax**, which occurs as an intended or inadvertent consequence of a diagnostic or therapeutic maneuver. Spontaneous pneumothoraces are further divided into **primary** and **secondary spontaneous pneumothoraces**. Primary spontaneous pneumothoraces occur in otherwise healthy individuals, whereas secondary spontaneous pneumothoraces occur as a complication of underlying lung disease, most commonly chronic obstructive pulmonary disease (COPD).

PRIMARY SPONTANEOUS PNEUMOTHORAX

Incidence

Probably, the most complete figures on the incidence of primary spontaneous pneumothorax come from a study of the residents of Olmsted County, Minnesota, where complete medical records are kept on all residents. Between 1959 and 1978, 77 cases of primary pneumothorax occurred among the county's population, which averaged 60,000 over this period. The age-adjusted incidence of primary spontaneous pneumothorax was 7.4/100,000/year for males and 1.2/100,000/year for females (1). If these figures are extrapolated to the entire population of 250 million in the United States, one can anticipate about 10,000 new cases of primary spontaneous pneumothorax per annum.

Etiologic Factors

Primary spontaneous pneumothorax results from rupture of subpleural emphysematous blebs that are usually located in the apices of the lung (2, 3). In one older study, Gobbel and coworkers operated on 31 patients with primary spontaneous pneumothorax and found subpleural blebs or bullae in each patient (2). In a more recent study Lesur and associates (3) obtained computed tomography (CT) scans on 20 young (mean age 27) patients with spontaneous pneumothorax and were able to demonstrate apical subpleural emphysematous lesions in 16 of the 20 (80%). In another recent study Bense and associates obtained CT scans on 27 nonsmoking patients with primary spontaneous pneumothorax and reported that 22 (81%) had emphysemalike changes, mostly in the upper lobes (4). It appears that the apical blebs present on direct visualization and the emphysemalike changes seen on CT scan represent the same abnormality.

The pathogenesis of these subpleural blebs is probably related to airway inflammation. One factor strongly associated with the development of a primary spontaneous pneumothorax is cigarette smoking, which certainly can produce airway inflammation. When the smoking habits of 505 patients from four separate studies are analyzed (5–8), 461 of the patients (91%), were smokers. Furthermore, the occurrence of a spontaneous pneumothorax appears to be related to the level of cigarette smoking. Compared to nonsmokers, the relative risk of a pneumothorax in men is 7 times higher in light smokers (1 to 12 cigarettes per day), 21 times higher in moderate smokers (13 to 22 cigarettes per day), and 102 times higher in heavy smokers (more than 22 cigarettes per day). For women the relative risk is 4, 14, and 68 times higher in light, moderate, and heavy smokers than in nonsmokers (8). Disease of the small airways related to the smoking probably contributes to the development of the subpleural blebs.

Spontaneous pneumothoraces are more likely to develop following days when there are broad swings in the atmospheric pressure

(9, 10). It is postulated that the air in the apical blebs is not in free communication with the airways. Therefore, when the atmospheric pressure falls, the distending pressure of the bleb may increase and could result in its rupture (9).

Patients with primary spontaneous pneumothorax are usually taller and thinner than control patients. Withers and associates, in a study of military recruits with pneumothorax, found that those with pneumothoraces were 2 inches taller and 25 pounds lighter than the average military recruit (11). Because the gradient in pleural pressure is greater from the lung base to the lung apex in taller individuals (see Chapter 2), the alveoli at the lung apex are subjected to a greater mean distending pressure in taller individuals. Over a long period, this phenomenon could lead to the formation of subpleural blebs in taller individuals who are genetically predisposed to bleb formation.

There seems to be some familial tendency for the development of primary spontaneous pneumothorax. In a recent study of primary spontaneous pneumothorax in the Israeli Defense Forces, 11.5% of 286 patients had a positive family history for primary spontaneous pneumothorax (12). A more in-depth analysis of 15 families suggested that the mode of inheritance for the tendency for pneumothorax was either autosomal-dominant with incomplete penetrance, or X-linked recessive (13). In another report of patients with familial pneumothorax, individuals with human lymphocyte antigen (HLA) haplotype A_2,B_{40} were found to be much more likely to have a pneumothorax (14). Other studies of familial pneumothorax have been unable to document any association with the HLA haplotypes (15). Yellin and coworkers reported a family (a father and two sons) inflicted with Marfan's syndrome who suffered multiple bilateral episodes of spontaneous pneumothorax (16).

There is a very high prevalence of bronchial abnormalities in nonsmoking patients with spontaneous pneumothorax. Bense and coworkers (17) performed fiberoptic bronchoscopy on 26 never-smokers with a history of spontaneous pneumothorax. They reported that 25 of 26 (96%) of the patients had bronchial abnormalities bilaterally. In comparison, only 1 of 41 control patients had such abnormalities (17). The bronchial abnormalities included disproportionate bronchial anatomy (smaller than normal dimensions and deviating anatomic arrangements of the airways at various locations), an accessory bronchus, or a missing bronchus. The most common abnormality was the disproportionate bronchial anatomy (17).

Pathophysiologic Features

The pressure in the pleural space is negative with reference to the atmospheric pressure during the entire respiratory cycle. The negative pressure is due to the inherent tendency of the lungs to collapse and of the chest wall to expand. The resting volume of the lung, the functional residual capacity (FRC), is the volume at which the outward pull of the chest wall is equal to, but opposite in direction to, the inward pull of the lung. In Figure 19.1, the FRC is at 36% of the vital capacity.

The alveolar pressure is always greater than the pleural pressure due to the elastic recoil of the lung. Therefore, if a communication develops between an alveolus and the pleural space, air will flow from the alveolus into the pleural space until a pressure gradient no longer exists or until the communication is sealed. Because the thoracic cavity is below its resting volume and the lung is above its resting volume, with a pneumothorax the thoracic cavity enlarges, and the lung becomes smaller.

The influence of a pneumothorax on the volumes of the hemithorax and lung is illustrated in Figure 19.1. In the example, enough air entered the pleural space to increase the pleural pressure from −5 to −2.5 cm H_2O at end expiration. The end-expiratory volume of the lung (point B) decreased from 36 to 11% of the vital capacity, whereas the end-expiratory volume of the hemithorax (point C) increased from 36 to 44% of the vital capacity. The total volume of the pneumothorax is equal to 33% of the vital capacity, of which 25% represents a decrease in lung volume, and 8% represents an increase in the volume of the hemithorax.

The main physiologic consequences of a pneumothorax are a decrease in the vital capacity and a decrease in PaO_2. In the otherwise healthy individual, the decrease in the vital capacity is well tolerated. If the patient's lung function is compromised prior to the pneumothorax, however, the decrease in the vital capacity may lead to respiratory insufficiency with alveolar hypoventilation and respiratory acidosis.

Most patients with a pneumothorax have a reduced PaO_2 and an increased alveolar-arterial oxygen difference ($AaDO_2$). In one series of 12 patients, the PaO_2 was below 80 mm Hg in 9 (75%) and was below 55 mm Hg in 2 patients (18). In the same series, 10 of the 12 patients (83%) had an increased $AaDO_2$. Patients with larger pneumothoraces had greater reductions in their PaO_2 (18).

Similar findings are present in animals with pneumothoraces. When a pneumothorax was induced in awake, standing dogs by the intrapleural injection of 50 ml/kg N_2, the mean PaO_2 fell from 86 to 51 mm Hg (19). The reduction in PaO_2 appears to be due to both anatomic shunts and areas of low ventilation-perfusion ratios in the partially atelectatic lung. When Norris and colleagues gave 100% oxygen to their 12 patients, the average anatomic shunt was over 10% (18). The larger pneu-

mothoraces were associated with greater shunts. Pneumothoraces occupying less than 25% of the hemithorax are not associated with increased shunts.

In the dog study of Moran and associates, the relative perfusion of the lungs was not altered when pneumothorax was induced, but the ventilation to the ipsilateral lung was reduced, resulting in low ventilation-perfusion ratios on the side with the pneumothorax (19). Anthonisen reported that lungs with pneumothorax demonstrated uniform airway closure at low lung volumes, and he suggested that airway closure is the chief cause of ventilation maldistribution in spontaneous pneumothorax (20).

The PaO_2 usually improves with treatment. In the animal study of Moran and associates in which the mean PaO_2 dropped from 86 to 51 mm Hg with the introduction of a pneumothorax, the PaO_2 returned to baseline immediately after re-expansion (19). In humans treated for pneumothorax, the normalization of the PaO_2 takes longer. Three patients with an initial anatomic shunt above 20% had a reduction of at least 10% in their shunt 30 to 90 minutes

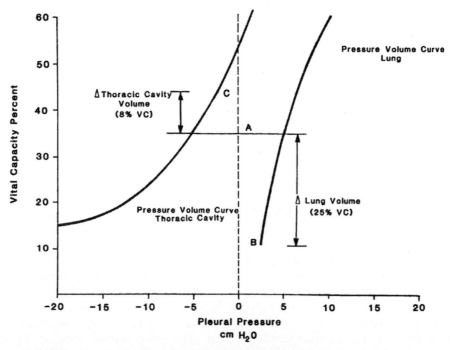

Figure 19.1. Influence of a pneumothorax on the volumes of the lung and hemithorax. See text for details.

after the removal of intrapleural air, but it still remained above 5% in all patients (18). Three additional patients with anatomic shunts of 10 to 20% had no change in their shunts when the air was removed (18). The delay in improvement in humans as compared to animals may be related to the duration of the pneumothorax.

The pathophysiologic features of tension pneumothorax are discussed later in this chapter.

Clinical Manifestations

The peak age for the occurrence of a primary spontaneous pneumothorax is in the early 20s and primary spontaneous pneumothorax rarely occurs after age 40. The main symptoms associated with the development of primary spontaneous pneumothorax are chest pain and dyspnea. In the series of 39 patients reported by Vail and coworkers, every patient had chest pain or dyspnea, and both symptoms were present in 25 of the 39 patients (64%) (21). Seremetis reported chest pain in 140 of 155 patients (90%) (7). The chest pain usually has an acute onset and is localized to the side of the pneumothorax. On rare occasions, the patient has neither chest pain nor dyspnea. In the series of Seremetis, 5 patients (3%) complained only of generalized malaise (7). Horner's syndrome has been reported as a rare complication of spontaneous pneumothorax and is thought to be due to traction on the sympathetic ganglion produced by shift of the mediastinum (22).

Primary spontaneous pneumothorax usually develops while the patient is at rest. In the series of 219 patients of Bense and associates (23) 87% of the patients were at rest at the onset of symptoms and no patients were exerting themselves heavily when symptoms began. Other series have reported comparable findings (5, 7).

Many patients with spontaneous pneumothorax do not seek medical attention immediately after the development of the symptoms. Eighteen percent of the patients in one series had symptoms for more than a week before seeking medical attention (7), whereas 46% in a second series waited more than 2 days before seeing a physician (5). Patients with symptoms for more than 3 days should not have negative pressure applied to their chest tubes in view of the higher incidence of re-expansion pulmonary edema with prolonged pneumothorax (see the final section of this chapter).

Physical Changes

Physical examination of patients with primary spontaneous pneumothorax reveals vital signs that are usually normal with the exception of a moderate tachycardia. If the pulse rate exceeds 140 or if hypotension, cyanosis, or electromechanical dissociation is present, a tension pneumothorax should be suspected (see the section later in this chapter on tension pneumothorax). Examination of the chest reveals that the side with the pneumothorax is larger than the contralateral side and moves less during the respiratory cycle. Tactile fremitus is absent, the percussion note is hyperresonant, and the breath sounds are absent or reduced on the affected side. The trachea may be shifted toward the contralateral side. With right-sided pneumothoraces, the lower edge of the liver may be shifted inferiorly.

Electrocardiographic Changes

Patients with spontaneous pneumothorax may show electrocardiographic changes due to the pneumothorax. In a study of 7 patients with spontaneous left pneumothorax, Walston and coworkers found that a rightward shift of the frontal QRS axis, a diminution of precordial R voltage, a decrease in QRS amplitude, and precordial T-wave inversion could all occur (24). These changes should not be mistaken for an acute subendocardial myocardial infarction.

Diagnosis

In a young, thin, tall male, the diagnosis is usually suggested by the clinical history and physical examination. The diagnosis is established by demonstrating a pleural line on the chest radiograph (see Figure 3.10.). Expiratory films are more sensitive at demonstrating pneumothoraces than are inspiratory films since the volume of the pneumothorax is proportionately higher on the expiratory films (25). Upright chest radiographs obtained on expiration are more sensitive than lateral decubitus films on expiration for detecting a pneumothorax (26). Approximately 10 to 20% of patients have an associated pleural effusion, which is usually small and is manifested radiographically as an air-fluid level (7, 21).

Quantitation

One should estimate the amount of lung collapse when treating a patient with a pneumothorax. The volume of the lung and the hemithorax are roughly proportional to the cube of their diameters. Thus, one can estimate the degree of collapse by measuring an average diameter of the lung and the hemithorax, cubing these diameters, and finding the ratios. For example, in Figure 3.10, the average diameter of the hemithorax is about 10 cm, and the distance between the lung and chest wall is 4 cm. Therefore, the ratio of the diameters cubed ($6^3/10^3$) equals 22% and about an 80% pneumothorax is present, although it appears substantially less severe at first glance.

Rhea and associates (27) have described an alternate method for estimating the percentage of collapse. With their method, the average interpleural distance is calculated. This is the mean of the maximum apical interpleural distance and two measurements of interpleural distances in the midpoints of the upper and lower halves of the lung. When this average interpleural distance is obtained, a nomogram is used to calculate the percentage of the lung that is collapsed.

Neither of the above methods is very accurate. If one wants to accurately quantitate the percentage of the hemithorax that is occupied by the pneumothorax, this is best done using CT scans in conjunction with computer programs, which are very accurate (28).

Recurrence Rates

A patient who has had a primary spontaneous pneumothorax is at risk of having a recurrence. Gobbel and coworkers followed a group of 119 patients with spontaneous pneumothorax for a mean of 6 years (2). These investigators found that, of the 110 patients who did not have a thoracotomy at the time of their initial pneumothorax, 57 (52%) had an ipsilat-

eral recurrence. Once a patient had second and third pneumothoraces without thoracotomy, the incidence of subsequent recurrence was 62% and 83%, respectively. In studies with a shorter follow-up period, Seremetis reported a recurrence rate of 41% after the initial spontaneous pneumothorax (7), whereas Larrieu and associates reported a recurrence rate of 23% during the 1st year following a pneumothorax in 63 patients treated by tube thoracostomy alone (29).

More recent studies have reported a lower rate of recurrence. Voge and Anthracite (30) sent questionnaires to 138 individuals with a history of spontaneous pneumothorax in the United States Air Force Waiver File at the United States Air Force School of Aerospace Medicine. They received 112 replies and only 28% had experienced a recurrence. Lippert and associates followed 122 patients with primary spontaneous pneumothorax for a mean of 5.2 years and reported that the recurrence rate within the first 12 months was only 13%, and that an additional 10% had a recurrence between the 1st and 5th year (31). Abolnik and coworkers studied 286 members of the Israeli Defense Forces who had a primary spontaneous pneumothorax and reported that 37.1% had an ipsilateral recurrence (12).

Older studies suggested that there is substantial risk of recurrence over many years. In the series of Gobbel and associates, the average interval between the first and the second pneumothorax was 2.3 years (2), although the average interval for recurrence in the series of Seremetis was 17 months (7). However, more recent studies have suggested that the majority of recurrences occur within the first year (31–33).

Attempts have been made to predict which patients with a primary spontaneous pneumothorax are more likely to have recurrence. If one could predict which patients are more likely to have a recurrence, then those patients could be treated more aggressively at the time of their first pneumothorax. Mitlehner and coworkers assessed the usefulness of the chest CT in predicting recurrence with the hypothesis being that those individuals with the most numerous and the largest bullae would be those who would be most likely to develop a recurrence (33). They obtained CT scans on 35 patients with primary spontaneous pneumothorax of whom 6 (17%) had a recurrence during the mean follow-up period of 9.6 months. They were unable to find a relationship between the size of blebs or the number of blebs and recurrences (33). Abolnik and associates did report that taller, thinner individuals were more likely to have a recurrence (12).

Treatment

Therapy for the patient with primary spontaneous pneumothorax has two goals: (*a*) to rid the pleural space of its air, and (*b*) to decrease the likelihood of a recurrence.

Several different treatments can be used for the management of a patient with a primary spontaneous pneumothorax. These include observation, supplemental oxygen, simple aspiration, tube thoracostomy with or without the instillation of a sclerosing agent, thoracoscopy with stapling of blebs, instillation of a sclerosing agent or pleural abrasion, and open thoracotomy. In selecting the appropriate treatment for any given patient, it should be remembered that a primary spontaneous pneumothorax is mainly a nuisance and is rarely life-threatening to the patient.

Observation

If the communication between the alveoli and the pleural space is eliminated, the air in the pleural space will be resorbed for the reasons discussed in Chapter 2. The rate of spontaneous absorption is slow, however. Kircher and Swartzel estimated that 1.25% of the volume of the hemithorax was absorbed each 24 hours (34). Therefore, a pneumothorax occupying 15% of the hemithorax would take 12 days to be completely resorbed.

It is recommended that only patients with pneumothoraces occupying less than 15% of the hemithorax be considered for this type of treatment. If the patient is hospitalized, supplemental oxygen should be administered to increase the rate of pleural air absorption.

Supplemental Oxygen

The administration of supplemental oxygen accelerates the rate of pleural air absorption in experimental and clinical situations. Chernick

and Avery (35) administered humidified 100% oxygen to rabbits with experimentally induced pneumothoraces and found that the oxygen increased the rate of air absorption by a factor of 6. Northfield (36) reported that the rate of absorption was increased 4-fold when patients were treated with high-flow supplemental oxygen via face mask. It is recommended that hospitalized patients with any type of pneumothorax who are not subjected to aspiration or tube thoracostomy be treated with supplemental oxygen at high concentrations.

Aspiration

The initial treatment for most patients with primary spontaneous pneumothoraces greater than 15% of the volume of the hemithorax should probably be simple aspiration (37–39). With this procedure, a 16-gauge needle with an internal polyethylene catheter is inserted into the second anterior intercostal space at the midclavicular line after local anesthesia. An alternate site is selected if the pneumothorax is loculated or if adhesions are present. After the needle is inserted, it is extracted from the cannula. Alternatively, one can use one of the commercially available thoracentesis trays such as the Arrow-Clark Thoracentesis Kit manufactured by Arrow International or the Argyle Turkel Safety Thoracentesis Set distributed by Sherwood. These kits have an outer cannula with an inner needle. If they are used, it is important to make a large enough incision in the skin such that the catheter does not become crumpled during its insertion.

A three-way stopcock and a 60-ml syringe are then attached to the catheter. Air is manually withdrawn until no more can be aspirated. If no resistance has been felt after a total of 4 L has been aspirated, it is assumed that no expansion has occurred, and a tube thoracostomy is performed. After no more air can be aspirated, the stopcock is closed and the catheter is secured to the chest wall. After 4 hours of observation, a chest radiograph should be obtained. If adequate expansion persists, Vallee and associates (39) recommend that the catheter be removed and the patient be observed for an additional 2 hours. If the lung remains expanded on a chest radiograph obtained at this time, the patient is then discharged and is instructed to return immediately if symptoms recur.

When three recent series are combined, 42 of 64 patients (64%) with primary spontaneous pneumothorax were successfully managed in this manner (37–39). The advantages to this technique are that it is simple and it is less traumatic than the insertion of a larger chest tube. Additionally, the patient need not be hospitalized and therefore this treatment is much less costly. It is unknown if the rate of recurrence with this technique is greater than when tube thoracostomy is performed.

Tube Thoracostomy

If simple aspiration is unsuccessful, then tube thoracostomy should be performed. This procedure permits the air in the pleural space to be evacuated rapidly. The chest tube should be positioned in the uppermost part of the pleural space, where residual air accumulates. The management of chest tubes in general is discussed in Chapter 24. Tube thoracostomy effectively evacuates the pleural air if the tube is properly inserted. In one series of 81 patients, only 3 patients (4%) had persistent air leaks after several days of chest tube drainage (7). The average duration of hospitalization in this series was only 4 days, with a range of 3 to 6 days. Although one might think that the placement of chest tubes would irritate the pleura and produce at least a partial pleurodesis, diminishing the likelihood of a recurrent pneumothorax, the incidence of recurrent pneumothorax is similar whether the initial episode is treated by bed rest alone or by tube thoracostomy (7).

When patients with spontaneous pneumothorax are managed with tube thoracostomy, several questions need to be addressed, such as what size of tube, whether to apply suction, when to remove the tube, and when to resort to more aggressive therapy. Although one older study (40) concluded that the success rates were poor when patients with spontaneous pneumothorax were treated with small chest tubes (13 FG), subsequent studies have reported that most pneumothoraces are effectively managed with small chest tubes. In a recent study Minami and associates treated 71 episodes of spontaneous pneumothorax using a small caliber catheter (5.5 or 7.0 FG) con-

nected to a Heimlich valve (41). They reported that the treatment was successful in 60 patients (84.5%) and ineffective in the remaining 11. Only six of these latter 11 patients were successfully managed when a large chest tube was placed (41). A total of 109 patients in two other series, mostly with iatrogenic pneumothoraces, were treated with small chest tubes (7 to 9.4 FG) and the treatment was successful in 101 (93%) (42, 43). In none of these three studies were difficulties encountered with the small tubes becoming obstructed. It is recommended that these small tubes (9–14 FG) be tried initially because their insertion is much less traumatic than that of a larger tube. They are best inserted using a guidewire technique as described in Chapter 24. If the lung does not re-expand with the small tube, then a larger tube can be inserted; however, it appears that most patients can be successfully managed with the small tube.

It is recommended that no suction be applied to chest tubes inserted for spontaneous pneumothorax. The chest tubes can either be connected to a Heimlich valve or an underwater seal. Most of the commercially available chest tube sets that use the guidewire technique come with a Heimlich valve. Two studies (40, 44) have concluded that the rate at which the lung re-expands is similar whether or not suction is applied. Because the risk of re-expansion pulmonary edema is greater when suction is applied to the chest tubes (45), and since the suction appears to offer no benefit, suction is not recommended. A Heimlich valve comes with some of the commercially available kits (see Chapter 24). It is important to hook the Heimlich valve up in the right direction or a tension pneumothorax can result (46).

If the chest tubes are removed too soon after the lung re-expands and the air leak ceases, there is a high likelihood of an early recurrence. Sharma and colleagues (44) reported a recollapse rate of 25% in 20 patients in whom the chest tubes were removed within 6 hours of lung expansion, but a recollapse rate of 0% in 20 patients in whom the chest tubes were removed 48 hours after lung expansion. We agree with the recommendations of So and Yu (40) that the chest tube be left in place for 24 hours after the lung has re-expanded and the air leak ceases. Then the chest tube should be clamped for an additional 24 hours and only removed if the lung does not recollapse.

The duration of the chest tube drainage can be reduced by using a device such as the Pleupump (47) to quantify the amount of air exiting the pleural space. When no air has exited the pleural space for 24 hours, the tube is clamped and removed if the lung remains expanded. Engdahl and Boe reported that the mean duration of chest tube drainage decreased from 8.1 to 4.8 days when this procedure was used (47).

Not all primary spontaneous pneumothoraces are treated successfully with a small chest tube. If the patient is initially treated with a small caliber chest tube and the lung does not expand within 48 hours, a larger chest tube should be placed. If the lung has not expanded after 5 days or if a bronchopleural fistula persists at 5 days, consideration should be given to more invasive therapy such as thoracoscopy or thoracotomy.

Tube Thoracostomy with Instillation of a Sclerosing Agent

Approximately 40% of patients with an inital primary spontaneous pneumothorax have a recurrence if they are treated with observation or tube thoracostomy. Efforts have been made to diminish the recurrence rates by injecting various agents into the pleural space in an attempt to create an intense inflammatory reaction that would obliterate the pleural space. Many different materials including quinacrine (29), talc, either insufflated (48, 49), or in a slurry (50), olive oil (51), and tetracycline (32, 52) have been instilled through the chest tube at the time of the initial pneumothorax in an effort to create a pleurodesis and prevent a recurrence.

The two agents that appear to be the best sclerosing agents are talc in a slurry and the tetracycline derivatives. Most commonly when talc is used as an agent to effect a pleurodesis, it is insufflated at the time of thoracoscopy or thoracotomy (see discussion below). There have been two reports (50, 53), however, with a total of 32 patients in which talc 5–10 g suspended in 250 ml saline was administered intrapleurally. The recurrence rate in these 32 patients was less than 10%. The primary drawback to talc is that there have been three reports of the acute development of the acute respiratory distress syndrome (ARDS) in patients soon after the intrapleural instillation of talc slurry for the treatment of malignant pleural effusion (54–56). There are no similar reports to my knowledge when talc, either insufflated or in a slurry, is used in the treatment of pneumothorax. Another concern about talc is its long-term side effects. Some have wondered whether talc might be contaminated by asbestos, and a case of adenocarcinoma of the lung occurring 2 years following talc pleurodesis has been reported (57). These fears appear largely unfounded in view of the report of the Research Committee of the British Thoracic Association, which reviewed 210 patients who had undergone pleurodesis with iodized talc or kaolin 14 to 40 years previously and found no mesotheliomas and no increased incidence of lung cancer (58).

An alternative agent for pleurodesis in patients with pneumothorax is the tetracycline derivatives. In the Veterans Affairs (VA) cooperative study on pneumothorax, 229 patients who were being treated with tube thoracostomy for spontaneous pneumothorax were randomized to receive 1500 mg tetracycline or nothing through their chest tube. During the 5-year study period, the 25% recurrence rate in the tetracycline group was significantly less than the 41% recurrence rate in the control group (32). Alfageme and associates recently reported their results using tetracycline to prevent recurrence of spontaneous pneumothorax (59). They reported that the recurrence rate was 9% in 66 patients treated with tetracycline intrapleurally while the recurrence rate was 36% for the 79 patients treated with observation or chest tubes only (59).

In summary, the evidence presented above suggests strongly that the intrapleural injection of talc in a slurry or tetracycline in patients with spontaneous pneumothorax significantly reduces the subsequent recurrence rates.

Which patients with spontaneous pneumothorax should receive the intrapleural injection of an agent in an attempt to produce a pleurodesis and decrease recurrence rates? It is recommended that all patients with primary or secondary spontaneous pneumothorax who are treated with tube thoracostomy receive an agent.

What agent should be used? At the present time the recommended agent for an attempted pleurodesis through a chest tube is a tetracycline derivative. If it were not for the reported cases of ARDS after the administration of talc in a slurry to patients with malignant pleural effusions, talc in a slurry would be the recommended agent. Parenteral tetracycline is no longer available due to increasingly stringent manufacturing requirements for parenteral antibiotics. Tetracycline derivatives appear comparable in effectiveness to tetracycline. In the rabbit model minocycline (60) or doxycycline (61) are as effective as tetracycline in producing a pleurodesis at approximately one-fourth the dose of tetracycline. Intrapleural doxycycline is also an effective treatment for malignant pleural effusion (62). Accordingly, doxycycline 500 mg intrapleurally is recommended for patients with spontaneous pneumothorax who are treated with chest tubes. An alternative agent is minocycline 300 mg intrapleurally. Bleomycin should not be used because it is ineffective in producing a pleurodesis in rabbits (63) and is very expensive.

The intrapleural injection of tetracycline derivatives is an intensely painful experience for many patients. In the VA cooperative study (32), over 50% of the patients reported severe pain at the time of the tetracycline injection, and 70% of the individuals stated that the pain was greater at the time of the tetracycline injection than at either the onset of the pneumothorax or at the time the chest tube was placed. The intrapleural administration of 100 mg xylocaine was not effective in ameliorating the intense chest pain. When tetracycline is administered intrapleurally for pneumothorax, it is recommended that the injection be preceded by 4 mg/kg of xylocaine up to a maximal dose of 250 mg (64). The patient should also be premedicated with an agent such as a short-acting benzodiazepine (e.g., midazolam).

It is recommended that the tetracycline derivative be injected as soon as the lung has re-expanded. The patient should be positioned such that the tetracycline comes into contact with the apical pleura. A persistent air leak is not a contraindication to tetracycline injection. There is, however, no evidence that the intrapleural injection of tetracycline leads to an earlier closure of the bronchopleural fistula (32, 65).

Thoracoscopy

Over the past few years thoracoscopy has become much more popular in this country due primarily to better instrumentation. With the advent of video-assisted thoracic surgery (VATS), there has been renewed interest in the use of thoracoscopy for the management of patients with pneumothorax. The visibility of the entire thoracic cavity obtained with VATS compares favorably with that obtained by direct view through a limited axillary, inframammary, or lateral thoracotomy (66). At the present time the same procedures can be done through the thoracoscope as can be done with a full thoracotomy, namely, wedge resection of bullae or blebs, ablation of blebs with laser or electrocoagulation, insufflation of talc, parietal pleurectomy, or pleural scarification. The advantages of the thoracoscopic surgical treatment over full thoracotomy are obvious: rapid full expansion of the lung, decreased postoperative pain, shorter postoperative hospital stay, and the avoidance of a painful thoracotomy wound. General anesthesia is recommended for VATS (66).

Thoracoscopy is effective in the treatment of spontaneous pneumothorax and the prevention of recurrent pneumothorax. With thoracoscopy there are two primary objectives: (a) to treat the bullous disease responsible for the pneumothorax and (b) to create a pleurodesis. The availability of an endoscopic stapling device and the Nd-YAG laser in the last few years have provided the means to achieve the first objective. Previously, the bullae were treated with electrocoagulation, which was associated with a higher recurrence rate (67). An alternative method of dealing with the apical bullae is to ligate the bullae with a Roeder loop (68). However, Inderbitzi and coworkers, who have reported the largest series using VATS for the treatment of pneumothorax, have reported a relatively high recurrence rate after use of the loop and recommend that it be abandoned in favor of wedge resection with the endo stapler (68). The primary disadvantage of the endo stapler is its expense. The Endo:GIA model costs about $500 and additional cartridges (of which an average of two per procedure are used) each cost $500 (69).

The largest series using VATS with wedge resection of the bullae with an endo stapler has been reported by Inderbicki and coworkers (68). They treated 79 patients between June 1990 and June 1993 for spontaneous pneumothorax. If the patients had a secondary spontaneous pneumothorax or if no bullous lesion was found, they also received an apical parietal pleurectomy. The recurrence rate in the 72 patients with follow-up was 8.3%. Since most of the recurrences occurred in patients who had not received the parietal pleurectomy, it appears that the pleurectomy does decrease the rate of recurrence (68). When four other series using VATS and endo staplers with a total of 84 patients are combined, there were only two recurrences (2%) (69–72).

An alternative to the endo stapler for resection of the bullae is the Nd-YAG laser. Torre and coworkers recently reported their experience with 85 patients with spontaneous pneumothorax in whom the bullae were ablated with the laser and the parietal pleura was abraded with the laser (73). The bullae in two of the patients could not be managed with the laser because they were larger than 2 cm in diameter, and these two patients were subjected to thoracotomy. There were three recurrences in the remaining 83 patients (4%) (73). This recurrence rate is comparable to that seen with the endo stapler or thoracotomy. In general both the endo stapler and the Nd-YAG laser are effective in treating spontaneous pneumothoraces and preventing recurrences. The endo stapler appears slightly superior since more complicated lesions can be managed with it.

Once the lesion in the lung is treated, some attempt should probably be made to create a pleurodesis. If the patient does not have a large (greater than 2-cm diameter) bullae, the intrapleural injection of a sclerosing agent can markedly decrease the recurrence rates. Olsen and coworkers performed thoracoscopy and administered 1 g tetracycline intrapleurally if no bullous lesions greater than 2 cm were found (74). The recurrence rate in this series was 16% and the authors attributed the recur-

rences to bullae that were missed at the time of the first thoracoscopy (which was not VATS).

Talc appears to be even more effective than tetracycline. Milanez and associates insufflated 2 g of sterile asbestos-free talc to 18 patients with recurrent pneumothorax and reported that the subsequent recurrence rate was 5.6% (75). Weissberg treated 122 patients with spontaneous pneumothorax with 2 g of insufflated talc and reported that excellent results were obtained in 86.8% (76).

There is still some worry about the long-term effects of talc. Although the incidence of mesothelioma or lung cancer does not appear to be increased after the insufflation of talc (58, 77), it does appear that the insufflation of talc is associated with significant pleural changes in a few patients. Viskum and associates (77) obtained chest radiographs on 50 patients who had received talc 20 to 30 years previously. They reported that the chest radiographs were normal in 11 patients, slightly abnormal in 37, and markedly abnormal in 2. The latter two patients had received talc bilaterally and had pronounced bilateral pleural thickening with calcification. Both patients complained of stiffness of the thorax. They also obtained spirometric values on the 50 patients and reported that the mean total lung capacity was 88% of predicted and the mean forced vital capacity (FVC) was 82% of predicted (77).

The ideal procedure for the creation of a pleurodesis at the time of thoracoscopy remains to be identified. Some authors have recommended that nothing be done if bullae are identified and ligated. However, it seems reasonable to me to try to create a pleurodesis while the patient is under general anesthesia. The simplest procedure to perform is a pleural abrasion with dry gauze. This is the recommended treatment since it is simple and effective (71). Other possibilities include parietal pleurectomy, laser abrasion of the parietal pleura, and the intrapleural instillation of talc or tetracycline.

Which patients with spontaneous pneumothorax should be subjected to thoracoscopy? In some centers, all patients with spontaneous pneumothorax are subjected to thoracoscopy to evaluate the status of the underlying lung (78). This approach seems overly aggressive since approximately 50% of patients with an initial pneumothorax will never have a recurrence with no treatment. In my opinion the indications for thoracoscopy in patients with primary spontaneous pneumothorax are the same as those I recommended for open thoracotomy in the previous edition of this book, namely, (*a*) an unexpanded lung after 5 days of tube thoracostomy, (*b*) a persistent bronchopleural fistula after 5 days, (*c*) a recurrent pneumothorax after chemical pleurodesis, or (*d*) an occupation or an avocation such as airplane piloting or deep sea diving in which the occurrence of the pneumothorax is dangerous to the patient.

Open Thoracotomy

The indications for open thoracotomy are the same as those for thoracoscopy. If videoassisted thoracoscopy is available, thoracotomy is recommended only after thoracoscopy has failed. The reason for this recommendation is that the hospitalization is shorter and the postoperative pain less after thoracoscopy (69, 79).

At thoracotomy, the apical pleural blebs are oversewn and the pleura is scarified. This procedure is effective in controlling the pneumothorax and diminishing the rate of recurrence. Maggi and associates followed 80 cases of spontaneous pneumothorax who were subjected to thoracotomy and reported no recurrences during a follow-up period of 7 to 91 months (80). However, recurrent pneumothoraces can occur after thoracotomy. Donahue and coworkers reviewed the experience at the Massachusetts General Hospital between 1965 and 1985 (81). During this period a total of 85 patients were subjected to thoracotomy for spontaneous pneumothorax. Five (5.6%) had an early recurrence following the removal of the chest tubes while an additional 3 patients (3.6%) had a late recurrence (80). In another large series in which 362 patients underwent parietal pleurectomy, only two documented ipsilateral recurrences were reported, with an average follow-up of 4.5 years in 310 patients (82). The low morbidity and mortality of the procedure are attested to in the same paper (82). Only one operative death was reported in the 362 operative procedures, and the average postoperative period of hospitaliza-

tion was only 6 days. Various methods proposed for scarification of the pleura range from visceral and parietal pleurectomy to mere abrasion of the pleura with dry sponges. All these procedures appear to be effective (5), but because pleural abrasion with dry gauze is less traumatic than pleurectomy and does not affect a potential later thoracotomy, it is the procedure of choice.

In summary, most patients with primary spontaneous pneumothorax should be initially managed with simple aspiration as outpatients. If the simple aspiration is ineffective or if the patient has a recurrent pneumothorax, tube thoracostomy with a small chest tube is recommended. The intrapleural injection of a tetracycline derivative at this time decreases the likelihood of a recurrence, but it is painful to the patient. If the lung does not re-expand or if an air leak persists for 5 days, thoracoscopy with endo stapling of bullae and pleural scarification is indicated. Thoracoscopy is also indicated if the patient has a recurrent pneumothorax after receiving intrapleural sclerotherapy. Thoracotomy with oversewing of the apical blebs and pleural scarification is indicated if thoracoscopy is not available or if it is unsuccessful.

SECONDARY SPONTANEOUS PNEUMOTHORAX

Secondary spontaneous pneumothoraces are more serious than primary spontaneous pneumothoraces because they decrease the pulmonary function of a patient with already compromised pulmonary function. The secondary spontaneous pneumothoraces that occur in patients with AIDS, cystic fibrosis, or tuberculosis are discussed in separate sections.

Incidence

The incidence of secondary spontaneous pneumothorax is similar to that of primary spontaneous pneumothorax. In the study from Olmsted County, Minnesota, the incidence was 6.3 and 2.0/100,000/year for males and females, respectively (1). If these figures are extrapolated to the entire population of the United States, about 10,000 new cases of secondary spontaneous pneumothorax will be seen each year.

Etiologic Factors

Most secondary spontaneous pneumothoraces are due to COPD or *Pneumocystis carinii* infection in patients with AIDS (83, 84), although almost every lung disease has been reported to be associated with secondary spontaneous pneumothorax. In one series of 45 cases of secondary spontaneous pneumothorax, the following underlying diseases were reported: COPD 22, blebs 8, tuberculosis 6, asthma 4, and miscellaneous 5 (83). Between 1983 and 1991 120 patients with a spontaneous pneumothorax were seen at Parkland Memorial Hospital in Dallas, Texas and 32 (27%) occurred in patients with AIDS (84).

There appears to be a tendency for patients with more severe COPD to develop spontaneous pneumothorax. In the VA cooperative study, which included 171 patients with secondary spontaneous pneumothorax, 51 of the patients (30%) had a 1-second forced expiratory volume (FEV_1) less than 1000 ml and 56 of the patients (33%) had an FEV_1/FVC less than 0.40 (32).

Clinical Manifestations

In general, the clinical symptoms associated with secondary spontaneous pneumothorax are more severe than those associated with primary spontaneous pneumothorax. Most patients with secondary spontaneous pneumothorax have dyspnea (85, 86), which frequently seems out of proportion to the size of the pneumothorax (87). In one series of 57 patients with COPD, all complained of shortness of breath, whereas 42 of 57 (74%) had chest pain on the side of the pneumothorax (85). In addition, 5 patients were cyanotic, and 4 patients were hypotensive.

The occurrence of a pneumothorax in a patient with underlying lung disease is a serious setback. Because the pulmonary reserve of these patients is already diminished, the partial or total loss of the function of a lung can be life-threatening. In one series of 18 patients in whom arterial blood gases were obtained at the time of admission, the mean Pao_2 was 48 mm Hg and the mean $Paco_2$ was 58 mm Hg

(85). In the VA cooperative study, the Pao_2 was below 55 mm Hg in 20 of 118 (17%) and was below 45 mm Hg in 5 of 118 (4%). The $Paco_2$ exceeded 50 mm Hg in 19 of 118 (16%) and exceeded 60 mm Hg in 5 of 118 (4%) (32).

Substantial mortality is associated with secondary spontaneous pneumothorax. When three series totaling 120 patients are combined, the mortality rate was 16% (85, 87, 88). Causes of death included sudden death before chest tubes could be inserted in 3 patients, respiratory failure within the first 24 hours of treatment in 3, late respiratory failure in 3, and massive gastrointestinal bleeding in 3 patients. In the VA cooperative study, none of the 185 patients with secondary spontaneous pneumothorax died from a recurrent ipsilateral pneumothorax. However, the overall mortality rate in the 5-year follow-up period was 43% (32). The high mortality rate probably reflects the severity of the underlying disease. The leading causes of death were COPD, lung cancer, pneumonia, and heart disease (32).

The physical examination of patients with secondary spontaneous pneumothorax is less helpful than in primary spontaneous pneumothorax. These patients already have hyperexpanded lungs, decreased tactile fremitus, hyperresonant percussion notes, and distant breath sounds over both lung fields. Accordingly, when a pneumothorax develops, side-to-side differences in the physical examination may not be apparent. The possibility of a pneumothorax should be considered in any patient with COPD who has increasing shortness of breath, particularly if chest pain is also present.

Diagnosis

As with primary spontaneous pneumothorax, the diagnosis of secondary spontaneous pneumothorax is established by the chest radiograph. In patients with COPD, the radiographic appearance of the pneumothorax is altered by the loss of elastic recoil of the lung and the presence of air trapping. Normal areas of the lung collapse more completely than diseased areas with large bullae or severe emphysema in the absence of adhesions. In addition, the deflation of the diseased lung is limited by its decreased elastic recoil.

The diagnosis of pneumothorax is established by the demonstration of a visceral pleural line. It is sometimes difficult to see this line because the lung is hyperlucent and little difference exists in radiodensity between the pneumothorax and the emphysematous lung. Frequently, the presence of the pneumothorax is overlooked on the initial chest radiograph. One must distinguish a spontaneous pneumothorax from a large, thin-walled, air-containing bulla. The pleural line with a pneumothorax is usually oriented in convex fashion toward the lateral chest wall, whereas the apparent pleural line with a large bulla is usually concave toward the lateral chest wall. If there is any doubt whether the patient has a pneumothorax or a giant bulla, computed tomography should be obtained because the two conditions are easily differentiated with this procedure (89). It is important to make the distinction between a large bulla and a pneumothorax, because only the pneumothorax should be treated with tube thoracostomy.

Occasionally, secondary spontaneous pneumothoraces result from primary carcinoma of the lung with bronchial obstruction. One must recognize the radiologic signs of bronchial obstruction in these patients because the insertion of chest tubes is contraindicated. When a patient has a totally collapsed lung, one should search for air bronchograms in the lung. Air bronchograms are absent when there is an endobronchial obstructing lesion, but otherwise they are present (90). If no air bronchograms are present, a bronchoscopic examination should be performed before a chest tube is inserted.

Recurrence Rates

The recurrence rates for secondary spontaneous pneumothorax appear to be somewhat higher than those for primary spontaneous pneumothorax (31, 32, 91). Videm and colleagues followed a total of 303 patients for a median period of 5.5 years and reported that 24 of the 54 patients (44%) with COPD had a recurrence. In patients without COPD, 96 of 249 (39%) had a recurrence (91). In the VA cooperative study, 92 patients with secondary spontaneous pneumothorax were treated with chest tubes without pleural sclerosis and the recurrence rate was 47% with a median follow-up of 3 years.

Treatment

The goals of treatment of the patient with secondary spontaneous pneumothorax, as with primary spontaneous pneumothorax, are to rid the pleural space of air and to decrease the likelihood of a recurrence. Achievement of these goals is more important in the patient with secondary spontaneous pneumothorax, however. A primary spontaneous pneumothorax or its recurrence is mostly just a nuisance. In contrast, the occurrence of a pneumothorax in a patient with lung disease may be life-threatening, even though the mortality rate from recurrent pneumothorax is low (32).

The treatment options for the patient with a secondary spontaneous pneumothorax are the same as those for a patient with a primary spontaneous pneumothorax as discussed earlier in this chapter. The recommendations for the treatment of the patient with a secondary spontaneous pneumothorax differ from those of the patient with a primary spontaneous pneumothorax in the following ways.

Nearly every patient with a secondary spontaneous pneumothorax should initially be managed by tube thoracostomy. Aspiration of the pneumothorax has only a limited role in the management of patients with secondary spontaneous pneumothorax. Aspiration is less likely to be successful in patients with secondary spontaneous pneumothorax (92, 93) and does nothing to prevent a future recurrence. Even if the pneumothorax is small, its evacuation can lead to a rapid improvement in symptoms. Arterial blood gases usually improve within 24 hours of instituting tube thoracostomy (88). If the patient has respiratory failure necessitating mechanical ventilation, a chest tube should definitely be placed because the pneumothorax is likely to enlarge during mechanical ventilation.

Tube thoracostomy is less efficacious in secondary than in primary pneumothorax, however. In primary spontaneous pneumothorax, the lung usually expands, and the air leak ceases within 3 days. In secondary spontaneous pneumothorax due to COPD, the mean time for the lung to expand is 5 days. In one series, 29% of the patients with COPD required more than one chest tube (87), whereas in another series, 35% of patients with cystic fibrosis required multiple chest tubes (94). In about 20% of patients with secondary spontaneous pneumothorax, the lung remains unexpanded, or the air leak persists after 7 days (84, 88, 89–91).

Once the lung has expanded, it is recommended that attempts be made to create a pleurodesis with a tetracycline derivative or talc in a slurry as described earlier in this chapter. The VA cooperative study (32) demonstrated that tetracycline intrapleurally decreased the recurrence rate from 47% (92 patients with only with tube thoracostomy) to 34% (93 patients treated with intrapleural tetracycline). Once the lung has been expanded and there has been no air leak for 24 hours, the chest tube can be removed.

When one contemplates injecting a sclerosing agent in patients with secondary spontaneous pneumothorax, one must consider the effect that the agent will have on a future lung transplant. In the past, patients were excluded from lung transplantation if attempts at pleurodesis had been made on the side of the proposed transplant due to the increased difficulty of the procedure and the risk of excessive bleeding. However, recently some centers have begun to accept patients for transplantation who have undergone attempts at pleurodesis on the side to be transplanted (95). It is recommended that patients with spontaneous pneumothorax who are transplant candidates be managed with thoracoscopy with stapling of blebs and bullae without any additional procedures such as pleural abrasion or the insufflation of talc.

If the lung does not expand within 72 hours or if there is a persistent air leak for more than 5 days, strong consideration should be given to performing thoracoscopy (96, 97). At thoracoscopy the blebs are excised with a stapling instrument and some other procedure is done to create a pleurodesis. Waller and coworkers recently reported their experience with 22 patients with secondary spontaneous pneumothorax due to COPD who were subjected to videothoracoscopy for either persistent air leak (18 patients) or recurrent pneumothorax (4 patients) (96). The mean age of the patients was 70 and the mean preoperative FEV_1 was 48% predicted. The mean duration of hospitalization prior to surgery was 18 days. They resected bullae and performed apical parietal pleurectomy in 20 of the 22 patients and performed apical parietal pleurectomy only in the remaining 2 patients because no leaking bulla was identified. The mean duration of the procedure was only 57 minutes. Only one patient required mechanical ventilation during the immediate postoperative period. The mean duration of postoperative hospitalization was 9 days. The videothoracoscopic procedure failed in 4 of the 22 patients (18%), in that there was a large air leak postoperatively, which necessitated thoracotomy. There were two deaths in this series; one patient developed a contralateral tension pneumothorax and a subsequent fatal myocardial infarction and the other developed bronchopneumonia after revisional thoracotomy and died in respiratory failure. None of the surviving patients had a recurrent pneumothorax (96).

The series of Waller and coworkers detailed above documents that elderly patients with severe COPD and pneumothorax can be managed successfully with videothoracoscopy with acceptable morbidity and mortality. It is interesting that the mean duration of the hospitalization prior to the videothoracoscopy was 18 days (96). Since videothoracoscopy has such good results, it is recommended that it be attempted if the lung remains unexpanded or if there is a persistent air leak after 5 days. If facilities are available for videothoracoscopy, it is advisable to attempt it relatively early rather than attempting to re-expand the lung with multiple chest tubes. Indeed, some authors have recommended that all patients with secondary spontaneous pneumothorax undergo videothoracoscopy (97).

The optimal protocol to follow during the videothoracoscopy remains to be determined. Deslauriers recommends a subtotal parietal pleurectomy with talc insufflation over the surfaces of the diaphragm and pericardium without removal of the bullae or blebs because their removal will produce prolonged air leaks (97). Comparative studies are necessary to identify the optimal procedure.

If videothoracoscopy fails or if it is unavailable, then a thoracotomy with a pleural abrasion and oversewing or removal of the bullae should be considered. Of course, these patients frequently have severe underlying lung disease, and thoracotomy carries a substantial risk. With COPD, the mortality rate from thoracotomy is about 10% (51). In general, the worse the underlying lung disease, the longer thoracotomy should be delayed. The lung reexpands and the air leak stops only after several weeks of tube thoracostomy in some patients (85, 87).

Pneumothorax Secondary to AIDS

Patients with AIDS and *Pneumocystis carinii* infection have a relatively high incidence of spontaneous pneumothorax. Most patients with AIDS who have a spontaneous pneumothorax have a history of *P. carinii* infection, are on prophylactic pentamidine, and have a recurrence of their *P. carinii* infection (98, 99). The reported prevalence of pneumothorax in patients who have a history of *P. carinii* infection and who receive prophylactic pentamidine has varied widely. In one series of 408 patients who were receiving prophylactic pentamidine therapy in San Francisco, there were 17 cases (4%) of spontaneous pneumothorax but only about one-fourth of the 408 patients had had *P. carinii* pneumonia previously (100). Renzi and coworkers reported that 5 of 48 patients (10%) with a history of *P. carinii* infection who were receiving prophylactic pentamidine therapy developed a spontaneous pneumothorax (101). In another small series of hemophiliacs receiving prophylactic pentamidine, 4 of 13 patients (31%) developed a spontaneous pneumothorax (102). At some medical centers where large numbers of patients with AIDS are treated, pneumothoraces in AIDS patients account for a sizeable percentage of all spontaneous pneumothoraces. For example, at Parkland Memorial Hospital in Dallas, Texas, 32 of 120 cases (27%) of all cases of spontaneous pneumothorax between 1983 and 1991 occurred in patients with AIDS (84).

The explanation for the high incidence of spontaneous pneumothorax in these patients appears to be the presence of multiple subpleural lung cavities, which are associated with subpleural necrosis (103–106). These bullous changes and pulmonary cysts develop due to repeated episodes of inflammation and cytotoxic effects of HIV on pulmonary macrophages (104). Most patients will have radiologic evidence of fibrocystic parenchymal disease (Fig. 19.2.) (103). If these patients are subjected to surgery, there is diffuse involvement of the lung parenchyma with greater involvement in the upper lobe than in the lower lobe regions. Areas of necrosis are usually present in consolidated areas of the lung and these areas are exceedingly friable and prone to laceration with the slightest manipulation. Emphysematous blebs are located on the surface of the lung and the apex of the lung contains multiple cysts based on consolidated parenchyma (107). Microscopically, the tissue specimens invariably reveal extensive necrosis with a complete loss of the inherent architecture (107). When patients are studied prospectively, those with a lower diffusion capacity are more likely to develop a spontaneous pneumothorax (101). The reason for the relationship between the aerosolized pentamidine and the occurrence of the pneumothorax is not clear, but it is probably related to the fact that the aerosolized pentamidine does not reach the periphery of the upper lobe. Accordingly, a low-grade infection persists and destroys the lung, leading to the development of the cysts and the bronchopleural fistulas.

The occurrence of a spontaneous pneumothorax in a patient with AIDS and *P. carinii* infection is ominous prognostically. In one series the mean survival of 5 patients who developed a spontaneous pneumothorax was 66 days, while only 5 of 31 patients who did not develop a spontaneous pneumothorax died during the study period (101). In a second series 17 of 22 patients (77%) with spontaneous pneumothorax died, with a mean survival of 147 days after the diagnosis of the pneumothorax (107). In another series, the in-hospital mortality was 10 of 35 (29%) for patients with spontaneous pneumothorax (108), while in a another series of 10 patients, the in-hospital mortality was 40% (109).

Once a patient with AIDS and *P. carinii* infection has a spontaneous pneumothorax, he is very likely to have a recurrent pneumothorax or a contralateral pneumothorax. In one

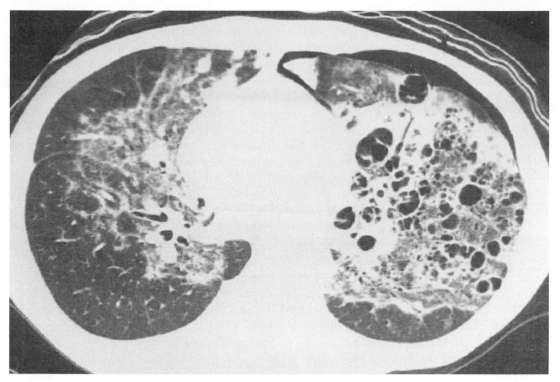

Figure 19.2. CT scan of patient with AIDS and *P. carinii* infection. Note the numerous cysts in the left lung and the large subpleural cyst anteriorly in the left lung, which is probably responsible for the pneumothorax seen anteriorly. (Courtesy of Dr. David P. Naidich.)

series of 20 patients, contralateral pneumothoraces occurred in 13 (65%) and ipsilateral recurrences occurred in 13 (65%) (98). In another series of 22 patients, 8 (36%) had synchronous or sequential bilateral pneumothoraces (107).

Due to the necrotic lung surrounding the ruptured cavity, the spontaneous pneumothorax associated with AIDS and *P. carinii* infection is notoriously difficult to treat. Conservative therapy consisting of tube thoracostomy is rarely successful. In one report of 20 patients, the median length of hospitalization was 42 days and a chest tube was required for a median of 20 days, but was successful in only 4 cases. In this series, the pneumothorax resolved in 11 patients with sclerotherapy, while five patients required thoracotomy (98). In a second series 35 patients were treated with chest tubes and tetracycline/doxycycline pleurodesis and this treatment was effective in only 9 (26%) (108).

In view of the poor results with tube thoracostomy alone, alternate procedures are necessary. It is recommended that alternate therapies be initiated if the patient still has an air leak after 3 days, because the leak will probably not close spontaneously. The simplest alternative is to attach a Heimlich valve to the chest tube and send the patient home while not worrying about the closure of the bronchopleural fistula (110, 111). This treatment gets the patient home fastest and is associated with the least morbidity. It is not always successful, however, in that in some patients the Heimlich valve cannot handle the air flow through the large bronchopleural fistula and the lung does not stay expanded.

If the patient cannot be managed with a Heimlich valve or if definitive treatment of the pneumothorax is desired, the treatment of choice is probably videothoracoscopy. The optimal procedure to perform with videothoracoscopy remains to be defined. Wait and Dal Nogare performed videothoracoscopy with the insufflation of 5 to 10 g of asbestos-free talc without treating the air leaks directly and reported success in 11 of 12 patients (92%) (108). The necrotic tissue may make wedge resection of the area of the air leak difficult.

An alternative aggressive approach is thoracotomy with stapling of blebs and pleural abrasion (109, 112, 113). Crawford et al. reported successful management for 13 of 14 patients using thoracotomy with direct closure of the bronchopleural fistula and parietal pleurectomy (112). Horowitz and Oliva reported the successful management of 7 of 7 patients with this procedure (113). Since the incidence of contralateral pneumothorax is so high in these patients, one group has recommended the use of a median sternotomy incision with bilateral pleurodesis for those patients who require surgery (109).

Pleurodesis has a limited role in the management of the secondary pneumothorax in these patients because it is usually ineffective (98, 108). The reason for its ineffectiveness is unknown, but it probably is related to the size of the bronchopleural fistula or the inability of the immunocompromised host to mount a brisk inflammatory response. If pleurodesis is attempted through a chest tube, talc in a slurry is recommended. There has been one report that suggested this approach was usually successful (112). Certainly aerosolized talc given at the time of thoracoscopy is usually successful (108).

Pneumothorax Secondary to Cystic Fibrosis

Secondary spontaneous pneumothorax is also frequent with cystic fibrosis, a disease with a high prevalence of severe chronic obstructive pulmonary disease. Spector and Stern (114) reviewed 1268 patients with cystic fibrosis who were followed between 1959 and 1987 in the University Hospitals of Cleveland. They reported that 99 of the patients (8%) had at least one episode of spontaneous pneumothorax. The median age of the patients at the time of their initial pneumothorax was 17 years (114). Approximately 16 to 20% of patients with cystic fibrosis above the age of 18 will experience a pneumothorax at some time in their lives.

The treatment of the secondary spontaneous pneumothorax associated with cystic fibrosis is similar to the treatment of that associated with COPD. Since the recurrence rate approaches 50% (115), consideration should be given to preventing a recurrence. Almost all patients should initially be treated with tube thoracostomy. If the air leak ceases and the lung remains expanded, consideration should be given to the injection of a sclerosant to produce a pleurodesis. However, if the patient is a candidate for lung transplantation, this procedure is not recommended since the pleurodesis can make the transplantation more difficult due to excessive bleeding (116).

If the air leak persists or the lung remains unexpanded for 5 days or the pneumothorax recurs, then more aggressive treatment is indicated (116). It is recommended that with any of the above three situations, videothoracoscopy should be performed. At the time of videothoracoscopy, the blebs should be resected with a stapler and the parietal pleura should be abraded. Neither parietal pleurectomy nor talc insufflation is recommended if the patient is a candidate for lung transplantation. If thoracoscopy is unavailable or if it is unsuccessful, then a thoracotomy can be performed.

Pneumothorax Secondary to Tuberculosis

Special mention should be made of the secondary spontaneous pneumothoraces that complicate pulmonary tuberculosis. Between 1 and 3% of patients hospitalized for pulmonary tuberculosis will have a pneumothorax (117). All patients with secondary spontaneous pneumothorax should be treated with tube thoracostomy. In one series of 28 patients, 11 were treated by observation or repeated pleural aspiration, and 7 of the 11 (64%) died. In contrast, of the 17 patients treated with chest tubes, only 1 (6%) died. Once chest tubes are placed in such patients, a long period of chest tube drainage can be anticipated. The duration of tube thoracostomy ranged from 5 days to 6 months, with a mean duration of 50 days in the above series (117). In general, open thoracotomy should not be considered until the patient has received antituberculous therapy for at least 6 weeks. To my knowledge, there are no published reports on the use of videothoracoscopy to treat pneumothoraces secondary to tuberculosis.

CATAMENIAL PNEUMOTHORAX

A catamenial pneumothorax occurs in conjunction with menstruation and is usually recurrent (118). It is unusual, with only 29 cases reported up to 1977 (119). The initial pneumothorax usually does not occur until the woman is at least 30; in only 1 of 20 (5%) of the cases reviewed by Lillington and associates did the initial pneumothorax occur before age 25 (118). Patients with catamenial pneumothorax classically develop respiratory symptoms within 24 to 48 hours of the onset of the menstrual flow (118). Catamenial pneumothorax may be more likely if the patient's menstrual period is preceded by mental or physical stress. These pneumothoraces are usually right-sided, but left-sided and even bilateral pneumothoraces have been reported (119).

Pathogenesis

The pathogenesis of catamenial pneumothorax is not definitely known. When Maurer and colleagues initially described the syndrome, they hypothesized that air gained access to the peritoneal cavity during menstruation and then entered the pleural cavity through a diaphragmatic defect, because their initial patient had a diaphragmatic defect (120). In Lillington's review of 18 patients who had undergone thoracotomy, however, only 3 had demonstrated diaphragmatic defects, whereas 6 of the 18 patients had pleural or diaphragmatic endometriosis (118). Stern and coworkers subsequently reported 5 additional patients with catamenial pneumothorax, all of whom had diaphragmatic defects (121). These investigators felt that diaphragmatic defects had been overlooked in many of the previously reported cases. If this is indeed the mechanism of the catamenial pneumothorax, why do more women not have free air in their peritoneal cavities during menstruation? There is one case report where a woman had simultaneous catamenial pneumothorax and air under her diaphragm on three different occasions (122).

Diagnosis and Treatment

The diagnosis of catamenial pneumothorax is not difficult if the possibility is considered. Any woman over the age of 25 who develops a pneumothorax during the first 48 hours of her menstrual flow should be considered to have a probable catamenial pneumothorax. The treatment of choice is the administration of ovulation-suppressing drugs (118, 121, 123). Most patients with catamenial pneumothorax do not have a recurrence as long as ovulation and menstruation are suppressed. There has been one report in which the ovulation was suppressed and there was no recurrence of the pneumothorax when the women were treated with analogues of gonadotropin-releasing hormones such as leuprolide (123). Interestingly, these drugs are very effective in the treatment of endometriosis. If for some reason the patient is unable to take these drugs or wishes to ovulate in order to become pregnant, one should consider thoracoscopy. At thoracoscopy, any subpleural blebs should be oversewn, and the diaphragm should be closely inspected for defects. Any such defects should be repaired. In addition, an attempt should be made to effect a pleurodesis with insufflated talc, pleural abrasion, or parietal pleurectomy. If facilities for thoracoscopy are not available, then the same procedures can be done with a thoracotomy (118, 121).

NEONATAL PNEUMOTHORAX

Spontaneous pneumothorax occurs more commonly in the newborn period than at any other age. In radiologic surveys, a pneumothorax is present shortly after birth in 1 to 2% of all infants (124), and a symptomatic pneumothorax is present in approximately 0.5% (124). Spontaneous neonatal pneumothorax is twice as common in males as in females, and the infants are usually full- or post-term (124). In most instances, the baby has a history of fetal distress requiring resuscitation or a difficult delivery with evidence of aspiration of meconium, blood, or mucus (124).

The incidence of pneumothorax in infants with the respiratory distress syndrome (RDS) is high (124, 125). The more severe the RDS, the more likely the infant is to develop a pneumothorax. In one series of 295 infants with RDS, 19% developed a pneumothorax (125). Pneumothorax developed in only 3.5% of those not requiring respiratory assistance, but occurred in 11% of those requiring continuous positive-airway pressure and in 29% of those requiring intermittent positive-pressure ventilation with positive-end-expiratory pressures (125).

Pathogenesis

The pathogenesis of neonatal pneumothorax in infants without RDS is related to the mechanical problems of first expanding the lung. Karlberg has demonstrated transpulmonary pressures averaging 40 cm H_2O during the first few breaths of life, with occasional transpulmonary pressures as high as 100 cm H_2O (126). At birth, the alveoli usually open in rapid sequence, but if bronchial obstruction occurs from the aspiration of blood, meconium, or mucus, high transpulmonary pressures may lead to rupture of the lung (124). A transpulmonary pressure of 60 cm H_2O ruptures an adult lung (124), whereas a transpulmonary pressure of 45 cm H_2O ruptures neonatal rabbit lungs (127).

In infants with RDS, the pneumothoraces also occur on account of high transpulmonary pressures. With the infant breathing spontaneously, abnormally negative transpulmonary pressures can be generated because of the reduced lung volumes and the noncompliant lung. Intermittent positive-pressure ventilation is even more likely to produce high transpulmonary pressures and pneumothorax.

Clinical Manifestations

Depending on the size of the pneumothorax, the signs vary from none to severe acute respiratory distress. In the infant with a small pneumothorax, no clinical signs or mild apneic spells with some irritability or restlessness may be present. Large pneumothoraces incur varying degrees of respiratory distress, and in severe cases, marked tachypnea (up to 120 per minute), grunting, retractions, and cyanosis are present (124). The detection of pneumothorax by physical examination is often difficult because abnormal physical signs are often not found. The most reliable sign is shift of the apical heart impulse away from the side of the pneumothorax. Because breath sounds are widely transmitted in the small neonatal thorax, appreciation of diminished breath sounds on the affected side is difficult (124).

In infants who develop pneumothorax as a complication of RDS, the onset of the pneumothorax is frequently heralded by a change in the vital signs (125). In the series of Ogata and associates of 49 infants with pneumothorax complicating RDS, cardiac arrest marked the development of the pneumothorax in 12 (24%) (125). Most of the other babies had a decrease in the pulse of 10 to 90 beats per minute, a decrease in the blood pressure of 8 to 22 mm Hg, or a decrease in the respiratory rate of 8 to 20 breaths per minute (125). Although the Po_2 decreased with the development of pneumothorax, no consistent changes were seen in the pH or Pco_2. The infant with the respiratory distress syndrome who develops hypotension as a result of a pneumothorax is at high risk of having an intraventricular hemorrhage. In one series 32 of 36 infants (89%) with pneumothorax associated with hypotension had a grade 3 or 4 intraventricular hemorrhage. In contrast only 3 of 31 (10%) of infants with pneumothorax and normal blood pressure developed an intraventricular bleed (128). It is hypothesized that the hypotension results in a cerebral infarction with the intraventricular hemorrhage occurring after the systemic blood pressure has been raised to normal values (128). The infants who developed hypotension had a higher mortality and more residual brain damage than did those who maintained their blood pressure (128).

Diagnosis

The diagnosis of pneumothorax should be entertained in any neonate with respiratory distress or in any infant with RDS who deteriorates clinically. A radiograph of the chest is essential to differentiate pneumothorax from pneumomediastinum, hyaline membrane disease, aspiration pneumonia, congenital cyst of the lung, lobar emphysema, and diaphragmatic hernia. A clinically significant pneumothorax should be evident on a high-quality anteroposterior or posteroanterior chest radiograph (124). In recent years, transillumination of the chest with a high-intensity transilluminating light has proved to be a rapid, accurate, and easy way to make the diagnosis of pneumothorax in the neonate (129).

Treatment

The neonate without RDS who is asymptomatic or is mildly symptomatic can be treated by close observation, and the pneumothorax resolves in the majority of patients over a few days. Close observation is necessary because of the possibility that the pneumothorax will enlarge or that a tension pneumothorax (see the section later in this chapter) will develop (124). Supplemental oxygen can increase the speed at which the pneumothorax is absorbed, but it should be administered with care, particularly in the preterm infant, because of the dangers of retrolental fibroplasia (124). A chest tube should be inserted in the neonate who is more than mildly symptomatic. With tube thoracostomy, the air leak almost always stops within 24 hours (124). When the leak has stopped for 24 hours, the chest tube can be safely removed.

Tube thoracostomy should almost always be performed in infants with RDS and pneumothorax because the pneumothorax compromises the patient's already poor ventilatory status and often increases in size. Usually, the air leak is small, and intermittent positive-pressure ventilation can maintain adequate gas exchange. In certain patients, however, air leaks are so large that most of the ventilation delivered by the respirator exits the lung through the bronchopleural fistula. In such patients, high-frequency ventilation may be the only method by which adequate gas exchange can be maintained (130). (See the discussion of bronchopleural fistula at the end of this chapter.)

IATROGENIC PNEUMOTHORAX

The incidence of iatrogenic pneumothorax is high and is likely to increase as the use of invasive procedures becomes more widespread. In Olmsted County, Minnesota between 1950 and 1974, 102 instances of iatrogenic pneumothorax were reported, as compared with 77 cases of primary and 64 cases of secondary spontaneous pneumothorax (1). In the recently completed VA cooperative study on spontaneous pneumothoraces, data were collected on the incidence of iatrogenic pneumothoraces at the same time (131). These investigators reported that during the 4-year study period, there were 538 instances of iatrogenic pneumothorax and 520 instances of spontaneous pneumothorax. This study probably underestimates the relative incidence of iatrogenic pneumothorax since some of the medical centers did not appear to be diligent in searching for iatrogenic pneumothoraces. The major causes of iatrogenic pneumothorax in this latter study are shown in Table 19.1.

There is substantial morbidity and even some mortality from iatrogenic pneumothorax. Despars and coworkers reviewed the cases of iatrogenic pneumothoraces at the VA Medical Center in Long Beach, California and reported that between October 1983 and December 1988, there were 105 cases of iatrogenic pneumothorax in comparison to 90 cases of spontaneous pneumothorax (132). The most common cause of iatrogenic pneumothorax was transthoracic needle aspiration (35) followed by thoracentesis (30), subclavian venipuncture (23), and positive pressure ventilation (7). There was substantial morbidity from the iatrogenic pneumothoraces in this series. The majority of patients (65 of 98) were treated with large chest tubes, which were in place 4.7 ± 3.9 days. Nine of the patients required a second chest tube. Two patients died from the iatrogenic pneumothorax (132).

At the present time, the leading cause of iatrogenic pneumothorax is transthoracic needle aspiration. The incidence of iatrogenic pneumothorax with this procedure in four

Table 19.1. Leading Causes of Iatrogenic Pneumothorax in the VA Cooperative Study

Procedure	Number	Percent
Transthoracic needle aspiration	128	24
Subclavian needle stick	119	22
Thoracentesis	101	20
Pleural biopsy	45	8
Positive pressure ventilation	38	7
Supraclavicular needle stick	24	5
Nerve block	16	3
Miscellaneous	5	1

separate studies (133–136), each with over 100 patients, was remarkably consistent, ranging from 32 to 37% with 9 to 11% of the patients with pneumothorax requiring chest tubes. The two primary factors related to the development of the pneumothorax may be the depth of the lesion and whether or not the patient has COPD. In one series (133), the incidence of pneumothorax was 13% if the lesion was 1 cm deep, 49% if the lesion was at 4 cm, and 86% if the lesion was at 7 cm. In a second study, however, there was no relationship between the depth of the lesion and the frequency of pneumothorax (137). Another study reported that pneumothorax only rarely occurred after needle aspiration of the lung with CT guidance if the needle did not traverse aerated lung (138). One study reported that the incidence of pneumothorax is directly related to the degree of pulmonary dysfunction, being approximately 70% if the FEV_1 is less than 1000 ml, 45% if the FEV_1 is between 1000 and 2000 ml, and 20% if the FEV_1 is greater than 3000 ml. However, a relationship between the level of pulmonary dysfunction and the incidence of pneumothorax could not be confirmed in two more recent series (137, 139). As of the present time, no method to decrease the incidence of the pneumothorax has been found. Positioning the patient with the biopsied lung inferior is not effective (136), even though it is in animals. Similarly, the use of a blood patch technique is ineffective in decreasing the incidence of pneumothorax (135, 140).

The second leading cause of iatrogenic pneumothorax is probably subclavicular and supraclavicular needle sticks (131). The reported incidence of iatrogenic pneumothorax following subclavian vein catheterization has varied from 1% (141, 142) to 12% (143). In the latter series the incidence of pneumothorax decreased dramatically once training programs were initiated (143). Since more than 1 million subclavian catheters are inserted annually in the United States, this procedure is responsible for a substantial number of pneumothoraces. The use of ultrasound to guide the subclavian catheter insertion does not decrease the incidence of complications (142). It is important to note that the pneumothorax following subclavian vein catheterization may not be apparent on the immediate postprocedure radiograph (144, 145).

Thoracentesis is probably the third leading cause of iatrogenic pneumothorax at the present time. In previous studies, the incidence of pneumothorax after thoracentesis has been about 10 to 20% (146–148) with about 20 to 30% of those with a pneumothorax requiring a chest tube. The incidence of pneumothorax is higher if the patients have COPD. Brandstetter and associates reported that the incidence of pneumothorax following thoracentesis was 41.7% in 36 patients with COPD while it was only 18.5% in 70 patients without COPD (149). Since two recent studies have demonstrated that there is a much lower rate of pneumothorax if the thoracentesis is done under ultrasound guidance (146, 150), consideration should be given to the wider use of ultrasound, particularly in individuals with small amounts of fluid.

Although mechanical ventilation was the leading cause of iatrogenic pneumothorax in the 1970s (151), it is probably now only the 3rd or 4th leading cause of iatrogenic pneumothorax. The relative decrease in the incidence of iatrogenic pneumothorax caused by mechanical ventilation probably is due to a combination of two factors. First, procedures such as transthoracic needle aspiration and subclavian vein catheterization were used much less commonly 20 years ago. Second, newer ventilatory modes have made it possible to ventilate patients with lower peak inspiratory pressures and lower mean airway pressures (132). The incidence of iatrogenic pneumothorax was 4% in a series of 553 patients requiring ventilatory support (152). The frequency of pneumothorax is increased if the patient has aspiration pneumonia (37%), chronic obstructive lung disease (8%), intubation of the right main stem bronchus (13%), or treatment with positive-end-expiratory pressure (15%) (152). The presence of mediastinal emphysema may precede the development of the pneumothorax. In one series of 20 patients who developed a pneumothorax while on mechanical ventilation, previous chest radiographs had shown the presence of mediastinal emphysema in 10 (50%) (153).

Other procedures associated with iatrogenic pneumothorax and an approximate incidence of pneumothorax with the procedure are pleural biopsy (10%) (154) and transbronchial lung biopsy (1–2%) (155, 156). The reported incidences are probably minimum percentages because the authors of articles are usually more experienced in the various procedures they describe than is the average physician. Iatrogenic pneumothorax may occur following tracheostomy, when air passes into the mediastinum and pleural space by the cervical fascial planes. Iatrogenic pneumothorax also frequently complicates cardiopulmonary resuscitation. In an autopsy series, 12 patients had tension pneumothoraces that were undiagnosed during life, and 9 of these patients had undergone cardiopulmonary resuscitation (157). Resuscitation-related rib fractures were found in only 3 of the 9 patients.

Clinical Manifestations

The clinical manifestations of iatrogenic pneumothorax depend both on the patient's condition and on the initiating procedure. If the pneumothorax occurs as a complication of mechanical ventilation, the patient is likely to demonstrate a sudden clinical deterioration. A sensitive indicator of the development of a pneumothorax in such patients is an increasing peak and plateau pressure on the respirator. The development of a pneumothorax during cardiopulmonary resuscitation is heralded by more difficulty ventilating the patient. In contrast, many patients who develop pneumothorax after thoracentesis, pleural biopsy, transbronchial biopsy, or percutaneous lung aspiration have no symptoms referable to the pneumothorax.

Diagnosis

The diagnosis of iatrogenic pneumothorax should be suspected in any patient treated by mechanical ventilation. The presence of mediastinal emphysema should serve as an indicator to closely look for a pneumothorax (154). Recognition of the pneumothorax in the patient on mechanical ventilation is more difficult because the chest radiographs are obtained with the patient supine or semisupine. When the patient is in this position, the most superior part of the chest (where the air accumulates) is the anterior costophrenic sul-

cus. In one series of 112 pneumothoraces seen on supine radiographs, the most common location of air was anteromedially (38%) followed by subpulmonic (26%), apicolateral (22%), and posteromedial (11%) (158). Air in the anterior costophrenic sulcus is manifested as hyperlucency over the upper abdominal quadrants (158). Pneumothoraces are frequently not recognized on the supine radiographs. Kollef prospectively reviewed all 464 medical ICU admissions at Fitzsimons Army Medical Center over a 1-year period and reported that 9 of 28 pneumothoraces (32%) were not originally recognized (159). Three of these 9 patients subsequently went on to develop a tension pneumothorax.

The occurrence of a iatrogenic pneumothorax should also be suspected in patients who become more short of breath after a medical or surgical procedure associated with the development of a iatrogenic pneumothorax. The signs and symptoms of the pneumothorax are similar to those of primary and secondary pneumothorax, and the diagnosis is confirmed by chest radiographs.

Treatment

The treatment of iatrogenic pneumothorax differs from that of spontaneous pneumothorax in that recurrence is not likely. When a pneumothorax occurs during positive-pressure ventilation, tube thoracostomy should be performed immediately if respiratory or cardiovascular deterioration is present or if immediate weaning from ventilatory support is not possible (160). Positive-pressure ventilation forces gas into the extrapulmonary planes and prevents sealing of the air leak; accordingly, a tension pneumothorax can rapidly develop. The chest tube(s) should be left in place for at least 48 hours after the air leak stops if the patient continues to receive mechanical ventilation. The bronchopleural fistula is sometimes so large that a great percentage of the total ventilation exits through the chest tubes. (See the discussion of bronchopleural fistula at end of this chapter.)

When a iatrogenic pneumothorax develops after a procedure, symptoms vary from none to severe respiratory distress. In general, if the patient has no symptoms or just mild symptoms and the pneumothorax occupies less than 40% of the hemithorax, the patient can be carefully observed. The administration of supplemental oxygen increases the rapidity with which the pneumothorax air is absorbed (see Chapter 2) (36). If the patient is more than mildly symptomatic, if the pneumothorax occupies more than 40% of the hemithorax, or if the pneumothorax continues to enlarge, however, one should consider removing the intrapleural air.

In general, most iatrogenic pneumothoraces should first be treated with aspiration. If the initial aspiration is unsuccessful, then a Heimlich valve should be attached to the catheter. Only when the lung does not expand and remain expanded with the Heimlich valve is a larger chest tube inserted. Delius and associates treated 79 needle-induced iatrogenic pneumothoraces by aspiration through an 8F radiopaque Teflon catheter. The initial aspiration was successful in 59 (75%) and an additional 9 patients (15%) were successfully managed with a Heimlich valve attached to this small catheter (161). In general, the patient is more likely to require a chest tube if he has COPD (137).

TRAUMATIC (NONIATROGENIC) PNEUMOTHORAX

Traumatic pneumothorax can result from both penetrating and nonpenetrating chest trauma.

Mechanism

The mechanism of the pneumothorax is easily understood with penetrating chest trauma because the wound allows air to enter the pleural space directly through the chest wall. In addition, the visceral pleura is frequently penetrated, allowing air to enter the pleural space from the alveoli. With nonpenetrating trauma, the ribs may become fractured or dislocated, and the visceral pleura may thereby be lacerated leading to a pneumothorax. In the majority of patients with pneumothorax secondary to nonpenetrating trauma, however, no associated rib fractures occur (162). The mechanism of the pneumothorax in such patients is thought to be as

follows (162). With sudden chest compression, the alveolar pressure increases and may cause alveolar rupture. Air then enters the interstitial spaces and dissects either toward the visceral pleura or toward the mediastinum, to produce mediastinal emphysema. A pneumothorax results when either the visceral or the mediastinal pleura ruptures.

Incidence and Diagnosis

The diagnosis of traumatic pneumothorax should be considered in any patient who suffers significant trauma. In most instances the initial chest radiograph on trauma patients is obtained in the supine position and small pneumothoraces may not be apparent. In recent years many small pneumothoraces are diagnosed only on the chest or abdominal CT scan. Pneumothoraces seen only on the CT scan are labeled as **occult** pneumothoraces. Overall about 5% of multiple trauma patients have a pneumothorax and about 40% of the pneumothoraces are occult. For example in one series of 2048 multiple trauma patients, the incidence of pneumothorax was 4.4% (163). Thirty-five (38.8%) of these pneumothoraces were not identified on the admission chest radiograph, but were subsequently identified on CT scan of the chest or abdomen (163). In a second series of 457 patients with multisystem injuries undergoing abdominal CT scans, the incidence of pneumothorax was 5.7% and none of the pneumothoraces was evident on the chest radiograph (164).

Pneumothorax is a frequent finding in blunt chest trauma. In one review of 515 patients with blunt chest trauma admitted to a trauma center, 206 patients (40%) had a pneumothorax (165), and 111 of those with pneumothorax had a hemopneumothorax (165). As might be expected, pneumothorax is also a frequent finding with stab wounds of the chest, even when they are asymptomatic (166). In a prospective study of 4106 consecutive cases of initially asymptomatic stab wounds of the chest, 493 (12%) developed a delayed pneumothorax (166).

Patients with abdominal trauma also have a significant incidence of pneumothorax. Wolfman and coworkers reported that the incidence of pneumothorax in 1086 consecutive patients with blunt abdominal trauma was 4.5%. Twenty-eight of the 49 pneumothoraces (57%) were seen on the abdominal CT scan but not on the supine chest radiograph (167) and were therefore occult pneumothoraces.

Treatment

Although most traumatic pneumothoraces should be treated with tube thoracostomy, tube thoracostomy may not be necessary for patients with small pneumothoraces or those with occult pneumothoraces. Knottenbelt and van der Spuy observed 333 patients with small (less than 1.5 cm from lung to chest wall) pneumothoraces due to chest trauma and reported that only 33 required subsequent drainage for enlarging pneumothorax (168). Ordog and coworkers observed 47 patients with small pneumothoraces (less than 20%) secondary to stab wounds of the chest and reported that only 32% required a chest tube or showed progression of the pneumothorax within 24 hours (166). They recommend that such patients be admitted to the hospital and have repeat radiographs at 6 hours, 24 hours, and again at 48 hours. The patients are then discharged if the pneumothorax is unchanged or shows evidence of resolving (166). If a hemopneumothorax is present, one chest tube should be placed in the superior part of the hemithorax to evacuate the air and another should be placed in the inferior part of the hemithorax to remove the blood (see Chapter 20). With traumatic pneumothorax, the lung expands and the air leak usually ceases within 72 hours.

Most patients with occult pneumothoraces need not be treated with tube thoracostomy (164, 167, 169). Some authors recommend that tube thoracostomy be performed only in those patients who have the larger occult pneumothoraces (164, 167) or those who are receiving mechanical ventilation (167). Some patients who have an occult pneumothorax and who receive mechanical ventilation have been managed without tube thoracostomy (169). Nevertheless, it is recommended that all patients with occult pneumothorax who receive mechanical ventilation be treated with tube thoracostomy due to the possibility of the development of a tension pneumothorax, which could be fatal. All other patients with occult pneumothoraces can probably be observed with tube thoracostomy being performed only if the pneumothorax is enlarging.

Whenever a patient with a traumatic pneumothorax is seen, two uncommon diagnostic possibilities, both indications for immediate thoracic operation, should be considered. One is fracture of the trachea or a major bronchus; the second is traumatic rupture of the esophagus. Bronchial rupture most commonly occurs in the presence of an anterior or lateral fracture of one or more of the first three ribs (162). In a patient with a traumatic pneumothorax, fiberoptic bronchoscopic examination should be done to assess the possibility of a bronchial tear if the patient has a persistent large air leak, fracture of one or more of the first three ribs, and hemoptysis (162, 170). Traumatic rupture of the esophagus usually produces a hydropneumothorax. Therefore, if a patient with a traumatic pneumothorax also has a pleural effusion, the possibility of esophageal rupture should be entertained. A reliable screening test for esophageal rupture is measurement of the pleural fluid amylase level (171). If the patient's pleural fluid amylase level is elevated, contrast radiographic studies of the esophagus should be performed.

Traumatic Pneumothorax Secondary to Drug Abuse

Intravenous drug abuse has become endemic in many urban areas. It appears that there is a high incidence of traumatic pneumothorax in intravenous drug users. Douglass and Levison (172) reviewed 525 diagnoses of pneumothorax between January 1, 1982 and December 31, 1984 at the Detroit Receiving Hospital. They reported that 113 (21.5%) occurred as a result of drug abuse. The user or a companion had attempted to inject the drug into the subclavian or internal jugular vein. It has been recommended that intravenous drug users with traumatic pneumothorax be managed with tube thoracostomy (172). In the series of Douglass and Levison, the average number of days for chest tube management was 4.4. It is probable, however, that many such cases could be managed with simple aspiration.

TENSION PNEUMOTHORAX

A tension pneumothorax is said to be present when the intrapleural pressure exceeds atmospheric pressure throughout expiration and often during inspiration as well. The mechanism by which a tension pneumothorax develops is probably related to some type of one-way valve process in which the valve is open during inspiration and closed during expiration. During inspiration, owing to the action of the respiratory muscles, the pleural pressure becomes negative, and air moves from the alveoli into the pleural space. Then, during expiration, with the respiratory muscles relaxed, the pleural pressure becomes positive. A one-way valve mechanism must be implicated; otherwise, on expiration, when the pleural pressure is positive with respect to the alveolar pressure, gas would flow from the pleural space into the alveoli, and no positive pressure would develop in the pleural space.

Pathophysiologic Features

The development of a tension pneumothorax is usually heralded by a sudden deterioration in the cardiopulmonary status of the patient. The precise explanation for sudden deterioration is not known, but it is probably related to the combination of a decreased cardiac output due to impaired venous return and marked hypoxemia (173). In animal experiments the contribution of a decreased cardiac output due to diminished venous return to the cardiopulmonary distress is minimal. Rutherford and coworkers induced tension pneumothoraces in goats and young monkeys (174). Both these species have mediastina comparable to the human mediastinum. Although the pressures in the inferior vena cava, superior vena cava, right atrium, right ventricle, and pulmonary artery all increased with the induction of the pneumothorax, the cardiac output did not fall at all in the goats and fell only minimally in the monkeys. Nevertheless, these animals developed marked distress, and many died. The genesis of the distress and the mortality seemed to be related

primarily to precipitous falls in the PaO_2. The mean PaO_2 fell from 85 to 28 mm Hg in the goats and from 90 to 22 mm Hg in the monkeys. Preterminally, the animals also developed carbon dioxide retention and respiratory acidosis, which these authors attributed to cerebral hypoxia (174). Although two subsequent studies (175, 176) demonstrated similar findings, one recent study in newborn piglets demonstrated more than a 50% reduction in the cardiac output when a tension pneumothorax was created (177).

In man, for obvious reasons, there have not been systematic studies of the blood gases or the hemodynamics associated with tension pneumothorax. In one recent report a 67-year-old man with COPD developed a tension pneumothorax while on mechanical ventilation. This patient's cardiac output fell from 7.11 to 3.80 L/minute and the stroke volume fell from 56 to 27 ml while the pulse increased from 127 to 142 (178). In the same patient the PaO_2 fell from 76 mm Hg to 47 mm Hg with the development of the tension pneumothorax.

In summary, the disastrous effect of a tension pneumothorax in patients appears to be the result of the combination of a marked decrease in the PaO_2 and in the cardiac output. A probable explanation for the decrease in cardiac output in the patient but not in the animals is that the patients have tachycardia initially and could therefore not compensate completely for the decreased stroke volume by a faster heart beat (173). Evidence to support this contention is provided by the observation that the stroke volumes do diminish when tension pneumothoraces are induced in animals (176).

Clinical Manifestations

Although tension pneumothorax occasionally evolves from a spontaneous pneumothorax, it is much more frequent in patients who develop pneumothorax while receiving mechanical ventilation or during cardiopulmonary resuscitation. The clinical status of patients with tension pneumothorax is striking. The patient appears distressed with rapid labored respirations, cyanosis, and usually profuse diaphoresis and marked tachycardia. Arterial blood gases reveal marked hypoxemia and sometimes respiratory acidosis. The physical findings are those of any large pneumothorax, but in addition, the involved hemithorax is larger than the contralateral hemithorax with the interspaces widened. The trachea is usually shifted toward the contralateral side.

Diagnosis and Treatment

The diagnosis of tension pneumothorax should be suspected in patients receiving mechanical ventilation, in those with a pneumothorax, or in patients whose condition suddenly deteriorates after a procedure known to cause a pneumothorax. If difficulty is encountered in the ventilation of a patient during cardiopulmonary resuscitation or the patient has electromechanical dissociation, a tension pneumothorax should also be suspected. In a series of 3500 autopsies, unsuspected tension pneumothorax was found in 12 patients; 10 of these had been supported by mechanical ventilators, and 9 had undergone cardiopulmonary resuscitation (157). There is one report of three cases of tension pneumothorax that occurred during hyperbaric oxygen therapy for acute carbon monoxide poisoning (179). There is another report of two cases of tension pneumothorax that occurred when the Heimlich valve used for treating pneumothorax was attached backward (180).

It is important to carefully assess the chest radiographs of patients who are receiving mechanical ventilation for the presence of a pneumothorax. Patients with unrecognized pneumothoraces who are receiving mechanical ventilation are those most likely to develop a pneumothorax. Kollef (159) reviewed 464 medical ICU admissions at Fitzsimons Army Medical Center over a 1-year period and reported that 28 patients acquired a pneumothorax during their ICU stay. The pneumothorax was not originally recognized in 9 of the patients and three of these (33%) subsequently developed a tension pneumothorax. In a second series, Tocino and coworkers reported that a pneumothorax was originally missed in 34 of 112 patients in an intensive care unit and 16 of these developed tension pneumothorax

(158). The diagnosis of pneumothorax on the supine chest radiograph is discussed earlier in this chapter in the section on iatrogenic pneumothorax.

Although the diagnosis of tension pneumothorax can be established radiographically by demonstrating severe contralateral mediastinal shift and ipsilateral diaphragmatic depression, tension pneumothorax is a medical emergency, and valuable time should not be wasted on radiologic studies because the clinical situation and the physical findings are usually sufficient to suggest the diagnosis. When the diagnosis is suspected, the patient should immediately be given a high concentration of supplemental oxygen to combat the hypoxia. Then, a large-bore needle should be inserted into the pleural space through the second anterior intercostal space. Optimally, the needle should be attached to a three-way stopcock and a 50-ml syringe partially filled with sterile saline solution. When the needle has been inserted into the pleural space, the plunger is withdrawn from the syringe. A rush of air bubbling outward through the fluid in the syringe establishes the diagnosis of tension pneumothorax. Tension pneumothoraces are easily managed with the needle-catheter units in some thoracentesis kits (see Chapter 23).

If a tension pneumothorax is confirmed, the needle should be left in place and in communication with the atmosphere until air ceases to exit through the syringe. If a needle-catheter unit has been used, the needle is withdrawn from the catheter and the catheter is left in the pleural space. Additional air can be withdrawn from the pleural space with the syringe and the three-way stopcock. If a tension pneumothorax is present, the patient should be prepared for the immediate insertion of a large chest tube. If no bubbles escape from the syringe, the patient does not have a tension pneumothorax, and the needle should be withdrawn from the pleural space.

RE-EXPANSION PULMONARY EDEMA

Re-expansion pulmonary edema is characterized by the development of unilateral pulmonary edema in a lung that has been rapidly reinflated following a variable period of collapse secondary to a pleural effusion or pneumothorax (181). The unilateral pulmonary edema is associated with a variable degree of hypoxia and hypotension, sometimes requiring intubation and mechanical ventilation and occasionally leading to death (182, 183).

Pathophysiologic Features

The exact mechanisms responsible for re-expansion pulmonary edema are not known. In the experimental animal, re-expansion pulmonary edema occurs only if the lung has been collapsed for several days and if negative pressure is applied to the pleural space. Miller and associates studied monkeys in which a pneumothorax had been present for 1 hour or 3 days (184). These researchers found that re-expansion pulmonary edema occurred only when the pneumothorax had been present for 3 days and the lung had been re-expanded with −10 mm Hg pleural pressure. If the lung was re-expanded by underwater-seal drainage after 3 days or by either underwater-seal drainage or negative pleural pressure after an hour, no pulmonary edema developed.

In a study of rabbits, Pavlin and Cheney found that re-expansion pulmonary edema was much more extensive in lungs that had been collapsed for 7 days than in those that had been collapsed for 3 days (181). Re-expansion with −20 mm Hg pleural pressure led to no more edema than did re-expansion with positive airway pressure, but re-expansion with −40 mm Hg or −100 mm Hg increased the amount of edema. In some of these animals, contralateral pulmonary edema also developed, but to a lesser extent than in the ipsilateral lung (181). Some cases of re-expansion pulmonary edema in humans, however, have occurred when no negative pressure was applied to the pleural space (185, 186). Almost all cases of re-expansion pulmonary edema occur when the pneumothorax or pleural effusion has been present for at least 3 days.

Re-expansion pulmonary edema appears to be due to increased permeability of the pulmonary vasculature. In both humans (187) and rabbits (188), the edema fluid has a high protein content, suggesting that it is leakiness of the capillaries rather than an increased hydrostatic pressure difference that leads to

the edema. Pavlin and co-workers have hypothesized that the mechanical stresses applied to the lung during re-expansion damage the capillaries and lead to the development of pulmonary edema (189). There is no evidence that the collapsed lung has increased permeability prior to reinflation (189).

Recently it has been hypothesized that re-expansion pulmonary edema is due to a reperfusion injury (190). With atelectasis, hypoxia of the atelectatic lung may be severe because oxygen delivery to the lung is reduced by absent ventilation and hypoperfusion. Then when the hypoxic areas are reperfused, O_2 free radical formation is promoted and lung injury can result. Mechanical stress is probably not the sole factor responsible for re-expansion pulmonary edema, because the edema is associated with neutrophil influx into the lung in both animals (191) and humans (192) and the fact that the edema fluid contains interleukin-8 and leukotriene B_4. Neutrophils are not responsible for the re-expansion edema, however, because neutrophil depletion in the animal model does not prevent its occurrence (191). The reperfusion injury hypothesis is supported by the observation that the administration of an increased FIO_2 (40%) for the duration of the pneumothorax prevents edema when lungs are re-expanded (193). The supplemental oxygen eliminates the systemic hypoxemia while the lung is collapsed. Additional support for this hypothesis is provided by the observation that the administration of antioxidants before re-expansion minimizes both the permeability edema and the degree of inflammation in rabbits (194).

Clinical Manifestations

Patients who develop re-expansion pulmonary edema typically develop pernicious coughing or chest tightness during or immediately following thoracentesis or chest tube placement. The symptoms progress for 24 to 48 hours, and the chest radiograph reveals pulmonary edema throughout the ipsilateral lung. Pulmonary edema may also develop in the contralateral lung (185). If the patient does not die within the first 48 hours, recovery is usually complete. The seriousness of the syndrome is emphasized by reports that it has been responsible for the death of healthy young people. In a recent review of the subject (185), the outcome was fatal in 11 of 53 reported cases (20%). The overall mortality rate is probably much less than 20% since fatal cases are more likely to be reported than are nonfatal cases.

The incidence of re-expansion pulmonary edema is not known, but it is thought to be uncommon. Until 1988, a total of only 53 cases had been reported (185). In the recent VA cooperative study on spontaneous pneumothorax there were no cases of re-expansion pulmonary edema among the 229 study subjects despite the use of suction in over 80% of the cases (32). However, another study from Japan reported an incidence of 14% in 146 cases of spontaneous pneumothorax (195). In this latter series the incidence was significantly higher in patients with primary as compared with secondary spontaneous pneumothoraces (195). There is no ready explanation for the marked differences in the incidences in the above two series.

Prevention

The possibility of re-expansion pulmonary edema should be considered in patients with large pneumothoraces or pleural effusions of more than a few days' duration who are undergoing tube thoracostomy or thoracentesis. When tube thoracostomy is performed for spontaneous pneumothorax, the tubes should be connected to an underwater-seal drainage apparatus rather than to negative pleural pressure in view of the animal studies of Miller and colleagues (184) and Pavlin and Cheney (181). If underwater-seal drainage does not effect re-expansion of the underlying lung within 24 to 48 hours, then negative pressure can be applied to the pleural space.

The amount of pleural fluid withdrawn during thoracentesis should be limited to 1000 ml unless pleural pressures are monitored. My coworkers and I have shown that during therapeutic thoracentesis, the pleural pressure sometimes falls rapidly, reaching levels of -50 cm H_2O or lower in some patients (see Figure 23.5) (196). The patient often has no immediate symptoms attributable to the low pleural

pressure, and the operator cannot appreciate the negative pleural pressure. I hypothesize that the large negative pleural pressures and the resulting mechanical stresses on the lung may lead to re-expansion pulmonary edema, and I therefore perform serial pleural pressure measurements in all patients undergoing thoracentesis of more than 1000 ml pleural fluid, and continue thoracentesis only as long as the pleural pressure remains above -20 cm H_2O (see Chapter 23). My colleagues and I have shown that as long as the pleural pressure does not fall below -20 cm H_2O, thoracentesis can be continued safely without the development of re-expansion pulmonary edema (196). Indeed, with pressure monitoring we have removed more than 5000 ml pleural fluid from some patients. Obviously, if the patient develops chest tightness or pernicious coughing at any time during a therapeutic thoracentesis, the procedure should be stopped.

BRONCHOPLEURAL FISTULAS

Bronchopleural fistula constitutes a serious and sometimes fatal disorder that usually occurs after pulmonary surgery or as a complication of an underlying pulmonary disease. Bronchopleural fistulas occurring concomitantly with spontaneous pneumothorax have been discussed earlier in this chapter. In this section the problem of bronchopleural fistulas in patients on mechanical ventilation and in patients after pulmonary surgery will be discussed.

Bronchopleural Fistulas and Mechanical Ventilation

The management of a patient on mechanical ventilation with a large bronchopleural fistula is frequently difficult. In general, hypoxia rather than hypercapnia is the main threat to the patient, because the air that leaves the bronchopleural fistula has a carbon dioxide level comparable to that in mixed expired air (197). In other words, the air that exits through the chest tube is effective in removing carbon dioxide from the patient. Indeed, Prezant and colleagues (198) reported a patient whose total ventilatory requirements could be maintained through a chronic bronchopleural fistula. At times, however, when a high percentage of the minute ventilation exits through the bronchopleural fistula, the patient's oxygenation may suffer (199).

The first question that must be addressed when dealing with a patient with a bronchopleural fistula who is receiving mechanical ventilation is the management of the chest tubes. How much suction? How many chest tubes? It appears that the level of flow through the fistula is decreased when the side with the fistula is placed in the dependent position (200). The number and size of the chest tubes should be sufficient to effect a complete expansion of the underlying lung. The amount of suction should probably be established on an individual basis. Powner and coworkers (201) have shown that the level of suction at which the flow through the bronchopleural fistula is minimized varies from patient to patient. In some patients the flow is minimized at no suction, whereas in others it is minimized at an intermediate level (10 to 15 cm H_2O), and in still others it is minimized with high suction (25 cm H_2O).

One approach to decreasing the flow through a bronchopleural fistula is to place the patient on a high-frequency jet ventilator. Although high-frequency ventilation appears to decrease the flow through the fistula and improve gas exchange in the experimental model (202), it is not recommended because it has not been demonstrated to be effective in patients. Two separate studies in adults (203, 204) demonstrated no benefits of high-frequency ventilation, compared with conventional mechanical ventilation with respect to the flow through the bronchopleural fistula or gas exchange. In infants, Gonzalez and associates (205) applied conventional ventilation at a rate of 60 and high-frequency jet ventilation with a rate of 420 to 6 infants with continuously bubbling chest tubes. They recommended that jet ventilation be used in such instances because the mean flow through the bronchopleural fistula dropped from 227 to 104 ml/minute as the infants were switched to the jet ventilator. The Pao_2 dropped from 49 to 44 mm Hg when the patients were switched to the jet ventilator, however. Therefore, it is difficult to agree with their recommendation.

Multiple agents and devices have been passed through a bronchoscope in attempts to occlude the fistula including silver nitrate, Gelfoam, cyanoacrylate-based agents, and fibrin agents (206). The cyanoacrylate agents have been recently improved with an additive that slows drying time to permit greater time for modeling of the agent into the fistula site (206) and show the most promise. There are, however, no sizable series on the use of any of these agents in the treatment of bronchopleural fistula in patients on mechanical ventilation.

Postoperative Bronchopleural Fistulas

A bronchopleural fistula is observed in approximately 1 to 4% of patients after a pneumonectomy or a lobectomy and less often after a segmentectomy or lesser procedure (207, 208). In patients with lung cancer, significant risk factors for the development of a bronchopleural fistula include residual carcinomatous tissue at the bronchial stump, preoperative irradiation, and diabetes mellitus (207). A bronchopleural fistula is more common after resections for inflammatory disease of the lung, especially in patients with active tuberculosis and positive sputum culture (208).

After pulmonary surgery, a bronchopleural fistula may develop immediately or weeks to months later. The early appearance of a fistula (1–6 days) frequently is due to a technically poor closure of the bronchial stump. After a pneumonectomy, the early fistula is massive and persistent. The patient frequently develops massive subcutaneous emphysema and may exhibit varying degrees of respiratory insufficiency (208).

When the bronchial leak occurs later in the postoperative course (7–10 days), it may be caused by failure of healing because of inadequate viable tissue coverage of the stump or as the result of infection of the fluid within the space and rupture of the empyema through the suture line of the bronchial stump. At this stage, the patient coughs up variable quantities of serosanguineous, frothy fluid from the respiratory tract. The patient should be placed with the affected side down to decrease the danger of flooding the remaining lung.

When a bronchopleural fistula occurs later than 2 weeks after pneumonectomy, it is most likely the result of rupture of a frank empyema through the bronchial stump, although at times, failure of healing of the bronchial stump may be the underlying cause (208). The patient appears chronically ill with a cough and fever. Thoracentesis reveals that the pleural fluid is infected.

The management of a postoperative bronchopleural fistula depends on the time of its development and its underlying cause. If the bronchopleural fistula occurs early in the postoperative period, it can sometimes be managed with reoperation and repair of the bronchial stump. If primary repair of the bronchial stump is attempted, it is imperative that the new bronchial suture line be covered. This can be done with a transposed muscle flap (209), the pericardial fat pad, or an omental pedicle flap (208). With direct closure, the bronchial stump should be shortened as much as possible (210).

If primary repair of the bronchopleural fistula is not attempted or is unsuccessful, the patient should be treated with a chest tube. Several articles have reported the implantation of different materials in the bronchus via a bronchoscope in an attempt to close the air leak. When the patient has undergone less than a pneumonectomy, a Fogarty balloon catheter is passed down the working channel of the bronchoscope, and systematic occlusion of all lung segments on the side of the air leak is undertaken. The segment or segments leading to the fistula can be noted by observing decreases or disappearance of the air leak (211). Materials placed in the appropriate bronchus to close the fistula have included Gelfoam (211), doxycycline and blood (212), tissue adhesives (213, 214) and vascular occlusion coils (215). Tissue adhesives appear to be the most promising material. Menard and associates instilled the tissue adhesive bucrylate in 5 dogs in whom a large bronchopleural fistula had been created approximately 1 month after a pneumonectomy. In all 5 the bronchopleural fistula closed and remained closed for 4 to 12 months of observation. These same workers reported the successful use of this method in 1 patient (213). More recently Scappaticci and coworkers reported their experience using the tissue glue adhesive methyl-2-cyanoacrylate in 12 consecutive patients with postresectional bronchopleural fistula. They reported that this treatment was successful in 10 (83%) (214). The ultimate place of this approach in the management of

patients with a postoperative bronchopleural fistula remains to be determined.

Bronchopleural fistulas that occur late after surgery are almost always associated with empyema. Such fistulas are discussed in Chapter 9 in the section on postpneumonectomy empyema.

REFERENCES

1. Melton LJ, Hepper NGG, Offord KP: Incidence of spontaneous pneumothorax in Olmsted County, Minnesota: 1950 to 1974. Am Rev Respir Dis 1979; 120:1379–1382.
2. Gobbel WG Jr, Rhea WG Jr, Nelson IA, Daniel RA Jr: Spontaneous pneumothorax. J Thorac Cardiovasc Surg 1963;46:331–345.
3. Lesur O, Delorme N, Fromaget JM, Bernadac P, Polu JM: Computed tomography in the etiologic assessment of idiopathic spontaneous pneumothorax. Chest 1990;98:341–347.
4. Bense L, Lewander R, Eklund G, Hedenstierna G, Wiman LG: Nonsmoking, non-alpha-1-antitrypsin deficiency-induced emphysema in nonsmokers with healed spontaneous pneumothorax, identified by computed tomography of the lungs. Chest 1993; 103:433–438.
5. O'Hara VS: Spontaneous pneumothorax. Milit Med 1978;143:32–35.
6. Jansveld CAF, Dijkman JH: Primary spontaneous pneumothorax and smoking. Br Med J 1975;4:559–560.
7. Seremetis MG: The management of spontaneous pneumothorax. Chest 1970;57:65–68.
8. Bense L, Eklund G, Wiman LG: Smoking and the increased risk of contracting spontaneous pneumothorax. Chest 1987;92:1009–1012.
9. Scott GC, Berger R, McKean HE: The role of atmospheric pressure variation in the development of spontaneous pneumothoraces. Am Rev Respir Dis 1989;139:659–662.
10. Bense L: Spontaneous pneumothorax related to falls in atmospheric pressure. Eur J Respir Dis 1985;65:544–546.
11. Withers JN, Fishback ME, Kiehl PV, Hannon JL: Spontaneous pneumothorax. Am J Surg 1964;108: 772–776.
12. Abolnik IZ, Lossos IS, Gillis D, Breuer R: Primary spontaneous pneumothorax in men. Am J Med Sci 1993;305:297–303.
13. Abolnik IZ, Lossos IS, Zlotogora J, Brauer R: On the inheritance of primary spontaneous pneumothorax. Am J Med Genetics 1991;40:155–158.
14. Sharpe IK, Ahmad M, Braun W: Familial spontaneous pneumothorax and HLA antigens. Chest 1980; 78:264–268.
15. Lenler-Petersen P, Grunnet N, Jespersen TW, Jaeger P: Familial spontaneous pneumothorax. Eur J Resp Dis 1990;3:342–345.
16. Yellin A, Shiner RJ, Lieberman Y: Familial multiple bilateral pneumothorax associated with Marfan syndrome. Chest 1991;100:577–578.

17. Bense L, Eklund G, Wiman LG: Bilateral bronchial anomaly. A pathogenetic factor in spontaneous pneumothorax. Am Rev Respir Dis 1992;146:513–516.

18. Norris RM, Jones JG, Bishop JM: Respiratory gas exchange in patients with spontaneous pneumothorax. Thorax 1968;23:427–433.

19. Moran JF, Jones RH, Wolfe WG: Regional pulmonary function during experimental unilateral pneumothorax in the awake state. J Thorac Cardiovasc Surg 1977;74:396–402.

20. Anthonisen NR: Regional function in spontaneous pneumothorax. Am Rev Respir Dis 1977;115:873–876.

21. Vail WJ, Alway AE, England NJ: Spontaneous pneumothorax. Dis Chest 1960;38:512–515.

22. Aston SJ, Rosove M: Horner's syndrome occurring with spontaneous pneumothorax. N Engl J Med 1972;287:1098.

23. Bense L, Wiman LG, Hedenstierna G: Onset of symptoms in spontaneous pneumothorax: correlations to physical activity. Eur J Resp Dis 1987;71:181–186.

24. Walston A, Brewer DL, Kitchens CS, Krook JE: The electrocardiographic manifestations of spontaneous left pneumothorax. Ann Intern Med 1974;80:375–379.

25. Aitchison F, Bleetman A, Munro P, McCarter D, Reid AW: Detection of pneumothorax by accident and emergency officers and radiologist on single chest films. Arch Emerg Med 1993;10:343–346.

26. Beres RA, Goodman LR: Pneumothorax: detection with upright versus decubitus radiography. Radiology 1993;186:19–22.

27. Rhea JT, DeLuca SA, Greene RE: Determining the size of pneumothorax in the upright patient. Radiology 1982;144:733–736.

28. Engdahl O, Toft T, Boe J: Chest radiograph—a poor method for determining the size of a pneumothorax. Chest 1993;103:26–29.

29. Larrieu AJ, Tyers GFO, Williams EH, et al: Intrapleural instillation of quinacrine for treatment of recurrent spontaneous pneumothorax. Ann Thorac Surg 1979;28:146–150.

30. Voge VM, Anthracite R: Spontaneous pneumothorax in the USAF aircrew population: a retrospective study. Aviat Space Environ Med 1986;57:939–949.

31. Lippert HL, Lund O, Blegvad S, Larsen HV: Independent risk factors for cumulative recurrence rate after first spontaneous pneumothorax. Europ Respir J 1991;4:324–331.

32. Light RW, O'Hara VS, Moritz TE, McElhinney AJ, Butz R, Haakenson CM, Read RC, Sassoon CS, Eastridge CE, Berger R, Fontenelle LJ, Bell RH, Jenkinson SG, Shure D, Merrill W, Hoover E, Campbell SC: Intrapleural tetracycline for the prevention of recurrent spontaneous pneumothorax. JAMA 1990;264:2224–2230.

33. Mitlehner W, Friedrich M, Dissmann W: Value of computer tomography in the detection of bullae and blebs in patients with primary spontaneous pneumothorax. Respiration 1992;59:221–227.

34. Kircher LT Jr, Swartzel RL: Spontaneous pneumothorax and its treatment. JAMA 1954;155:24–29.

35. Chernick V, Avery ME: Spontaneous alveolar rupture at birth. Pediatrics 1963;32:816–824.

36. Northfield TC: Oxygen therapy for spontaneous pneumothorax. Br Med J 1971;4:86–88.

37. Bevelaqua FA: Management of spontaneous pneumothorax with small lumen catheter manual aspiration. Chest 1982;81:693–694.

38. Archer GJ, Hamilton AAD, Upadhyay R, et al: Results of simple aspiration of pneumothoraces. Br J Dis Chest 1985;79:177–182.

39. Vallee P, Sullivan M, Richardson H, et al: Sequential treatment of a simple pneumothorax. Ann Emerg Med 1988;5:45–47.

40. So SY, Yu DYC: Catheter drainage of spontaneous pneumothorax: suction or no suction, early or late removal. Thorax 1982;37:46–48.

41. Minami H, Saka H, Senda K, Horio Y, Iwahara T, Nomura F, Sakai S, Shimokata K: Small caliber catheter drainage for spontaneous pneumothorax. Am J Med Sci 1992;404:345–347.

42. Conces DJ Jr, Tarver RD, Gray WC, Pearcy EA: Treatment of pneumothoraces utilizing small caliber chest tubes. Chest 1988;94:55–57.

43. Casola G, van Sonnenberg E, Keightley A, Ho M, Withers C, Lee AS: Pneumothorax: radiologic treatment with small catheters. Radiology 1988;166:89–91.

44. Sharma TN, Agnihotri SP, Jain NK, et al: Intercostal tube thoracostomy in pneumothorax: factors influencing re-expansion of lung. Indian J Chest Dis Allied Sci 1988;30:32–35.

45. Shaw TJ, Caterine JM: Recurrent re-expansion pulmonary edema. Chest 1984;86:784–786.

46. Lizotte PE, Whitlock WL, Prudhomme JC, Brown CR, Hershon JL, Mainini SE, Johnson FE: Tension pneumothorax complicating small-caliber chest tube insertion. Chest 1990;97:759–760.

47. Engdahl O, Boe J: Quantification of aspirated air volume reduces treatment time in pneumothorax. Europ Resp J 1990;3:649–652.

48. Adler RH: A talc powder aerosol method for the prevention of recurrent spontaneous pneumothorax. Ann Thorac Surg 1968;5:474–477.

49. Nandi P: Recurrent spontaneous pneumothorax: an effective method of talc poudrage. Chest 1980;77:493–495.

50. Almind M, Lange P, Viskum K: Spontaneous pneumothorax: comparison of simple drainage, talc pleurodesis, and tetracycline pleurodesis. Thorax 1989;44:627–630.

51. Ofoegbu RO: Pleurodesis for spontaneous pneumothorax: experience with intrapleural olive oil in high risk patients. Am J Surg 1980;140:679–681.

52. Goldszer RC, Bennett J, VanCampen J, Rudnitzky J: Intrapleural tetracycline for spontaneous pneumothorax. JAMA 1979;241:724–725.

53. Spector ML, Stern RC: Pneumothorax in cystic fibrosis: A 26-year experience. Ann Thorac Surg 1989;47:204–207.

54. Kennedy L, Rusch VW, Strange C, Ginsberg RJ, Sahn SA: Pleurodesis using talc slurry. Chest 1994; 106:342-346.

55. Bouchama A, Chastre J, Gaudichet A, et al: Acute pneumonitis with bilateral effusion after talc pleurodesis. Chest 1984;86:795-797.

56. Rinaldo JE, Owens GR, Rogers RM: Adult respiratory distress syndrome following intrapleural instillation of talc. J Thorac Cardiovasc Surg 1983;85: 523-526.

57. Jackson JW, Bennett MH: Chest wall tumour following iodized talc pleurodesis. Thorax 1969;28:788-793.

58. Research Committee of the British Thoracic Association: a survey of the long-term effects of talc and kaolin pleurodesis. Br J Dis Chest 1979;73:285-288.

59. Alfageme I, Moreno L, Huetas C, Vargas A, Hernandez J, Beizteggui A: Spontaneous pneumothorax. Long-term results with tetracycline pleurodesis. Chest 1994;106:347-350.

60. Light RW, Wang N-S, Sassoon CSH, Gruer SE, Vargas FS: Comparison of the effectiveness of tetracycline and minocycline as pleural sclerosing agents in rabbits. Chest 1994;106:577-582.

61. Hurewitz AD, Lidonicci K, Wu CL, Reim D, Zucker S: Histologic changes of doxycycline pleurodesis in rabbits. Effect of concentration and pH. Chest 1994;106:1241-1245.

62. Heffner JE, Standerfer RJ, Torstveit J, Unruh L: Clinical efficacy of doxycycline for pleurodesis. Chest 1994;105:1743-1747.

63. Vargas FS, Wang N-S, Lee HM, Gruer SE, Sassoon CSH, Light RW: Effectiveness of bleomycin in comparison to tetracycline as pleural sclerosing agent in rabbits. Chest 1993;104:1582-1584.

64. Sherman S, Ravikrishnan KP, Patel AS, Seidman JC: Optimum anesthesia with intrapleural lidocaine during chemical pleurodesis with tetracycline. Chest 1988;93:533-536.

65. Wang YT, Ng KY, Poh SC: Intrapleural tetracycline for spontaneous pneumothorax with persistent air leak. Singapore Med J 1988;29:72-73.

66. Landreneau RJ, Hazelrigg SR, Mack MJ, Keenan RJ, Ferson PF: Video-assisted thoracic surgery for pulmonary and pleural disease. In: Shields TW, ed. General Thoracic Surgery. Malvern, PA: Williams & Wilkins, 1994:4;508-528.

67. Takeno Y: Thoracoscopic treatment of spontaneous pneumothorax. Ann Thorac Surg 1993;56:688-690.

68. Inderbitzi RGC, Leiser A, Furrer M, Althaus U: Three years experience in video-assisted thoracic surgery (VATS) for spontaneous pneumothorax. J Thorac Cardiovasc Surg 1994;107:1410-1415.

69. Hazelrigg SR, Landreneau RJ, Mack M, Acuff T, Seifert PE, Auer JE, Magee M: Thoracoscopic stapled resection for spontaneous pneumothorax. J Thorac Cardiovasc Surg 1993;105:389-393.

70. Bagnato VJ: Treatment of recurrent spontaneous pneumothorax. Surg Laparosc Endosc 1992;2:100-103.

71. Fosse E, Fjeld NB, Brockmeier V, Buanes T: Thoracoscopic pleurodesis. Scand J Thorac Cardiovasc Surg 1993;27:117-119.

72. Waller DA, Yoruk Y, Morritt GN, Forty J, Dark JH: Videothoracoscopy in the treatment of spontaneous pneumothorax: an initial experience. Ann Royal College Surg Eng 1993;75:237-240.

73. Torre M, Grassi M, Nerli FP, Maioli M, Belloni PA: Nd-YAG laser pleurodesis via thoracoscopy. Endoscopic therapy in spontaneous pneumothorax Nd-YAG laser pleurodesis. Chest 1994;106:338-341.

74. Olsen PS, Andersen HO: Long-term results after tetracycline pleurodesis in spontaneous pneumothorax. Ann Thorac Surg 1992;53:1015-1017.

75. Milanez JRC, Vargas FS, Filomeno LTB, Fernandez A, Jatene A, Light RW: Intrapleural talc for the prevention of recurrent pneumothorax. Chest 1994; 106:1162-1165.

76. Weissberg D, Ben-Zeev I: Talc pleurodesis. Experience with 360 patients. J Thorac Cardiovasc Surg 1993;106:689-695.

77. Viskum K, Lange P, Mortensen J: Long term sequelae after talc pleurodesis for spontaneous pneumothorax. Pneumologie 1989;43:105-106.

78. Janssen JP, van Mourik J, Cuesta Valentin M, Sutedja G, Gigengack K, Postmus PE: Treatment of patients with spontaneous pneumothorax during videothoracoscopy. Europ Respir J 1994;7:1281-1284.

79. Urschel JD: Thoracoscopic treatment of spontaneous pneumothorax. A review. J Cardiovasc Surg 1993;34:535-537.

80. Maggi G, Ardissone F, Oliaro A, Ruffini E, Cianci R: Pleural abrasion in the treatment of recurrent or persistent spontaneous pneumothorax. Results of 94 consecutive cases. Internat Surg 1992;77:99-101.

81. Donahue DM, Wright CD, Viale G, Mathisen DJ: Resection of pulmonary blebs and pleurodesis for spontaneous pneumothorax. Chest 1993;104:1767-1769.

82. Deslauriers J, Beaulieu M, Després J-P, et al: Transaxillary pleurectomy for treatment of spontaneous pneumothorax. Ann Thorac Surg 1980;30:569-574.

83. O'Rourke JP, Yee ES: Civilian spontaneous pneumothorax. Treatment options and long-term results. Chest 1989;96:1302-1306.

84. Wait MA, Estrera A: Changing clinical spectrum of spontaneous pneumothorax. Am J Surg 1992;164: 528-531.

85. Dines DE, Clagett OT, Payne WS: Spontaneous pneumothorax in emphysema. Mayo Clin Proc 1970;45:481-487.

86. Tanaka F, Itoh M, Esaki H, Isobe J, Ueno Y, Inoue R: Secondary spontaneous pneumothorax. Ann Thorac Surg 1993;55:372-376.

87. Shields TW, Oilschlager GA: Spontaneous pneumothorax in patients 40 years of age and older. Ann Thorac Surg 1966;2:377-383.

88. George RB, Herbert SJ, Shames JM, et al: Pneumothorax complicating pulmonary emphysema. JAMA 1975;234:389-393.

89. Bourgouin P, Cousineau G, Lemire P, Hebert G: Computed tomography used to exclude pneumothorax in bullous lung disease. J Can Assoc Radiol 1985;36:341-342.

90. Fraser RG, Pare JAP: Diagnosis of Diseases of the Chest. 2nd Ed. Philadelphia: WB Saunders, 3:1977.

91. Videm V, Pillgram-Larsen J, Ellingsen O, Andersen G, Ovrum E: Spontaneous pneumothorax in chronic obstructive pulmonary disease: complications, treatment and recurrences. Eur J Respir Dis 1987;71: 365-371.

92. Ng AW, Chan KW, Lee SK: Simple aspiration of pneumothorax. Singapore Med J 1994;35:50-52.

93. Seaton D, Yoganathan K, Coady T, Barker R: Spontaneous pneumothorax: marker gas technique for predicting outcome of manual aspiration. BMJ 1991; 302:262-265.

94. Boat TF, De Sant'Agnese PA, Warwick WJ, Handwerger SA: Pneumothorax in cystic fibrosis. JAMA 1969;209:1498-1504.

95. Schidlow DV, Taussig LM, Knowles MR: Cystic Fibrosis Foundation consensus conference report on pulmonary complications of cystic fibrosis. Pediatr Pulmonol 1993;15:187-198.

96. Waller DA, Forty J, Soni AK, Conacher ID, Morritt GN: Videothoracoscopic operation for secondary spontaneous pneumothorax. Ann Thorac Surg 1994;57:1612-1615.

97. Deslauriers J: The management of spontaneous pneumothorax [Editorial]. Can J Surg 1994;37:182.

98. Sepkowitz KA, Telzak EE, Gold JW, Bernard EM, Blum S, Carrow M, Dickmeyer M, Armstrong D: Pneumothorax in AIDS. Ann Intern Med 1991;114: 455-459.

99. Coker RJ, Moss F, Peters B, McCarty M, Nieman R, Claydon E, Mitchell D, Harris JR: Pneumothorax in patients with AIDS. Respir Med 1993;87:43-47.

100. Leoung GS, Feigal DW Jr, Montgomery AB, Corkery K, Wardlaw L, Adams M, et al: Aerosolized pentamidine for prophylaxis against Pneumocystis carinii pneumonia. N Engl J Med 1990;323:769-775.

101. Renzi PM, Corbeil C, Chasse M, Braidy J, Matar N: Bilateral pneumothoraces hasten mortality in AIDS patients receiving secondary prophylaxis with aerosolized pentamidine. Association with a lower Dco prior to receiving aerosolized pentamidine. Chest 1992;102:491-496.

102. Cuthbert AC, Wright D, McVerry BA: Pneumothorax in pentamidine-treated haemophiliacs [letter]. Lancet 1991;13:337-918.

103. Newsome GS, Ward DJ, Pierce PF: Spontaneous pneumothorax in patients with acquired immunodeficiency syndrome treated with prophylactic aerosolized pentamidine. Arch Intern Med 1990;150: 2167-2168.

104. Shanley DJ, Luyckx BA, Haggerty MF, Murphy TF: Spontaneous pneumothorax in AIDS patients with recurrent Pneumocystis carinii pneumonia despite aerosolized pentamidine prophylaxis. Chest 1991; 99:502-504.

105. Scannell KA: Pneumothoraces and Pneumocystis carinii pneumonia in two AIDS patients receiving aerosolized pentamidine. Chest 1990;97:479-480.

106. Beers MF, Sohn M, Swartz M: Recurrent pneumothorax in AIDS patients with pneumocystis pneumonia. A clinicopathologic report of three cases and review of the literature. Chest 1990;98:266-270.

107. Gerein AN, Brumwell ML, Lawson LM, Chan NH, Montaner JS: Surgical management of pneumothorax in patients with acquired immunodeficiency syndrome. Arch Surg 1991;126:1272-1276.

108. Wait MA, Dal Nogare AR: Treatment of AIDS-related spontaneous pneumothorax. Chest 1994;106:693-696.

109. Byrnes TA, Brevig JK, Yeoh CB: Pneumothorax in patients with acquired immunodeficiency syndrome. J Thorac Cardiovas Surg 1990;98:546-550.

110. Driver AG, Peden JG, Adams HG, Rumley RL: Heimlich valve treatment of Pneumocystis carinii-associated pneumothorax. Chest 1991;100:281-282.

111. Walker WA, Pate JW, Amundson D, Kennedy C: AIDS-related bronchopleural fistula. Ann Thorac Surg 1993;55:1048.

112. Crawford BK, Galloway AC, Boyd AD, Spencer FC: Treatment of AIDS-related bronchopleural fistula by pleurectomy. Ann Thorac Surg 1992;212-213.

113. Horowitz MD, Oliva H: Pneumothorax in AIDS patients: operative management. Am Surg 1993;59: 200-204.

114. Spector ML, Stern RC: Pneumothorax in cystic fibrosis: a 26-year experience. Ann Thorac Surg 1989;47:204-207.

115. Luck SR, Raffensperger JG, Sullivan HJ, Gibson LE: Management of pneumothorax in children with chronic pulmonary disease. J Thorac Cardiovasc Surg 1977;74:834-839.

116. Noyes BE, Orenstein DM: Treatment of pneumothorax in cystic fibrosis in the era of lung transplantation. Chest 1992;101:1187-1188.

117. Wilder RJ, Beacham EG, Ravitch MM: Spontaneous pneumothorax complicating cavitary tuberculosis. J Thorac Cardiovasc Surg 1962;43:561-573.

118. Lillington GA, Mitchell SP, Wood GA: Catamenial pneumothorax. JAMA 1972;219:1328-1332.

119. Wilhelm JL, Scommegna A: Catamenial pneumothorax: bilateral occurrence while on suppressive therapy. Obstet Gynecol 1977;50:223-231.

120. Maurer ER, Schaal JA, Mendez FL: Chronic recurrent spontaneous pneumothorax due to endometriosis of the diaphragm. JAMA 1958;168: 2013-2014.

121. Stern H, Toole AL, Merino M: Catamenial pneumothorax. Chest 1980;78:480-482.

122. Downey DB, Towers MJ, Poon PY, Thomas P: Pneumoperitoneum with catamenial pneumothorax. Am J Roentgenol 1990;155:29-30.

123. Dotson RL, Peterson CM, Doucette RC, Quinton R, Rawson DY, Jones KP: Medical therapy for recurring catamenial pneumothorax following pleurodesis. Ob Gynecol 1993;82(4 Pt 2 Suppl):656-658.

124. Chernick V, Reed MH: Pneumothorax and chylothorax in the neonatal period. J Pediatr 1970;76:624-632.

125. Ogata ES, Gregory GA, Kitterman JA, et al: Pneumothorax in the respiratory distress syndrome: incidence and effect on vital signs, blood gases, and pH. Pediatrics 1976;58:177–183.

126. Karlberg P: Respiratory studies in newborns. II. Pulmonary ventilation and mechanics of breathing in the first minutes of life including the onset of respiration. Acta Paediatr 1962;51:121–136.

127. Adler SM, Wyszogrodski I: Pneumothorax as a function of gestational age: clinical and experimental studies. J Pediatr 1975;87:771–775.

128. Mehrabani D, Gowen CW Jr, Kopelman AE: Association of pneumothorax and hypotension with intraventricular haemorrhage. Arch Dis Child 1991; 66:48–51.

129. Kuhns LR, Bednarek FJ, Wyman ML, et al: Diagnosis of pneumothorax or pneumomediastinum in the neonate by transillumination. Pediatrics 1975;56: 355–360.

130. Carlon GC, Kahn RC, Howland WS, et al: Clinical experience with high frequency jet ventilation. Crit Care Med 1981;9:1–6.

131. Sassoon CSH, Light RW, O'Hara VS, Moritz TE: Iatrogenic pneumothorax: etiology and morbidity. Respiration 1992;59:215–220.

132. Despars JA, Sassoon CSH, Light RW: Significance of iatrogenic pneumothoraces. Chest 1994;105:1147–1150.

133. Poe RH, Kallay MC, Wicks CM, Odoroff CL: Predicting risk of pneumothorax in needle biopsy of the lung. Chest 1984;85:232–235.

134. Miller KS, Fish GB, Stanley JH, Schabel SI: Prediction of pneumothorax rate in percutaneous needle aspiration of the lung. Chest 1988;93:742–745.

135. Bourgouin PM, Shepard JA, McLoud TC, et al: Transthoracic needle aspiration biopsy: evaluation of the blood patch technique. Radiology 1988;166: 93–95.

136. Berger R, Smith D: Efficacy of the lateral decubitus position in preventing pneumothorax after needle biopsy of the lung. South Med J 1988;81:1140–1143.

137. Anderson CLV, Crespo JCA, Lie TH: Risk of pneumothorax not increased by obstructive lung disease in percutaneous needle biopsy. Chest 1994;105: 1705–1708.

138. Haramati LB, Austin JHM: Complications after CT-guided needle biopsy through aerated versus nonaerated lung. Radiology 1991;181:778.

139. Hill PC, Spagnolo SV, Hockstein MJ: Pneumothorax with fine-needle aspiration of thoracic lesions. Is spirometry a predictor? Chest 1993;104:1017–1020.

140. Herman SJ, Weisbrod GL: Usefulness of the blood patch technique after transthoracic needle aspiration biopsy. Radiology 1990;176:395–397.

141. Conces DJ Jr, Holden RW: Aberrant locations and complications in initial placement of subclavian vein catheters. Arch Surg 1984;119:293–295.

142. Mansfield PF, Hohn DC, Fornage BD, Gregurich MA, Ota DM: Complications and failures of subclavian vein catheterization. N Engl J Med 1994;331: 1735–1738.

143. Lockwood AH: Percutaneous subclavian vein catheterization. Too much of a good thing? Arch Intern Med 1984;144:1407–1408.

144. Tyburski JG, Joseph AL, Thomas GA, Saxe JM, Lucas CE: Delayed pneumothorax after central venous access: a potential hazard. Am Surg 1993;59:587–589.

145. Plaus WJ: Delayed pneumothorax after subclavian vein catheterization. J Par Ent Nutrit 1990;14:414–415.

146. Raptopoulos V, Davis LM, Lee G, Umali C, Lew R, Irwin RS: Factors affecting the development of pneumothorax associated with thoracentesis. Am J Roentgenol 1991;156:917–920.

147. Collins TR, Sahn SA: Thoracocentesis: Clinical value, complications, technical problems and patient experience. Chest 1987;91:817–822.

148. Seneff MG, Corwin RW, Gold LH, Irwin RS: Complications associated with thoracocentesis. Chest 1986;90:97–100.

149. Brandstetter RD, Karetzky M, Rastogi R, Lolis JD: Pneumothorax after thoracentesis in chronic obstructive pulmonary disease. Heart Lung 1994;23: 67–70.

150. Grogan DR, Irwin RS, Channick R, Raptopoulos V, Curley FJ, Bartter T, Corwin RW: Complications associated with thoracentesis. A prospective, randomized study comparing three different methods. Arch Intern Med 1990;150:873–877.

151. Steier M, Ching N, Bonfils-Roberts E, Nealon JF Jr. Iatrogenic cause of pneumothorax: increasing incidence with advances in medical care. NY State J Med 1973;173:1296–1298.

152. De Latorre FJ, Tomasa A, Klamburg J, et al: Incidence of pneumothorax and pneumomediastinum in patients with aspiration pneumonia requiring ventilatory support. Chest 1977;72:141–144.

153. Gammon RB, Shin MS, Buchalter SE: Pulmonary barotrauma in mechanical ventilation. Patterns and risk factors. Chest 1992;102:568–572.

154. Poe RH, et al: Sensitivity, specificity, and predictive values of closed pleural biopsy. Arch Intern Med 1984;144:325–328.

155. Frazier WD, Pope TL Jr, Findley LJ: Pneumothorax following transbronchial biopsy. Chest 1990;97: 539–540.

156. Blasco LH, Hernandez IMS, Garrido VV, Poch EM, Delgado MN, Abrea JA: Safety of the transbronchial biopsy in outpatients. Chest 1991;99:562–565.

157. Ludwig J, Kienzle GD: Pneumothorax in a large autopsy population. Am J Clin Pathol 1978;70:24–26.

158. Tocino IM, Miller MH, Fairfax WR: Distribution of pneumothorax in the supine and semirecumbent critically ill adult. AJR 1985;144:901–905.

159. Kollef MH: Risk factors for the misdiagnosis of pneumothorax in the intensive care unit. Crit Care Med 1991;19:906–910.

160. Pollack MM, Fields AI, Holbrook PR: Pneumothorax and pneumomediastinum during pediatric mechanical ventilation. Crit Care Med 1979;7:536–539.

161. Delius RE, Obeid FN, Horst HM, Sorensen VJ, Fath JJ, Bivins BA: Catheter aspiration for simple pneu-

mothorax. Experience with 114 patients. Arch Surg 1989;124:833-836.

162. Pierce AK: Pleural disease. In: Guenter CA, Welch MH, eds. Pulmonary Medicine. Philadelphia: JB Lippincott, 1977.

163. Bridges KG, Welch G, Silver M, Schinco MA, Esposito B: CT detection of occult pneumothorax in multiple trauma patients. J Emerg Med 1993;11: 179-186.

164. Garramone RR Jr, Jacobs LM, Sahdev P: An objective method to measure and manage occult pneumothorax. Surg Gynecol Obstet 1991;173:257-261.

165. Shorr RM, Crittenden M, Indeck M, et al: Blunt thoracic trauma: Analysis of 515 patients. Ann Surg 1987;206:200-205.

166. Ordog GJ, Wasserberger J, Balasubramanium S, Shoemaker W: Asymptomatic stab wounds of the chest. J Trauma 1994;36:680-684.

167. Wolfman NT, Gilpin JW, Bechtold RE, Meredith JW, Ditesheim JA: Occult pneumothorax in patients with abdominal trauma: CT studies. J Comp Assist Tomog 1993;17:56-59.

168. Knottenbelt JD, van der Spuy JW: Traumatic pneumothorax: a scheme for rapid patient turnover. Brit J Acc Surg 1990;21:77-80.

169. Collins JC, Levine G, Waxman K: Occult traumatic pneumothorax: immediate tube thoracostomy versus expectant management. Am Surg 1992;58:743-746.

170. Guest JL, Anderson JN: Major airway injury in closed chest trauma. Chest 1977;72:63-66.

171. Sherr HP, Light RW, Merson MH, et al: Origin of pleural fluid amylase in esophageal rupture. Ann Intern Med 1972;76:985-986.

172. Douglass RE, Levison MA: Pneumothorax in drug abusers: an urban epidemic. Am Surg 1986;52:377-380.

173. Light RW: Tension pneumothorax. Intensive Care Med 1994;20:468-469.

174. Rutherford RB, Hurt HH, Brickman RD, Tubb JM: The pathophysiology of progressive, tension pneumothorax. J Trauma 1968;8:212-227.

175. Gustman P, Yerger L, Wanner A: Immediate cardiovascular effects of tension pneumothorax. Am Rev Respir Dis 1983;127:171-174.

176. Hurewitz AN, Sidhu U, Bergofsky EH, et al: Cardiovascular and respiratory consequences of tension pneumothorax. Bull Eur Physiopathol Respir 1986; 22:545-549.

177. Brann BS IV, Mayfield SR, Goldstein M, Oh W, Stonestreet BS: Cardiovascular effects of hypoxia/hypercarbia and tension pneumothorax in newborn piglets. Crit Care Med 1994;22:1453-1460.

178. Connolly JP: Hemodynamic measurements during a tension pneumothorax. Crit Care Med 1993;21:294-296.

179. Murphy DG, Sloan EP, Hart RG, Narasimhan K, Barreca RS: Tension pneumothorax associated with hyperbaric oxygen therapy. Am J Emerg Med 1991; 9:176-179.

180. Mainini SE, Johnson FE: Tension pneumothorax complicating small-caliber chest tube insertion. Chest 1990;97:759-760.

181. Pavlin J, Cheney FW Jr: Unilateral pulmonary edema in rabbits after re-expansion of collapsed lung. J Appl Physiol 1979;46:31-35.

182. Trapnell DH, Thurston JGB: Unilateral pulmonary edema after pleural aspiration. Lancet 1970;1:1367-1369.

183. Peatfield RC, Edwards PR, Johnson NM: Two unexpected deaths from pneumothorax. Lancet 1979;1: 356-358.

184. Miller WC, Toon R, Palat H, Lacroix J: Experimental pulmonary edema following re-expansion of pneumothorax. Am Rev Respir Dis 1973;108:664-666.

185. Mahfood S, Hix WR, Aaron BI, et al: Re-expansion pulmonary edema. Ann Thorac Surg 1988;45:340-345.

186. Olcott EW: Fatal reexpansion pulmonary edema following pleural catheter placement. J Vasc Intervent Radiol 1994;5:176-178.

187. Waqaruddin M, Bernstein A: Re-expansion pulmonary edema. Thorax 1975;30:54-60.

188. Sprung CL, Loewenherz JW, Baier H, Hauser MJ: Evidence for increased permeability in re-expansion pulmonary edema. Am J Med 1981;71:497-500.

189. Pavlin DJ, Nessly ML, Cheney FW: Increased pulmonary vascular permeability as a cause of re-expansion edema in rabbits. Am Rev Respir Dis 1981;124:422-427.

190. Pavlin DJ: Lung re-expansion: for better or worse. Chest 1986;89:2-3.

191. Jackson RM, Veal CF, Alexander CB, Brannen AL, Fulmer JO: Neutrophils in reexpansion pulmonary edema. J Appl Physiol 1988;65:228-234.

192. Nakamura H, Ishizaka A, Sawafuji M, Urano T, Fujishima S, Sakamaki F, Sayama K, Kawamura M, Kato R, Kikuchi K, et al: Elevated levels of interleukin-8 and leukotriene B4 in pulmonary edema fluid of a patient with reexpansion pulmonary edema. Am J Respir Crit Care Med 1994;149: 1037-1040.

193. Pavlin DJ, Nessly ML, Cheney FW: Hemodynamic effects of rapidly evacuating prolonged pneumothorax in rabbits. J Appl Physiol 1987;62:477-484.

194. Jackson RM, Veal CF, Alexander CB, et al: Re-expansion pulmonary edema: a potential role for free radicals in its pathogenesis. Am Rev Respir Dis 1988;137:1165-1171.

195. Matsuura Y, Nomimura T, Murakami H, Matsushima T, Kakehashi M, Kajihara H: Clinical analysis of reexpansion pulmonary edema. Chest 1991;100: 1562-1566.

196. Light RW, Jenkinson SG, Minh VD, George RB: Observations on pleural fluid pressure as fluid is withdrawn during thoracentesis. Am Rev Respir Dis 1980;121:799-804.

197. Bishop MJ, Benson MS, Pierson DJ: Carbon dioxide excretion via bronchopleural fistulas in adult respiratory distress syndrome. Chest 1987;91:400-402.

198. Prezant DJ, Aldrich TK, Fell SC, et al: The maintenance of total ventilatory requirements through a chronic bronchopleural cutaneous fistula. Am Rev Respir Dis 1987;136:1001-1002.

199. Feeley TW, Keating D, Nishimura T: Independent lung ventilation using high-frequency ventilation in

the management of a bronchopleural fistula. Anesthesiology 1988;69:420–422.

200. Lau KY: Postural management of bronchopleural fistula. Chest 1988;94:1122.

201. Powner DJ, Cline CD, Rodman GH: Effect of chest-tube suction on gas flow through a bronchopleural fistula. Crit Care Med 1985;13:99–101.

202. Orlando R III, Gluck EH, Cohen M, Mesologites CG: Ultra-high-frequency jet ventilation in a bronchopleural fistula model. Arch Surg 1988;123:591–593.

203. Albelda SM, Hansen-Flaschen JH, Taylor E, et al: Evaluation of high frequency jet ventilation in patients with bronchopleural fistulas by quantitation of the air leak. Anesthesiology 1985;63:551–554.

204. Bishop MJ, Benson MS, Sato P, Pierson DJ: Comparison of high frequency jet ventilation with conventional mechanical ventilation for bronchopleural fistula. Anesth Analg 1987;66:833–838.

205. Gonzalez F, Harris T, Black P, Richardson P: Decreased gas flow through pneumothoraces in neonates receiving high-frequency jet versus conventional ventilation. J Pediatr 1987;110:464–466.

206. Baumann MH, Sahn SA: Medical management and therapy of bronchopleural fistulas in the mechanically ventilated patient. Chest 1990;97:721–728.

207. Asamura H, Naruke T, Tsuchiya R, Goya T, Kondo H, Suemasu K: Bronchopleural fistulas associated with lung cancer operations. Univariate and multivariate analysis of risk factors, management, and outcome. J Thorac Cardiovasc Surg 1992;104:1456–1464.

208. Shields TW: General features and complications of pulmonary resections. In: General Thoracic Surgery. Shields TW, ed. Baltimore: Williams & Wilkins, 1994:4;407–409.

209. Arnold PG, Pairolero PC: Intrathoracic muscle flaps. An account of their use in the management of 100 consecutive patients. Ann Surg 1990;211:656–662.

210. De Maeseneer N, Van Hee R, Schoofs E, Vaneerdeweg W: The management of bronchopleural fistulas. Acta Chir Belg 1987;87:269–274.

211. Jones DP, David I: Gelfoam occlusion of peripheral bronchopleural fistulas. Ann Thorac Surg 1986;42:334–335.

212. Lan R-S, Lee C-H, Tsai Y-H, et al: Fiberoptic bronchial blockade in a small bronchopleural fistula. Chest 1987;92:944–946.

213. Menard JW, Prejean CA, Tucker WY: Endoscopic closure of bronchopleural fistulas using a tissue adhesive. Am J Surg 1988;155:415–416.

214. Scappaticci E, Ardissone F, Ruffini E, Baldi S, Mancuso M: Postoperative bronchopleural fistula: endoscopic closure in 12 patients. Ann Thorac Surg 1994;57:119–122.

215. Salmon CJ, Ponn RB, Westcott JL: Endobronchial vascular occlusion coils for control of a large parenchymal bronchopleural fistula. Chest 1990;98:233–234.

CHAPTER 20
Hemothorax

Hemothorax is the presence of significant amounts of blood in the pleural space. Most hemothoraces result from penetrating or nonpenetrating chest trauma. An occasional hemothorax results from iatrogenic manipulation such as the placement of central venous catheters percutaneously by the subclavian or internal jugular route or from translumbar aortography. On rare occasions, a hemothorax results from a medical condition such as pulmonary embolism or rupture of an aortic aneurysm.

Blood may enter the pleural space from injury to the chest wall, diaphragm, lung, or mediastinum. Blood entering the pleural space coagulates rapidly but, presumably as a result of physical agitation produced by movement of the heart and the lungs, the clot may be defibrinated. Loculation occurs early in the course of hemothorax, as with empyema.

When a diagnostic thoracentesis in a medical patient reveals pleural fluid that appears to be pure blood, a hematocrit should always be obtained on the pleural fluid. Frequently, even though the pleural fluid appears to be blood, the hematocrit on the pleural fluid is under 5%. A hemothorax should be considered to be present only when the hematocrit of the pleural fluid is at least 50% that of the peripheral blood.

TRAUMATIC HEMOTHORAX

Traumatic hemothoraces are a frequent occurrence, particularly in centers that treat victims of trauma. In one Houston hospital, over 300 patients with hemothorax due to penetrating trauma were seen in a 1-year period (1). The relative incidence of hemothorax due to penetrating and blunt thoracic trauma depends on whether the medical center cares primarily for victims of automobile accidents or of stab and gunshot wounds.

There is a high incidence of hemothorax with blunt trauma. In a retrospective analysis of 515 cases of blunt chest trauma, 193 pa-

tients (37%) had hemothoraces (2). A hemopneumothorax was present in 111 of the 193 patients (58%) (2). Interestingly, the 35% incidence of hemothorax in the 127 patients without rib fractures was comparable to the 38% incidence of hemothorax in the 388 patients with fractures 35% (2). In patients with rib fractures, hemothorax is more common if the fracture is displaced (3).

Diagnosis

The diagnosis of a traumatic hemothorax should be suspected in any patient with penetrating or nonpenetrating trauma to the chest. The diagnosis is usually established by the demonstration of a pleural effusion with a chest radiograph in a patient with thoracic trauma. The hemothorax may not be apparent on the initial chest radiograph. In one series of 130 patients with hemothorax secondary to nonpenetrating trauma, the hemothorax was not appreciated on the initial film in 31 (24%) (4). These authors felt that obtaining the chest radiograph with the patient supine led to the failure to recognize the hemothorax in some patients and recommended that upright chest radiographs be obtained whenever possible in trauma victims. Some of the patients in this series had no evidence of a hemothorax on the original upright radiograph, however (4). In another study ultrasonic examination in the emergency room failed to detect pleural fluid in 11 of 58 (19%) trauma victims who eventually needed a chest tube for hemothorax (5). Therefore, patients with severe chest trauma should have a follow-up chest radiograph 3–6 hours after the accident (6). The incidence of pneumothorax occurring concomitantly with hemothorax is high whether the trauma is blunt or penetrating (Fig. 20.1). In a series of 114 patients with hemothorax secondary to blunt trauma, 71 (62%) also had pneumothorax (4). In another series of 373 patients with hemothorax secondary to penetrating trauma, 307 (83%) had pneumothorax (1).

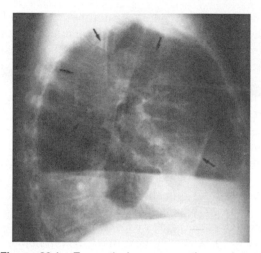

Figure 20.1. Traumatic hemopneumothorax. Lateral chest radiograph, obtained from a patient shortly after he was stabbed in the chest, that shows a pleural effusion and a pneumothorax. The pleural line (*arrows*) is easily seen outlining the lung. (Courtesy of Dr. Harry Sassoon.)

Treatment

The treatment of choice for patients with traumatic hemothorax is the immediate insertion of a chest tube. In the past it was felt by some that the insertion of a chest tube would decrease pleural pressure and would thereby augment the pleural bleeding. If the bleeding originates from lacerated pleura, however, apposition of the pleural surfaces will produce a tamponade and will stop the bleeding (7). If the bleeding is from larger vessels, the slight decrease in the pleural pressure with a chest tube is insignificant in comparison to the transvascular pressure (7). The advantages of the immediate institution of tube thoracostomy are as follows: (*a*) it allows more complete evacuation of the blood from the pleural space; (*b*) it stops the bleeding if the bleeding is from pleural lacerations; (*c*) it allows one to easily quantitate the amount of continued bleeding; (*d*) it may decrease the incidence of subsequent empyema because blood is a good culture medium (8); (*e*) the blood drained from the pleural space may be autotransfused (1); and (*f*) the rapid evacuation of pleural blood decreases the incidence of subsequent fibrothorax (9).

Large-bore chest tubes (size 36 to 40 FG) should be inserted in patients with hemothorax because the blood frequently clots. Beall

and coworkers recommend inserting the chest tube high (4th or 5th intercostal space) in the midaxillary line because the diaphragm may have been elevated by the trauma (8). Immediate thoracotomy is indicated for suspected cardiac tamponade, vascular injury, pleural contamination, debridement of devitalized tissue, sucking chest wounds, or major bronchial air leaks (10).

Continued pleural hemorrhage is another indication for immediate thoracotomy. There are no precise criteria for the amount of pleural bleeding that should serve as an indication for thoracotomy, because each case must be considered individually (7); however, if the bleeding is more than 200 ml/hour and shows no signs of slowing, thoracotomy should be seriously considered. Approximately 20% of patients with hemothorax require thoracotomy (1, 3, 4, 8). Chest tubes should be removed as soon as they stop draining or cease to function because they can serve as conduits for pleural infection. The majority of patients with a traumatic hemothorax can be discharged from the hospital within 48 hours if no other serious injuries are present (8).

One must ensure that the bleeding is not from a misplaced central venous catheter (11). Mattox and Fisher reported 7 patients with a traumatic hemothorax in whom continued bleeding originated from a misplaced central venous catheter (11). This diagnosis is readily established by examining the appearance of the pleural drainage when the character of the infusion fluid is changed. If blood is obtained when fluid is withdrawn from the central catheter, the catheter may still be misplaced in the pleural space (12).

Videothoracoscopy may replace thoracotomy in some patients with traumatic hemothorax who otherwise would have been subjected to thoracotomy. Thoracotomy rather than thoracoscopy should be performed if there is exsanguinating hemorrhage through the chest tubes (13). Smith and coworkers performed videothoracoscopy for continued hemorrhage in five patients with continued bleeding from the chest tube after gunshot wounds. They found that a laceration of an intercostal artery was the source of the continued blood loss in all five patients. The hemorrhage could be controlled in three of the five patients at thoracoscopy, but two patients had to undergo a limited thoracotomy for the control of their hemorrhage (13).

It is recommended that patients who are treated with tube thoracostomy for hemothorax be given antibiotics. Brunner and coworkers randomly allotted 90 such patients to receive cefazolin or nothing immediately before and then every 6 hours until tube removal. They reported that there were six empyemas and three pneumonias in the control group but only one pneumonia and no empyema in the antibiotic group (14).

It appears that prehospital autotransfusion has a role in the management of life-threatening hemothorax. Barriot and coworkers (15) developed a system by which autotransfusions could be administered in ambulances. The system consists of a 28- to 30-F plastic chest tube and an autotransfusion device. The latter is basically a 750 ml bag with filters. The blood drains by gravity into the collection bag and then is reinfused without anticoagulation into a central line. They reported the use of their system on 18 patients in Paris with life-threatening traumatic hemothorax. During transfer to the hospital the patients received 4.1 ± 0.6 L of autotransfused blood, without anticoagulation. Thirteen of the 18 patients (72%) survived and there were no complications. They believed that the 13 patients would have died had it not been for the autotransfusions.

Complications

The four main pleural complications of traumatic hemothorax are the retention of clotted blood in the pleural space, pleural infection, pleural effusion, and fibrothorax. Several researchers have recommended that thoracotomy be performed to remove residual blood if it cannot be removed by chest tubes (1, 4, 16). These researchers feel that the presence of large amounts of clotted blood in the pleural space increases the incidence of subsequent empyema and fibrothorax. One study, however, suggested that thoracotomy is not necessary for removal of clotted blood (10). In this study, 290 patients with no residual hemothorax were compared with 118 patients who had some residual hemothorax

after treatment with chest tubes. The incidence of empyema was comparable in both groups, and 84% of the patients with residual hemothorax had no pleural abnormalities on follow-up examination. This study indicates that not all patients with residual hemothorax need be subjected to exploratory thoracotomy. If more than 30% of the hemithorax is occupied by clotted blood, consideration should be given to its removal. Traditionally, the clotted blood has been removed via a thoracotomy, but there have been two recent reports in which the clotted blood was removed successfully with videothoracoscopy (12, 17). Some authors have recommended the intrapleural injection of streptokinase to dissolve the blood clots (7, 16), but no controlled studies of this therapeutic technique have been reported. One possible problem with the use of these agents is that the clot over the bleeding source will dissolve and the intrathoracic bleeding will resume (17). A second problem reported in one case was the development of hypoxemic respiratory failure after the intrapleural administration of both urokinase and streptokinase (18). The authors attributed the respiratory failure to the effects of the products of fibrinolysis on the pulmonary circulation (18).

The second complication following hemothorax is empyema, occurring in 1 to 4% of cases (1, 8, 10). As mentioned above, the administration of antibiotics to patients with hemothorax who are treated with tube thoracostomy significantly reduces the subsequent development of empyema and pneumonia (14). Patients who are admitted in shock are more likely to develop empyema, as are those with gross contamination of the pleural space at the time of the original injury. Empyema is also more common with associated abdominal injuries (9) and with prolonged pleural drainage (10). The treatment of empyema complicating hemothorax is similar to that of any bacterial infection of the pleural space (see Chapter 9). Because many of the patients with empyema complicating hemothorax are young and physically fit, decortication should be considered if tube thoracotomy does not rapidly resolve the pleural infection.

The third complication of hemothorax is the occurrence of a pleural effusion when the chest tubes are removed. In the series reported by Wilson and associates, 37 of 290 patients (13%) with no residual hemothorax developed pleural effusions after removal of the chest tubes, and 40 of 118 patients with residual hemothorax (34%) had pleural effusions at the time of discharge from hospital (10). Of these 77 patients with pleural effusion after tube thoracostomy, 20 (26%) had empyema, but the pleural effusions resolved in the other 57, leaving no or minimal residual disease (10). This series indicates that pleural effusions are common after tube thoracostomy for hemothorax. When such effusions occur, a diagnostic thoracentesis should be performed to rule out the possibility of a pleural infection. If no pleural infection is present, the pleural effusion usually clears by itself and leaves no residual disease.

The fourth complication of hemothorax is the development of diffuse pleural thickening producing a fibrothorax weeks to months after the hemothorax. This complication occurs in less than 1% of patients, even if residual blood is not removed by exploratory thoracotomy (10). Fibrothorax appears to be more common with hemopneumothorax or when pleural infection is present in addition to the hemothorax. The definitive treatment for fibrothorax is decortication of the lung (see Chapter 22). Decortication should be postponed for several months following the injury in most cases because the pleural thickening frequently diminishes with time.

IATROGENIC HEMOTHORAX

When a hemothorax is discovered, the possibility of iatrogenic origin should be considered. The most common causes of iatrogenic hemothorax are the perforation of a central vein by a percutaneously inserted catheter (11, 19) or leaking from the aorta after translumbar aortographic study (20). Iatrogenic hemothorax can also follow thoracentesis or pleural biopsy. Iatrogenic pneumothoraces have also been reported after many other procedures, including percutaneous lung aspiration or biopsy, transbronchial biopsy, and sclerotherapy for esophageal varices (21). Patients with iatrogenic hemothorax should be managed with chest tubes for the same reasons as for traumatic hemothorax.

NONTRAUMATIC HEMOTHORAX

Nontraumatic hemothoraces are distinctly uncommon. The most common cause is metastatic malignant pleural disease (22), the second most common cause is a complication of anticoagulant therapy for pulmonary emboli (23) and the third leading cause is probably catamenial hemothorax (24). Other causes of spontaneous hemothorax include complication of a bleeding disorder such as hemophilia or thrombocytopenia (25), complication of spontaneous pneumothorax, ruptured thoracic aorta, pancreatic pseudocyst (26), rupture of a patent ductus arteriosus (27), rupture of a coarctation of the aorta (27), rupture of a splenic artery aneurysm through the diaphragm (28), rupture of a pulmonary arteriovenous fistula (29), hereditary hemorrhagic telangiectasia (Osler-Rendu-Weber syndrome) (30), intrathoracic extramedullary hematopoiesis (31), chickenpox (32), osteochondroma of the rib (33), and bronchopulmonary sequestration (34). In some patients, the cause of the hemothorax remains unknown despite exploratory thoracotomy (25, 30).

Diagnosis and Treatment

When bloody-appearing pleural fluid is obtained during a diagnostic thoracentesis, the hematocrit of the pleural fluid should be determined. If the hematocrit of the pleural fluid is greater than 50% that of the peripheral blood, the patient has a hemothorax. Regardless of how bloody the pleural fluid looks, a hematocrit should be obtained because pleural fluid with a hematocrit under 5% may appear to be blood. A chest tube should be inserted into patients with a spontaneous hemothorax to evacuate the blood and to assess the rate of continued bleeding. Thoracotomy should be performed if brisk (more than 100 ml/hour) bleeding persists.

Hemothorax Complicating Anticoagulant Therapy

Eleven cases of hemothorax complicating anticoagulant therapy had been reported by

1977 (23). Usually, the hemothorax becomes apparent 4 to 7 days after anticoagulant therapy is initiated, but it may occur only after several months (23). Of the 11 patients reported, 5 were receiving heparin only, 4 were receiving heparin and warfarin, and 2 were receiving only warfarin. The coagulation studies in patients with this complication are usually within an acceptable therapeutic range. The spontaneous hemothorax is almost always on the side of the original pulmonary embolus (23). The treatment for spontaneous hemothorax complicating anticoagulant therapy is immediate discontinuance of the anticoagulant therapy and insertion of chest tubes in an attempt to remove all the blood in the pleural space (23).

Catamenial Hemothorax

Catamenial hemothorax is an unusual cause of hemothorax. By 1993 there had only been 16 cases reported (24). The majority of patients with catamenial hemothorax have associated pelvic and abdominal endometriosis. The right hemithorax is universally involved, and diaphragmatic fenestrations with communication of pleural and peritoneal fluid have been documented in some of the patients. Most patients with catamenial hemothorax have endometriosis of the pleura if surgical exploration is undertaken. The treatment of choice is total hysterectomy with bilateral oophorectomy (24). If the patient refuses surgery, an alternative treatment is hormonal suppression.

REFERENCES

1. Graham JM, Mattox KL, Beall AC Jr: Penetrating trauma of the lung. J Trauma 1979;19:665–669.
2. Shorr RM, Crittenden M, Indeck M, Hartunian S, Rodriguez A: Blunt Thoracic Trauma. Analysis of 515 patients. Ann Surg 1987;206:200–205.
3. Quick G: A randomized clinical trial of rib belts for simple fractures. Am J Emerg Med 1990;8:277–281.
4. Drummond DS, Craig RH: Traumatic hemothorax: complications and management. Am Surg 1967;33: 403–408.
5. Rothlin MA, Naf R, Amgwerd M, Candinas D, Frick T, Trentz O: Ultrasound in blunt abdominal and thoracic trauma. J Trauma 1993;34:488–495.
6. Kiev J, Kerstein MD: Role of three hour roentgenogram of the chest in penetrating and nonpenetrating injuries of the chest. Surg Gynecol Obstet 1992;175: 249–253.
7. Weil PH, Margolis IB: Systematic approach to traumatic hemothorax. Am J Surg 1981;142:692–694.
8. Beall AC Jr, Crawford HW, DeBakey ME: Considerations in the management of acute traumatic hemothorax. J Thorac Cardiovasc Surg 1966;52:351–360.
9. Griffith GL, Todd EP, McMillin RD, et al: Acute traumatic hemothorax. Ann Thorac Surg 1978;26: 204–207.
10. Wilson JM, Boren CH, Peterson SR, Thomas AN: Traumatic hemothorax: is decortication necessary? J Thorac Cardiovasc Surg 1979;77:489–495.
11. Mattox KL, Fisher RG: Persistent hemothorax secondary to malposition of a subclavian venous catheter. J Trauma 1977;17:387–388.
12. Kollef MH: Fallibility of persistent blood return for confirmation of intravascular catheter placement in patients with hemorrhagic thoracic effusions. Chest 1994;106:1906–1908.
13. Smith RS, Fry WR, Tsoi EK, Morabito DJ, Koehler RH, Reinganum SJ, Organ CH Jr: Preliminary report on videothoracoscopy in the evaluation and treatment of thoracic injury. Am J Surg 1993;166:690–693.
14. Brunner RG, Vinsant GO, Alexander RH, Laneve L, Fallon WF Jr: The role of antibiotic therapy in the prevention of empyema in patients with an isolated chest injury (ISS 9-10): a prospective study. J Trauma 1990;30:1148–1153.
15. Barriot P, Riou B, Viars P: Prehospital autotransfusion in life-threatening hemothorax. Chest 1988;93:522–526.
16. Coselli JS, Mattox KL, Beall AC Jr: Reevaluation of early evacuation of clotted hemothorax. Am J Surg 1984;148:786–790.
17. Mancini M, Smith LM, Nein A, Buechter KJ: Early evacuation of clotted blood in hemothorax using thoracoscopy: case reports. J Trauma 1993;34:144–147.
18. Frye MD, Jarratt M, Sahn SA: Acute hypoxemic respiratory failure following intrapleural thrombolytic therapy for hemothorax. Chest 1994;105: 1595–1596.
19. Krauss D, Schmidt GA: Cardiac tamponade and contralateral hemothorax after subclavian vein catheterization. Chest 1991;99:517–518.
20. Bilbrey GL, Hedberg CL: Hemorrhagic pleural effusion secondary to aortography: a case report. J Thorac Cardiovasc Surg 1967;54:85–89.
21. Hussain A, Raja AJ: Occurrence of hemothorax (unilateral) after sclerotherapy. Am J Gastroenterol 1991; 86:1553–1554.
22. Berliner K: Hemorrhagic pleural effusion: an analysis of 120 cases. Ann Intern Med 1941;14:2266–2284.
23. Rostand RA, Feldman RL, Block ER: Massive hemothorax complicating heparin anticoagulation for pulmonary embolus. South Med J 1977;70:1128–1130.
24. Shepard MK, Mancini MC, Campbell GD, Geroge RB: Right-sided hemothorax and recurrent abdominal pain in a 34-year-old woman. Chest 1993;103:1239–1240.

25. Slind RO, Rodarte JR: Spontaneous hemothorax in an otherwise healthy young man. Chest 1974;66:81.

26. Cochran JW: Pancreatic pseudocyst presenting as massive hemothorax. Am J Gastroenterol 1978;69:84-87.

27. Dippel WF, Doty DB, Ehrenhaft JL: Tension hemothorax due to patent ductus arteriosus. N Engl J Med 1973;288:353-354.

28. DeFrance JH, Blewett JH Jr, Ricci JA, Patterson LT: Massive hemothorax: two unusual cases. Chest 1974;66:82-84.

29. Spear BS, Sully L, Lewis CT: Pulmonary arteriovenous fistula presenting as spontaneous hemothorax. Thorax 1975;30:355-356.

30. Martinez FJ, Villanueva AG, Pickering R, Becker FS, Smith DR: Spontaneous hemothorax. Report of 6 cases and review of the literature. Medicine 1992;71:354-368.

31. Smith PR, Manjoney DL, Teitcher JB, et al: Massive hemothorax due to intrathoracic extramedullary hematopoiesis in a patient with thalassemia intermedia. Chest 1988;94:603-608.

32. Rodriguez E, Martinez MJ, Javaloyas M, et al: Haemothorax in the course of chickenpox. Thorax 1986;41:491.

33. Harrison NK, Wilkinson J, O'Donohue J, Hansell D, Sheppard MN, Goldstraw PG, Davison AG, Newman Taylor AJ: Osteochondroma of the rib: an unusual cause of haemothorax. Thorax 1994;49:618-619.

34. Laurin S, Aronson S, Schuller H, Henrikson H: Spontaneous hemothorax from bronchopulmonary sequestration. Pediatr Radiol 1980;10:54-56.

CHAPTER 21
Chylothorax and Pseudochylothorax

At times, pleural fluid is milky or at least turbid. When the milkiness or turbidity persists after centrifugation, it is almost always due to a high lipid content of the pleural fluid. High levels of lipid accumulate in the pleural fluid in two situations. First, when the thoracic duct is disrupted, chyle can enter the pleural space to produce a **chylous pleural effusion**. In this situation, the patient is said to have a **chylothorax**. Second, in long-standing pleural effusions, large amounts of cholesterol or lecithin-globulin complexes can accumulate in the pleural fluid to produce a **chyliform pleural effusion**. The patient is then said to have a **pseudochylothorax**. It is important to differentiate between these two conditions because the prognosis and management are completely different.

CHYLOTHORAX

A chylothorax is formed when the thoracic duct is disrupted and chyle enters the pleural space.

Pathophysiologic Features

Dietary fats in the form of long-chain triglycerides are transformed into chylomicra and very low-density lipoproteins. These are secreted into the intestinal lacteals and lymphatics and are then conveyed to the cisterna chyli, which overlies the anterior surface of the second lumbar vertebra, posterior to and to the right of the aorta (1). Usually, one major lymphatic vessel, the thoracic duct, leaves the cisterna chyli and passes through the esophageal hiatus of the diaphragm into the thoracic cavity. The thoracic duct ascends extrapleurally in the posterior mediastinum along the right side of the anterior surface of the vertebral column and lies between the azygos vein and the descending aorta in close proximity to the esophagus and the pericardium. At the level of the 4th to 6th thoracic vertebrae, the duct crosses to the left of the vertebral column

and continues cephalad to enter the superior mediastinum between the aortic arch and the subclavian artery and the left side of the esophagus.

Once the thoracic duct passes the thoracic inlet, it arches 3 to 5 cm above the clavicle and passes anterior to the subclavian artery, vertebral artery, and thyrocervical trunk to terminate in the region of the left jugular and subclavian veins. Wide anatomic variations may exist in all portions of the thoracic duct. More than one thoracic duct may leave the cisterna chyli. The duct may continue on the right side of the vertebral column to enter the veins in the right subclavian region. Multiple anastomoses usually exist between various lymphatic channels, and direct lymphaticovenous communications with the azygos vein may be present (2, 3).

The drainage from the thoracic duct is called chyle. Chyle appears grossly as a milky, opalescent fluid that usually separates into three layers upon standing: a creamy uppermost layer containing chylomicrons, a milky intermediate layer, and a dependent layer containing cellular elements, most of which are small lymphocytes (3). If the patient has not eaten, however, chyle may be only slightly turbid because its lipid content will be reduced. Chyle is bacteriostatic and does not become infected even when it stands at room temperature for several weeks (3). Lampson reported that *Escherichia coli* and *Staphylococcus aureus* were unable to grow in 100% chyle (4). Chyle that is extravasated into the pleural cavity is not irritating and usually does not evoke the formation of a pleural peel or a fibroelastic membrane.

Each day between 1500 and 2500 ml chyle normally empty into the venous system (2). The ingestion of fat can increase the flow of lymph in the thoracic duct by 2 to 10 times the resting level for several hours (3). Ingestion of liquid also increases the chyle flow, whereas the ingestion of protein or carbohydrates has little effect on the lymph flow (3). The protein content of chyle is usually above 3 g/dl, and the electrolyte composition of chyle is similar to that of serum (3).

The primary cell in chyle is the small lymphocyte, and lymphocyte counts range from 400 to 6800/mm^3 (5). Prolonged drainage of a chylous pleural effusion can result in profound T lymphocyte depletion. Breaux and Marks (6) reported that in one patient with a chylothorax the total peripheral lymphocyte count fell from 1665/mm^3 to 264/mm^3 with 14 days of chest tube drainage, during which time the total drainage was approximately 35 L. Almost all the lymphocytes in the pleural fluid were T lymphocytes.

A chylothorax results when the lymphatic duct becomes disrupted. Ligation of the thoracic duct at any point in its course does not produce chylothorax in experimental animals (2), presumably on account of the many collateral vessels and lymphaticovenous anastomoses. Ligation of the superior vena cava produces chylothorax about half the time in experimental animals. In the experimental animal, laceration or transection of the thoracic duct does not always produce a chylothorax. Hodges and associates produced a 2.5-cm longitudinal laceration of the thoracic duct in three dogs at the level of T-9 and transected the thoracic duct at this level in another three dogs. They reported that all animals developed a pleural effusion, but that the effusion ceased to form after 2 to 5 days in the animals with lacerations and after 4 to 10 days in the animals with transections (7). Lymphangiograms demonstrated that there was no continuity of the thoracic duct in the animals with the transections and the researchers concluded that the lymph was being conveyed by collaterals (7).

Etiologic Factors

The causes of 143 chylothoraces from five separate series (2, 3, 8-10) are tabulated in Table 21.1. For convenience, the causes of chylothorax can be grouped into four different categories. The cause of over 50% of chylothoraces is tumor, which is in the lymphoma group about 75% of the time. Chylothorax may be the presenting symptom of lymphoma

Table 21.1.   Causes of 143 Chylothoraces From Five Separate Series

		Number	Percentage
Tumor		76	54
Lymphoma	57		
Other	19		
Trauma		36	25
Surgical	31		
Other	5		
Idiopathic		22	15
Congenital	8		
Other	14		
Miscellaneous		9	6

(3, 9, 11). Therefore, a nontraumatic chylothorax is an indication for a diligent search for a lymphoma. In the series of Roy and associates, the diagnosis of lymphoma was not established until 6 to 12 months after the appearance of the chylothorax in four patients (9).

The second leading cause of chylothorax is trauma. This trauma is usually a cardiovascular, pulmonary, or esophageal surgical procedure. Chylothorax appears particularly frequently following operations in which the left subclavian artery is mobilized (10). The incidence of chylothorax after most thoracic surgeries is less than 1.0%. The incidence of chylothorax was 0.5% in one series of 2660 cardiovascular operations (12) while it was 0.74% in a series of 1744 pleuropulmonary surgeries (13). The incidence of chylothorax following esophageal resection is relatively high; it was 4.0% in one series of 255 cases (14). Dougenis and associates reported that the incidence of chylothorax following esophageal surgery was significantly higher when the main thoracic duct was not ligated at the time of the resection. Accordingly, they recommend ligation of the main thoracic duct when esophageal resections are performed (14).

Thrombosis of the superior vena cava or the subclavian vein is becoming one of the more common causes of chylothorax. Berman and coworkers reviewed the case histories of 37 infants and children with thrombosis of their superior vena cava in a newborn and pediatric intensive care unit and reported that nine (24%) had a chylothorax (15). There is one report of a patient who developed thrombosis of the superior vena cava and bilateral chylothoraces as a complication of the LeVeen shunt (16). Chylothorax has also been reported as a complication of coronary artery bypass surgery when the internal mammary artery is harvested (17), heart transplant (18), high translumbar aortography (19), sclerotherapy for esophageal varices (20), and cervical node dissection (21).

Of course, penetrating trauma to the chest or neck such as gunshot or knife wounds can also sever the thoracic duct and may lead to chylothorax. Trauma in which the spine is hyperextended or a vertebra is fractured is most likely to cause chylothorax, particularly if the injury occurs after the recent ingestion of a fatty meal (22). A chylothorax secondary to closed trauma is usually on the right side and the site of rupture is most commonly in the region of the 9th or 10th thoracic vertebra (22). Such trauma includes falls from a height, motor vehicle accidents, compression injuries to the trunk, heavy blows to the back or stomach, and childbirth (23). The injury may be less impressive, and chylothoraces have been attributed to coughing, vomiting, and weightlifting. In one well-documented case report, an episode of vigorous stretching while yawning was followed by swelling in the left supraclavicular fossa and the development of bilateral chylothoraces (24).

The third leading cause of chylothorax is idiopathic, including most cases of congenital chylothorax. One should exclude lymphoma as a cause of the chylothorax before it is labeled as idiopathic. Most cases of idiopathic chylothorax in the adult are probably due to minor trauma, such as coughing or hiccuping, after the ingestion of fatty meals.

Chylothorax is the most common form of pleural effusion encountered in the first few days of life (25). The fetal pleural effusion discussed in Chapter 18 is probably also a chylothorax. Neonatal chylothorax is relatively uncommon; during a 22-year period 12 cases were diagnosed at the Hospital for Sick Children, which is a large pediatric tertiary care center (26). The babies are usually born at full term after normal labor and delivery. The etiology of congenital chylothorax is unknown (27). Abnormalities of the thoracic duct have not been found in most babies who have undergone exploratory thoracotomy (25).

Several cases of generalized pleural oozing have been described during surgery (26). It is possible that birth trauma may result in a tear of a major lymphatic channel in at least some individuals. In some cases a congenital chylothorax is associated with Turner's syndrome, Noonan's syndrome, or Down's syndrome (27). Congenital chylothorax is also more common in infants who are hydropic or who have polyhydramnios (26).

Miscellaneous etiologies comprise the fourth group of chylothoraces. Many other causes of chylothorax have been reported, but even when all are grouped together, they account for only a small percentage of chylothoraces. The most interesting of these is pulmonary lymphangiomyomatosis, which has associated interstitial parenchymal infiltrates and is discussed later in this chapter. Other causes include Gorham's syndrome (28) (also discussed later in this chapter), Kaposi's sarcoma in patients with AIDS (29, 30), filariasis, lymph node enlargement, cirrhosis, heart failure, lymphangitis of the thoracic duct, obstruction of the superior vena cava secondary to Behçet's syndrome (31, 32), tuberculosis (33) or sarcoidosis (34) involving the intrathoracic lymph nodes, aneurysms of the thoracic aorta that erode the duct, abnormalities of the lymphatic vessels such as intestinal lymphangiectasis or reticular hyperplasia (10, 35), and hypothyroidism (36).

Clinical Manifestations

The initial symptoms of chylothorax are usually related to the presence of the space-occupying fluid in the thoracic cavity, and therefore patients have dyspnea. Pleuritic chest pain and fever are rare because chyle is not irritating to the pleural surface. With traumatic chylothorax, a latent period of 2 to 10 days usually occurs between the trauma and the onset of the pleural effusion (22). There is one case report where the latent period was 11 weeks (37). Lymph collects extrapleurally in the mediastinum after the initial thoracic duct disruption, forms a chyloma, and produces a posterior mediastinal mass (1). The mediastinal pleura eventually ruptures, chyle gains access to the pleural space, and dyspnea is produced by the chyle compressing the lung.

At times, hypotension, cyanosis, and extreme dyspnea occur when the chyloma ruptures into the pleural space. The ruptured chyloma is no longer visible radiographically.

With nontraumatic chylothorax, the onset of symptoms is usually gradual. In congenital chylothorax, the infant develops respiratory distress in the first few days of life; 50% of patients have symptoms within the first 24 hours, whereas 75% have symptoms by the end of the first week (25). The chyle production in a neonate may exceed 250 ml/day (27).

The main threat to life from chylothorax is malnutrition and a compromised immunologic status. Because the thoracic duct carries 2500 ml fluid daily that contains substantial amounts of protein, fats, electrolytes, and lymphocytes, the patient can become cachectic rapidly if this amount of chyle is removed daily through chest tubes or repeated thoracentesis. In addition, the patients develop lymphopenia and a compromised immunologic status due to the removal of large numbers of lymphocytes with the chyle. Over a 14-day period, 1 patient had over 35 L of fluid withdrawn, which contained 2.3 kg fat and 0.7 kg protein (6). Indeed, until Lampson initially described successful ligation of the thoracic duct in 1948 (4), the mortality rate from chylothorax was 50%. When managing a patient with chylothorax, one should abandon conservative treatment before the patient becomes too malnourished and immunocompromised.

Diagnosis

The diagnosis of chylothorax is usually not difficult because chyle has a distinctive white, odorless, milky appearance. When such fluid is found, the main differentiation is between empyema and a pseudochylothorax. The milkiness with empyema is caused by the suspended white blood cells, and if such fluid is centrifuged, the supernatant will be clear. The cloudiness of the chyliform pleural effusion from a pseudochylothorax is also caused by high lipid levels, either cholesterol or lecithin-globulin complexes. Chylous and chyliform pleural fluids remain opaque after centrifugation.

If cholesterol crystals are responsible for the turbidity, they may be easily demonstrated by examination of the pleural fluid sediment (Fig. 21.1). If the turbidity is due to high levels of cholesterol, the turbidity will clear when 1 to 2 ml ethyl ether is added to a test tube of the fluid; if the turbidity is due to chylomicrons or lecithin complexes, the turbidity will not clear (38).

Triglyceride Measurement

The best way to establish the diagnosis of chylothorax is by measuring the triglyceride levels in the pleural fluid (see Figure 4.4). If the pleural fluid triglyceride level is above 110 mg/dl, the patient probably has a chylothorax, whereas if the triglyceride level is below 50 mg/dl, the patient does not have a chylothorax (8). Some patients with chyliform pleural effusions will also have triglyceride levels above 110 mg/dl, but they will also have cholesterol levels above 200 mg/dl (39). In patients with triglyceride levels between 50 and 110 mg/dl, lipoprotein analysis of the pleural fluid should be performed. The demonstration of chylomicrons in the pleural fluid by lipoprotein analysis establishes the diagnosis of chylothorax (8). One should usually be able to differentiate chylothorax and pseudochylothorax by the clinical course. A chylothorax has an acute onset with normal pleural surfaces while a pseudochylothorax occurs in a patient with a long-standing pleural effusion with thickened pleura (40). If any doubt exists, the pleural fluid should be analyzed for chylomicrons.

Not all chylous pleural effusions have the typical, milky appearance. With congenital chylothorax, the pleural fluid is initially serous and only turns chylous when milk feedings are started (25). Because congenital chylothorax is the most common cause of pleural effusion in the newborn (25), pleural fluid triglyceride and lipoprotein analyses should be performed in all newborns with pleural effusion.

In adults, the pleural fluid does not always look like typical chyle. Staats and coworkers reported that 20 of 38 cases of chylothorax (53%) were described as other than chylous (8). All 20 that were not described as chylous were bloody or turbid, however. To establish the diagnosis of chylothorax, all turbid or bloody pleural fluids should be subjected to centrifugation. If turbidity persists in the su-

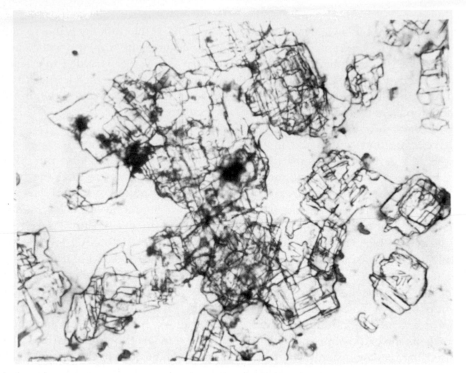

Figure 21.1. Cholesterol crystals. Typical large polyhedric crystals from a patient with a cholesterol pleural effusion. This patient had a rheumatoid pleural effusion.

pernatant, pleural fluid triglyceride levels should be determined.

Lipophilic Dye Ingestion

Another test for the diagnosis of chylothorax is ingestion of a fatty meal with a lipophilic dye, followed by a thoracentesis 30 to 60 minutes later, to ascertain whether the pleural fluid has changed in color (41). The most commonly used dye is Drug and Cosmetic Green No. 6, a coal-tar dye. One gram of this dye is mixed thoroughly with a quarter pound of butter, and the mixture is spread on a slice of bread. The patient eats the bread, and a thoracentesis performed 30 to 60 minutes later should yield green fluid if a chylothorax is present. I have attempted this test in about 6 different patients. The greatest problem I have encountered is in maintaining a straight face when I ask the patient to eat the disgusting green mess. Because the diagnosis is usually easily established with triglyceride and lipoprotein analysis, I no longer ask my patients with suspected chylothorax to eat dark green sandwiches.

Treatment

The main dangers to patients with chylothorax are malnourishment and immunocompromise due to the removal of large amounts of protein, fat, electrolytes, and lymphocytes from the body with repeated thoracentesis or chest tube drainage. In the past, the mortality rate from chylothorax approached 50%. When managing a patient with chylothorax, one must treat the chylothorax definitively, such as with thoracic duct ligation or pleuroperitoneal shunt implantation, before the patient becomes too cachectic to tolerate the operation. Because the management of chylothorax differs for traumatic, nontraumatic, and congenital chylothoraces, treatment regimens are described separately.

Traumatic Chylothorax

The general aims in treating the patient with traumatic chylothorax are relief of dyspnea by removing the chyle, prevention of dehydration, maintenance of nutrition, and a reduction in the rate of chyle formation. The defect in the thoracic duct frequently closes spontaneously in traumatic chylothorax. If the thoracic duct is transected in dogs, chyle will cease to enter the pleural space within 10 days as collateral lymphatic channels are formed (7). In a recent series of 26 children with postoperative chylothorax, 19 (73.1%) closed spontaneously (42). The average drainage duration of these 19 patients was 11.9 days with a range of 4 to 30 (42). In another recent series of 29 patients with posttraumatic chylothorax that included both children and adults, the chylothorax resolved with tube thoracostomy in 23 patients (79%) with a mean duration of drainage of 13.3 days (43).

The insertion of a pleuroperitoneal shunt is the best way to remove the chyle and alleviate the dyspnea (44–46). The advantage of the pleuroperitoneal shunt is that the lymph is not removed from the body and therefore the patient does not become malnourished or immunocompromised. It appears that when the chyle is shunted to the peritoneal cavity, it is absorbed without creating significant ascites (44). A second advantage of the shunt is that more time is provided for the defect to close spontaneously because the patient is not becoming nutritionally depleted. When the chyle ceases to enter the pleural space, the shunt is removed. The shunt should not be inserted if chylous ascites is present. Little and coworkers (44) inserted pleuroperitoneal shunts in two patients with chylothoraces postoperatively and reported that the patients had complete resolution of their effusions with subsequent removal of the shunts. In the largest series using the pleuroperitoneal shunt, 16 infants were treated with the shunt and excellent results were obtained in 12 (45). The only patients who did not have favorable outcomes were those whose chylothoraces were from central venous thrombosis (45). Murphy and associates recommend placing the shunt if the drainage persists beyond 5 days (45). Since there is no reason to subject a patient to both tube thoracostomy and shunt insertion, I recommend that the initial procedure be insertion of the shunt. The pleuroperitoneal shunt is discussed in more detail in Chapter 7.

In the past, much effort was devoted toward reducing the flow of chyle in patients with chylothorax. If the flow of chyle was reduced, then the patient would become nu-

tritionally and immunologically depleted less rapidly. In addition, it was felt that the disruption in the thoracic duct was more likely to close if chyle formation was minimized. The flow of chyle is minimized if all nourishment by mouth is halted and if the patient's gastrointestinal tract is maintained as empty as possible by constant gastric suction (47). The patient's nutritional status can be maintained with intravenous hyperalimentation (48). In the past attempts have been made to decrease the lymph flow by providing the fat calories in the diet with medium-chain triglycerides (48). These triglycerides have ten or fewer carbon atoms and are absorbed directly into the portal vein and thus gain entrance to the circulatory system without ever entering the thoracic duct (49). Since they are relatively unpalatable and hyperalimentation decreases the flow of chyle much more, hyperalimentation rather than medium-chain triglycerides is recommended when one wishes to reduce the flow of chyle. The flow of chyle is also decreased if the patient stays in bed because any activity of the lower extremities increases the flow of lymph (49). It is not known how important it is to slow the flow of lymph if a pleuroperitoneal shunt is inserted. Presently, I place no dietary restrictions on my patients who have chylothoraces and who are being treated with pleuroperitoneal shunts.

An alternative to the pleuroperitoneal shunt is tube thoracostomy. Because chyle is bacteriostatic (4), the likelihood of the patient developing a pleural infection from the chest tube is low. The placement of the chest tube also permits the underlying lung to remain constantly expanded and allows the wide apposition of the visceral and parietal pleura, and may result in a pleurodesis (22). In addition, the rate of chyle leakage can be accurately measured and recorded if a chest tube is in place. The prime disadvantage of tube thoracostomy is that the patient is likely to become nutritionally and immunologically depleted very rapidly. If a patient is treated with tube thoracostomy, it is recommended that the gastrointestinal tract be put to rest and the nutrition of the patient be maintained with hyperalimentation.

If a chylothorax is treated with tube thoracostomy, consideration should be given to recycling the chyle. Thomson and Simms reported one case in which the chyle was reinfused directly from the chest tube into the subclavian vein for a total of 18 days (50). There have been no large series evaluating this procedure and in the first half of the century a couple of patients died from "anaphylaxis" soon after chyle infusion was started (50). In most instances of traumatic chylothorax, the leakage of chyle into the pleural space slows or stops completely within 10 to 14 days. If the patient has a chest tube and the drainage of chyle persists beyond 7 to 10 days or does not progressively decrease, a more aggressive treatment regimen should be initiated, so the patient does not become malnourished and immunocompromised. The alternatives at this juncture are (*a*) to insert a pleuroperitoneal shunt, (*b*) to attempt to create a pleurodesis to obliterate the pleural space, (*c*) to perform thoracoscopy with insufflation of talc, (*d*) to perform thoracoscopy with attempted ligation of the thoracic duct, or (*e*) to perform a thoracotomy with ligation of the thoracic duct.

The insertion of a pleuroperitoneal shunt is recommended if the patient is not in good condition medically, as long as he/she does not have ascites. The basis for this recommendation is discussed above. Rheuban and associates inserted pleuroperitoneal shunts into 10 infants with postoperative chylothoraces who were still draining chyle 14 to 64 days after the initial operation. They reported successful management in 9 of the 10 patients and in 8 of the 9 successes, the shunt could be removed a median of 7 months after its insertion (51).

There are a limited number of reports where pleurodesis has been attempted by injecting a sclerosing agent through a chest tube. Adler and Levinsky reported the successful treatment of one patient with a postoperative chylothorax with 10 g talc in a slurry (52). Akaogi and coworkers reported that two patients with postoperative chylothorax were successfully managed with fibrin glue injected through the chest tube (53). Others have had a less satisfactory experience with tetracycline (54), nitrogen mustard, or atabrine (55). Tetracycline was ineffective in three patients on whom I attempted pleurodesis. In view of these experiences, pleurodesis by injecting a material through the chest tube is not generally recommended for chylothorax. If one wishes to attempt a pleurodesis by this route, then talc 5 g in a slurry is recommended.

There are at least three reports in which more than five patients were treated with talc insufflation at the time of thoracoscopy for chylothorax. Weissberg reported that the intrapleural insufflation of 2 g talc controlled the chylothorax in seven of nine patients (56). Vargas and associates recently reported the successful treatment of five patients with 2 g insufflated talc at the time of thoracoscopy (57). Graham and coworkers insufflated talc in eight patients with pneumothorax and reported that the treatment was successful in all, although four of the patients experienced a prolonged course of high output from their chest tubes with relatively slow resolution of the effusions. All had completely resolved by 12 days after the procedure (58). Therefore, thoracoscopy with the insufflation of talc appears to be a viable alternative for the management of chylothorax.

A definitive treatment for postoperative chylothorax is ligation of the thoracic duct. Lampson first demonstrated that a chylothorax could be controlled by ligation of the thoracic duct (4). Ligation of the thoracic duct causes no ill effects, probably on account of the multiple anastomoses among various lymphatic channels and direct lymphaticovenous communications (2, 3). If the chylothorax is unilateral, the thoracotomy should be performed on the side of the fluid (47). If the chylothorax is bilateral, a right thoracotomy should be performed because the duct is more readily approached from that side (47).

It has been recommended that a preoperative lymphangiogram be obtained in every case of chylothorax that does not respond to nonoperative management because the site of leak or obstruction can usually be demonstrated by this technique (59). At the time of operation, one should attempt to find the actual point of leakage from the duct and ligate the duct on both sides of the leak (47). In many instances, however, the leak cannot be localized, and the thoracic duct should therefore be ligated. Several aids for identifying the thoracic duct intraoperatively have been suggested. Probably, the best method is to inject Evans blue dye at a dose of 0.7 to 0.8

mg/kg, the total dose not exceeding 25 mg, into the subcutaneous tissue of the leg. Within 5 minutes, the chyle will be stained blue (47). The patient may also be given butter or cream to eat 3 to 4 hours preoperatively. The objection to this method is that the stomach may not be empty before the induction of anesthesia, although stomach contents may be removed by nasogastric suction (47). If for some reason the thoracic duct cannot be successfully ligated at thoracotomy, a parietal pleurectomy should be performed in order to obliterate the pleural space (3).

If the chylous drainage from the chest tubes persists and the nutritional status of the patient is deteriorating, one must not delay thoracotomy too long. In one series, all three patients with traumatic chylothorax who underwent thoracotomy died in the postoperative period (9). These deaths were attributed to the debilitation of the patients by the time the operation was performed.

With the advent of video-assisted thoracic surgery (VATS), one would expect that ligation of the thoracic duct would be tried with the videothoracoscope. Thoracoscopy permits the entire pleural space to be visualized, as well as to allow direct suture of a lymphatic leak. Although this technique has not been widely employed for the control of chylothorax, there are anecdotal reports documenting its successful use (60–62). Kent and Pinson successfully ligated the thoracic duct in one patient who developed a chylothorax after a radical neck dissection (60). Shirai and coworkers performed thoracoscopy on a patient who developed a chylothorax postoperatively. They were able to identify the site of leakage and the leakage stopped with the application of fibrin glue (61). Zoetmulder and associates (62) reported a 51-year-old patient who developed a chylothorax 4 years after treatment of a soft tissue sarcoma. At thoracoscopy, the thoracic duct leak could be identified and oversewn. The patient also had talc insufflated into her pleural space. The patient had no recurrence of her pleural effusion. It is unclear whether the procedure would have been effective if only the talc insufflation had been performed. It remains to be seen whether the endoscopic closure of chylous leaks is more successful or better tolerated than current open techniques (63).

Nontraumatic Chylothorax

In general, the goals of management of nontraumatic chylothorax are the same as for traumatic chylothorax. With nontraumatic chylothorax, however, one must also attempt to establish a cause. Because, as is shown in Table 21.1, lymphoma is the most common cause of nontraumatic chylothorax, and because lymphoma is now treatable by chemotherapy or radiotherapy, every effort should be made to establish this diagnosis in a patient with a nontraumatic chylothorax. Frequently, the patient with lymphoma and chylothorax has no evidence of lymphoma outside the thorax. Computed tomographic (CT) studies of the mediastinum should be done in all patients with nontraumatic chylothorax to ascertain whether mediastinal lymphadenopathy is present. In women with chylothorax and parenchymal infiltrates, another possibility is pulmonary lymphangiomyomatosis (see the section later in this chapter).

Another test that should be obtained on all patients with nontraumatic chylothoraces is a lymphangiogram. With the lymphangiogram a total or partial obstruction of lymph flow and the position of the obstacle can be demonstrated. In addition, the lymphangiogram can demonstrate the presence of enlarged lymph nodes or lymphangiectasis, which may give a clue as to the etiology of the chylothorax.

The initial management of a patient with a nontraumatic chylothorax should be similar to that of a patient with a traumatic chylothorax. In most cases a pleuroperitoneal shunt should be inserted. If tube thoracostomy is performed, the gastrointestinal tract should be put at rest, and the patient's nutritional status should be maintained by parenteral hyperalimentation. If the chylothorax is due to minor trauma, these measures are usually curative within a week. If CT examination of the mediastinum reveals no lymphadenopathy or other masses, and the chylothorax is controlled, no further treatment is indicated. In one series of 35 patients with chylothorax due to tumors, none were successfully managed with chest tubes or repeated pleural aspiration (9). If the chylothorax is not controlled with the pleuroperitoneal shunt, or if the CT study of the mediastinum is positive, the patient should undergo a videothoracoscopy or an exploratory thoracotomy. The mediastinum should then be carefully examined for masses, with lymphoma in mind. In addition, the thoracic duct should be ligated.

If the patient is known to have lymphoma or metastatic carcinoma, then neither chest tube insertion nor exploratory thoracotomy is indicated because the chylothorax usually responds to mediastinal radiation. Roy and coworkers (9) reported that radiation therapy to the mediastinum adequately controlled the chylothorax for the remainder of the patient's life in 68% of those with lymphoma and in 50% of those with metastatic carcinoma. If radiotherapy or chemotherapy does not control the chylothorax in patients with known lymphoma or metastatic carcinoma, exploratory thoracotomy is probably not indicated in view of these patients' dismal prognosis (9). If these patients are symptomatic from the chylothorax, however, one should insert a pleuroperitoneal shunt unless the patient also has ascites.

There are special aspects to the treatment of chylothorax associated with some entities. Since patients with chylothorax secondary to the nephrotic syndrome are likely to have chylous ascites, it is important not to place a pleuroperitoneal shunt or ligate the thoracic duct until this possibility is evaluated (64). The chylothorax associated with sarcoidosis is likely to disappear if the patient is treated with corticosteroids (34).

Congenital Chylothorax

Chylothorax in infancy can be fatal. The mortality rate was 30% in one series of 10 patients with congenital chylothorax (59). The three deaths in this series were all ascribed to malnutrition and secondary infection, and the babies who died were the only ones in the series who were subjected to more than 14 thoracenteses. On the other hand, five of the babies (50%) had no recurrence of their chylothorax after one to three thoracenteses, and all seven babies who survived were apparently normal (59). The recommended management of congenital chylothorax, in view of these findings, is as follows. Initially, the baby should be treated conservatively with repeated thoracenteses. If the chylothorax recurs after the third pleural aspiration, a pleuroperitoneal shunt should be inserted (65). Milson and associates (65) implanted pleuroperitoneal shunts in seven infants, one of whom was 7 days old, and reported that the shunt cured the chylothorax in six of the seven patients. Thoracic duct ligation is indicated if the pleuroperitoneal shunting fails to resolve the chylous leak. The advantage of the shunt over the thoracic duct ligation is that it is a much simpler procedure.

Pulmonary Lymphangiomyomatosis

Pulmonary lymphangiomyomatosis is a rare condition characterized by widespread proliferation of immature smooth muscle throughout the peribronchial, perivascular, and perilymphatic regions of the lung (66–68). Only 67 cases had been reported by 1977 (68). The perilymphatic proliferation of smooth muscle results in lymphatic obstruction and a chylothorax in the majority of affected individuals (68). The lymph nodes in the mediastinum and retroperitoneal space may also be infiltrated with immature smooth muscle cells, further impairing lymphatic flow. The thoracic duct may be either obliterated or dilated (66). The proliferation of smooth muscle in the perivascular spaces may obstruct the pulmonary venules and may produce pulmonary hemorrhage, hemoptysis, and pulmonary hemosiderosis. The proliferation of the peribronchial smooth muscles can partially or completely obstruct the airways to cause air trapping, cyst and bullae formation, and a high incidence of pneumothorax (68).

Clinical Manifestations

Pulmonary lymphangiomyomatosis occurs almost exclusively in women of reproductive age (67). In one series of 32 patients, however, two women who were postmenopausal developed the disease (69). Both of these women had undergone hysterectomy and bilateral oophorectomy and were taking maintenance estrogens (69). The onset of symptoms can occur from age 18 to 70, but most patients are between the ages of 25 and 50 when symptoms begin. Most patients have increasing shortness of breath, but hemoptysis, pneu-

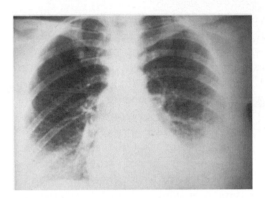

Figure 21.2. Posteroanterior radiograph from a 37-year-old woman with pulmonary lymphangiomyomatosis. Note the reticulonodular pattern and the wide distance between the ribs, suggesting hyperinflation. The pleural effusion on the left was a chylothorax. (Courtesy of Dr. Harry Sassoon.)

mothorax, or an incidentally discovered chylothorax can be the presenting manifestation. During the course of their disease, almost all patients have parenchymal infiltrates, about 50% have chylothorax, and about 50% have pneumothorax (68, 69).

Pulmonary lymphangiomyomatosis is at times part of the syndrome of pulmonary tuberous sclerosis. This uncommon, genetically transmitted disease has a classic triad of seizures, adenoma sebaceum, and mental retardation. Only a small percentage of patients with tuberous sclerosis have pulmonary involvement. Clinically, pulmonary tuberous sclerosis is similar to pulmonary lymphangiomyomatosis. The radiographic and pathologic findings in the lung are identical in both disorders. Lymph nodes are less commonly involved and chylothorax occurs much less commonly with pulmonary tuberous sclerosis, however (66, 67). Further support for the relationship between tuberous sclerosis and lymphangiomyomatosis comes from one report in which estrogen receptors were demonstrated in a woman with tuberous sclerosis and the lymphangiomyomatosis syndrome (70).

The chest radiograph usually suggests the diagnosis of lymphangiomyomatosis (Fig. 21.2). A coarse reticulonodular pattern similar to that with fibrosing alveolitis is seen; however, the lung volumes in lymphangiomyomatosis are increased rather than decreased, as in fibrosing alveolitis and almost every other

cause of interstitial lung disease (68). The interstitial lung infiltrates vary in extent, and their distribution may be primarily basal or diffuse. The pleural effusion from the chylothorax may be unilateral or bilateral and is typically large and recurrent. All have been chylous on direct examination. CT scans of the chest and abdomen are useful in demonstrating the lung cysts, lymphangiectasis, and soft tissue masses representing the angioleiomyomata (71). Serial CT scans may be useful in assessing the response to therapy.

Pulmonary function tests in the patient with lymphangiomyomatosis reveal a normal or reduced vital capacity, but an increased total lung capacity. Evidence of moderate to severe obstructive ventilatory dysfunction usually exists, and the diffusing capacity for carbon monoxide is markedly reduced (68). Arterial blood gases reveal hypoxia and hypocapnia.

Diagnosis

The diagnosis of pulmonary lymphangiomyomatosis is frequently delayed. In the series of 32 patients from Stanford and the Mayo clinic, the diagnosis was delayed an average of 44 months after the initial manifestation of the disease. Only one patient was given a diagnosis of lymphangiomyomatosis during her initial medical evaluation (69). This diagnosis should be suspected in any woman between the ages of 25 and 50 with a chylothorax, particularly if interstitial infiltrates and increased lung volumes are also present.

The diagnosis can probably be established by transbronchial biopsy. In one retrospective review of four transbronchial biopsies in women with lymphangiomyomatosis, the biopsies were thought to be diagnostic in three patients and suggestive in the fourth (69). The diagnosis was not made via the transbronchial lung biopsy in any of these four patients (69). The diagnosis is usually established at open thoracotomy with the demonstration of the typical histologic pattern of widespread proliferation of immature smooth muscle. When the thoracotomy is performed, tissue should be obtained for progesterone- and estrogen-receptor assay for the reason discussed in the following paragraph. Macroscopically, the lungs have diffuse interstitial thickening and multiple cystlike spaces of varying size sub-pleurally and within the parenchyma (66). Microscopically, the most characteristic feature is the widespread smooth muscle proliferation in the region of the normal lymphatic distribution. This perilymphatic smooth muscle proliferation is generally regarded as a hamartomatous rather than a neoplastic process (66). Characteristically, clefts or spaces between the smooth muscle bundles are lined by endothelium. Microscopic changes in involved lymph nodes are similar to those in the lung: interlacing bundles of smooth muscle proliferation demarcated by endothelial-lined clefts (66).

Treatment

In the past it was felt that the prognosis of women with pulmonary lymphangiomyomatosis was dismal and that most patients died within 10 years of the onset of symptoms (67). The recently reported series of 32 patients from Stanford and the Mayo Clinic had a much better prognosis (69). In this series 26 of the 32 patients (78%) were alive at the time of the report and the mean interval since the onset of the lymphangiomyomatosis was 10 years. Although pleurodesis or thoracic duct ligation can control the chylothorax, these patients nonetheless die of progressive respiratory insufficiency (72).

Several researchers have suggested that hormonal manipulation may be of value in treating this disease (70, 73–77). The exclusive occurrence of the disease in women of reproductive age has suggested that the smooth muscle proliferation may be hormonally dependent. McCarty and coworkers reported a patient with lymphangiomyomatosis in which the involved lung tissue had high levels of high-affinity, low-capacity progestin binding sites (73). When this patient was treated with medroxyprogesterone acetate, 400 mg intramuscularly each month, the disorder went into remission. Adamson and colleagues (75) described a case of a woman who had received multiple human chorionic gonadotropin injections before developing lymphangiomyomatosis. Treatment with medroxyprogesterone 400 mg every month was initiated and the patient improved and remained in good health over the following 3 years. Luna and

coworkers (70) reported a case in which estrogen receptors were demonstrated and whose disease stabilized with tamoxifen (antiestrogen) therapy. There is one case report of a woman who responded to a gonadotropin-releasing hormonal analog (78). In a meta-analysis of 30 cases of lymphangiomyomatosis treated with various hormonal manipulations it was concluded that the administration of progesterone or oophorectomy or both are the most effective treatments, resulting in improvement or stabilization of the disease in the majority of cases (79).

There is just about as much evidence that hormonal manipulation has no effect on the course of the disease. In the series of Taylor, 16 patients underwent oophorectomy and none improved while 11 worsened (69). Nine patients took tamoxifen for at least 6 months and none had improvement (69). Nineteen patients took medroxyprogesterone acetate for at least 6 months; two had a clear improvement in their dyspnea, and six additional patients had stabilization of their dyspnea during an average observation length of 32 months (69). When Taylor and coworkers reviewed the literature they concluded that there was no apparent correlation between the status of progesterone and estrogen receptors and the response to therapy (69). Urban and associates treated eight patients with anti-estrogen therapy and reported clinical deterioration or death in all (80). Since there were no controls, it is possible that the anti-estrogen therapy slowed the progression of the disease (80). Shen and associates (77) reported a case where estrogen therapy led to a rapid downhill course. When the estrogen therapy was stopped and tamoxifen initiated, the disease stabilized (77). Other reports (76, 81), however, have demonstrated that medroxyprogesterone therapy is not always beneficial even when progestin receptors are present (76).

It therefore appears that hormonal manipulations may favorably influence the course of at least some patients. When the diagnosis of lymphangiomyomatosis is suspected, lung tissue should be obtained for progesterone- and estrogen-receptor assay if possible if for no other reason than to ascertain if there is a relationship between the presence of receptors and the response to therapy. It is recommended that all patients be treated initially with medroxyprogesterone. If the disease progresses, then consideration should be given to performing an oophorectomy or possibly manipulating the estrogen therapy, particularly if estrogen receptors were present.

In the future, lung transplantation may prove to be the best therapy for this disease, since the disease affects young women and carries a poor prognosis (82). Given the relatively good prognosis of the patients in the combined Stanford and Mayo Clinic study, lung transplantation is not recommended until the patient becomes debilitated from her disease. To my knowledge, there are no long-term follow-up studies of patients who received lung transplantation for lymphangiomyomatosis.

Gorham's Syndrome

Gorham's syndrome is a rare disease that can occur at any age but is most often recognized in children or young adults. Other names for Gorham's syndrome include hemangiomatosis, disappearing bone disease, and massive osteolysis. The characteristic lesion of Gorham's syndrome is an intraosseous proliferation of vascular or lymphatic channels that leads to the disappearance of bones. There is a propensity for involvement of the maxilla, shoulder girdle, and pelvis (28).

Patients with Gorham's syndrome have a high incidence of chylothorax. Chylothorax was present in 25 of the 146 cases (17%) of Gorham's syndrome in the literature up until 1994 (28). All the patients with Gorham's syndrome and chylothorax had either rib, scapular, clavicular, or thoracic vertebral bony involvement. Patients with Gorham's syndrome and chylothorax should be treated with a pleuroperitoneal shunt or thoracic duct ligation (28).

CHYLIFORM PLEURAL EFFUSIONS AND PSEUDOCHYLOTHORAX

A **chyliform** pleural effusion resulting in a **pseudochylothorax** is a pleural effusion that is turbid or milky from high lipid content not resulting from disruption of the thoracic duct. Some authors have separated pseudochylothoraces into those with cholesterol crystals, designated pseudochylous effusions, and those without cholesterol crystals, designated chyliform pleural effusions (38). Because no practical reason exists for making this distinction, I designate all high-lipid nonchylous effusions chyliform pleural effusions. Pseudochylothoraces with their associated chyliform pleural fluid are uncommon. Until 1961, only 99 cases had been reported in the international literature (40). Pseudochylothoraces are much less common than chylothoraces. In a series of 53 nontraumatic high-lipid effusions, only 6 (11%) were chyliform pleural effusions (9).

Pathogenesis

The precise pathogenesis of chyliform pleural effusions is not known (39). Most patients with chyliform pleural effusions have long-standing pleural effusions (mean 5 years) and have thickened and sometimes calcified pleura. Most of the cholesterol in chyliform pleural effusions is associated with high density lipoproteins in contrast to the cholesterol in acute exudates, which is mostly bound to low density lipoproteins (LDL) (39). It has been hypothesized that the cholesterol that enters the pleural space with acute pleural inflammation becomes trapped in the pleural space and undergoes a change in lipoprotein binding characteristics (39). The diseased pleura may result in an abnormally slow transfer of cholesterol and other lipids out of the pleural space and may lead to the accumulation of cholesterol in the pleural fluid (40). The origin of the cholesterol and other lipids is not definitely known, but one possibility is from degenerating red and white blood cells in the pleural fluid (40). Most patients with chyliform pleural effusions do not appear to have disturbed cholesterol metabolism because the serum cholesterol levels are usually within normal limits and the patients have no signs of altered cholesterol metabolism, such as xanthomas.

Some chyliform pleural effusions contain cholesterol crystals. The factors that dictate whether cholesterol crystals will be present are unknown. Cholesterol crystals have been seen in pleural fluid with cholesterol levels below 150 mg/dl, whereas other pleural fluids with cholesterol levels above 800 mg/dl have had none (40).

Clinical Manifestations

Chyliform pleural effusions are seen in patients with long-standing pleural effusions (40). The mean duration of the effusion is 5 years before it turns chyliform, but a few chyliform effusions have been known to develop within a year of onset. The two most common causes of the effusion initially are rheumatoid pleuritis and tuberculosis (40, 83, 84). Patients who have had artificial pneumothoraces for pulmonary tuberculosis and in whom the lung remains atelectatic with a resultant pleural effusion are particularly prone to chyliform pleural effusions (84). In many patients, the etiology of the original pleural effusion remains undetermined. Many of the pleural fluids secondary to paragonimiasis have cholesterol crystals (85).

Many patients with chyliform pleural effusions are asymptomatic, or at least are no more symptomatic than when they initially developed the pleural effusion. Because the visceral pleura is usually thickened, the underlying lung contributes minimally to the total ventilation, and the patient may have dyspnea on exertion. Chyliform pleural effusions are usually unilateral.

Diagnosis

The diagnosis of chyliform pleural effusion is not usually difficult. When a patient with a long-standing pleural effusion is found to have turbid or milky pleural fluid, the two other diagnostic possibilities are empyema and chylothorax. In an empyema, centrifugation results in a clear supernatant. The differentiation between chylothorax and pseudochylothorax is not usually difficult; the patient with chylothorax has an acute pleural effusion and normal pleural surfaces, whereas the patient with pseudochylothorax has a chronic pleural effusion and a thickened or calcified pleura.

Analysis of the pleural fluid is useful in the differentiation of chylothorax and pseudochylothorax. If cholesterol crystals are seen on smears of the sediment, the patient has a chyliform pleural effusion. The cholesterol crystals give a distinct, satin-like sheen to the pleural fluid. Microscopically, the cholesterol crystals present a typical rhomboid configuration (Fig. 21.1). If no cholesterol crystals are seen, the patient may still have a chyliform effusion. Pleural fluid cholesterol levels above 200 mg/dl strongly suggest a chyliform effusion (39). The cholesterol levels in the pleural fluid are elevated in high-lipid pleural effusions due to high numbers of cholesterol crystals or lecithin-globulin complexes (38), but cholesterol levels may also be elevated in chylous pleural effusions (8). Lipoprotein analysis should be performed if any doubt exists as to whether the fluid is chylous or pseudochylous because only chylous pleural fluid contains chylomicrons (8, 40). Some chyliform effusions have high (greater than 250 mg/dl) triglyceride levels (40), so this finding is not diagnostic of chylothorax.

Treatment

When a patient is diagnosed as having a chyliform pleural effusion, the possibility of tuberculosis should always be entertained. If the patient has a history of tuberculosis and has never been treated with antituberculous therapy, isoniazid and rifampin should be given for at least 9 months. Similarly, if the patient has a positive purified protein derivative (PPD) test, he should be treated with these drugs unless he has been treated previously or has received bacille Calmette-Guérin (BCG).

If the patient's exercise capacity is limited by shortness of breath, a therapeutic thoracentesis should be performed. Hillerdal (84) reported that the removal of several hundred milliliters of pleural fluid from patients with pseudochylothorax resulted in a markedly improved exercise tolerance (84). Decortication should be considered if the patient is symptomatic and the underlying lung is believed to be functional (86). The decortication may result in a markedly improved functional status for the patient (86).

REFERENCES

1. Sassoon CS, Light RW: Chylothorax and Pseudochylothorax. Clin Chest Med 1985;6:163–171.
2. Bower GC: Chylothorax: observations in 20 cases. Dis Chest 1964;46:464–468.
3. Williams KR, Burford TH: The management of chylothorax. Ann Surg 1964;160:131–140.
4. Lampson RS: Traumatic chylothorax: a review of the literature and report of a case treated by mediastinal ligation of the thoracic duct. J Thorac Surg 1948;17:778–791.

5. Teba L, Dedhia HV, Bowen R, Alexander JC: Chylothorax review. Crit Care Med 1985;13:49-52.

6. Breaux JR, Marks C: Chylothorax causing reversible T-cell depletion. J Trauma 1988;28:705-707.

7. Hodges CC, Fossum TW, Evering W: Evaluation of thoracic duct healing after experimental laceration and transection. Veterin Surg 1993;22:431-435.

8. Staats BA, Ellefson RW, Budahn LL, et al: The lipoprotein profile of chylous and non-chylous pleural effusions. Mayo Clin Proc 1980;55:700-704.

9. Roy PH, Carr DT, Payne WS: The problem of chylothorax. Mayo Clin Proc 1967;42:457-467.

10. Strausser JL, Flye MW: Management of non-traumatic chylothorax. Ann Thorac Surg 1981;31:520-526.

11. Bruneau R, Rubin P: The management of pleural effusions and chylothorax in lymphoma. Radiology 1965;85:1085-1092.

12. Maloney JV, Spencer FC: The non-operative treatment of traumatic chylothorax. Surgery 1956;40:121-128.

13. Terzi A, Furlan G, Magnanelli G, Terrini A, Ivic N: Chylothorax after pleuro-pulmonary surgery: a rare but unavoidable complication. Thorac Cardiovasc Surg 1994;42:81-84.

14. Dougenis D, Walker WS, Cameron EW, Walbaum PR: Management of chylothorax complicating extensive esophageal resection. Surg Gynecol Obstet 1992;174:501-506.

15. Berman W Jr, Fripp RR, Yabek SM, Wernly J, Corlew S: Great vein and right atrial thrombosis in critically ill infants and children with central venous lines. Chest 1991;99:963-967.

16. Warren WH, Altman JS, Gregory SA: Chylothorax secondary to obstruction of the superior vena cava: a complication of the LeVeen shunt. Thorax 1990;45:978-979.

17. Smith JA, Goldstein J, Oyer PE: Chylothorax complicating coronary artery by-pass grafting. J Cardiovasc Surg 1994;35:307-309.

18. Twomey CR: Chylothorax in the adult heart transplant patient: a case report. Am J Crit Care 1994;3:316-319.

19. Dupont PA: Chylothorax after high translumbar aortography. Thorax 1975;30:110-112.

20. Nygaard SD, Berger HA, Fick RB: Chylothorax as a complication of oesophageal sclerotherapy. Thorax 1992;47:134-135.

21. Thomas TV: Upper abdominal mass following cervical node dissection. Chest 1975;67:93-94.

22. Thorne PS: Traumatic chylothorax. Tubercle 1958;39:29-34.

23. Cammarata SK, Brush RE Jr, Hyzy RC: Chylothorax after childbirth. Chest 1991;99:1539-1540.

24. Reilly KM, Tsou E: Bilateral chylothorax: a case report following episodes of stretching. JAMA 1975;233:536-537.

25. Chernick V, Reed MH: Pneumothorax and chylothorax in the neonatal period. J Pediatr 1970;76:624-632.

26. Van Aerde J, Campbell AN, Smyth JA, et al: Spontaneous chylothorax in newborns. Am J Dis Child 1984;138:961-964.

27. van Straaten HL, Gerards LJ, Krediet TG: Chylothorax in the neonatal period. Europ J Ped 1993;152:2-5.

28. Tie MLH, Poland GA, Rosenow EC III: Chylothorax in Gorham's syndrome. A common complication of a rare disease. Chest 1994;105:208-213.

29. Pennington DW, Warnock ML, Stulbarg MS: Chylothorax and respiratory failure in Kaposi's sarcoma. West J Med 1990;152:421-422.

30. Judson MA, Postic B: Chylothorax in a patient with AIDS and Kaposi's sarcoma. South Med J 1990;83:322-324.

31. Konishi T, Takeuchi H, Iwata J, Nakano T: Behcet's disease with chylothorax—case report. Angiology 1988;39:68-71.

32. Coplu L, Emri S, Selcuk ZT, Kalyoncu F, Balkanci F, Sahin AA, Baris YI: Life threatening chylous pleural and pericardial effusion in a patient with Behcet's syndrome. Thorax 1992;47:64-65.

33. Vennera MC, Moreno R, Cot J, et al: Chylothorax and tuberculosis. Thorax 1983;38:694-695.

34. Parker JM, Torrington KG, Phillips YY: Sarcoidosis complicated by chylothorax. South Med J 1994;87:860-862.

35. Bresser P, Kromhout JG, Reekers JA, Verhage TL: Chylous pleural effusion associated with primary lymphedema and lymphangioma-like malformations. Chest 1993;103:1916-1918.

36. Kollef MH: Recalcitrant chylothorax and chylous ascites associated with hypothyroidism. Milit Med 1993;158:63-65.

37. Milano S, Maroldi R, Vezzoli G, Bozzola G, Battaglia G, Mombelloni G: Chylothorax after blunt chest trauma: an unusual case with a long latent period. Thorac Cardiovasc Surg 1994;42:187-190.

38. Hughes RL, Mintzer RA, Hidvegi DF, et al: The management of chylothorax. Chest 1979;76:212-218.

39. Hamm H, Pfalzer B, Fabel H: Lipoprotein analysis in a chyliform pleural effusion: Implications for pathogenesis and diagnosis. Respiration 1991;58:294-300.

40. Coe JE, Aikawa JK: Cholesterol pleural effusion. Arch Intern Med 1961;108:763-774.

41. Klepser RG, Berry JF: The diagnosis and surgical management of chylothorax with the aid of lipophilic dyes. Dis Chest 1954;25:409-426.

42. Bond SJ, Guzzetta PC, Snyder ML, Randolph JG: Management of pediatric postoperative chylothorax. Ann Thorac Surg 1993;56:469-472.

43. Marts BC, Naunheim KS, Fiore AC, Pennington DG: Conservative versus surgical management of chylothorax. Am J Surg 1992;164:532.

44. Little AG, Kadowaki MH, Ferguson MK, et al: Pleuroperitoneal shunting: alternative therapy for pleural effusions. Ann Surg 1988;208:443-450.

45. Murphy MC, Newman BM, Rodgers BM: Pleuroperitoneal shunts in the management of persistent chylothorax. Ann Thorac Surg 1989;48:195-200.

46. Rheuban KS, Kron IL, Carpenter MA, Gutgesell HP, Rodgers BM: Pleuroperitoneal shunts for refractory chylothorax after operation for congenital heart disease. Ann Thorac Surg 1992;53:85-87.

47. Ross JK: A review of the surgery of the thoracic duct. Thorax 1961;16:12-21.

48. Valentine VG, Raffin TA: The management of chylothorax. Chest 1992;102:586-591.

49. Lichter I, Hill GL, Nye ER: The use of medium-chain triglycerides in the treatment of chylothorax in a child. Ann Thorac Surg 1968;4:352-355.

50. Thomson IA, Simms MH: Postoperative chylothorax: a case for recycling? Cardiovasc Surg 1993;1:384-385.

51. Rheuban KS, Kron IL, Carpenter MA, Gutgesell HP, Rodgers BM: Pleuroperitoneal shunts for refractory chylothorax after operation for congenital heart disease. Ann Thorac Surg 1992;53:85-87.

52. Adler RH, Levinsky L: Persistent chylothorax. J Thorac Cardiovasc Surg 1978;76:859-863.

53. Akaogi E, Mitsui K, Sohara Y, Endo S, Ishikawa S, Hori M: Treatment of postoperative chylothorax with intrapleural fibrin glue. Ann Thorac Surg 1989; 48:116-118.

54. Meurer MF, Cohen DJ: Current treatment of chylothorax: a case series and literature review. Texas Med 1990;86:82-85.

55. Robinson CLN: The management of chylothorax. Ann Thorac Surg 1985;39:90-95.

56. Weissberg D, Ben-Zeev I: Talc pleurodesis. experience with 360 patients. J Thorac Cardiovasc Surg 1993;106:689-695.

57. Vargas FS, Milanez JRC, Filomenao LTB, Fernandez A, Jatene A, Light RW: Intrapleural talc for the prevention of recurrence in benign or undiagnosed pleural effusions. Chest 1994;106:1771-1775.

58. Graham DD, McGahren ED, Tribble CG, Daniel TM, Rodgers BM: Use of video-assisted thoracic surgery in the treatment of chylothorax. Ann Thorac Surg 1994;57:1507-1511.

59. Perry RE, Hodgman J, Cass AB: Pleural effusion in the neonatal period. J Pediatr 1963;62:838-843.

60. Kent RB 3d, Pinson TW: Thoracoscopic ligation of the thoracic duct. Surg Endoscopy 1993;7:52-53.

61. Shirai T, Amano J, Takabe K: Thoracoscopic diagnosis and treatment of chylothorax after pneumonectomy. Ann Thorac Surg 1991;52:306-307.

62. Zoetmulder F, Rutgers E, Baas P: Thoracoscopic ligation of a thoracic duct leakage. Chest 1994;106:1233-1234.

63. Ferguson MK: Thoracoscopy for empyema, bronchopleural fistula, and chylothorax. Ann Thorac Surg 1993;56:644-645.

64. Moss R, Hinds S, Fedullo AJ: Chylothorax: A complication of the nephrotic syndrome. Am Rev Respir Dis 1989;140:1436-1437.

65. Milson JW, Kron IL, Rheuban KS, Rodgers BM: Chylothorax: an assessment of current surgical management. J Thorac Cardiovasc Surg 1985;89:221-227.

66. Silverstein EF, Ellis K, Wolff M, Jaretzki A: Pulmonary lymphangiomyomatosis. AJR 1974;120:832-850.

67. Corrin B, Liebow AA, Friedman PJ: Pulmonary lymphangiomyomatosis. Am J Pathol 1975;79:348-367.

68. Carrington CB, Cugell DW, Gaensler EA, et al: Lymphangioleiomyomatosis. Am Rev Respir Dis 1977; 116:977-995.

69. Taylor JR, Ryu J, Colby TV, Raffin TA: Lymphangioleiomyomatosis: clinical course in 32 patients. N Engl J Med 1990;323:1254-1260.

70. Luna CM, Gene R, Jolly EC, et al: Pulmonary lymphangiomyomatosis associated with tuberous sclerosis. Chest 1985;88:473-475.

71. Merchant RN, Pearson MG, Rankin RN, Morgan WKC: Computerized tomography in the diagnosis of lymphangioleiomyomatosis. Am Rev Respir Dis 1985; 131:295-297.

72. Miller WT, Cornog JL, Sullivan MA: Lymphangiomyomatosis. AJR 1972;111:565-572.

73. McCarty KS Jr, Mossler JA, McLelland R, Sieker HO: Pulmonary lymphangiomyomatosis responsive to progesterone. N Engl J Med 1980;303:1461-1465.

74. Banner AS, Carrington CB, Emory WB, et al: Efficacy of oophorectomy in lymphangioleiomyomatosis and benign metastasizing leiomyoma. N Engl J Med 1981; 305:204-208.

75. Adamson D, Heinrichs WL, Raybin DM, Raffin TA: Successful treatment of pulmonary lymphangiomyomatosis with oophorectomy and progesterone. Am Rev Respir Dis 1985;132:916-921.

76. Brentani MM, Varvalho CR, Saldiva PH, et al: Steroid receptors in pulmonary lymphangiomyomatosis. Chest 1984;85:96-98.

77. Shen A, Iseman MD, Waldron JA, King TE: Exacerbation of pulmonary lymphangioleiomyomatosis by exogenous estrogens. Chest 1987;91:782-785.

78. Eysvogel MMM, Page PS: Lymphangiomyomatosis. Chest 1990;98:1945-1946.

79. Eliasson AH, Phillips YY, Tenholder MF: Treatment of lymphangioleiomyomatosis. A meta-analysis. Chest 1989;196:1352-1355.

80. Urban T, Kuttenn F, Gompel A, Marsue J, Lacronique J: Pulmonary lymphangiomyomatosis. Follow-up and long- term outcome with antiestrogen therapy: A report of eight cases. Chest 1992;102:472-476.

81. Bevelaqua FA, Epstein H: Pulmonary lymphangiomyomatosis: long-term survival in a patient with poor response to medroxyprogesterone. Chest 1985;87:552-553.

82. Lizotte PE, Whitlock WL, Prudhomme JC, Brown CR, Hershon JL: Lymphangiomyomatosis. Chest 1990;98:1044-1045.

83. Ferguson GC: Cholesterol pleural effusion in rheumatoid lung disease. Thorax 1966;21:577-582.

84. Hillerdal G: Chyliform (cholesterol) pleural effusion. Chest 1985;86:426-428.

85. Johnson RJ, Johnson JR: Paragonimiasis in Indochinese refugees: roentgenographic findings with clinical correlations. Am Rev Respir Dis 1983;128:534-538.

86. Goldman A, Burford TH: Cholesterol pleural effusion: a report of three cases with a cure by decortication. Dis Chest 1950;18:586-594.

CHAPTER 22
Other Pleural Diseases

PLEURAL DISEASE DUE TO ASBESTOS EXPOSURE

Exposure to asbestos can cause several different types of pleural disease. First, it can lead to a diffuse malignant mesothelioma, as described in Chapter 8; second, it can lead to a benign pleural effusion, as described in Chapter 18; third, it can bring about the development of pleural plaques or calcification, discussed in this chapter; fourth, it can lead to massive pleural fibrosis, also discussed in this chapter; and fifth, it can produce a localized pleural abnormality called "rounded atelectasis," which is easily confused with a parenchymal tumor and is discussed in this chapter.

Pleural Plaques

These hyalinized fibrous tissue collections are located on the parietal pleura of the chest wall, diaphragm, or mediastinum and are usually associated with a history of asbestos exposure (1). Pleural plaques do not appear to develop into malignant mesotheliomas (1).

Prevalence

The prevalence of pleural plaques is somewhat dependent upon the population studied. Hillerdal reviewed the chest radiographs of a sizeable proportion of the residents of Uppsala, Sweden and found that the prevalence of pleural plaques in those individuals above the age of 40 had increased from 0.2% in 1965 to 2.7% in 1985 (2). The prevalence of pleural plaques was 22% in 91 elevator construction workers who probably had been exposed to low levels of asbestos in their work (3). The incidence of pleural plaque at autopsy has varied from 0.5 to 58% (4, 5). When 16 separate studies with a total of 7085 routine autopsies are combined, the prevalence of pleural plaques was 12.2% (4). The standard chest radiograph is able to identify between 50 and 80% of the pleural plaques that are actually present (4).

Pleural plaques slowly develop in patients exposed to asbestos. Epler and coworkers reviewed the chest radiographs of 1135 patients who had been exposed to asbestos and reported that none of the patients developed pleural plaques during the 10 years after the initial exposure, and the incidence was still only about 10% 20 years after the initial exposure (6). Forty years after the initial exposure, however, over 50% of the patients had radiologically visible pleural plaques. The mean duration between the initial exposure to asbestos and the development of pleural plaques was 33 years in the series of Hillerdal (2). These plaques usually calcify within several years of becoming evident radiologically. Calcification of the pleural plaques rarely occurs within the first 20 years of initial exposure to asbestos, but by 40 years, over one-third of these individuals have calcified pleural plaques (6).

Pleural plaques can also develop in individuals who are not occupationally exposed to asbestos. Kilburn and associates (7) reported that the prevalence of pleural abnormalities was 5.4% in the chest radiographs of 280 wives of asbestos workers who were initially exposed to asbestos at least 20 years previously. Churg and DePaoli (8) reported 4 cases of pleural plaques found at autopsy in individuals who resided in or near the chrysotile mining town of Thetford Mines, Quebec, but who did not work with asbestos. Mineral analysis of the lungs revealed that the individuals with pleural plaques had higher levels of tremolite, but comparable levels of chrysotile, than did the lungs of nine control subjects without pleural plaques. Constantopoulos and colleagues (9) reported the prevalence of pleural calcification was 47% in 688 inhabitants of the Metsovo area in northwest Greece, an area where a solution containing tremolite was used to whitewash the houses.

Pathogenesis

Convincing evidence links pleural plaques to previous asbestos exposure. Kiviluoto reviewed the place of residence of all individuals with bilateral pleural calcification in Finland and demonstrated that almost all such subjects lived near open asbestos pits (10). Hillerdal reported that 88% of 1596 adults over the age of 40 with pleural plaques had an occupational exposure to asbestos (2). Many patients who have pleural plaques at autopsy have a work history in which asbestos exposure would be expected (11, 12).

Ferruginous bodies (asbestos bodies), the histologic hallmark of exposure to asbestos (1), consist of fibers coated by complexes of hemosiderin and glycoproteins and are believed to be formed by macrophages that have phagocytized the particles. Although these bodies have been shown to form from foreign inorganic and organic fibers of many different types, ferruginous bodies in most human lungs have asbestos as a core and are commonly known as **asbestos bodies** (1). Patients with pleural plaques have much higher numbers of asbestos bodies in their lungs than do patients without pleural plaques (11, 13, 14). Conversely, the higher the number of asbestos bodies in the lungs, the more likely the presence of pleural plaques (1, 14). Finally, most pleural plaques contain many submicroscopic asbestos fibers that can be demonstrated by transmission electron microscopic examination, selective area electron diffraction, and microchemical analysis of particles (15, 16).

It appears that the various types of asbestos fibers differ in their ability to induce pleural plaques. Churg and coworkers correlated the presence of pleural plaques with the fiber type, concentration, and size as determined by analytic electron microscopy in 94 long-term chrysotile miners. They found that patients with pleural plaques had a significantly higher aspect ratio for the tremolite fibers than did those without plaques (17). It is felt by some that a substance other than chrysotile is responsible for pleural plaques in the asbestos mines in Canada (18).

Not all pleural plaques are due to asbestos exposure. Zeolite minerals are aluminum silicates widespread in the earth's crust. Erionite is a zeolite that is found in old volcanic sites such as Turkey, New Zealand, areas of Japan, and in the southwestern United States. In a few villages in Turkey, the mineral has been used in buildings and for roads, and a large percentage of the population has fiber-related pleural changes (19). One case of diffuse pleural thickening has been attributed to this fiber in Nevada (20). Wollastonite, a silicate that can be fibrous and which is used in ceramics, has been reported to cause pleural plaques (21). Talc, another mineral that is a flaky silicate, has been reported to be associated with plaque formation, but this mineral is often contaminated with amphiboles, so the relationship remains to be proven (22).

The mechanism by which asbestos fibers produce pleural plaques is unknown. Kiviluoto proposed that pleural plaques are formed in response to inflammation of the parietal pleura (10). When an asbestos fiber is inhaled, it passes toward the periphery of the lung. Kiviluoto suggested that the fiber pierces the visceral pleura and then rubs against and irritates the parietal pleura during respiratory movements. The resulting parietal pleural inflammation then gradually evolves into the hyaline plaque, which eventually calcifies. If this theory were correct, however, one would expect to find adhesions between the visceral and parietal pleura in the areas of pleural plaques, as well as long asbestos fibers in the parietal pleura.

Hillerdal has suggested that short submicroscopic fibers are primarily responsible for the pleural plaques because these fibers can be demonstrated in the plaques (23). He proposes that these short fibers reach the pleural space by penetrating the pulmonary parenchyma and the visceral pleura. These fibers are then removed from the pleural space, as is all particulate matter, by the lymphatic vessels that lie in the parietal pleura. Some fibers are caught in the lymphatic vessels, however, and the presence of the fiber, in conjunction with the appropriate inflammatory cell, causes pleural plaques to form over many years. This hypothesis does not explain several important characteristics of the pleural plaques such as the bilaterality, the symmetric shape, the orientation parallel to the ribs, and sparing of the apices and costophrenic angle (4).

A third hypothesis for the pathogenesis of pleural plaques is that the microfibrils embolize to the parietal pleura by either the parenchymal lymphatic plexus or via the costal vascular supply. Then, once present in the parietal pleura, the fiber itself or agents carried by the fiber appear to be responsible for initiating and promoting the inflammatory response. This hypothesis is very compatible with the peculiar characteristics of circumscribed pleural plaques (bilateral, symmetric, and oriented parallel to the ribs) (4).

If asbestos is injected intratracheally, it migrates to the pleura. In one study in rats (24), the asbestos fibers appeared in the pleural space by 3 days after intratracheal injection. Over a 30-day period, there were two peaks in the appearance of the asbestos fibers in the pleural space. The first peak occurred on day 7 at which time the mean length of the fiber was 1.2 μm. The second peak occurred on day 21 when the mean length of the fiber was only 0.3 μm (24).

The intrapleural injection of either crocidolite or chrysotile asbestos fibers leads to the development of a pleural effusion (25, 26). Sahn and Antony injected chrysotile asbestos fibers into normal rabbits who developed exudative pleural effusions within 4 hours. Over the next 120 hours, there was increasing metabolic activity in the pleural fluid as evidenced by a falling pH and an increasing Pco_2. The animals developed pleural plaques that were evident by 7 days and completely developed by 1 month. Interestingly, if the rabbits were made neutropenic, they still developed the pleural effusion, but subsequently developed marked pleural fibrosis and did not develop pleural plaques. The neutropenic rabbits did not have a macrophage influx as did the normal rabbits. These workers concluded that the pleural macrophage is important in localizing the asbestos fiber and in the ultimate formation of the pleural plaque. When a critical number of macrophages is not present, disorganization and widespread fibrosis occur (26).

Several studies have demonstrated that the exposure of mesothelial cells in cell culture to asbestos particles can induce the cells to produce substances associated with the development of fibrosis. If rat pleural mesothelial cells are exposed to crocidolite or chrysotile asbestos fibers, the asbestos fibers are actively phagocytosed and are incorporated within the phagosomes. Both types of asbestos also stimulate the mesothelial cells to produce fibronectin, a substance with fibroblast chemoattractant activity (27). In contrast, quartz and carbonyl iron particles do not induce similar changes (27). When human pleural mesothelial cells are cultured with suspensions of amosite, chrysotile, or crocidolite asbestos in concentrations as low as 5 μg/ml, the cells avidly phagocytize the particles and release interleukin-8 (IL-8) (28). IL-8 is a neutrophil chemoattractant.

Pathologic Features

Macroscopically, pleural plaques appear as discrete, raised, irregularly shaped areas separated by normal or slightly thickened pleura (13). These plaques are always on the parietal pleura and are found most commonly on the posterior wall of the lower half of the pleural space. Pleural plaques on the costal pleura usually have an elliptical shape, running parallel to the ribs superiorly and inferiorly (13). Pleural plaques usually do not occur in the apices of the pleural cavities or in the costophrenic angles (13). The thinner plaques are only slightly raised above the pleural surface and are grayish white in color, whereas the thicker plaques are ivory or cream-colored. The diameter of the plaques varies from a few millimeters to 10 cm (13). The pleural plaques are usually multiple, and the costal pleura can look like an archipelago of different-sized plaques (22).

Microscopically, the plaques consist of collagenous connective tissue containing few cells (13, 16). The connective tissue is arranged in a coarse, basket weave pattern and contains only a few capillaries. Normal mesothelium covers the plaques. The boundary between a plaque and the surrounding normal pleura is always sharply demarcated (13). Elastin stains show the continuity of the lamellae beneath the plaque with the surrounding normal parietal pleural connective tissue. Some calcium deposition is present in a high proportion of plaques (13). Although no asbestos fibers are visible by light microscopy, electron microscopic study demonstrates many submicroscopic fibers in almost all plaques (16).

Radiologic Features

Noncalcified pleural plaques are frequently not visible radiologically (11, 12). The earliest radiologically visible change is a line of increased density adjacent to a rib (Fig. 22.1), usually the seventh or eighth rib (15, 16, 23, 29). As the plaque enlarges, it becomes elliptical and protuberant, with tapering superior and inferior margins typical of an extrapleural lesion (Fig. 22.2). A plaque rarely extends vertically for more than four interspaces. The thickness of the plaque varies from 1 to more than 10 mm, but is usually in the range of 1 to 5 mm. Pleural plaques are usually bilateral and are often symmetric. When the pleural plaques are unilateral, they are left-sided about 75% of the time (30). In addition, if the disease is bilateral, there tends to be more disease on the left side (31). The explanation for this left-sided predominance is unknown. Involvement of the apices or the costophrenic angles by pleural plaques is rare.

On a standard chest radiograph, pleural plaques are most clearly defined when viewed tangentially, that is, in profile along their long

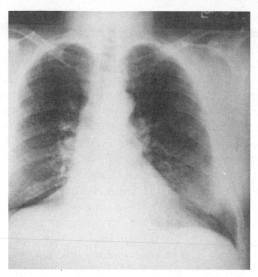

Figure 22.2. Posteroanterior radiograph of a patient with advanced pleural plaques.

axes. A routine posteroanterior chest radiograph distinctly demonstrates a plaque located on the inner surface of the lateral chest wall because the x-ray beam passes through more of the plaque. Noncalcified pleural plaques are best visualized by radiography at 110 to 140 kV, whereas calcification within plaques is best demonstrated at 80 kV.

When the x-ray beam is perpendicular to the plaque, the plaque is presented in a frontal or "en face" orientation. When viewed en face, small, noncalcified plaques are difficult to see and are perceived as ill-defined, irregular densities adjacent to the ribs. The en face plaque rarely appears uniformly rounded; rather, it shows a peripheral irregularity of contour that has been likened to the fringe of a map or a lily leaf (15). Because of its faintness in outline, the plaque is often overlooked or is dismissed as an artifact. I recommend the use of oblique views for the detection of pleural plaques (15, 29). In the oblique view, plaques seen en face on the posteroanterior projection are viewed in profile.

Conventional and high-resolution computed tomography (HRCT) scans are more sensitive at detecting pleural plaques than is the standard chest radiograph. In one study of 159 asbestos-exposed workers with a normal chest radiograph, pleural plaques were detected in 59 (37.1%). The conventional CT scan detected pleural plaques in 58 of the patients,

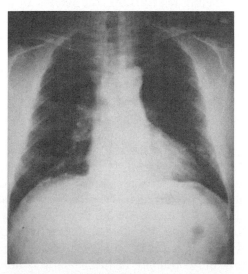

Figure 22.1. Pleural plaques. Posteroanterior radiograph of a patient with a history of asbestos exposure 30 years previously demonstrating bilateral pleural plaques of moderate size. Note the diaphragmatic calcification. A moderate degree of interstitial fibrosis secondary to asbestosis is also present.

while the HRCT scan detected the pleural plaques in only 48 cases (32). On CT, plaques appear as discrete soft-tissue or calcific thickening of the pleural surface. Focal plaques are commonly observed in the posterior and paraspinous regions of the thorax, areas that are poorly seen on chest radiographs (33).

Differential Radiologic Diagnosis

At times, it is difficult to distinguish pleural plaques from normal anatomic shadows. Close examination is necessary to distinguish normal fat collections from plaques caused by asbestos inhalation. At autopsy some degree of fat accumulation is almost always visible on gross examination along the chest wall in the reflections of the parietal pleura, oriented parallel to the long axes of the ribs on the subpleural osseous surfaces (34). More extensive fat deposits tend to form pads and folds concentrated at the level of the midthoracic wall in the region of the fourth to eighth ribs. Subpleural fat and pleural plaques are frequently indistinguishable on standard chest radiographs (34). The chest CT scan is efficient at distinguishing pleural plaques from subpleural fat. If a pleural abnormality is not calcified, a CT scan should probably be obtained to verify that the pleural abnormalities are indeed plaques, particularly if litigation is involved. When two series are combined (34, 35) 87 patients were thought to have pleural plaques on their standard chest radiographs. When they underwent CT examination, however, only 48 of the patients (55%) had pleural plaques, whereas the remainder had fat pads.

On the normal posteroanterior chest radiograph, a vertical line of water density may parallel the medial surface of the first three or four ribs along the lateral thoracic wall (15). This line is formed by a combination of muscles, the areolar tissue of the endothoracic fascia, and fat, but it is distinguishable from pleural plaques because plaques rarely extend superior to the third rib and are most prominent at the level of the seventh and eighth ribs. Below the level of the fourth rib, 1 mm is generally considered the maximal acceptable thickness for this normal pleural shadow (16).

The costal slips of origin of the serratus anterior and external abdominal oblique muscles have been confused with pleural plaques because they produce a characteristic rhythmic sequence of shadows between successive intercostal spaces. These anatomic structures are most commonly visible over the eighth rib, but the fifth through the ninth ribs may be involved. These costal slips of muscular origin appear either as one or two distinct triangular shadows or a combination of two opacities superimposed, and they can usually be differentiated from pleural plaques in that the muscle shadow has one sharply defined border and elsewhere fades into the surrounding soft tissues. At times, oblique radiographic views are necessary to make the distinction (15, 29); the shadows of these muscle structures disappear on oblique views.

The diaphragm is also a common site for pleural plaques (29). In the posteroanterior projection, the plaques usually affect the middle third of each diaphragm and rarely occur within 2.5 cm of the lateral chest wall. Most fibrous plaques are rounded or buttonlike and may easily be confused with the normal polycyclic outline of the diaphragm because of uneven muscle contraction.

Pleural Calcification

As mentioned earlier in this chapter, pleural plaques often become calcified. Forty years after the initial exposure to asbestos, nearly 40% of individuals have radiologically demonstrable pleural calcification (6). In general, calcified plaques are more striking than uncalcified plaques on the radiograph. When the x-ray beam strikes a plaque tangentially, the calcification is seen as a dense white line, usually discontinuous, paralleling the chest wall, diaphragm, or cardiac border (Fig. 22.3). Because the calcium is deposited near the center of the typical subpleural hyalinized plaque, it is separated from the inner surface of the rib by a line of water density. If the x-ray beam strikes the surface of the calcified plaque en face, it presents an irregular and unevenly dense pattern (Fig. 22.3). Oblique radiographic views are recommended for better delineating calcified pleural plaques (Fig. 22.3*B* and *C*).

Differential Diagnosis

Asbestos exposure is not the only cause of localized pleural thickening or pleural calcification. Discrete, localized, noncalcified pleu-

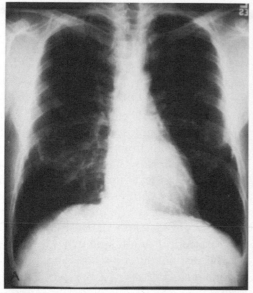

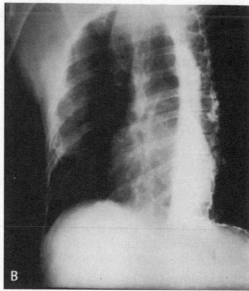

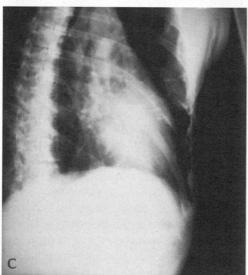

Figure 22.3. Calcified pleural plaques. **A.** Posteroanterior radiograph of a patient with heavy asbestos exposure 35 years previously. Diaphragmatic calcification is present, along with ill-defined densities bilaterally in the midlung fields and some pleural calcification. **B**, Right anterior oblique, and **C**, left anterior oblique, radiographs of the same patient. Note how much more evident the pleural calcification is on the oblique views. Note also the irregular configuration of the calcified pleural plaques.

ral thickening may occur with localized mesothelioma, metastatic disease, lymphoma, or myeloma (15). Pleural thickening from these diseases is usually unilateral. Localized pleural thickening and callus formation simulating asbestos pleural plaques may occur following rib fractures. The changes in such patients are usually unilateral, and the overlying rib deformity suggests the diagnosis (15). Pleural plaques that may or may not be calcified occur in other pneumoconioses including those caused by tremolite talc, mica, Bakelite, calcimine, tin, barite, and silica. Concomitant exposure to asbestos is probably responsible for the pleural plaques seen with such diseases, however (15).

The other main causes of diffuse pleural calcification are long-standing inflammatory diseases, particularly hemothorax, empyema, or repeated pneumothorax for tuberculosis. In such instances, the pleural thickening is unilateral, and the calcification is often extensive and sheetlike. The thickening is usually on the visceral pleura, and the calcification occurs in the inner aspect of the pleural thickening (Fig. 22.4).

Significance

Bilateral pleural plaques or calcifications are significant as an index of previous exposure to asbestos. It is controversial whether the presence of the pleural plaques increases the risk

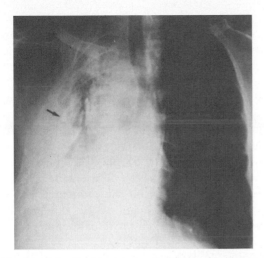

Figure 22.4. Posteroanterior chest radiograph showing marked pleural thickening on the right. The inner border of the pleural thickening is calcified (*arrow*). This patient had a history of advanced tuberculosis of the right lung. (Courtesy of Dr. Harry Sassoon.)

of lung cancer if the level of smoking is taken into consideration (36). Weiss reviewed the English language literature in 1993 and concluded that the weight of evidence favors the conclusion that persons with asbestos-related pleural plaques do not have an increased risk of lung cancer in the absence of parenchymal asbestosis (37). Hillerdal more recently reviewed the incidence of bronchial carcinoma and mesothelioma in 1596 men with pleural plaques initially detected between 1963 and 1985. He found that 50 bronchial carcinomas occurred while 32.1 were expected, and that 9 mesotheliomas occurred whereas only 0.8 were expected (38). The risk of cancer and mesotheliomas therefore is probably somewhat increased in patients with pleural plaques, and they should be encouraged to stop smoking.

The presence of pleural plaques does produce mild abnormalities of pulmonary function (39–41). Schwartz and associates performed spirometry on 1211 sheet metal workers (39). They reported that the forced vital capacity (FVC) in the 258 individuals with circumscribed plaque was 3.75 L compared to an FVC of 4.09 in 877 workers without pleural fibrosis. In a subsequent study, this same group was able to demonstrate a significant relationship between the volume of the pleural fibrosis as computed from the three-dimensional reconstruction of the HRCT scan and the total

lung capacity (40). The mean total lung capacity, however, of 24 patients with pleural fibrosis was 106% of predicted (40). Fridriksson and coworkers (42) studied 45 men with asbestos-related pleural plaques of at least 5-mm thickness without parenchymal abnormalities. They found that when the level of smoking was taken into consideration, the mean total lung capacity was 16% below predicted, whereas the vital capacity was 15% below predicted. The lung compliance was decreased by approximately 40%. Patients with calcified pleural plaques had more severe changes in lung physiology than those who had only hyaline plaques. They attributed the functional abnormalities to subclinical parenchymal disease. Certainly, the functional abnormalities produced by pleural plaques alone are not sufficient to produce symptoms. Shih and coworkers demonstrated that the maximal work capacity was 91.4% of predicted in 20 patients with pleural plaques and no asbestosis of the lung (43).

Diffuse Thickening

In addition to the occurrence of parietal pleural plaques, exposure to asbestos may be followed by the development of diffuse pleural fibrosis. Although some authors consider this diffuse pleural fibrosis to be part of the spectrum of parenchymal asbestosis (16), it appears to be a distinct entity (2, 44–46). In contrast to pleural plaques, diffuse pleural fibrosis commonly involves the costophrenic angles, is associated with involvement of the visceral pleura with pleural symphysis (Fig. 22.5), and sometimes involves a marked loss of pulmonary function that can lead to hypercapnic respiratory failure (44–46).

The incidence of diffuse pleural fibrosis is much lower than that of pleural plaques. Hillerdal (44), in surveying a group of asbestos workers, found 827 individuals with pleural plaques, but only 27 with progressive pleural thickening. Schwartz and coworkers reviewed the chest radiographs of 1211 sheet metal workers and reported that 260 had circumscribed plaques while 74 had diffuse thickening (39). One report suggested that the development of pleural fibrosis was more common with HLA phenotype DQ2 (47).

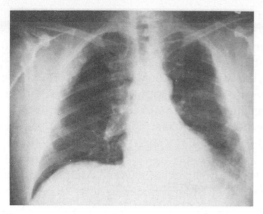

Figure 22.5. Posteroanterior chest radiograph demonstrating diffuse pleural thickening and blunting of the left costophrenic angle from a patient with a history of asbestos exposure.

The pathogenesis of diffuse pleural thickening is unknown. However, its locale and strong association with interstitial fibrosis suggest that it may be a direct extension of parenchymal fibrosis to the visceral pleura (4). Subpleural interstitial fibrosis has been a constant feature in the limited studies using HRCT in subjects with diffuse pleural disease (33). This does not explain the observation that diffuse pleural fibrosis associated with asbestos exposure frequently follows a benign asbestos pleural effusion (see Chapter 18). Epler and coworkers reviewed 1135 asbestos workers and found that of the 44 patients with diffuse thickening greater than 5 mm, almost 50% had had a previous asbestos pleural effusion (6). Of 35 workers with asbestos effusion, 54% had residual diffuse pleural thickening. Hillerdal documented that the initiating event in 4 of 27 patients with progressive pleural thickening was a benign pleural effusion (44). Diffuse pleural thickening secondary to asbestos exposure almost always involves the costophrenic angle and invariably becomes bilateral, although it may be unilateral at first. This diffuse pleural thickening starts at the bases and progresses at a variable rate. Thickening of the pleural cap may be considerable (44). Although routine radiographs do not demonstrate pleural calcification in the majority of patients, CT scanning often demonstrates pleural calcification (45). Many patients with diffuse pleural fibrosis have no evidence of intrapulmonary fibrosis on a CT scan (45).

Patients with diffuse pleural thickening have a significant decrease in their FVC (45, 46). In one study the mean FVC was 3.16 L in 74 patients with diffuse pleural thickening, which can be compared to a mean FVC of 4.09 in 877 similarly exposed individuals without pleural changes (39). Serial pulmonary function testing demonstrates a much faster decrease in the vital capacity than would be expected from aging alone (45, 48). The elastic recoil of the lungs of patients with diffuse pleural thickening is increased, and the reduction in the vital capacity is thought to be due to the pleural fibrosis, which prevents the lung from expanding (45). The diffusing capacity of these patients is reduced, but when the diffusing capacity is corrected for the patient's lung volume, it is above normal in the majority of patients (45). The exercise capacity of some patients with diffuse pleural fibrosis is diminished (43, 49). In one study the work capacity of 12 patients with diffuse pleural thickening was 82.7% of predicted. The intense dyspnea during exercise has been attributed to the rapid shallow breathing pattern that these patients exhibit during exercise. Oxygen desaturation does not occur and there is no definite evidence that the patients develop respiratory muscle fatigue (49).

The diagnosis of diffuse pleural thickening secondary to asbestos exposure is usually based primarily on the history of exposure. Pleural plaques are present in the majority of patients with diffuse pleural thickening secondary to asbestos exposure (50). In addition, the diffuse thickening secondary to asbestos exposure is usually bilateral and does not have nodular invasion of the lung (50). One must worry about the possibility of mesothelioma in patients with diffuse thickening from asbestos exposure. Features that suggest neoplasm are the presence of pleural nodularity or ring, parietal pleural thickening greater than 1 cm, or involvement of the mediastinal pleural surfaces (33).

The optimal management of patients with progressive pleural fibrosis due to asbestos exposure is unknown. Wright and coworkers suggested that because these patients have an increased elastic recoil and a normal diffusing capacity when corrected for lung volume, they might benefit from decortication (45).

Hillerdal, however, performed decortication on four patients and reported that only one of them improved subjectively (44). He attributed the lack of improvement to concomitant parenchymal fibrosis.

Rounded Atelectasis

Rounded atelectasis refers to atelectasis of the peripheral lung resulting from pleural adhesions and fibrosis. Rounded atelectasis can mimic a pulmonary neoplasm because it presents as a peripheral mass. Rounded atelectasis consists of a peripheral part of the lung that has become atelectatic secondary to the pleural inflammation. At thoracotomy, fibrous tissue can always be peeled off in several layers. After extensive dissection, the lung fully expands. The most probable explanation for rounded atelectasis is that an inflammatory reaction starts in the visceral pleura and leads to formation of fibrous tissue on the lung surface. This tissue subsequently shrinks and causes atelectasis of the underlying lung (51).

Rounded atelectasis is usually due to asbestos exposure. Dernevik and Gatzinsky (51) reported pleural plaques in 29 of 37 cases (78%) of rounded atelectasis. Hillerdal and Ozesmi (52) reported that 6 of 60 (10%) patients with benign asbestos-related pleural effusion developed rounded atelectasis. Rounded atelectasis has also been reported in conjunction with tuberculosis, parapneumonic effusions, pulmonary embolization, and Dressler's syndrome (53). It is likely that any disease that produces localized inflammation of the visceral pleura can lead to rounded atelectasis.

The main importance of rounded atelectasis is that it must be differentiated from a malignant lung lesion. The rounded atelectasis itself does not produce symptoms. The roentgenologic picture is often suggestive of the diagnosis, whereas a CT scan is frequently diagnostic. On the standard chest radiograph, rounded atelectasis appears as a spherical, sharply marginated mass abutting the pleura. Pleural thickening is always present and frequently is thickest near the mass. The comet-tail sign is produced by the crowding together of bronchi and blood vessels that extend from the lower border of the mass to the hilum. Although these features may be appreciated on standard radiographs, CT shows the characteristic features, including the associated pleural thickening and peripheral location of the mass to better advantage (54). Fine-needle biopsy can be performed easily because the lesion is pleural-based, but its utility is limited since malignancy cannot be excluded (53). Thoracotomy is definitive, but should rarely be necessary (22).

DIFFUSE BILATERAL PLEURAL THICKENING UNRELATED TO ASBESTOS

Although asbestos exposure accounts for most cases of diffuse bilateral pleural thickening, there are other causes. These include drugs (see Chapter 17), collagen vascular disease (Chapter 16), and infectious diseases, which usually produce unilateral pleural thickening. Nevertheless, there are some cases for which no etiology is apparent. Buchanan and coworkers (55) described four patients with bilateral pleural effusions progressing to diffuse pleural thickening for which there was no evidence of an infective, embolic, or occupational cause. Histology showed that in all cases both layers of the pleura were thickened by fibrous tissue and frequently the pleural space was obliterated. Interestingly, all four cases were HLA-B44 positive. Pleural decortication was successful in the three patients on whom this procedure was attempted (55).

FIBROTHORAX

When pleural inflammation is intense, its resolution may be associated with the deposition of a thick layer of dense fibrous tissue on the visceral pleura. The patient is then said to have a fibrothorax. As a result of the marked pleural thickening, the hemithorax becomes contracted, and its mobility is reduced (56). As the fibrothorax progresses, the intercostal spaces may narrow, the size of the involved hemithorax may diminish, and the mediastinum may be displaced ipsilaterally. Radiologically, a peel of uniform thickness surrounds the lung. Calcification occurs frequently on the inner aspect of the peel (Fig. 22.4) and provides an indicator by which the thickness of the peel may be accurately measured (56).

The three main causes of fibrothorax are hemothorax, tuberculosis, and bacterial lung infection (56), but pancreatitis (57), collagen vascular disease (58), and uremia (59) can all lead to fibrothorax.

Clinical Manifestations

Pulmonary function is severely compromised in fibrothorax. The degree of functional abnormality is much greater than one would expect from the degree of pleural disease (60). Pleural thickening in the costophrenic angle can cause profound alterations in the ventilation of, and blood flow to, the entire lung. Routine pulmonary function testing reveals mild-to-severe restrictive ventilatory dysfunction. Surprisingly, the blood flow is reduced more than the ventilation of the affected side (61). In a study of 127 patients (61), the mean O_2 uptake on the affected side was 19% of the total, whereas the mean ventilation was 33% of the total. This finding is in contrast to parenchymal diseases, in which the O_2 uptake and ventilation are reduced to the same degree (61). In severe disease, there is no ventilation or perfusion to the affected side (61).

Treatment

The only treatment available for fibrothorax is decortication, which involves removing the fibrous peel from the visceral pleura. The functional improvement following decortication has been variable (56, 60, 61). The most important clinical factor is the extent of the disease in the underlying lung (60, 61). The vital capacity may improve more than 50% following decortication if no underlying parenchymal disease is present, but the vital capacity may even decrease following decortication in patients with extensive parenchymal disease. In patients with long-standing fibrothorax, decortication can still lead to functional improvement. One case report noted a marked subjective improvement in a patient who had had a fibrothorax for 44 years (60).

Which patients should have decortication? Patients with recent hemothorax (see Chapter 21), recent empyema in which the infection is controlled (see Chapter 9), or recent tuberculous pleuritis (see Chapter 10) should not have a decortication because the pleural thickening frequently resolves by itself over several months. Therefore, decortication should be considered only if the pleural thickening has been stable or progressive over at least a 6-month period. If the pleural thickening has been present for several months and if the patient's way of life is compromised by exertional dyspnea, decortication should probably be performed unless previous chest radiographs demonstrated extensive parenchymal disease. Decortication is a major surgical procedure and should not be performed on patients debilitated by other diseases. In one series of 141 patients, the mortality rate with decortication was 3.5% (56).

INTRATHORACIC SPLENOSIS

Splenosis is defined as the autotransplantation of splenic tissue, usually after rupture of the spleen. Most commonly, it is discovered as innumerable purple nodules coating the mesentery, omentum, and peritoneal surfaces of the abdominal cavity. When the diaphragm and spleen are lacerated simultaneously, seeding of the pleural cavities can occur.

Intrathoracic splenosis can present with solitary or multiple pleural-based nodules (62). The presentation may be 15 years or more after the spleen was injured. A clue to the diagnosis is the absence of Howell-Jolly bodies, pitted erythrocytes, and siderocytes in the peripheral blood of asplenic individuals. Normally asplenic individuals have these abnormalities in their peripheral blood smear. However, if there is functional splenic tissue elsewhere such as in the chest, these cells will be absent. Technetium-99m-labeled sulfur colloid radionucleotide scanning can identify residual splenic tissue. If the patient is asymptomatic, no therapy is indicated.

REFERENCES

1. Craighead JE, Mossman BT: The pathogenesis of asbestos-associated diseases. N Engl J Med 1982;306: 1446–1455.
2. Hillerdal G: Pleural plaques in the general population. Ann NY Acad Sci 1991;643:430–437.
3. Bresnitz EA, Gilman MJ, Gracely EJ, Airoldi J, Vogel E, Gefter W: Asbestos-related radiographic abnormalities in elevator construction workers. Am Rev Respir Dis 1993;147:1341–1344.
4. Schwartz DA: New developments in asbestos-induced pleural disease. Chest 1991;99:191–198.
5. Karjalainen A, Karhunen PJ, Lalu K, Penttila A, Vanhala E, Kyyronen P, Tossavainen A: Pleural plaques and exposure to mineral fibres in a male

urban necropsy population. Occupat Environ Med 1994;51:456-460.

6. Epler GR, McLoud TC, Gaensler EA: Prevalence and incidence of benign asbestos pleural effusion in a working population. JAMA 1982;247:617-622.

7. Kilburn KH, Warshaw R, Thornton JC: Asbestos diseases and pulmonary symptoms and signs in shipyard workers and their families in Los Angeles. Arch Intern Med 1986;146:2213-2220.

8. Churg A, DePaoli L: Environmental pleural plaques in residents of a Quebec chrysotile mining town. Chest 1988;94:58-69.

9. Constantopoulos SH, Theodoracopoulos P, Dascalopoulos G, et al: Tremolite whitewashing and pleural calcifications. Chest 1987;92:709-712.

10. Kiviluoto R: Pleural calcification as a roentgenologic sign of non-occupational endemic anthophyllite-asbestosis. Acta Radiol 1960;194(Suppl):1-67.

11. Hourihane DO'B, Lessof L, Richardson PC: Hyaline and calcified pleural plaques as an index of exposure to asbestos: a study of radiological and pathological features of 100 cases with a consideration of epidemiology. Br Med J 1966;1:1069-1074.

12. Hillerdal G, Lindgren A: Pleural plaques: correlation of autopsy findings to radiographic findings and occupational history. Eur J Respir Dis 1980;61:315-319.

13. Roberts GH: The pathology of parietal pleural plaques. J Clin Pathol 1971;24:348-353.

14. Kishimoto T, Ono T, Okada K, Ito H: Relationship between number of asbestos bodies in autopsy lung and pleural plaques on chest x-ray film. Chest 1989;95:549-552.

15. Sargent EN, Jacobson G, Gordonson JS: Pleural plaques: a signpost of asbestos dust inhalation. Semin Roentgenol 1977;12:287-297.

16. Becklake MR: Asbestos-related diseases of the lung and other organs: their epidemiology and implications for clinical practice. Am Rev Respir Dis 1976;114:187-227.

17. Churg A, Wright JL, Vedal S: Fiber burden and patterns of asbestos-related disease in chrysotile miners and millers. Am Rev Respir Dis 1993;148:25-31.

18. Gibbs GW: Etiology of pleural calcification: a study of Quebec chrysotile miners and millers. Arch Environ Health 1979;34:76-83.

19. Baris I, Simonato L, Artivinli M, et al: Epidemiological and environmental evidence of the health effects of exposure to erionite fibres: a four-year study in the Cappadocian region of Turkey. Int J Cancer 1987;39:10-17.

20. Casey KR, Shigeoka JW, Rom WN, Moatamed F: Zeolite exposure and associated pneumoconiosis. Chest 1985;87:837-840.

21. Huuskonen MS, Tossavainen A, Koskinen H, et al: Wollastonite exposure and lung fibrosis. Environ Res 1983;30:291-304.

22. Hillerdal G: Nonmalignant pleural disease related to asbestos exposure. Clin Chest Med 1985;6:141-152.

23. Hillerdal G: The pathogenesis of pleural plaques and pulmonary asbestosis: possibilities and impossibilities. Eur J Respir Dis 1980;61:129-138.

24. Viallat JR, Raybuad F, Passarel M, Boutin C: Pleural migration of chrysotile fibers after intratracheal injection in rats. Arch Environ Health 1986;41:282-286.

25. Shore BL, Daughaday CC, Spilberg I: Benign asbestos pleurisy in the rabbit. Am Rev Respir Dis 1983;128:481-485.

26. Sahn SA, Antony VB: Pathogenesis of pleural plaques: relationship of early cellular response and pathology. Am Rev Respir Dis 1984;130:884-887.

27. Kuwahara M, Kuwahara M, Verma K, Ando T, Hemenway DR, Kagan E: Asbestos exposure stimulates pleural mesothelial cells to secrete the fibroblast chemoattractant, fibronectin. Am J Respir Cell Mol Biol 1994;10:167-176.

28. Griffith DE, Miller EJ, Gray LD, Idell S, Johnson AR: Interleukin-1-mediated release of interleukin-8 by asbestos-stimulated human pleural mesothelial cells. Am J Respir Cell Mol Biol 1994;10:245-252.

29. Fletcher DE, Edge JR: The early radiological changes in pulmonary and pleural asbestosis. Clin Radiol 1970;21:355-365.

30. Withers BF, Ducatman AM, Yang WN: Roentgenographic evidence for predominant left-sided location of unilateral pleural plaques. Chest 1989;95:1262-1264.

31. Hu H, Beckett L, Kelsey K, Christiani D: The left-sided predominance of asbestos-related pleural disease. Am Rev Respir Dis 1993;148:981-984.

32. Gevenois PA, De Vuyst P, Dedeire S, Cosaert J, Vande Weyer R, Struyven J: Conventional and high-resolution CT in asymptomatic asbestos-exposed workers. Acta Radiolog 1994;35:226-229.

33. Aberle DR, Balmes JR: Computed tomography of asbestos-related pulmonary parenchymal and pleural diseases. Clin Chest Med 1991;12:115-131.

34. Sargent EN, Boswell WD Jr, Ralls PW, Markovitz A: Subpleural fat pads in patients exposed to asbestos: distinction from non-calcified pleural plaques. Radiology 1984;152:273-277.

35. Friedman AC, Fiel SB, Fisher MS, et al: Asbestos-related pleural disease and asbestosis: a comparison of CT and chest radiography. AJR 1988;150:269-275.

36. Edelman DA: Asbestos exposure, pleural plaques and the risk of lung cancer. Int Arch Occup Environ Health 1988;60:389-393.

37. Weiss W: Asbestos-related pleural plaques and lung cancer. Chest 1993;103:1854-1859.

38. Hillerdal G: Pleural plaques and risk for bronchial carcinoma and mesothelioma. Chest 1994;105:144-150.

39. Schwartz DA, Fuortes LJ, Galvin JR, Burmeister LF, Schmidt LE, Leistikow BN, LaMarte FP, Merchant JA: Asbestos-induced pleural fibrosis and impaired lung function. Am Rev Respir Dis 1990;141:321-326.

40. Schwartz A, Galvin JR, Yagla SJ, Speakman SB, Merchant JA, Hunninghake GW: Restrictive lung function and asbestos-induced pleural fibrosis. A quantitative approach. J Clin Invest 1993;91:2685-2692.

41. Hillerdal G, Malmberg P, Hemmingsson A: Asbestos-related lesions of the pleura: parietal plaques compared to diffuse thickening studied with chest roent-

genography, computed tomography, lung function, and gas exchange. Am J Indust Med 1990;18:627-639.

42. Fridriksson HV, Hedenstrom H, Hillerdal G, Malmberg P: Increased lung stiffness in persons with pleural plaques. Eur J Respir Dis 1981;62:412-424.

43. Shih J-F, Wilson JS, Broderick A, Watt JL, Galvin JR, Merchant JA, Schwartz DA: Asbestos-induced pleural fibrosis and impaired exercise physiology. Chest 1994;105:1370-1376.

44. Hillerdal G: Non-malignant asbestos pleural disease. Thorax 1981;36:669-675.

45. Wright PH, Hanson A, Kreel L, Capel LH: Respiratory function changes after asbestos pleurisy. Thorax 1980;35:31-36.

46. Miller A, Teirstein AS, Selikoff I: Ventilatory insufficiency due to asbestos-induced pleural disease. Am Rev Respir Dis 1982;125:114A.

47. Shih J-F, Hunninghake GW, Goeken NE, Galvin JR, Merchant JA, Schwartz DA: The relationship between HLA-A, B, DQ, and DR antigens and asbestos-induced lung disease. Chest 1993;104:26-31.

48. Schwartz DA, Davis CS, Merchant JA, et al: Longitudinal changes in lung function among asbestos-exposed workers. Am J Respir Crit Care Med 1994;150:1243-1249.

49. Picado C, Laporta D, Grassino A, et al: Mechanisms affecting exercise performance in subjects with asbestos-related pleural fibrosis. Lung 1987;165:45-57.

50. Leung AN, Muller NL, Miller RR: CT in differential diagnosis of diffuse pleural disease. Am J Roentgenol 1990;154:487-492.

51. Dernevik L, Gatzinsky P: Pathogenesis of shrinking pleuritis with atelectasis: "rounded atelectasis." Eur J Respir Dis 1987;71:244-249.

52. Hillerdal G, Ozesmi M: Benign asbestos pleural effusion: 73 exudates in 60 patients. Eur J Respir Dis 1987;71:113-121.

53. Szydlowski GW, Cohn HE, Steiner RM, Edie RN: Rounded atelectasis: a pulmonary pseudotumor. Ann Thorac Surg 1992;53:817-821.

54. McLoud TC, Flower CD: Imaging the pleura: sonography, CT, and MR imaging. AJR 1991;156:1145-1153.

55. Buchanan DR, Johnston ID, Kerr IH, et al: Cryptogenic bilateral fibrosing pleuritis. Br J Dis Chest 1988;82:186-193.

56. Morton JR, Boushy SF, Guinn GA: Physiological evaluation of results of pulmonary decortication. Ann Thorac Surg 1970;9:321-326.

57. Shapiro DH, Anagnostopoulos CE, Dineen JP: Decortication and pleurectomy for the pleuropulmonary complications of pancreatitis. Ann Thorac Surg 1970;9:76-80.

58. Brunk JR, Drash EC, Swineford O: Rheumatoid pleuritis successfully treated with decortication. Report of a case and review of the literature. Am J Med Sci 1966;251:545-551.

59. Gilbert L, Bribot S, Franked H, et al: Fibrinous uremic pleuritis: a surgical entity. Chest 1975;67:53-56.

60. Hughes R, Jensik RJ, Faber LP, Bliss K: Evaluation of unilateral decortication: a patient successfully treated 44 years after onset of tuberculosis. Ann Thorac Surg 1975;19:704-715.

61. Gaensler EA: Lung displacement: abdominal enlargement, pleural space disorders, deformities of the thoracic cage. In: Fenn WD, Rahn H, eds: Handbook of Physiology: Section 3, Respiration. Washington, DC: American Physiological Society, 1965;2:1623-1661.

62. Yousem SA: Thoracic splenosis. Ann Thorac Surg 1987;44:411-412.

CHAPTER 23

Thoracentesis (Diagnostic and Therapeutic) and Pleural Biopsy

DIAGNOSTIC THORACENTESIS

Indications

A diagnostic thoracentesis should be performed on almost all patients with a pleural effusion of unknown origin. Empirically, I have found it difficult to obtain fluid with a diagnostic thoracentesis if the thickness of the fluid on the decubitus chest radiograph is less than 10 mm, and I usually do not attempt thoracentesis in such patients. If thoracentesis is to be attempted with small amounts of fluid, the proper location can be identified by ultrasound (1).

Contraindications

The main contraindication to a diagnostic thoracentesis is a hemorrhagic diathesis. One should hesitate to perform a thoracentesis in a patient who is receiving anticoagulants, particularly thrombolytic agents. Depending on the urgency of the situation, however, diagnostic thoracentesis using a small needle can be performed on almost any patient if one is careful. McVay and coworkers demonstrated that there was no increased risk of bleeding if the prothrombin time or the partial thromboplastin time was not more than two times the normal value (2). Likewise there was no increased risk of bleeding with moderately low platelet counts (25,000/mm^3) (2). Accordingly, these authors recommend that prophylactic blood product transfusions are not needed prior to thoracentesis in patients with mild coagulopathy and no clinical evidence of bleeding (2). These authors did note an increased risk of bleeding if the creatinine was elevated above 6 mg/dl (2).

It appears that thoracentesis can be performed on patients who are undergoing mechanical ventilation. McCartney and associates reported a series of 31 patients who underwent thoracentesis while they were receiving mechanical ventilation; 25 patients were receiving positive end expiratory pressure (PEEP) between 5 and 20 cm H_2O. All thoracenteses were performed with patients in the lateral decubitus position. Only three of the patients (10%) developed a pneumothorax and all were managed with a chest tube (3). In a second series 2 of 32 patients (6%) developed a pneumothorax after undergoing a thoracentesis while on mechanical ventilation (4).

A thoracentesis should not be attempted through an area affected by a local cutaneous condition such as pyoderma or Herpes zoster infection.

Positioning of Patient

For a diagnostic thoracentesis, and particularly for a therapeutic thoracentesis, the patient and the operator must be comfortable. I find that the patient is most comfortable when he sits on the side of the bed with his arms and head resting on one or more pillows on a bedside table (Fig. 23.1). A footstool is placed on the floor for the patient to have some place to rest his feet. The bed is elevated so that the operator does not have to stoop over. The patient sits near the foot of the bed with the side containing the fluid toward the foot of the bed. With the patient in this position, the operator does not have to reach across the entire bed, yet the foot of the bed can be covered with sterile drapes to provide a sterile area from which to work. The patient should be positioned with his back vertical so that the lowest part of his hemithorax is posterior. If the patient leans forward too far, the lowest part of the hemithorax may move anteriorly, and no fluid will remain posteriorly.

Some patients are too debilitated to assume a sitting position. The thoracentesis may then be performed with the patient lying on the

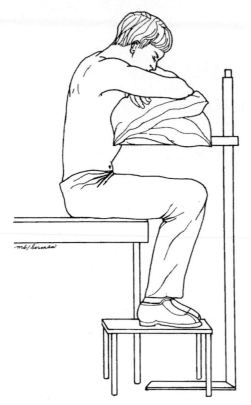

Figure 23.1. Recommended position of the patient for diagnostic or therapeutic thoracentesis.

side of the pleural effusion in the lateral decubitus position, with his back near the edge of the operating table or bed. Alternately, the patient may sit in bed with the head of the bed maximally elevated. With the patient in this position, the thoracentesis is performed in the midaxillary line.

Selection of Site

The site for the attempted thoracentesis should be selected with care. Most thoracenteses that fail to yield fluid are performed too low (5). A review of the chest radiographs will indicate an approximate location. The physical examination of the patient's chest is most important in determining the site, however. When fluid is present between the lung and the chest wall, tactile fremitus is lost, and the light percussion note becomes dull. Accordingly, thoracentesis should be attempted one interspace below the spot where tactile fremitus is lost and the percussion note becomes dull. Thoracentesis should usually be per-

formed posteriorly several inches from the spine, where the ribs are easily palpated. The exact location for the thoracentesis attempt should be just superior to a rib. The rationale for this location is that the arteries, veins, and nerves run just inferior to the ribs (Fig. 23.2), so that if the needle is just superior to a rib, the danger of damage to these structures is minimized.

Ultrasound has been proposed as being superior to chest roentgenography in identifying pleural fluid and choosing the optimal site for thoracentesis (6). One study (7), however, has demonstrated that it is not cost effective to obtain ultrasound routinely prior to thoracentesis. Kohan and coworkers randomly allocated 205 patients to undergo or not undergo chest ultrasonography prior to thoracentesis. They reported that the incidence of dry attempts was significantly higher without ultrasound (33%) than with ultrasound (10%) in patients with small effusions, but there was no difference with large effusions. Moreover, there was no difference in the rate of complications with either small or large effusions (7). Based on this study it is recommended that thoracentesis initially be attempted without ultrasound unless the amount of pleural fluid is very small. If no fluid is obtained after two or three attempts, then the fluid should be localized with ultrasound before additional attempts are made to obtain fluid. It should be noted, however, that in a smaller study (8), the incidence of pneumothorax was much less if the thoracentesis was done with ultrasound guidance (8).

Thoracentesis Kits

The materials required to perform the diagnostic thoracentesis are listed in Table 23.1, and these should be assembled before the procedure is initiated. What is done more commonly, however, is to use a thoracentesis kit where all the materials have been preassembled. There are several thoracentesis kits available commercially, including the Pharmaseal, distributed by Baxter; the Arrow-Clark Thoracentesis Kit, distributed by Arrow; and the Argyle Turkel, distributed by Sherwood. The kit that is used by far the most frequently is the Pharmaseal (Baxter), and this kit is

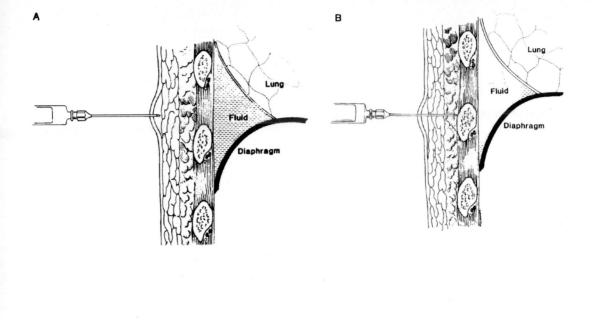

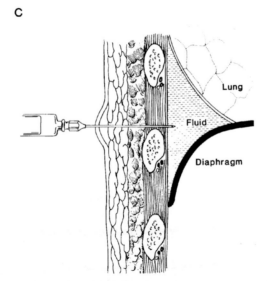

Figure 23.2. Diagnostic thoracentesis. **A.** The skin is injected using a 25-gauge needle with a local anesthetic agent. **B.** The periosteum is injected with the local anesthetic. **C.** The pleural space is entered, and pleural fluid is obtained. **D.** The thoracentesis attempt is too high, and air bubbles are obtained. **E.** The thoracentesis attempt is too low, and neither bubbles nor fluid is obtained.

unsatisfactory in my opinion. The primary needle for the aspiration is a 3-inch, 16-gauge needle. A needle this large should never be used for a diagnostic thoracentesis. If a diagnostic thoracentesis is going to be performed, there is no need to use such a large needle. If a therapeutic thoracentesis is going to be performed, it should not be done with a sharp needle because the sharp needle may lacerate the lung.

One excellent thoracentesis kit is the Arrow-Clark Thoracentesis Kit manufactured by Arrow International, Reading, Pennsylvania. The basic thoracentesis apparatus in this kit is an 8 French-gauge catheter over an 18-gauge needle with a three-way stopcock and self-sealing valve. With this apparatus one constantly aspirates as the needle is advanced through the chest wall. Then when a free flow of fluid is encountered, the catheter is advanced about

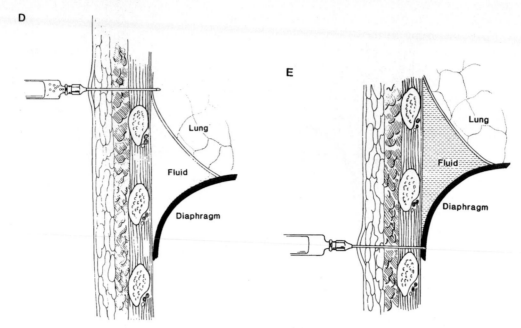

Figure 23.2D–E.

Table 23.1 Materials Needed for Diagnostic Thoracentesis

Basic Materials
  Lidocaine 1 or 2%
  Aqueous heparin, 1000 U/ml
  Atropine
  Antiseptic solution
  Alcohol swabs
  Sterile gloves
  6 4 x 4-inch gauze pads
  Sterile drape with center hole
  Sterile drape (to cover bed)
  Adhesive tape
  2 5- to 10-ml syringes
  1 50-ml syringe
  1 No. 25 needle, ⅝ inch long
  2 No. 20 to No. 22 needles, 1½ inches long
  Bandaids
Additional Materials for Therapeutic Thoracentesis
  2 No. 14 needles and catheters
  1 3-way stopcock
  1 sterile container for pleural fluid
  1 50-ml syringe (additional)
Additional Materials for Pleural Biopsy
  Pleural biopsy needle
  Scalpel
  Formalin

1 cm and the needle is withdrawn completely. One nice feature of this set is that there is a self-sealing valve so that air does not leak into the pleural space when the needle is withdrawn; however, the needle cannot be reinserted through the catheter. With this system, small amounts of fluid can be withdrawn by aspirating directly through the side port on the catheter. Another nice feature of this set is that one may easily withdraw large amounts of fluid either with a syringe or via vacuum bottles. If a syringe is used, aspiration is done through a Y connector, which has one-way valves such that no stopcocks need be turned with each aspiration. If vacuum bottles are used, there is vacuum bottle tubing included, which attaches directly to the side port of the catheter. There is also a roller clamp to control the flow of fluid into the vacuum bottles. The cost of this thoracentesis kit is approximately $31.00.

Another excellent set is the Argyle Turkel Safety Thoracentesis Set manufactured by Sherwood Medical, St. Louis, Missouri. This system incorporates a blunt, multi-side-holed, spring-loaded inner cannula coaxially housed within a 16-gauge conventional sharp-beveled hollow needle. The advantage of this system is as the needle and blunt cannula penetrate the chest wall, the blunt cannula is forced into the shaft of the needle. Then when the tip of the needle encounters low resistance, such as an area of pleural effusion within the pleural space, the spring-loaded cannula automatically extends beyond the bevel, thus helping to protect the underlying tissue from further, inadvertent penetration. Another advantage of this system is an indicator in the needle housing, which identifies the position of the blunt cannula; if resistance is being met such that the sharp end of the needle is exposed, then the indicator is red. In contrast, if no resistance is being met, then the indicator is green. Therefore, when the pleural space is entered, the indicator turns green. If a diagnostic thoracentesis is being performed, the pleural fluid can be withdrawn through the needle. If a therapeutic thoracentesis is being performed, the catheter assembly is advanced and then the needle assembly is withdrawn completely. There is a one-way valve such that there is no possibility of air leaking into the pleural space when the needle is withdrawn. There is a side port for fluid removal. The cost of these kits is approximately $33.00.

When comparing the two kits described above, the Argyle Turkel kit has the advantage of the spring-loaded inner cannula, which should decrease the incidence of lung laceration. The advantage of the Arrow-Clark system is the ease with which a therapeutic thoracentesis can be performed with either a syringe or with vacuum bottles.

Technique

The procedure should be carefully explained to the patient, and a signed consent form should be obtained. I do not routinely administer atropine to prevent vasovagal reactions as advocated by some (9), because I find such reactions to be uncommon. I do have atropine available, however, and I administer 1.0 mg subcutaneously or intramuscularly at the first sign of such a reaction. Similarly, I do not administer an analgesic, a sedative, or a tranquilizer routinely prior to the procedure unless the patient shows excessive anxiety. To those I administer intravenous midazolam (Versed) just before the procedure.

Once the site for thoracentesis is identified, the skin over the site is cleansed thoroughly with an antiseptic solution over an area extending at least 4 inches in all directions from the proposed thoracentesis site. The sterile drape with the center hole is then taped to the patient's back, and another sterile drape is placed on the bed.

The next step is to obtain local anesthesia. It is necessary to anesthetize the skin, the periosteum of the rib, and the parietal pleura. The skin is anesthetized using a short No. 25 needle by injecting enough lidocaine, about 0.5 ml, to raise a small wheal (Fig. 23.2A). The small needle is then replaced by a No. 22 needle 1½ inches long. This needle is inserted to the periosteum of the underlying rib and is moved up and over the rib with the frequent injection of small amounts (0.1 to 0.2 ml) of lidocaine (Fig. 23.2B). Once this needle is superior to the rib, it is slowly advanced toward the pleural space with aspiration followed by the injection of 0.1 to 0.2 ml lidocaine every 1 to 2 mm (Fig. 23.2C). This frequent aspiration and the injection of lidocaine guarantee anesthesia of the parietal pleura. When pleural fluid is obtained through this needle into the syringe containing lidocaine, the needle should be withdrawn from the pleural space and should be reattached to a 50- to 60-ml syringe containing 1 ml heparin. Heparin is added to the syringe to prevent clotting of the pleural fluid. It is difficult to obtain differential white blood cell counts or pH determinations if the pleural fluid is clotted. The same needle is reintroduced along the same tract slowly with constant aspiration until pleural fluid is obtained. Aspiration is then continued until the syringe is filled. The needle is then withdrawn, and the procedure is finished. Most commonly one uses one of the commercially available thoracentesis sets to perform a diagnostic thoracentesis. The special needles that come with these kits offer very few advantages over a syringe and a needle for a diagnostic thoracentesis; however, they should always be used for a therapeutic thoracentesis.

At times, no pleural fluid is obtained when the 1½-inch No. 22 needle is inserted all the way to its hub. In such a situation, the needle should be slowly withdrawn with constant aspiration. The rim of the pleural fluid is sometimes thin and may be missed as the needle is inserted. If no pleural fluid is obtained either as the needle is inserted or withdrawn, one of four possibilities exists: (*a*) the needle was too short; (*b*) placement of the needle was too far superior; (c) placement of the needle was too far inferior; or (d) no pleural fluid is present. If the patient is abnormally muscular or obese and if no air is obtained on the initial attempt, the 1½-inch needle should be replaced with a longer needle, and the attempt should be repeated. If air bubbles are obtained on the initial attempt with the local anesthetic, the lung parenchyma has been penetrated, and the needle was inserted too far superiorly (Fig. 23.2D). Therefore, the procedure should be repeated one interspace inferiorly. If no fluid or air bubbles are obtained on the initial attempt, the needle was inserted too far inferiorly (Fig. 23.2E) and the procedure should be repeated one interspace superiorly. Penetration of the lung with a small needle is not a catastrophe, and only occasionally does a pneumothorax result. Pleural fluid is almost never too thick to be aspirated through a No. 20 or a No. 22 needle.

Processing of Pleural Fluid

The main purpose of a diagnostic thoracentesis is to examine the pleural fluid. The recommended distribution of the pleural fluid to various laboratories is outlined in Table 23.2. For determination of pleural fluid pH, the sample should be maintained anaerobically and should be packed in ice in the original syringe and sent to the laboratory. Interpretation of the results of the various tests obtained in Table 23.2 is discussed in Chapters 4 and 5.

If there is a good chance that the patient has a transudative pleural effusion, the most cost-effective approach is to measure only the lactic acid dehydrogenase (LDH) and protein in the pleural fluid until these measurements demonstrate that the patient does not have a transudative pleural effusion (10).

Complications

The most common complication of thoracentesis is pneumothorax. When three different series (7, 11, 12) involving 459 patients are combined, 51 of the patients (11%) developed a pneumothorax and chest tubes were necessary in 9 (2%). The incidence of pneumothorax following thoracentesis is reduced if experienced individuals such as pulmonary fellows or pulmonologists perform the procedure (13). The incidence of iatrogenic pneumothorax may be also be lower if the procedure is performed under sonographic guidance. Raptopoulos and associates reported that the incidence of pneumothorax was 18% for 154 thoracenteses done with conventional techniques while it was only 3% for 188 done with sonographic guidance (14). A second study with a comparable number of patients reported that the incidence of pneumothorax was comparable whether or not the procedure was performed with ultrasound guidance (7). This difference in the incidence of complications in the first study is at least partially explained by the fact that the sonographers

Table 23.2.   Laboratory Distribution of Pleural Fluid Obtained with Diagnostic Thoracentesis

Laboratory	Amount (ml)	Test Ordered
Chemistry	5	Protein Lactic acid dehydrogenase (LDH) Glucose Amylase
Hematology	5	White blood cell count (WBC) Wright's stain Hematocrit (if pleural fluid is bloody)
Bacteriology	10	Aerobic and anaerobic cultures Gram stain
Tuberculosis and mycology	5	Tuberculosis and fungal cultures Acid-fast stain
Cytology	5–25	Cytologic examination
Blood gas	5	pH P_{CO_2}

were more experienced in catheter placement (14).

It appears that the likelihood of the development of a pneumothorax may be higher in patients with chronic obstructive pulmonary disease (COPD). Brandstetter and associates performed thoracentesis in 106 patients, of whom 36 had COPD. The incidence of pneumothorax was significantly higher (41.7%) in those patients with COPD than in those without COPD (18.5%) (15). Nine of the 106 patients were treated with chest tubes and 7 of them had COPD (15). The explanation of the very high incidence of pneumothorax in this series is not clear. In contrast, Raptopoulos and associates were unable to find a relationship between the occurrence of a pneumothorax and the presence of underlying lung disease (14).

There are two different reasons that patients develop pneumothorax after a thoracentesis. First, air may flow from the atmosphere into the pleural space if the pleural space, with its negative pressure, communicates freely with the atmosphere. This most commonly happens when a syringe is removed from a needle or catheter and the air then flows from the atmosphere into the pleural space and produces a pneumothorax. This can be prevented if the special needles with one way valves (such as the Arrow-Clark or Argyle Turkel) are used during thoracentesis. Second, the needle for thoracentesis may lacerate the lung and permit air to enter the pleural space from the alveoli. This can be prevented if catheters rather than sharp needles are used to perform therapeutic thoracenteses. I do not recommend obtaining chest radiographs routinely after diagnostic thoracentesis because the incidence of pneumothorax is relatively low. Rather, I check for tactile fremitus on the side of the procedure superior to the level of the pleural fluid. I only obtain a chest radiograph if the tactile fremitus is diminished following the procedure or if the patient complains of symptoms. The treatment of iatrogenic pneumothorax is discussed in Chapter 19.

Other common complications of thoracentesis are cough and chest pain (13). Cough most frequently complicates thoracentesis when it is done for therapeutic reasons and

usually occurs toward the end of the thoracentesis (13). Indeed if excessive coughing occurs during a thoracentesis, it should serve as an indication to stop the procedure. The chest pain that complicates thoracentesis is of three types. Firstly, the patient may experience sharp pain when the skin is anesthetized or when the parietal pleura is pierced. This pain should not be persistent if the parietal pleura is adequately anesthetized. Secondly, the patient may experience chest tightness or dull pain as fluid is removed during a therapeutic thoracentesis. This type of pain usually indicates that the patient's lung is not expanding rapidly and should serve as an indication for stopping the procedure. Thirdly, the patient may develop pleuritic chest pain after the procedure, which is usually due to the roughened pleural surfaces rubbing on each other after some of the fluid has been withdrawn.

At times, a diagnostic thoracentesis provokes a vasovagal reflex characterized by bradycardia, a decreased stroke volume, and a resultant fall in cardiac output and blood pressure. This reaction is blocked by the intramuscular administration of 1 mg atropine. A similar syndrome may be provoked by various noxious, emotional, and physical stimuli such as apprehension, pain, or the sight of blood, and is characterized by the sudden loss of peripheral vascular resistance without significant bradycardia. The patient develops hypotension, pallor, cold and clammy skin, and faintness. This syndrome is not blocked by atropine. The recommended treatment is termination of the procedure and the immediate placement of the patient in a reverse Trendelenburg position (16).

Another complication of thoracentesis is infection of the pleural space. Approximately 2% of all pleural infections are due to contamination of the pleural space at the time of thoracentesis. For this reason, sterile technique must be strictly followed during thoracentesis, and the skin must be thoroughly cleansed before the procedure is started. The treatment of pleural infections is discussed in Chapter 9.

Diagnostic thoracentesis can also produce a hemothorax if an intercostal artery is lacerated. This complication can usually be avoided if the thoracentesis is performed just superior to a rib, as previously described. In older patients, however, the intercostal arteries may be tortuous, and a hemothorax can result even with proper technique (17). The treatment of iatrogenic hemothorax is described in Chapter 20. Other rare complications of diagnostic thoracentesis include splenic or hepatic laceration, soft tissue infection secondary to seeding of the needle tract with bacteria, seeding of the needle tract with tumor cells, and adverse reactions to the local anesthetic.

Another uncommon complication of which one should be aware is HIV infection with seroconversion. Oksenhendler and associates (18) reported an instance where a nurse received a superficial self-inflicted needlestick injury to the finger while recapping a needle contaminated by the bloody pleural fluid of a patient with persistent generalized lymphadenopathy, pleural effusion, and seropositivity for HIV and hepatitis B surface antigen. Anicteric hepatitis developed 53 days later, and serum samples became HIV antibody positive by day 68. This case emphasizes the need for strict precautions regarding the handling of needles and body fluids from patients infected with HIV.

THERAPEUTIC THORACENTESIS

Indications

The two main indications for therapeutic thoracentesis are to relieve the symptom of dyspnea secondary to a pleural effusion and to remove the pleural fluid so that the status of the lung underlying a pleural effusion can be evaluated. Although the thoracentesis in the second instance is really diagnostic, it is classified as therapeutic because large amounts of pleural fluid are removed. In general, the role of therapeutic thoracentesis in the management of patients with pleural effusions is limited. The thoracentesis itself does not alter the basic condition that produced the pleural effusion, but it does remove substantial amounts of protein from the patient. If 2000 ml pleural fluid with a protein level of 5 g/dl are removed, the patient will lose 100 g protein. A therapeutic thoracentesis should be performed in an acutely dyspneic patient with a large pleural effusion, however, particularly if the

mediastinum is shifted toward the contralateral side.

Serial therapeutic thoracenteses can be performed in patients dyspneic from malignant pleural effusions with mediastinal shift toward the contralateral side in whom a pleurodesis cannot be successfully effected. It is recommended, however, that such patients have a pleuroperitoneal shunt placed. A therapeutic thoracentesis is also indicated in a patient with a malignant pleural effusion and dyspnea to see whether the dyspnea can be relieved by the thoracentesis. This procedure should be performed before a chest tube is inserted and pleurodesis is attempted (see Chapter 7). The contraindications for therapeutic thoracentesis are the same as for diagnostic thoracentesis.

Technique

The positioning of the patient and the selection of the site for the thoracentesis are the same as for a diagnostic thoracentesis. The most important difference between a therapeutic and a diagnostic thoracentesis is that one must not use a sharp needle for the therapeutic thoracentesis. As the fluid is removed, the lung expands and can easily be lacerated if a sharp needle is present in the pleural space. Therefore, either a plastic catheter or a blunt pleural biopsy needle should be used. If a pleural biopsy is also indicated, the therapeutic thoracentesis can be performed through the pleural biopsy needle once the biopsy specimens have been obtained.

The additional materials required for the procedure are listed in Table 23.1. In most instances a commercially available kit such as the Arrow-Clark Thoracentesis Kit or the Argyle Turkel Safety Thoracentesis Kit is used. It is important use a kit with a catheter over a needle set rather than one like the Pharmaseal that only has a sharp needle. The Arrow-Clark or the Argyle Turkel thoracentesis kits are recommended because they each contain the catheter and they each have a device that prevents air from entering the pleural space when the needle is withdrawn (see discussion of these kits earlier in this chapter).

It is recommended that the Arrow-Clark or the Argyle Turkel thoracentesis kits be used

A

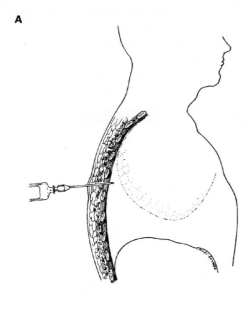

B

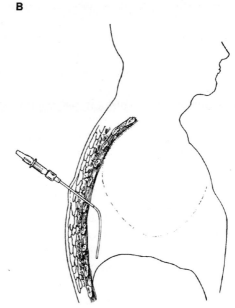

C

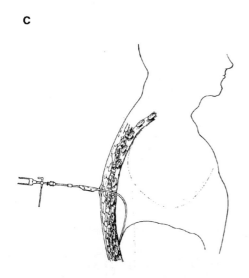

Figure 23.3. Therapeutic thoracentesis. **A.** A standard 14-gauge needle attached to a syringe is introduced into the pleural space. **B.** A 14-gauge catheter is threaded through the needle and is directed down toward the costodiaphragmatic recess. **C.** The needle is withdrawn from the pleural space, and its end is covered immediately with the guard. Fluid can be withdrawn from the pleural space using the three-way stopcock and the syringe.

for therapeutic thoracentesis. Directions for their use come with the kits. When these kits are used, it is important to make a large enough incision in the skin to allow easy passage for the needle with its overlying catheter. If the incision is too small, the catheter may be damaged during the insertion.

If these kits are not available, the procedure can be performed with a plastic catheter (Intracath) as outlined in Figure 23.3. When the fluid has been localized and identified by means of the lidocaine-filled syringe, as in diagnostic thoracentesis, a standard 16-gauge (Intracath) needle is attached to a plastic syringe. With gentle constant suction on the syringe, the needle is carefully and evenly advanced until pleural fluid is obtained. When the pleural fluid has been obtained, the syringe is disconnected from the needle, and the needle is temporarily occluded by a finger to prevent the development of a pneumothorax. Then, the 16-gauge (Intracath) catheter is inserted through the needle and is directed inferiorly toward the costodiaphragmatic recess. The catheter should not be advanced against resistance or its end may become traumatized and occluded. When the catheter has been advanced all the way to the hilt of the needle or when resistance is encountered, the needle is withdrawn carefully from the chest, and the plastic catheter is left in the pleural space.

Immediately after withdrawing the needle, one should place the guard over the end of the needle so that the needle does not shear off the end of the catheter. The catheter should not be pulled back through the needle because the needle's sharp point may cut off a portion of the catheter. Once the needle is withdrawn from the pleural space, it should be taped to the patient's skin so that the catheter is not inadvertently removed from the pleural space.

The advantage of the plastic catheter system for therapeutic thoracentesis is that no sharp needle is present in the pleural space to lacerate the lung as it re-expands. Moreover, the patient can be repositioned with the catheter in place to allow more complete pleural fluid removal.

When the catheter has been positioned in the pleural space, the needle has been withdrawn, and the needle's end has been covered with the guard, a syringe with a three-way stopcock is attached to the end of the catheter, and the pleural fluid is withdrawn. Alternatively, the fluid can be drained by vacuum bottles. There are no studies comparing the side effects with syringe versus vacuum bottle drainage.

A chest radiograph should be obtained after a therapeutic thoracentesis to verify that no pneumothorax has occurred. If the therapeutic thoracentesis was performed mainly for diagnostic purposes, it is sometimes useful to obtain bilateral decubitus radiographs after the procedure to delineate the amount of fluid remaining and to distinguish the remaining fluid from parenchymal infiltrates or masses. Similarly, it may be useful to inject 200 to 400 ml air into the pleural space at the end of the procedure before obtaining the radiographs. By means of this intentional iatrogenic pneumothorax, the thickness of the visceral and parietal pleura can be determined.

How Much Pleural Fluid Can Be Withdrawn?

Not more than 1000 to 1500 ml pleural fluid should be removed with a single thoracentesis (9, 19). The reason for this recommen-

dation is that an occasional patient develops re-expansion pulmonary edema (see Chapter 19) or hypovolemia after a thoracentesis.

My colleagues and I hypothesize that the development of these complications is related to the development of negative pleural pressure during therapeutic thoracentesis. We have demonstrated that larger amounts of pleural fluid can be removed safely if the pleural pressure is monitored during thoracentesis and if thoracentesis is terminated when the pleural pressure falls below -20 cm H_2O (19). Pleural pressure can be monitored by a "U"-shaped manometer, as illustrated in Figure 23.4. The change in the pleural pressure as fluid is withdrawn varies from patient to patient (Fig. 23.5). Frequently, neither the operator nor the patient is aware of the development of abnormally negative pleural pressure (19). In our series of 52 patients, 13 procedures (25%) were stopped because the patient's pleural pressures dropped below -20 cm H_2O. We have now removed more than 4000 ml pleural fluid in a single thoracentesis from eight separate patients with no adverse consequences. Of course, the procedure should be terminated if the patient develops unwarranted symptoms. The symptoms for which we most commonly terminate therapeutic thoracentesis are pernicious coughing and

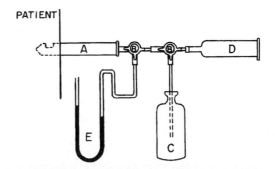

Figure 23.4. Schematic diagram of apparatus used to measure pleural pressures and to aspirate pleural fluid. To measure the pleural pressure, the stopcock (*B*) adjacent to the Abram's needle (*A*) is turned so that the pleural space is in communication with the manometer (*E*). It is important in measuring the pressure not to let fluid enter the plastic catheter between the tube and the manometer. *C*, Bottle; *D*, 60-ml syringe. (From Light RW, Jenkinson SG, Minh V, George RB: Observations on pleural pressures as fluid is withdrawn during thoracentesis. Am Rev Respir Dis 1980;121:799–804.)

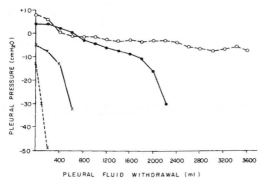

Figure 23.5. Changes in pleural pressure as fluid is withdrawn during therapeutic thoracentesis in two patients with malignant pleural disease (*circles*) and in two patients with trapped lung (*x's*). Note how rapidly the pleural pressures fall in the patients with trapped lung. (From Light RW, Jenkinson SG, Minh V, George RB: Observations on pleural pressures as fluid is withdrawn during thoracentesis. Am Rev Respir Dis 1980;121:799–804.)

chest tightness or chest pain. In our series of 52 thoracenteses, five procedures (10%) were stopped because of symptoms. Little correlation exists between the development of these symptoms and the decrease in pleural pressures.

Complications

Therapeutic thoracentesis is associated with the same complications as diagnostic thoracentesis, including vasovagal reaction, pneumothorax, pleural infection, and hemothorax. In addition, re-expansion pulmonary edema (see Chapter 19) and hypovolemia may complicate therapeutic thoracentesis, and as mentioned earlier, these complications may be related to the development of abnormally negative pleural pressures. Pneumothorax is more common with therapeutic than with diagnostic thoracentesis for two reasons (14). First, if a sharp needle is used for therapeutic thoracentesis, the lung is likely to be lacerated as it re-expands, leading to a bronchopleural fistula and a pneumothorax. Second, because the pleural pressure at times becomes abnormally negative during a therapeutic thoracentesis, air is more likely to enter the pleural space through faulty technique or even through the thoracentesis tract. The treatment of iatrogenic pneumothorax is discussed in Chapter 19. Pleural infection is probably more com-

mon after therapeutic than after diagnostic thoracentesis because the needles and catheters remain in the pleural space longer. In view of the much higher incidence of pneumothorax after therapeutic thoracentesis, a chest radiograph should be routinely obtained immediately following the procedure.

NEEDLE BIOPSY OF THE PLEURA

Indications

A small piece of parietal pleura is obtained for microscopic and/or microbiologic evaluation with needle biopsy of the pleura. Pleural biopsy should be performed in almost all patients with exudative pleural effusion of undetermined origin. Although some advocate the performance of a pleural biopsy every time a diagnostic thoracentesis is performed, I recommend that pleural biopsy be performed only if the patient has an undiagnosed exudative pleural effusion. Pleural biopsy causes more morbidity and is more expensive than simple diagnostic thoracentesis and rarely yields useful information if the patient has a transudative pleural effusion. One can use a refractometer (20) at the patient's bedside at the time of a diagnostic thoracentesis to estimate the pleural fluid protein level and to determine whether the patient has an exudative pleural effusion and is therefore a candidate for pleural biopsy. Pleural biopsy may also be performed in patients with pleural thickening of unknown origin without pleural effusion (21). Most pleural biopsies are performed in the presence of pleural fluid, however.

Contraindications

The main contraindication to pleural biopsy is a bleeding diathesis. Pleural biopsy should not be performed in patients who are taking anticoagulants or whose bleeding parameters are prolonged. If the platelet count is below 50,000/mm^3, platelet transfusion should be given before the procedure is attempted. If the patient has borderline respiratory failure, one should hesitate to perform a pleural biopsy because the production of a pneumothorax could precipitate respiratory failure.

Another contraindication to needle biopsy is the presence of an empyema. In one series, subcutaneous abscesses developed at the biopsy site in two of five patients with empyema in whom pleural biopsy was attempted (21). Other contraindications include an uncooperative patient and local cutaneous lesions such as pyoderma or Herpes zoster infection.

Technique

The materials necessary for pleural biopsy are listed in Table 23.1. Most frequently one uses a thoracentesis kit plus the pleural biopsy needle. The patient is positioned, and the site is selected as for diagnostic thoracentesis. The skin is cleaned, and the local anesthetic is administered as for diagnostic thoracentesis (described earlier in this chapter). Liberal amounts of lidocaine should be injected once the rib is passed to ensure adequate anesthesia of the parietal pleura. In general, if no fluid is obtained with the local anesthetic, the biopsy should not be attempted. When pleural fluid has been obtained with the lidocaine syringe and needle, a pleural biopsy can be performed with an Abram's or a Cope needle.

A biopsy is sometimes attempted without free pleural fluid. If there is no fluid, the procedure should be performed with fluoroscopic or ultrasonic guidance (21).

Abram's Needle

The Abram's needle (Fig. 23.6) consists of three parts: a large outer trocar, an inner cutting cannula, and an inner solid stylet. The end of the outer trocar is blunt so that the instrument will not lacerate the lung, but the bluntness of the instrument requires one to make a small scalpel incision in the anesthetized skin and subcutaneous tissue to permit

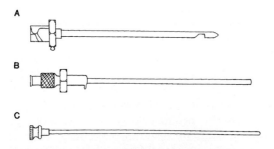

Figure 23.6. Abram's pleural biopsy needle. **A.** Large outer trocar. **B.** Inner cutting cannula. **C.** Stylet.

insertion of the biopsy needle without undue force. This incision should be made along the lines of cleavage to minimize postoperative scarring. The inner cutting cannula (Fig. 23.6*B*) fits tightly in the outer trocar (Fig. 23.6*A*) and can be locked in one of two positions: a closed position, in which the inner cannula obstructs the notch on the outer trocar to make the needle airtight; and an open position, in which the inner cannula is slightly withdrawn so that the notch on the outer trocar is not occluded. An indicator knob in the hexagonal grip of the larger outer trocar indicates the position of the notch in the distal end of the trocar.

To insert the Abram's pleural biopsy needle, the stylet is placed in the inner cannula, which in turn is placed in the outer trocar. The inner cannula (Fig. 23.6*B*) is twisted clockwise to close the distal notch of the outer trocar. The needle is pushed into the pleural space by exerting firm pressure on the stylet. Because the needle has a large diameter and is blunt, a substantial amount of pressure is needed. Usually, a "pop" is heard as the needle enters the pleural space. The inability to pass the needle into the pleural space is usually due to an insufficiently large skin incision. At times, the ribs are too close together to allow the needle to pass. In such situations, rotation of the patient's arm and shoulder over his/her head frequently separates the ribs sufficiently.

Once the tip of the needle is thought to be in the pleural space, the inner stylet (Fig. 23.6*C*) is removed, and with the inner cannula in the closed position, a syringe is attached to the connection on the inner cannula. Then, the inner cannula is rotated counterclockwise in the outer trocar so that the distal notch is locked open (Fig. 23.7*A*). At this time, pleural fluid may be aspirated for diagnostic studies. When the desired fluid has been obtained, the inner cannula of the needle is rotated clockwise to occlude the distal notch so that the syringe can be changed without creating a pneumothorax. A 10- to 20-ml syringe is then attached to the needle, and the inner cannula is rotated to open the distal notch. The entire needle is then rotated so that the knob on the outer trocar is inferior. The biopsy needle is then slowly withdrawn with constant aspiration until it hooks onto the pleura (Fig. 23.7*B*). When the needle hooks, one can be sure that

A

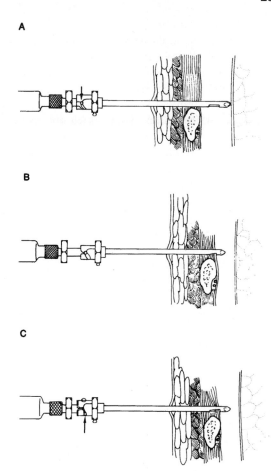

B

C

Figure 23.7A. Abram's needle in pleural space with notch open so that fluid can be aspirated. **B.** Abram's needle snagging the parietal pleura. **C.** The biopsy is obtained when the inner cutting cannula closes the notch in the outer trocar and shears off parietal pleura and anything else that remains in the notch. *Arrows* point to the pin on the inner cannula that locks into the outer trocar in either the open or closed position.

parietal pleura is in the notch of the needle if pleural fluid can still be aspirated through the syringe. When the needle is hooked on the pleura, the outer trocar is held firmly with one hand while the inner cannula is rotated into the closed position with the other hand to cut off a small piece of parietal pleura (Fig. 23.7*C*). Usually, mild resistance is met immediately before the needle is completely closed, and this resistance is due to the inner cannula's severing the entrapped pleura for the biopsy specimen.

Once the initial biopsy specimen is obtained, the needle can either be withdrawn from the pleural space in the closed position

or reinserted into the pleural space. If the needle is withdrawn from the chest, the pleural biopsy specimen is found in the tip of the needle and can be closely examined, but the needle then has to be reinserted. Reinsertions of the needle are through the same tract, however, and are easier than the original insertion. If the needle is reinserted into the pleural space without a complete withdrawal, the tissue specimen can be aspirated through the syringe. The biopsy procedure can be repeated without removing the biopsy needle. The difficulty in not withdrawing the needle is that the biopsy specimen sometimes becomes lodged in the syringe or is confused with a pleural fluid clot. I prefer to remove the pleural biopsy needle after obtaining each biopsy specimen. Whenever the Abram's pleural biopsy needle is withdrawn from the pleural space, the biopsy tract should be occluded with a finger immediately after the needle is withdrawn to decrease the likelihood of a pneumothorax.

At least four separate biopsy specimens should be obtained. Three of the four should be placed in formalin and taken to the pathology laboratory, and the fourth should be placed in a sterile tube and sent to the tuberculosis laboratory to be ground up and cultured for mycobacterium and fungus. Once the biopsy specimens are obtained, a therapeutic thoracentesis can be performed through the Abram's needle. The pleural fluid should be removed only after obtaining the biopsy specimens because the pleural fluid separates the parietal and visceral pleura and increases the safety of the procedure.

When the Abram's needle is withdrawn for the last time, a small adhesive bandage should be placed over the biopsy incision in a crosswise fashion to act as a butterfly-type dressing. The biopsy site should be massaged for a short time prior to placement of the bandage to eradicate the needle tract. Occasionally, pleural fluid exits or air enters through the biopsy tract after the procedure, particularly in patients who are debilitated and thin with poor tissue turgor. If this should happen, the biopsy site should be closed with a purse-string suture. Chest radiographs should be obtained on all patients after pleural biopsies.

Raja Needle

Since the last edition of this book, the Raja needle has been developed. The Raja needle is very similar in design to the Abram's needle except that it has a self-opening stainless steel biopsy flap mounted on the inner tube (22, 23). When the Raja needle is withdrawn from the pleural space, the biopsy flap catches the parietal pleural. In the hands of the inventor, the Raja needle provides larger biopsy specimens in the experimental situation (22). In addition, the developer has reported that there is a significantly higher diagnostic yield with the Raja needle compared with the Abram's needle (22). Until these findings are confirmed by investigators without a personal interest in the Raja needle, the Raja needle is not recommended.

Cope Needle

The Cope needle (Fig. 23.8) consists of four separate parts: a large outer cannula with a square but sharp end, a hollow, blunt-tipped, hooked biopsy trocar, a hollow-beveled trocar, and a solid, thin obturator or stylet. To insert the outer cannula (Fig. 23.8*A*) into the pleural space, the stylet (Fig. 23.8*D*) is inserted into the hollow-beveled trocar (Fig. 23.8*C*) which in turn is placed in the large outer cannula. Then, this apparatus is inserted through the small skin incision into the pleural space. The stylet and the hollow-beveled trocar must then be removed from the outer cannula and replaced by the hollow, blunt-tipped, hooked biopsy trocar (Fig. 23.8*B*). This maneuver is performed at the end of a normal expiration

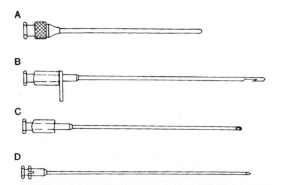

Figure 23.8. Cope pleural biopsy needle. **A.** Outer cannula. **B.** Hollow, blunt-tipped, hooked biopsy trocar. **C.** Hollow-beveled trocar. **D.** Obturator or stylet.

while the patient is holding his breath, by removing the hollow-beveled trocar and the stylet and by placing the operator's thumb over the end of the outer cannula to prevent a pneumothorax. A syringe may be attached to the outer cannula to obtain fluid for diagnostic studies at this time. Then, with the patient again holding his breath, the hooked biopsy trocar, to which a 10- to 20-ml syringe has been attached, is inserted through the large outer cannula into the pleural space. If a syringe is not attached to the hooked biopsy trocar, it should be occluded with a stopcock or the operator's thumb.

The right-angled projection on the proximal end of the hooked biopsy trocar indicates the direction of the distal biopsy hook. To obtain a biopsy, the apparatus is withdrawn with the hook directed inferiorly so as not to ensnare any nerves, veins, or arteries until the hooked biopsy trocar engages the parietal pleura (Fig. 23.9*A*). Then, with one hand, the engaged hook is held steady with a continual outward pulling motion, while the other hand advances the large outer cannula toward the pleural space using a rotary motion to sever the engaged piece of pleura (Fig. 23.9*B*). Then, the hooked biopsy trocar containing the tissue specimen is removed while the patient holds his breath, and is replaced with the beveled trocar and obturator before the procedure is repeated for an additional biopsy specimen. Once the required biopsy specimens have been obtained, a therapeutic thoracentesis may be performed by attaching a large syringe and a three-way stopcock to the outer cannula.

The biopsy site and the biopsy specimens are handled identically with both Abram's and Cope pleural biopsy needles.

Abram's versus Cope Needles

The rate of success in obtaining a pleural biopsy specimen depends more upon the skill of the operator than upon the choice of instruments (24). Morrone and associates obtained pleural biopsies simultaneously with the Abram's and Cope needles and reported that the diagnostic yields were virtually identical (25). The Abram's needle provided slightly larger specimens and was slightly superior in detecting mesothelial cells. The Cope needle provided larger specimens of intercostal

A

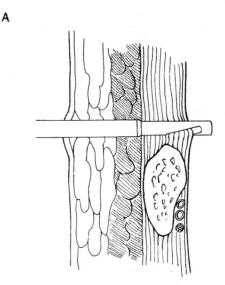

B

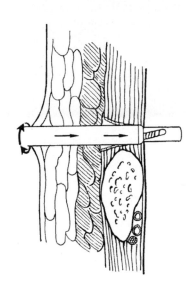

Figure 23.9A. The parietal pleura is hooked with the hollow, blunt-tipped biopsy trocar. **B.** The biopsy specimen is obtained by advancing the outer cannula with a rotary motion (*arrows*) to sever the engaged piece of pleura.

muscle. The Abram's needle is generally preferred over the Cope needle, however, because it is easier to use, it is a closed system and hence the likelihood of a pneumothorax is decreased, it provides a larger biopsy specimen, and it is safer for concomitant therapeutic thoracentesis because the end of the outer cannula is blunt.

Complications

Pleural biopsy has the same complications as diagnostic thoracentesis. One might expect pneumothorax to be more common with pleural biopsy than with thoracentesis for two reasons. First, the atmosphere has much more opportunity to be in communication with the pleural space with the biopsy, particularly when the Cope needle is used. Second, when the biopsy specimen is obtained, the visceral pleura may be inadvertently incised, leaving a small bronchopleural fistula that can lead to a large pneumothorax. The incidence of pneumothorax and the requirement for tube thoracostomy are comparable after thoracentesis and pleural biopsy, however (26). This is probably because more experienced individuals are performing the pleural biopsy.

The second major complication of pleural biopsy is bleeding. If an intercostal artery or vein is inadvertently biopsied, a hemothorax can result (21, 27). There is one case report of an arteriovenous fistula from an intercostal artery to an intercostal vein developing after pleural biopsy (28). The fistula subsequently ruptured, causing a hemothorax. The pleural biopsy needle can also be mistakenly inserted into the liver, spleen, or kidney. Even though hepatic or kidney tissue may be demonstrated in the biopsy specimen, the patient usually suffers no significant adverse effects. Penetration of the spleen frequently requires splenectomy (29), however, and one should therefore be careful not to perform pleural biopsy or thoracentesis too far inferiorly on the left side.

REFERENCES

1. Adams FV, Galati V: M-mode ultrasonic localization of pleural effusion. JAMA 1978;239:1761–1764.
2. McVay PA, Toy PT: Lack of increased bleeding after paracentesis and thoracentesis in patients with mild coagulation abnormalities. Transfusion 1991;31:164–171.
3. McCartney JP, Adams JW, Hazard PB: Safety of thoracentesis in mechanically ventilated patients. Chest 1993;103:1920–1921.
4. Godwin JE, Sahn SA: Thoracentesis: a safe procedure in mechanically ventilated patients. Ann Intern Med 1990;113:800–802.
5. Weingardt JP, Guico RR, Nemcek AA Jr, Li YP, Chiu ST: Ultrasound findings following failed, clinically directed thoracenteses. J Clin Ultrasound 1994;22:419–426.

6. Lipscomb DJ, Flower CDR, Hadfield JW: Ultrasound of the pleura: an assessment of its clinical value. Clin Radiol 1981;32:289–290.

7. Kohan JM, Poe RH, Israel RH, et al: Value of chest ultrasonography versus decubitus roentgenography for thoracentesis. Am Rev Respir Dis 1986;133:1124–1126.

8. Grogan DR, Irwin RS, Channick R, Raptopoulos V, Curley FJ, Bartter T, Corwin RW: Complications associated with thoracentesis. A prospective, randomized study comparing three different methods. Arch Intern Med 1990;150:873–877.

9. Rhodes ML: Thoracentesis. In: Jay SJ, Stonehill RB, eds. Manual of Pulmonary Procedure. Philadelphia: WB Saunders, 1980:1–11.

10. Peterman TA, Speicher CE: Evaluating pleural effusion: a two-stage laboratory approach. JAMA 1984;252:1051–1053.

11. Seneff MG, Corwin RW, Gold LH, Irwin RS: Complications associated with thoracocentesis. Chest 1986;90:97–100.

12. Collins TR, Sahn SA: Thoracocentesis: clinical value, complications, technical problems and patient experience. Chest 1987;91:817–822.

13. Bartter T, Mayo PD, Pratter MR, Santarelli RJ, Leeds WM, Akers SM: Lower risk and higher yield for thoracentesis when performed by experienced operators. Chest 1993;103:1873–1876.

14. Raptopoulos V, Davis LM, Lee G, Umali C, Lew R, Irwin RS: Factors affecting the development of pneumothorax associated with thoracentesis. AJR 1991;156:917–920.

15. Brandstetter RD, Karetzky M, Rastogi R, Lolis JD: Pneumothorax after thoracentesis in chronic obstructive pulmonary disease. Heart Lung 1994;23:67–70.

16. Kiblawi S: Pharmacologic agents. In: Jay SJ, Stonehill RB, eds. Manual of Pulmonary Procedures. Philadelphia: WB Saunders, 1980:83–101.

17. Carney M, Ravin CE: Intercostal artery laceration during thoracentesis. Increased risk in elderly patients. Chest 1979;75:520–521.

18. Oksenhendler E, Harzic M, Le Roux JM, et al: HIV infection with seroconversion after a superficial needlestick injury to the finger. N Engl J Med 1986;315:582.

19. Light RW, Jenkinson SG, Minh V, George RB: Observations on pleural pressures as fluid is withdrawn during thoracentesis. Am Rev Respir Dis 1980;121:799–804.

20. Light RW: Falsely high refractometric readings for the specific gravity of pleural fluid. Chest 1979;76:300–301.

21. Levine H, Cugell DW: Blunt-end needle biopsy of pleura and rib. Arch Intern Med 1971;109:516–525.

22. Ogirala RG, Agarwal V, Aldrich TK: Raja pleural biopsy needle. A comparison with the Abrams needle in experimental pleural effusion. Am Rev Respir Dis 1989;139:984–987.

23. Ogirala RG, Agarwal V, Vizioli LD, Pinsker KL, Aldrich TK: Comparison of the Raja and the Abrams pleural biopsy needles in patients with pleural effusion. Am Rev Respir Dis 1993;147:1291–1294.

24. Walsh LJ, Macfarlane JT, Manhire AR, Sheppard M, Jones JS: Audit of pleural biopsies: an argument for a pleural biopsy service. Respir Med 1994;88:503–505.

25. Morrone N, Algranti E, Barreto E: Pleural biopsy with Cope and Abram's needles. Chest 1987;92:1050–1052.

26. Poe RH, Israel RH, Utell MJ, et al: Sensitivity, specificity, and predictive values of closed pleural biopsy. Arch Intern Med 1984;144:325–328.

27. Ali J, Summer WR: Hemothorax and hyperkalemia after pleural biopsy in a 43-year-old woman on hemodialysis. Chest 1994;106:1235–1236.

28. Lai JH, Yan HC, Kao SJ, Lee SC, Shen CY: Intercostal arteriovenous fistula due to pleural biopsy. Thorax 1990;45:976–978.

29. Mearns AJ: Iatrogenic rupture of the spleen. Br Med J 1973;1:395–396.

CHAPTER 24
Chest Tubes

Chest tubes are frequently used in the practice of pulmonary medicine, but many physicians do not appear to understand how the drainage system for chest tubes functions and how to troubleshoot problems with chest tubes. In this chapter, the various methods of inserting chest tubes are discussed, followed by a more in-depth discussion of the different drainage systems used with chest tubes, as well as recommendations for troubleshooting-related problems. The indications for chest tube insertion with pneumothorax, hemothorax, empyema, and malignant pleural effusion are discussed in the respective chapters on these entities.

CHEST TUBE INSERTION

In general, chest tubes are inserted into the pleural space by three methods: tube thoracostomy with a guidewire and dilators, tube thoracostomy with a trocar, and operative tube thoracostomy. If the chest tube is inserted to drain blood, pus, or another fluid from the pleural space, the patient should be seated when the tube is inserted to ensure that the diaphragm is in the most dependent position and the fluid is collected in the lower part of the chest. When an anterior chest tube is placed for a pneumothorax, the patient should be recumbent, whereas if the chest tube is placed in the axillary line, the patient should be in the decubitus position.

Guidewire Tube Thoracostomy

This is probably the easiest way to insert a chest tube. Commercial kits are available for guidewire tube thoracostomy. This procedure uses the Seldinger technique with guidewires and dilators (1). In general, after the skin, periosteum, and parietal pleura are anesthetized as is done for pleural biopsy (Chapter 23), an incision is made in the skin that is ample to permit passage of the desired size chest tube (Fig. 24.1*A*). Then an 18-gauge needle attached to a syringe is introduced into the pleural space. Fluid or air is aspirated to confirm the intrapleural position (Fig. 24.1*B*). The syringe is removed and the "J" wire is threaded through the needle in the desired direction into the pleural space. The needle is then removed and more local anesthetic is injected into the intercostal muscles surrounding the wire (Fig. 24.1*C*). The smallest dilator is inserted and with a rotating movement is advanced into the pleural space over the guidewire (Fig. 24.1*D*). The wire should always project out beyond the end of the dilator or inserter. The first dilator is removed. Leaving the wire in place, the next size dilator is advanced over the guidewire into the pleural space and removed. Finally, the chest tube containing the inserter is threaded over the guidewire (Fig 24.1*E*). The tube should readily pass, following the path that is made by the dilators and guided by the wire (1).

Once the tube is in place, the inserter and the guidewire are withdrawn (Fig 24.1*F*). The tube is then clamped until it is attached to the chest drainage system. The tube is anchored in place by means of a long suture through the skin and around the tube. The incision is sutured without tension to avoid necrosis of the skin next to the tube. The operative area is cleaned and is covered with plain 4×4 gauze pads. The gauze is then covered with tape, and additional fixation of the tube is obtained by the tape.

There are many different types of chest tubes that can be inserted with the above technique. Kits are made so that chest tubes from 8.0 to 36.0 French can be inserted. The kits with the smaller chest tubes (less than 12 French) have no dilators. Some of the catheters have different characteristics. For example, with the Wayne Pneumothorax Set (Cook Critical Care) a 14.0 French catheter is inserted over a 19-gauge needle; the catheter with this set is curved at the end like a pig's tail, and hence the name pigtail catheter.

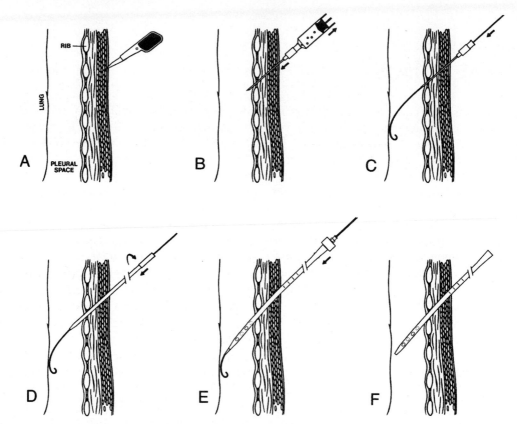

Figure 24.1. Guidewire tube thoracostomy. **A.** Making a small skin incision slightly larger than the diameter of the chest tube. **B.** Introduction of 18-gauge needle into the pleural space. **C.** Insertion of wire with "J" end into the pleural space. **D.** With guidewire in place, the tract is enlarged by advancing progressively larger dilators over the wire guide. Introduction of the dilators is facilitated by rotating and advancing the dilators in the same plane of the wire guide. **E.** Introduction of the chest tube inserter/chest tube assembly over the guidewire. **F.** Guidewire and the chest tube inserter have been removed, leaving the chest tube positioned within the pleural space.

Trocar Tube Thoracostomy

This method is similar to the guidewire tube thoracostomy, except that there are no guidewire and no dilators. In general, it is not recommended. This method initially requires a 2- to 4-cm incision parallel to the superior border of the rib through the skin and subcutaneous tissues after local anesthesia is obtained. The trocar can then be inserted between the ribs into the pleural cavity, with the flat edge of the stylet tip cephalad to prevent damage to the intercostal vessels (Fig. 24.2*A*). Because significant force is often required to insert the trocar, the hand not applying the force should be placed next to the patient's chest wall to control the depth of penetration. Once the trocar is in the pleural space, the stylet is removed, and the operator should immediately cover the trocar with his thumb to prevent a pneumothorax. Then, the chest tube, with its distal end clamped, is quickly inserted into the pleural space as the operator's thumb is removed (Fig. 24.2*B*). The trocar is removed by sliding it back over the tube. When the trocar has been removed from the chest, the chest tube is clamped between the trocar and the chest wall so that the clamp on the distal end of the chest tube can be removed. This maneuver allows the trocar to be withdrawn from around the tube. The chest tube must remain clamped until it is attached to an underwater seal to prevent air from entering the pleural space.

The chest tube is managed identically to that with the guidewire tube thoracostomy as described above.

An alternate trocar method uses a chest tube with a trocar positioned inside the tube.

A

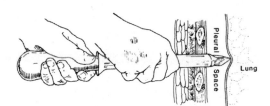

B

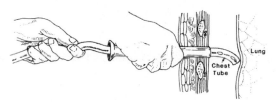

Figure 24.2. Trocar tube thoracostomy. **A.** Insertion of trocar into the pleural space. Note the position of the hands, the position of the trocar relative to the ribs, and the cephalad position of the flat edge of the trocar. **B.** Insertion of chest tube through the trocar.

The procedure with this apparatus is similar to that already detailed. Once the pleural cavity is entered, the inner trocar is gradually removed from the chest tube. When the proximal end of the trocar clears the chest wall, a clamp is placed between the trocar and the chest wall until the trocar can be completely withdrawn and the tube attached to a water-seal drainage system.

Operative Tube Thoracostomy

With this method, the incision, coupled with blunt dissection with the hemostat, allows the operator to place his finger into the pleural space, to break adhesions between the lung and chest wall, and to ascertain the position of the chest tube. It is a more extensive procedure than trocar tube thoracostomy, but it is probably safer. The most serious complications of tube thoracostomy are insertion of the tube ectopically, namely, into the lung, stomach, spleen, liver, or heart. These complications are more likely when a trocar chest tube is used. With the operative method, digital exploration of the insertion site delineates whether the tract leads into the pleural space and whether any tissue or organ is adherent to the parietal pleura at the planned site of tube insertion (2).

A 3- to 4-cm incision is made in the skin parallel to the chosen intercostal space. The incision should be made down to the fascia overlying the intercostal muscle. This fascia is then incised throughout the length of the incision, with care taken not to cut the muscle. Once the fascia has been incised, the muscle fibers are spread with a blunt-tipped hemostat until the intercostal interspace is identified. Then, an incision is made in the intercostal fascia just above the superior border of the inferior rib over which the tube will pass. The parietal pleura is then penetrated by pushing a blunt-tipped hemostat through it. The hole in the parietal pleura is then enlarged by means of the operator's index finger (Fig. 24.3A). At this time, the operator should palpate the adjacent pleural space to detect any adhesions. Then, the chest tube with its distal end clamped is inserted into the pleural space. A hemostat is used to guide the tube into the pleural space as the operator's finger is withdrawn (Fig. 24.3B). The last hole in the chest tube should be at least 2 cm inside the pleural space. The tube is sutured in place, and the incision is cleaned as in guidewire tube thoracostomy.

Interestingly, the chest tubes frequently end up in the fissures, even with operative tube thoracostomy. Curtin and associates reviewed the posteroanterior (PA) and lateral chest radiographs in 50 patients who had 66 chest tubes placed in the emergency room for trauma. They reported that 38 of the 66 chest tubes (58%) were within a fissure. There was no evidence, however, that the presence of the tube within the fissure decreased its functional effectiveness (3).

PLEURAL DRAINAGE SYSTEMS

Chest tubes are inserted into the pleural space in order to evacuate air or fluid. Because the pleural pressure is usually negative, at least during part of the respiratory cycle, various methods have been developed to prevent air from entering the pleural space when the pleural pressure is negative, but to permit air and fluid to drain from the pleural space continuously. When managing patients with

A

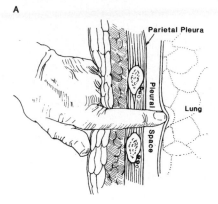

B

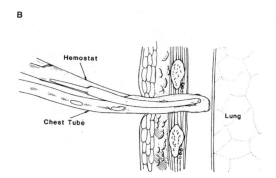

Figure 24.3. Operative tube thoracostomy. **A.** The physician's index finger is used to enlarge the opening and to explore the pleural space. **B.** Placement of chest tube intrapleurally using a large hemostat.

chest tubes, one must understand how these various drainage systems operate. In the past, the bottle system (described below) was used for pleural drainage. Commercially manufactured collection systems subsequently replaced the bottle system. Nevertheless, the bottle system is described in detail because all the commercially manufactured systems are based on the same principles as the bottle system.

One-Way (Heimlich) Valve

This drainage system is by far the simplest. The chest tube is attached to a one-way flutter valve assembly, which is constructed so that the flexible tubing is occluded whenever the pressure inside the tubing is less than atmospheric pressure and is patent whenever the pressure inside the tubing is above atmospheric pressure. Therefore, when the pleural pressure, and hence the pressure in the tube, are negative (Fig. 24.4A), the flutter valve is closed, and no air enters the pleural space. When the pleural pressure becomes positive (Fig. 24.4B), however, the tube is patent, and air or fluid can egress from the pleural space. This drainage system is only useful when the chest tube is placed for pneumothorax because with it there is no good manner by which fluid, blood, or pus can be collected. The main advantages of the flutter valve are its simplicity and the freedom of the patient from a bulky drainage apparatus. When using the Heimlich valve, it is important to attach it with the correct orientation. Cases have been reported where tension pneumothorax developed because the Heimlich valve was attached backward (4).

A

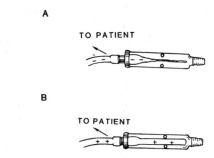

TO PATIENT

B

TO PATIENT

Figure 24.4. Heimlich valve. **A.** When the pleural pressure, and hence the intratube pressure, is negative (inspiration), the flexible tube is occluded because the pressure outside the tube is greater than the pressure inside the tube. **B.** When the pleural pressure is positive (expiration), the flexible tube is held open by the positive pressure allowing the egress of air from the pleural space.

One-Bottle Collection System

This system consists of one bottle that serves as both a collection container and a water seal (Fig. 24.5). The chest tube is connected to a rigid straw inserted through a stopper into a sterile bottle. Enough sterile saline solution is instilled into the bottle so that the tip of the rigid straw is about 2 cm below the surface of the saline solution. The bottle's stopper must have a vent to prevent pressure from building up when air or fluid coming from the pleural space enters the bottle. The bottle usually is provided with a cap on the vent, and it is crucial to remove this cap before the system is connected to the patient.

This system works as follows. When the pleural pressure is positive, the pressure in the rigid straw becomes positive, and if the pres-

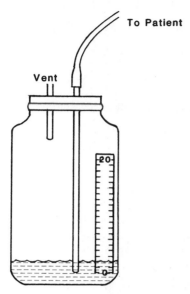

Figure 24.5. One-bottle collection system. See text for details.

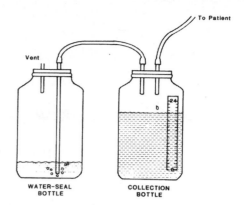

Figure 24.6. Two-bottle collection system. See text for details.

sure inside the rigid straw is greater than the depth to which the straw is inserted into the saline solution, air (or liquid) will enter the bottle and will be vented to the atmosphere. If the pleural pressure is negative, fluid will be drawn from the bottle into the rigid straw, and no extra air will enter the system of the pleural space and the rigid straw. This system is called a **water seal** because the water in the bottle seals the pleural space from air or fluid from outside the body. Obviously, if the straw is above the fluid level in the bottle, the system will not operate, and a large pneumothorax will develop.

This one-bottle system works well for uncomplicated pneumothorax. If substantial amounts of pleural fluid are draining from the patient's pleural space, however, the level of fluid will rise in the one-bottle system, and therefore, the pressure will have to be greater in the rigid straw to allow additional air or fluid to exit from the pleural space. Another disadvantage of this system is that if the bottle is inadvertently placed above the level of the patient's chest, fluid can run back into the pleural cavity.

Two-Bottle Collection System

This system (Fig. 24.6) is preferred over the one-bottle collection system when substantial amounts of liquid are draining from the pleural space. With this system, the bottle adjacent to the patient acts as a **collection bottle** for the drainage, and the second bottle provides the water seal and the air vent. Therefore, the degree of water seal does not increase as the drainage accumulates. The water-seal bottle functions identically in both one- and two-bottle systems.

Suction and Three-Bottle Collection Systems

At times, it is desirable to apply negative pressure to the pleural space in order to facilitate re-expansion of the underlying lung or to expedite the removal of air or fluid from the pleural space. Suction at a fixed level, usually -15 to -20 cm H_2O, can be applied to the vent on a one- or two-bottle collection system with an Emerson pump. In many facilities, however, suction is provided by wall suction or other pumps in which the level of suction is not easily controlled. Because uncontrolled high levels of suction are considered dangerous, it is necessary to have some means of controlling the amount of suction.

Controlled amounts of suction can be readily applied to the system if a third **suction control** bottle is added to the system, as illustrated in Figure 24.7. A vent on the suction control bottle is connected to a vent on the water-seal bottle. The suction control bottle has a rigid straw similar to that of the water-seal bottle. The suction is connected to a second vent on the suction control bottle. When suction is applied to the suction control bottle, air enters this bottle through its rigid straw if the pressure in the bottle is more

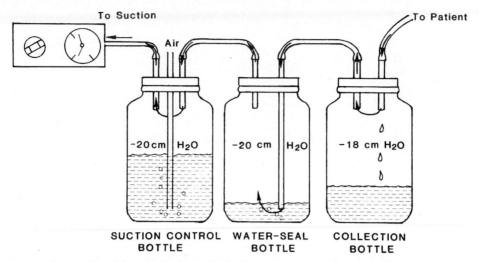

Figure 24.7. Three-bottle collection system. *Arrows* describe the pathway for air to leave the pleural space. See text for details.

negative than the depth to which the straw is submerged. Therefore, the amount of negative pressure in the system is equal to the depth to which the rigid straw in the suction control bottle is submerged below the surface as long as bubbles are entering the suction control bottle through its rigid straw. In the example in Figure 24.7, air enters the suction control bottle from the atmosphere and its rigid straw is submerged in 20 cm H_2O. Therefore, the pressure in the suction control bottle is −20 cm H_2O. The same pressure exists in the water-seal bottle because these two bottles are in direct communication. The pressure in the drainage collection bottle is less negative than that in the other bottles, however, on account of the intervening water seal. In this case, the depth of the water seal is 2 cm, so the pressure in the drainage collection bottle and the pleural space (if no liquid is present in the chest tube) is −18 cm H_2O.

The amount of negative pressure in the system can be changed by adjusting the position of the rigid straw in the suction control bottle or by changing the depth of the water in the suction control bottle. Bubbles must come continuously from the bottom of the suction control straw if one is to have the expected degree of suction. The bubbling does not need to be vigorous, just continuous; vigorous bubbling only creates more noise and hastens evaporation of the saline solution in the control bottle.

Intrinsic Negative Pressure in Chest Tubes

The presence of liquid in the chest tubes can markedly influence the negative pressure that is applied to the pleural space, as illustrated in Figure 24.8. The liquid in the tube that runs from the patient to the floor basically produces the effects of a siphon (5, 6). If the distance from the patient's chest to the top of the collection apparatus is 50 cm and the tube is filled with liquid, there will be a negative pressure of 50 cm H_2O in the pleural space if no suction is applied. The actual negative pressure applied to the pleural space from the entire system is the net vertical distance that the liquid occupies in the tube ($A − B$) minus the level of fluid in the water seal (C) plus the negative pressure applied via the suction (D). Of course, if there is no liquid in the tube, the actual applied pressure will be the suction pressure minus the depth of the water seal.

COMMERCIALLY AVAILABLE DRAINAGE SYSTEMS

As can be appreciated from Figure 24.7, three-bottle systems are unhandy to set up and are cumbersome to move if the patient needs to be transported. Therefore, a number of more compact and convenient chest drainage units are commercially available. The main disadvantage of these units is that they are more expensive than the older systems. The

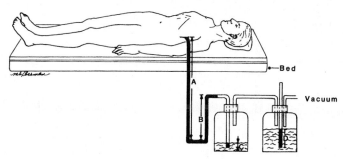

Figure 24.8. The presence of liquid in the tube can affect the amount of negative pressure applied to the pleural space. The actual negative pressure in the chest = $A - B - C + D$.

average cost is about $75. The most popular system is a one-piece disposable, molded plastic unit called the Pleur-Evac. Other available systems include the Atrium Total Recovery Water-Seal Chest Drains, Sentinel Seal, the Thora-Klex, Argyle Double-Seal unit, and the Compact 2002. An acceptable drainage system should have the following characteristics: (*a*) the water seal should be easily visualized, so one can determine whether the chest tube is patent and whether a bronchopleural fistula is present; (*b*) the tube should be functional when no suction is applied; (*c*) the volume of the collection chamber should be adequate and the markings should be such that the drainage is easily quantitated; and (*d*) there should be a pop-off valve to provide a safety factor if pressure builds up in the system. If the patient has a large amount of blood in the pleural space, consideration should be given to using a unit with autotransfusion capabilities such as the Atrium Blood Recovery Water-Seal Chest Drain or the Davo Thora-Klex Chest Drainage System with Autotransfusion.

Pleur-Evac Unit

The Pleur-Evac system is a disposable, molded plastic unit with three chambers duplicating the classic three-bottle system (Fig. 24.9). The chamber to the right is equivalent to the drainage collection bottle, whereas the middle chamber is equivalent to the water-seal bottle, and the chamber on the left is equivalent to the suction control bottle. The height of water in the suction control chamber minus the height of water in the water-seal compartment again determines the amount of pressure applied to the pleural space when suction is being applied. A valve located in the water-

seal portion of the Pleur-Evac unit also vents air whenever the pressure in the system is greater than +2 cm H_2O.

The advantages of the Pleur-Evac unit are that it is simple to use, the amount of drainage can be easily measured, and the amount of negative pressure can be easily controlled. If the suction rate is turned up too high, the fluid will evaporate from the suction control chamber, and the system will be exceedingly noisy. If no suction is applied and the suction port is vented to room air, the system functions as a two-bottle collection system. When the patient is not receiving suction, the patency of the chest tube can be assessed by observing oscillations in the water-seal chamber with respiratory movements. In addition, if the patient is not receiving suction, the pressure in the chest tube can be calculated as the difference in the level of water in the two arms of the water-seal chamber.

Other Chest Drainage Systems

Most of the other commercially available units are similar in design to the Pleur-Evac unit. Autotransfusion can be performed with the Atrium Blood Recovery Water-Seal Chest Drain or the Davo Thora-Klex Chest Drainage System with Autotransfusion. The Thora-Klex Chest Drainage System is somewhat unique in that it does not require water for either the water seal or the suction control. For the water seal, this system uses a one-way valve rather than a water seal and there is a relatively large chamber in which air leaks can be observed. The suction can be set between 0 and 40 cm H_2O with a suction control knob. The advantage of this system is that one need

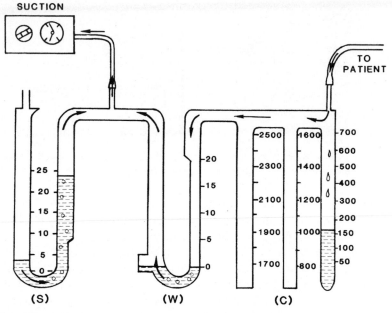

Figure 24.9. Pleur-Evac collection system, analogous to a three-bottle collection system. *C*, calibrated collection system; *W*, water-seal chamber; *S*, suction control chamber. *Arrows* demonstrate the pathway for air to leave the pleural space. If the suction vent is left open to atmospheric pressure, the Pleur-Evac system functions as a two-bottle collection system. When suction is applied, atmospheric air enters through *S* and leaves through the suction apparatus.

not worry about it tipping over, since it contains no water.

INJECTION OF MATERIALS THROUGH CHEST TUBES

There are circumstances in which one would like to inject various materials through the chest tubes. For example, one might want to inject urokinase or streptokinase through the chest tube in a patient with a complicated parapneumonic effusion, or one might want to inject talc in a slurry or a tetracycline derivative through the chest tube in a patient with a malignant pleural effusion. This is usually done by taking the chest tube apart and injecting the material through a Toomey syringe. This procedure is less than ideal since the sterility of the system is compromised if the tubes are disconnected, and there is always the possibility of a pneumothorax if the tubes are not clamped properly.

There is a commercially available adapter called a Thal-Quick Chest Tube Adapter (Cook Critical Care, Bloomington, IN) that will fit in any chest tube. This unit (Fig. 24.10) consists

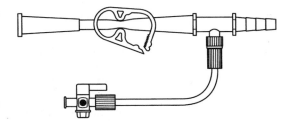

Figure 24.10. Thal-Quick Chest Tube Adapter. This adapter provides an easy means by which materials can be injected into the pleural space through chest tubes. See text for details.

of two adapters separated by flexible tubing with a clamp. On the proximal end there is a side port with a short segment of connecting tubing to which is attached a three-way stopcock. When one wishes to inject anything through the chest tube, the tube is clamped and the material is injected via the three-way stopcock.

CARE OF A CHEST TUBE

The following three questions should be answered each time the condition of a patient with a chest tube is evaluated:

1. Is there bubbling through the water-seal bottle or the water-seal chamber on the disposable unit?
2. Is the tube functioning?
3. What is the amount and type of drainage from the tube?

Bubbling Through Water-Seal Chamber

If air bubbles are escaping through the water seal, it means that air is entering the chest tube between the pleural space and the water seal. If the patient is receiving water-seal drainage without suction, the presence of bubbling in the water seal usually indicates a persistent air leak from the lung into the pleural space. If no air bubbles are seen on the initial inspection of the water seal, the patient should be asked to cough, and the water seal should be observed for bubbling. The coughing maneuver increases the patient's pleural pressure and should demonstrate small air leaks into the pleural space.

If the patient is receiving suction, disconnection or partial disconnection anywhere between the water seal and the patient will lead to bubbling through the water seal. For example, if the cap on the collection bottle in Figure 24.7 is not airtight, air will be pulled into the collection bottle by the negative pressure and will exit through the water-seal bottle, producing bubbling. Leaks in the system may be detected by clamping the chest tube at the point where it exits from the chest. If bubbling through the water seal persists, the drainage system itself is responsible for the leak, and the system should be examined thoroughly for leaks. If the bubbling stops when the chest tube is clamped, then the air is coming from the pleural space.

The presence of bubbling through the water seal does not necessarily indicate a communication between the lung and the pleural space. If the chest tube is not inserted far enough into the pleural space, one or more of the holes in the chest tube may lie outside the pleural space. Obviously, in such a situation, air enters the chest tube directly from the atmosphere. The possibility is evaluated by inspecting the chest tube. At times, particularly in debilitated patients with poor tissue turgor, air leaks into the pleural space around the chest tube insertion site. At times it may be difficult to tell whether the air is leaking around the chest tube or whether it is due to a bronchopleural fistula. One may make this differentiation by measuring the level of P_{CO_2} in the air coming from the chest tube. The air from the chest tube is collected in a syringe and analyzed with the regular blood gas analyzer. Usually a simple modification must be made on the analyzer so that it can analyze gas rather than liquid. If the air came from the lung via a bronchopleural fistula, then the P_{CO_2} should be greater than 20 mm Hg. Alternatively, if the air leaked around the chest tube, it will not have participated in gas exchange in the lung, and the P_{CO_2} should be less than 10 mm Hg. In such patients, additional sutures are necessary to make the chest tube insertion site airtight.

Bubbling through the water-seal chamber should not be confused with bubbling through the suction control chamber. If suction is working properly, bubbling through the suction control chamber or the suction control bottle will always be present.

Is The Chest Tube Functioning?

Each time the condition of a patient with a chest tube is evaluated, the functional status of the chest tube itself should be evaluated. If the patient is not receiving suction, one should observe the level of the liquid in the water seal. If the chest tube is patent and in the pleural space, the level of the liquid should rise in the tube on inspiration when the pleural pressure is more negative and should fall on expiration. When no fluctuations are observed with spontaneous respiration, the patient should be asked to make a maximal inspiratory effort, and if still no movement is observed, the chest tube is not functioning.

When the patient is receiving suction, it may be more difficult to ascertain chest tube function. If large bubbles of air are entering the suction control chamber, the level of liquid in the water-seal chamber will fluctuate, depending on the number and size of bubbles in the chamber. These fluctuations should not be mistaken for evidence that the tube is functional. When the patient is receiving suction, the negative pressure in the suction control chamber should be transmitted to the pleural space continuously to keep the pleural pressure constant. Therefore, to detect changes in pleural pressures with respiration, the suction must be temporarily discontinued. When suction is discontinued, the volume of air and liquid between the water seal and the pleural space should not change, and therefore, the level of liquid in the water-seal chamber should rise to be equivalent to the suction previously applied. This initial rise occurs whether or not the chest tube is patent, but respiratory fluctuations should occur in the level of the fluid in the water-seal chamber only if the chest tube is patent.

If a chest tube is not functioning, its functional status should be restored, or it should be removed. The patency of a chest tube obstructed by clots in the extrathoracic portion of the tube can frequently be restored by "stripping" the tube. The usual technique is to grip and stabilize the tubing adjacent to the chest with the thumb and index finger of one hand and then to slide the other hand toward the drainage unit to compress a section of the tubing. Then, the first hand is repositioned adjacent to the second hand, and the procedure is repeated until the entire length of the tubing is cleared. A special chest tube roller is sometimes used. Stripping may relieve the obstruction in the tube. An alternate strategy is to instill the fibrinolytic enzyme streptokinase into the chest tube. The utility of streptokinase in clearing obstructed peritoneal catheters has been documented. The instillation of 250,000 IU streptokinase successfully relieved the obstruction in 13 of 19 episodes of catheter failure (7). In my hands, the injection of streptokinase into chest tubes successfully unplugged the tubes in three of four patients.

Chest tubes that are no longer patent and are no longer draining fluid should be removed because they serve as conduits for bacterial infection of the pleural space. In general, it is not advisable to inject air or liquid through the chest tube into the pleural space in an effort to restore the patency of the tube. Chest tubes frequently become colonized with bacteria, and when the tube becomes obstructed with a clot, the clot may well contain bacteria. Pleural infection is likely if these clots are forced back into the pleural space. At times, chest tubes function only intermittently in that pleural drainage continues to accumulate, but the chest tube does not always appear to be patent. In such situations, the chest tubes need not be removed.

Amount and Type of Drainage

The amount and the character of the drainage from the chest tube should be recorded for each 24-hour period. The amount of drainage is most easily quantitated by marking the level of the liquid in the collection chamber each day. This record keeping is important because many therapeutic decisions are based on the quantity of the drainage. The character of the drainage is best described by quantitating the percentage of solid drainage material. This quantitation is easily done by marking the level of the sediment in the collection chamber each day. If the increase in volume of the entire collection system is known and if the increase in volume of the solid sediment is known, it is simple to calculate what percentage of the daily drainage is solid.

COMPLICATIONS OF TUBE THORACOSTOMY

There are numerous complications of tube thoracostomy. Many of the complications occur when the tube is first inserted and include insertion of the chest tube into the lung, stomach, spleen, liver, or heart (2). These complications occur very rarely and are more likely when a trocar chest tube is used or when the tube is inserted before digital exploration of the insertion site is performed to determine whether indeed the tract leads into the pleural space. There is one case report where a patient developed reversible cardiogenic shock due to chest tube compression of the right ventricle (8). There is another report of two patients that developed tension pneumothoraces because the Heimlich valves were hooked up backward to the chest tube (4).

Pleural infection is another complication of tube thoracostomy. The administration of antibiotics to patients who have chest tubes for thoracic trauma may decrease the prevalence of empyema. Brunner and coworkers randomly allocated 90 such patients to receive cefazolin or nothing immediately before and then every 6 hours until tube removal. They reported that there were six empyemas and three pneumonias in the control group but only one pneumonia and no empyema in the antibiotic group (9). In a later study, Nichols and coworkers administered placebo or 1 g cefonicid daily to 119 patients requiring chest tubes for thoracic trauma and reported that four patients got empyema in the placebo group and no patient got empyema in the antibiotic group (10).

The insertion of a chest tube creates inflammation in the pleural space. Carvalho and associates (11) studied the pleural fluid characteristics of sheep with an experimental pleural effusion and an Argyle 32-Fr tube in the pleural space. The white count in the pleural effusion increased from 125 to over 6000/mm^3 within 6 hours. In this model the pleural fluid protein level increased from 0 to 3.7 g/dl by 48 hours and the pleural fluid lactate dehydrogenase increased from 44 IU/L to 638 IU/L by 24 hours.

AUTOTRANSFUSION

Autotransfusion involves the collection, filtration, and reinfusion of the patient's shed blood for repletion of intravascular volume and the diminution of transfusion requirements. Postoperative patients with chest tubes and patients with hemothorax should be considered as candidates for autotransfusion. Several autotransfusion systems are commercially available. Atrium Medical Corporation manufactures a system capable of continuous infusion.

CHEST TUBE REMOVAL

The indications for the discontinuance of the tube thoracostomy for various conditions are discussed in the respective chapters on these conditions. In general, chest tubes for pneumothorax are removed when the lung has re-expanded and no air leaks are present. Chest tubes for hemothorax and empyema are removed when pleural drainage of blood or pus, respectively, has ceased.

Before chest tube removal is attempted, the procedure should be explained to the patient.

In addition, petrolatum-impregnated gauze and an occlusive bandage should be prepared for use in a sterile field. Then, the dressing covering the thoracostomy site is removed, and the suture restraining the chest tube is cut. Petrolatum-impregnated gauze is placed around the tube on the patient's chest wall so that it can be moved to cover the wound when the tube is removed. Then, while the patient performs a Valsalva maneuver in order to create positive pleural pressure and to decrease the likelihood that air may enter the pleural space, the tube is quickly pulled out of the chest, and the wound is covered immediately with the gauze. The wound usually closes sufficiently without using sutures. The procedure is completed by placing an occlusive dressing over the gauze.

REFERENCES

1. Thal AP, Quick KL: A guided chest tube for safe thoracostomy. Surg Gyn Obstet 1988;167:517.
2. Symbas PN: Chest drainage tubes. Surg Clin North Am 1989;69:41–46.
3. Curtin JJ, Goodman LR, Quebbeman EJ, Haasler GB: Thoracostomy tubes after acute chest injury: relationship between location in a pleural fissure and function. AJR 1994;163:1339–1942.
4. Mainini SE, Johnson FE: Tension pneumothorax complicating small-caliber chest tube insertion. Chest 1990;97:759–760.
5. Enerson DM, McIntyre J: A comparative study of the physiology and physics of pleural drainage systems. J Thorac Cardiovasc Surg 1966;52:40–46.
6. Kam AC, O'Brien M, Kam PC: Pleural drainage systems. Anaesthesia 1993;48:154–161.
7. Wiegmann TB, Stuewe B, Duncan KA, Chonko A, Diederich DA, Grantham JJ, Savin VJ, MacDougall ML: Effective use of streptokinase for peritoneal catheter failure. Am J Kid Dis 1985;6:119–123.
8. Kollef MH, Dothager DW: Reversible cardiogenic shock due to chest tube compression of the right ventricle. Chest 1991;99:976–980.
9. Brunner RG, Vinsant GO, Alexander RH, Laneve L, Fallon WF Jr: The role of antibiotic therapy in the prevention of empyema in patients with an isolated chest injury (ISS 9-10): a prospective study. J Trauma 1990;30:1148–1153.
10. Nichols RL, Smith JW, Muzik AC, Love EJ, McSwain NE, Timberlake G, Flint LM: Preventive antibiotic usage in traumatic thoracic injuries requiring closed tube thoracostomy. Chest 1994;106:1493–1498.
11. Carvalho P, Kirk W, Butler J, Charan NB: Effects of tube thoracostomy on pleural fluid characteristics in sheep. J Appl Physiol 1993;74:2782–2787.

CHAPTER 25
Thoracoscopy

Although thoracoscopy has been a part of thoracic surgical practice for many years, the advent of video-assisted techniques has greatly expanded the indications and the uses of this procedure. Where previously, thoracoscopy was performed mainly for diagnostic purposes, video-assisted thoracic surgery (VATS) now has assumed a major role in the therapy of chest pathology. Indeed in some institutions it is now the most commonly used operative approach in general thoracic surgical practices (1). The primary advantage of VATS is that it produces less morbidity and mortality and shorter hospitalization times than does thoracotomy. Presently VATS is used for many surgical procedures in the chest other than those related to pleural disease including pulmonary nodule removal, lobectomy, lung biopsy, exploration of the mediastinum, myotomy for achalasia, sympathectomy, and pericardial window creation. In this chapter we will only discuss those procedures that deal with pleural disease. We will use the term videothoracoscopy to refer to VATS throughout this chapter.

HISTORY

Thoracoscopy was developed by Jacobaeus in the early 1900s because a method was needed to break down adhesions in patients with pulmonary tuberculosis, so that an artificial pneumothorax could be produced (2). Thoracoscopy was used extensively for this purpose up until 1945, at which time streptomycin was introduced for the treatment of tuberculosis (3). In one report the results in 1000 cases where thoracoscopy was used to break down adhesions were detailed (4). Jacobaeus also published an early report on the use of thoracoscopy to localize and diagnose benign and malignant lesions of the pleura and pulmonary parenchyma (5).

After 1950 thoracoscopy was rarely performed in the United States, although some physicians in Europe continued to perform the procedure. During this period thoracoscopy was used primarily to assist in diagnosing undiagnosed pleural effusions, although pleurodesis was sometimes attempted with talc (6, 7) or silver nitrate (8, 9). A number of instruments were employed including rigid bronchoscopes, mediastinoscopes, flexible bronchoscopes, and specialized rigid fiberoptic thoracoscopes (10). Two books published in the past 10 years provide state-of-the-art discussions on thoracoscopy before the advent of VATS (11, 12).

The recent revival of thoracoscopy was made possible by the tremendous advances in endoscopic technology (13). The development of the charged coupling device, a silicon chip that is light sensitive, led to the sufficient miniaturization of a video camera. When attached to a fiberoptic telescope, the video camera produces a well-defined, magnified image on a video monitor that allows the operating surgeon to work with an assistant. Previously, the surgeon had to hold the thoracoscope, and only he was able to look into it while working, which did not allow for the aid of an assistant and thus, limited the complexity of the procedure (10).

PROCEDURE

Most VATS procedures are done under general anesthesia so that endoscopic surgical manipulation can be done safely and expeditiously (1). It is imperative that the anesthesia personnel be experienced in open thoracic procedures. In addition, they must be well-versed with the principles of selective one-lung ventilation. Ventilation for the patient is provided via the contralateral lung. It is most convenient to work with two video monitors, one on each side, so that both the operator and the assistant may have an unobstructed view.

The patient is placed on the operating table and the chest is prepared and draped as for a thoracotomy. After general anesthesia is induced, the thoracoscope is inserted and the ipsilateral lung collapsed for unimpaired visibility of the intrathoracic structures. At this time the thoracic cavity is systematically examined. After the initial thoracoscopic exploration of the pleural cavity is concluded, further intercostal access for VATS instrumentation is achieved under direct thoracoscopic vision. Usually three incisions are made to create a triangular configuration, an arrangement that facilitates instrument placement and allows one to work in coordination with an assistant. The incisions are placed along a line of the proposed thoracotomy incision so that if a thoracotomy is required, the incisions simply are joined. At the completion of the VATS procedure, a single chest tube is placed into the pleural space.

Instrumentation for videothoracoscopy is slowly improving. Initially, instruments designed for laparoscopy were used but were less than ideal, particularly for grasping lung parenchyma, which has a tendency to tear. The most significant advance in instrumentation was the development of an endoscopic linear stapler, which simultaneously cuts while laying down parallel rows of staples that are both hemostatic and aerostatic (Endo:GIA, U.S. Surgical Corporation, Norwalk, CT).

CONTRAINDICATIONS TO THORACOSCOPY

The two primary contraindications to videothoracoscopy are inability to tolerate one-lung ventilation and pleural adhesions of sufficient density to preclude entry into the chest (10). Of course the patient must be able to tolerate general anesthesia and must not have bleeding abnormalities, which would preclude other surgical procedures.

INDICATIONS AND RESULTS

Undiagnosed Pleural Effusion

Frequently, the etiology of a pleural effusion remains uncertain after the initial diagnostic workup, which includes a diagnostic thoracentesis with pleural fluid cytology and a needle biopsy of the pleura with repeat pleural fluid cytology. Such patients are possible candidates for videothoracoscopy to establish the etiology of the pleural effusion.

Videothoracoscopy is an excellent means by which malignant disease of the pleura can be diagnosed. Recently two separate studies, each with 102 patients, were published that reported diagnostic yields of 93% (14) and 80% (15). However, when these two studies are examined in detail, one finds that the only diagnosis that was definitely established is malignancy. When the above two studies are combined, the diagnosis of malignancy was established in 99 of the 117 patients (85%) with malignancy, including 51 of 56 (91%) with mesothelioma. It should be noted that neither of these two studies used VATS (14, 15). One would expect that the diagnostic yield would be better with videothoracoscopy than with classical thoracoscopy since videothoracoscopy allows a better view of the parietal pleura, especially in the otherwise difficult-to-examine costodiaphragmatic recess of the pleura (16).

Where is the rightful place of videothoracoscopy in the management of the patient with an undiagnosed pleural effusion? In the diagnosis of pleural disease VATS procedures should only be used when the less invasive methods of diagnosis, such as pleural aspiration for cytological, bacteriological, and chemical examinations, and needle biopsy of the pleura, have not yielded a diagnosis. In one series of 620 patients with pleural effusions, only 48 (8%) remained without a diagnosis and were subjected to thoracoscopy (17). In these 48 patients, a diagnosis of malignancy was established in 24 (50%) and in an additional 16 patients the diagnosis of benign disease was established when the thoracoscopic and clinical findings were considered jointly. In the remaining 8 patients (16%), no diagnosis was established at thoracoscopy, but 6 of the patients were subsequently diagnosed as having malignancy (17).

Videothoracoscopy is best at diagnosing malignant pleural effusions, but what is the hurry to establish this diagnosis? No definitive treatment exists for most malignant pleural effusions, and this diagnosis can usually be established by pleural fluid cytologic study, immunohistochemical tests, or pleural biopsy. Thoracoscopy is recommended for the patient with an undiagnosed pleural effusion in whom the diagnosis of malignancy is strongly suspected, and in whom at least two pleural fluid cytologic studies and one needle biopsy of the pleura have been negative. When one does thoracoscopy for diagnostic purposes, it is important to be prepared to perform a procedure to create a pleurodesis at the time of surgery. Our preferred method is the insufflation of 2–5 g of talc (18–20). If a patient has a recurrent benign effusion, consideration should also be given to creating a pleurodesis with the insufflation of talc (21).

Malignant Pleural Effusion

If a patient with an undiagnosed pleural effusion undergoes videothoracoscopy and if malignancy is discovered, 2–5 g of talc should be insufflated into the pleural space because this method is very effective at preventing a recurrence (see Chapter 7). If the lung does not fully re-expand at the time of thoracoscopy, it is still probably worthwhile to insufflate talc, because this might reduce the size of subsequent pleural effusions and decrease the need for therapeutic thoracentesis (20).

If the patient has a known malignancy, should videothoracoscopy be done to effect a pleurodesis? The most effective therapy for creating a pleurodesis for a malignant pleural effusion appears to be talc (22), and most of the series evaluating talc have used insufflated talc (22). However, in a recent review, the rate of success with talc in a slurry (overall 91%) was identical to that with insufflated talc (23). Therefore it does not seem reasonable to subject a patient to general anesthesia and the extra expense of videothoracoscopy when he could be managed just as effectively with tube thoracostomy and talc in a slurry. The only reservation I have about this recommendation is that it appears that the incidence of respiratory distress might be more common after talc slurry than after insufflated talc.

If the patient has a malignant pleural effusion that is loculated, it is possible that the loculations could be broken down and the pleural space cleared with videothoracoscopy.

Parapneumonic Pleural Effusion

Videothoracoscopy should be considered for the patient with a loculated parapneumonic effusion that does not respond to the intrapleural administration of thrombolytic agents (24). With thoracoscopy, the loculations in the pleural space can be disrupted and the pleural space can be completely drained (25). The chest tube can be positioned optimally with thoracoscopic guidance. In addition, the pleural surfaces can be inspected to determine the necessity for further intervention, such as decortication. In one recent report, eight patients who had posttraumatic empyemas were subjected to thoracoscopy for debridement, and none required any additional surgical procedures (26). If at thoracoscopy the patient is found to have a very thick pleural peel with a large amount of debris and entrapment of the lung, the thoracoscopy incision can be enlarged to allow for decortication (27). It should be emphasized, however, that frequently thoracoscopy does not cure the patient. In one series, 12 of 30 patients (40%) had to have an additional surgical procedure following thoracoscopy (28). In view of this, one should be ready to extend the thoracoscopic procedure to a decortication.

Chylothorax

It appears that chylothoraces can be managed effectively with thoracoscopy. It is unclear whether talc pleurodesis or thoracic duct ligation should be done to treat the chylothorax. When three reports with a total of 22 patients are combined, talc insufflation at the time of thoracoscopy controlled the chylothorax in 20 (90%) (7, 21, 29). Some patients do have a high-volume output from their chest tubes for more than 10 days after the procedure (29). Again one might ask whether or not it would be preferable to instill talc slurry through the chest tube.

With the advent of VATS, one would expect that ligation of the thoracic duct would be tried with the videothoracoscope. Thoracoscopy permits the entire pleural space to be visualized, and allows the lymphatic leak to be directly sutured. Although this technique has not been widely used for the control of chylothorax, there are anecdotal reports documenting its successful use (30–32). Kent and Pinson successfully ligated the thoracic duct in one patient who developed a chylothorax after a radical neck dissection (30). Shirai and coworkers performed thoracoscopy on a patient who developed a chylothorax postoperatively. They were able to identify the site of leakage, and the leakage stopped with the application of fibrin glue (31). Zoetmulder and associates (32) reported a 51-year-old patient who developed a chylothorax 4 years after treatment of a soft tissue sarcoma. At thoracoscopy, the thoracic duct leak was identified and oversewn, and talc was insufflated into her pleural space. The patient had no recurrence of her pleural effusion. It is unclear whether the procedure would have been effective if only the talc insufflation had been performed. It remains to be seen whether the endoscopic closure of chylous leaks is more successful or better tolerated than current open techniques (25).

Hemothorax

Videothoracoscopy may replace thoracotomy in some patients with traumatic hemothorax who otherwise would have been subjected to thoracotomy. Thoracotomy rather than thoracoscopy should be performed if there is exsanguinating hemorrhage through the chest tubes (33). Smith and coworkers performed videothoracoscopy for continued hemorrhage in five patients with continued bleeding from the chest tube after gunshot wounds. They found that a laceration of an intercostal artery was the source of the continued blood loss in all five patients. The hemorrhage could be controlled in three of the five patients at thoracoscopy, but two patients had to undergo a limited thoracotomy for the control of their hemorrhage (33).

If more that 30% of the hemothorax is occupied by clotted blood, removal of the blood is usually recommended. Traditionally, the clotted blood has been removed via a thoracotomy, but there have been two recent reports in which the clotted blood was removed successfully with videothoracoscopy (33, 34).

Pneumothorax

Thoracoscopy is effective in the treatment of spontaneous pneumothorax and the prevention of recurrent pneumothorax. With thoracoscopy there are two primary objectives: (a) to treat the bullous disease responsible for the pneumothorax and (b) to create a pleurodesis. The availability of an endoscopic stapling device and the Nd-YAG laser in the last few years have provided the means to achieve the first objective. Previously, the bullae were treated with electrocoagulation, which was associated with a higher recurrence rate (35). An alternative method of dealing with the apical bullae is to ligate the bullae with a Roeder loop (36). However, Inderbitzi and coworkers, who have reported the largest series using VATS for the treatment of pneumothorax, have reported a relatively high recurrence rate after use of the loop, and recommend that it be abandoned in favor of wedge resection with the endo stapler (36). The primary disadvantage of the endo stapler is its expense. The Endo:GIA model costs about $500, and additional cartridges (of which an average of two per procedure are used) each cost $500 (37).

The largest series using VATS with wedge resection of the bullae with an endo stapler has been reported by Inderbitzi and coworkers. They treated 79 patients between June 1990 and June 1993 for spontaneous pneumothorax. If the patients had a secondary spontaneous pneumothorax or if no bullous lesion was found, they also received an apical parietal pleurectomy. The recurrence rate in the 72 patients with follow-up was 8.3%. Since most of the recurrences occurred in patients who had not received the parietal pleurectomy, it appears that the pleurectomy does decrease the rate of recurrence. When four other series using VATS and endo staplers with a total of 84 patients are combined, there were only two recurrences (2%) (37–40).

An alternative to the endo stapler for resection of the bullae is the Nd-YAG laser. Torre and coworkers (41) recently reported their experience with 85 patients with spontaneous pneumothorax in whom the bullae were ablated with the laser and parietal pleura was abraded with the laser. The bullae in two of the patients could not be managed with the laser because they were larger than 2 cm in diameter, and these two patients were subjected to thoracotomy. There were three recurrences in the remaining 83 patients (4%) which is a rate similar to that seen with the endo stapler or thoracotomy. In general both the endo stapler and the Nd-YAG laser are effective in treating spontaneous pneumothoraces and preventing recurrences. The endo stapler appears to be slightly superior since more complicated lesions can be managed with it.

Once the lesion in the lung is treated, some attempt should probably be made to create a pleurodesis. The ideal procedure for the creation of a pleurodesis at the time of thoracoscopy remains to be identified. Some authors have recommended that nothing be done if bullae are identified and ligated. However, it seems reasonable to me to try to attempt something to create a pleurodesis while the patient is under general anesthesia. The simplest procedure to perform is a pleural abrasion with dry gauze. To me it is the procedure of choice since it is simple and effective (10, 39). Other possibilities include parietal pleurectomy, laser abrasion of the parietal pleura, and the intrapleural instillation of talc or a tetracycline derivative.

The sclerosing agent of choice is probably insufflated talc. Milanez and associates insufflated 2 g of sterile asbestos-free talc to 18 patients with recurrent pneumothorax and reported that the subsequent recurrence rate was 5.6% (42). Weissberg treated 122 spontaneous pneumothorax patients with 2 g of insufflated talc and reported that excellent results were obtained in 86.8% (7). Daniel and associates recommend that patients with secondary spontaneous pneumothorax be treated with talc pleurodesis, since in their experience they have found that attempts at staple closure of air leaks in these patients rarely succeed (43). In the dog the insufflation of talc produces a better pleurodesis than does tetracycline, Nd-Yag laser, photocoagulation, or argon beam coagulation (44).

There is still some worry about the long-term effects of talc. Although the incidence of mesothelioma or lung cancer does not appear to be increased after the insufflation of talc (45, 46), it does appear that the insufflation of talc is associated with significant pleural changes in a few patients. Viskum and associates (45) obtained chest radiographs on 50 patients who had received talc 20 to 30 years previously. They reported that the chest radiographs were normal in 11 patients, slightly abnormal in 37, and markedly abnormal in 2. The latter two patients had received talc bilaterally and had pronounced bilateral pleural thickening with calcification. Both patients complained of stiffness of the thorax. They also obtained spirometric values on the 50 patients and reported that the mean total lung capacity was 88% of predicted, and the mean forced vital capacity was 82% of predicted (45).

Which patients with spontaneous pneumothorax should be subjected to thoracoscopy? In some centers, all patients with spontaneous pneumothorax are subjected to thoracoscopy to evaluate the status of the underlying lung (47). This approach seems overly aggressive since approximately 50% of patients with their initial pneumothorax will never have a recurrence without any treatment. In my opinion, the indications for thoracoscopy in patients with primary spontaneous pneumothorax are the same as those for open thoracotomy, as described in the previous edition of this book; namely, (a) an unexpanded lung after 5 days of tube thoracostomy, (b) a persistent bronchopleural fistula after 5 days, (c) a recurrent pneumothorax after chemical pleurodesis, or (d) an occupation or an avocation such as airplane piloting or deep sea diving, in which the occurrence of the pneumothorax is dangerous to the patient.

COMPLICATIONS OF THORACOSCOPY

Videothoracoscopy has a relatively low rate of complications. Data collected on 1820 patients from the Video-Assisted Thoracic Surgical Study Group Registry revealed that the overall mortality was 2%. Prolonged air leak was the most frequent complication, and occurred in 3.2%; significant bleeding resulting in transfusion occurred in only 1%. Pneumonia and empyema occurred in 1.1 and 0.6%, respectively (48). VATS is tolerated relatively well by the patient with chronic obstructive pulmonary disease (COPD). In the above study, there were 59 patients who had an FEV_1 below 1 liter who underwent VATS. There was one death (1.7%), and the average postprocedure hospital stay was only 5.4 days (48). Kaiser and Bavaria (49) reviewed the rate of complications in the initial 266 VATS procedures at their institution. There were no deaths, but ten of the patients had air leaks lasting longer than 7 days. Bleeding requiring blood transfusion occurred in five patients, and there were five patients who developed superficial wound infections. There have also been at least ten instances of tumor seeding of VATS incisions.

REFERENCES

1. Landreneau RJ, Mack MJ, Hazelrigg SR, Dowling RD, Keenan RJ, Ferson PF: The role of thoracoscopy in the management of intrathoracic neoplastic processes. Sem Thorac Cardiovasc Surg 1993;5:219-228.

2. Jacobaeus HC: Ueber die Môglichkeit die Zystoskopie bei untersuchung serôser hôhlungen anzuwenden. München Med Wochenschr 1910;57:2090-2092.

3. Braimbridge MV: The history of thoracoscopic surgery. Ann Thorac Surg 1993;56:610-614.

4. Day JC, Chapman PT, O'Brien EJ: Closed intrapleural pneumonolysis: an analysis of 1000 consecutive operations. J Thorac Surg 1948;17:537-554.

5. Jacobaeus HC: The practical importance of thoracoscopy in surgery of the chest. Surg Gynecol Obstet 1922;34:289-296.

6. Adler RH, Rappole BW: Recurrent malignant pleural effusions and talc powder aerosol treatment. Surgery 1967;62:1000-1006.

7. Weissberg D, Ben-Zeev I: Talc pleurodesis. experience with 360 patients. J Thorac Cardiovasc Surg 1993;106:689-695.

8. Andersen I, Poulsen T: Surgical treatment of spontaneous pneumothorax. Acta Chir Scandinav 1959;118:105-112.

9. Wied U, Andersen K, Schultz A, Rasmussen E, Watt-Boolsen S: Silver nitrate pleurodesis in spontaneous pneumothorax. Scand J Thor Cardiovasc Surg 1981;15:305-307.

10. Kaiser LR: Video-assisted thoracic surgery. Current state of the art. Ann Surg 1994;220:720-734.

11. Brandt H-J, Loddenkemper R, Mai J: Atlas of Diagnostic Thoracoscopy. New York: Thieme, 1985.

12. Boutin C, Viallat JR, Aelony Y: Practical Thoracoscopy. Berlin: Springer-Verlag, 1991.

13. Loddenkemper R, Boutin C: Thoracoscopy: present diagnostic and therapeutic indications. Eur Respir J 1993;6:1544-1555.

14. Hucker J, Bhatnagar NK, al-Jilaihawi AN, Forrester-Wood CP: Thoracoscopy in the diagnosis and management of recurrent pleural effusions. Ann Thorac Surg 1991;52:1145-1147.

15. Menzies R, Charbonneau M: Thoracoscopy for the diagnosis of pleural disease. Ann Intern Med 1991;114:271-276.

16. Linder A, Friedel G, Toomes H: Prerequisites, indications, and techniques of video-assisted thoracoscopic surgery. Thorac Cardiovasc Surg 1993;41:140-146.

17. Kendall SW, Bryan AJ, Large SR, Wells FC: Pleural effusions: is thoracoscopy a reliable investigation? A retrospective review. Resp Med 1992;86:437-440.

18. Aelony Y, King R, Boutin C: Thoracoscopy talc poudrage for chronic recurrent pleural effusions. Ann Intern Med 1991;115:778-782.

19. Hartman DL, Gaither JM, Kesler KA, Mylet DM, Brown JW, Mathur PN: Comparison of insufflated talc under thoracoscopic guidance with standard tetracycline and bleomycin pleurodesis for control of malignant pleural effusions. Cardiovasc Surg 1993;105:743-748.

20. Milanez RC, Vargas FS, Filomeno LB, Teixeira LR, Fernandez A, Jatene F, Light RW: Intrapleural talc for the treatment of malignant pleural effusions secondary to breast cancer. Cancer 1995, in press.

21. Vargas FS, Milanez JR, Filomeno LT, Fernandez A, Jatene A, Light RW: Intrapleural talc for the prevention of recurrence in benign or undiagnosed pleural effusion. Chest 1994;106:1771-1775.

22. Walker-Renard PB, Vaughan LM, Sahn SA: Chemical pleurodesis for malignant pleural effusions. Ann Intern Med 1994;120:56-64.

23. Kennedy L, Sahn SA: Talc pleurodesis for the treatment of pneumothorax and pleural effusion. Chest 1994;106:1215-1222.

24. Shields TW: Parapneumonic empyema. In: Shields TW, ed. General Thoracic Surgery. Baltimore: Williams & Wilkins, 1994;4:684-693.

25. Ferguson MK: Thoracoscopy for empyema, bronchopleural fistula, and chylothorax. Ann Thorac Surg 1993;56:644-645.

26. O'Brien J, Cohen M, Solit R, Solit R, Lindenbaum G, Finnegan J, Vernick J: Thoracoscopic drainage and decortication as definitive treatment for empyema thoracis following penetrating chest injury. J Trauma 1994;36:536-539.

27. Moores DWO: Management of acute empyema. [Editorial]. Chest 1992;102:1316-1317.

28. Ridley PD, Braimbridge MV: Thoracoscopic debridement and pleural irrigation in the management of empyema thoracis. Ann Thorac Surg 1991;51:461-464.

29. Graham DD, McGahren ED, Tribble CG, Daniel TM, Rodgers BM: Use of video-assisted thoracic surgery in the treatment of chylothorax. Ann Thorac Surg 1994;57:1507-1511.

30. Kent RB 3d, Pinson TW: Thoracoscopic ligation of the thoracic duct. Surg Endoscopy 1993;7:52-53.

31. Shirai T, Amano J, Takabe K: Thoracoscopic diagnosis and treatment of chylothorax after pneumonectomy. Ann Thorac Surg 1991;52:306-307.

32. Zoetmulder F, Rutgers E, Baas P: Thoracoscopic ligation of a thoracic duct leakage. Chest 1994;106:1233-1234.

33. Smith RS, Fry WR, Tsoi EK, Morabito DJ, Koehler RH, Reinganum SJ, Organ CH Jr: Preliminary report on videothoracoscopy in the evaluation and treatment of thoracic injury. Am J Surg 1993;166:690-693.

34. Mancini M, Smith LM, Nein A, Buechter KJ: Early evacuation of clotted blood in hemothorax using thoracoscopy: case reports. J Trauma 1993;34:144-147.

35. Takeno Y: Thoracoscopic treatment of spontaneous pneumothorax. Ann Thorac Surg 1993;56:688-690.

36. Inderbitzi RGC, Leiser A, Furrer M, Althaus U: Three years' experience in video-assisted thoracic surgery (VATS) for spontaneous pneumothorax. J Thorac Cardiovasc Surg 1994;107:1410–1415.

37. Hazelrigg SR, Landreneau RJ, Mack M, Acuff T, Seifert PE, Auer JE, Magee M: Thoracoscopic stapled resection for spontaneous pneumothorax. J Thorac Cardiovasc Surg 1993;105:389–393.

38. Bagnato VJ: Treatment of recurrent spontaneous pneumothorax. Surg Laparosc Endosc 1992;2:100–103.

39. Fosse E, Fjeld NB, Brockmeier V, Buanes T: Thoracoscopic pleurodesis. Scand J Thorac Cardiovasc Surg 1993;27:117–119.

40. Waller DA, Yoruk Y, Morritt GN, Forty J, Dark JH: Videothoracoscopy in the treatment of spontaneous pneumothorax: an initial experience. Ann R Coll Surg Engl 1993;75:237–240.

41. Torre M, Grassi M, Nerli FP, Maioli M, Belloni PA: Nd-YAG laser pleurodesis via thoracoscopy. Endoscopic therapy in spontaneous pneumothorax Nd-YAG laser pleurodesis. Chest 1994;106:338–341.

42. Milanez JRC, Vargas FS, Filomeno LTB, Fernandez A, Jatene A, Light RW: Intrapleural talc for the prevention of recurrent pneumothorax. Chest 1984;106:1162–1165.

43. Daniel TM, Kern JA, Tribble CG, Kron IL, Spotnitz WB, Rodgers BM: Thoracoscopic surgery for diseases of the lung and pleura. Effectiveness, changing indications, and limitations. Ann Surg 1993;217:566–574.

44. Bresticker MA, Oba J, LoCicero J 3d, Greene R: Optimal pleurodesis: a comparison study. Ann Thorac Surg 1993;55:364–366.

45. Viskum K, Lange P, Mortensen J: Long term sequelae after talc pleurodesis for spontaneous pneumothorax. Pneumologie 1989;43:105–106.

46. Research Committee of the British Thoracic Association: a survey of the long-term effects of talc and kaolin pleurodesis. Br J Dis Chest 1979;73:285–288.

47. Janssen JP, van Mourik J, Cuesta Valentin M, Sutedja G, Gigengack K, Postmus PE: Treatment of patients with spontaneous pneumothorax during videothoracoscopy. Europ Respir J 1994;7:1281–1284.

48. Hazelrigg SR, Nunchuck SK, LoCicero J, and the Video-Assisted Thoracic Surgery Study Group. Video-assisted thoracic surgery study group data. Ann Thorac Surg 1993;56:1039–1044.

49. Kaiser LR, Bavaria JE: Complications of thoracoscopy. Ann Thorac Surg 1993;56:796–798.

INDEX

Page numbers in *italics* denote figures; those followed by "t" denote tables.